MANUAL OF SMALL ANIMAL **SURGICAL EMERGENCIES**

Filippo Cinti
Matteo Rossanese
Marie Burneko

edra
PUBLISHING

Manual of Small Animal Surgical Emergencies
F. Cinti, M. Rossanese, M. Burneko

ISBN: 9781962679459
eISBN: 9781962679428

Book Publishing Manager: Costanza Smeraldi
Project Manager: Elisa Bechi
Paper, Printing and Binding Manager: Paolo Ficicchia
Cover: Ursula Giusti
Copyediting: Jorge Viejo Adiego
Layout: Daniela Manunza

Edra Publishing US LLC
3309 Northlake Boulevard, Suite 203
Palm Beach Gardens, FL, 33403
EIN: 844113980
info@edrapublishing.com
www.edrapublishing.com

edra
PUBLISHING

Printed in Italy by "Erregiemme printing" S.r.l., June 2024

Editors

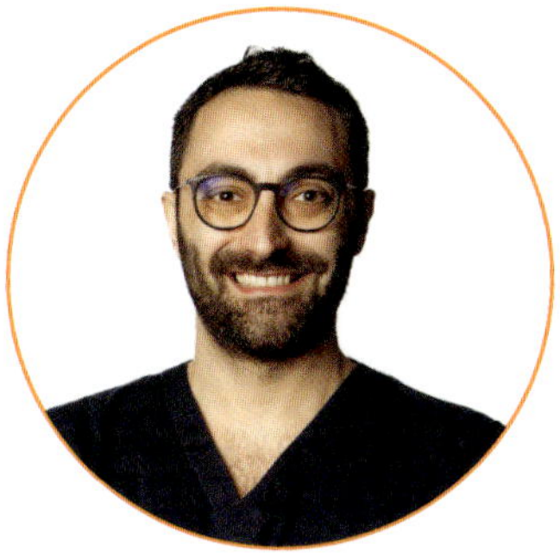

Filippo Cinti

DVM, PhD, GPCert(SASTS), DECVS, MRCVS,
EBVS® and RCVS Specialist in Small Animal Surgery

Filippo Cinti is the head of Soft Tissue and Mini-invasive Surgery at San Marco Veterinary Clinic and Laboratory. He also collaborates at Vet Hospital h24 Firenze as a specialist surgeon. Filippo graduated from the University of Bologna, Italy, in 2009. In 2014 he successfully gained a PhD in Veterinary Science (Surgery) at the University of Bologna, and in 2018 he achieved the Certificate in Small Animal Soft Tissue Surgery. Filippo completed a three-year European College of Veterinary Surgeons approved residency program in small animal surgery at Centro Veterinario Luni Mare and Clinica Veterinaria Vezzoni. After the residency program, Filippo worked with his ECVS co-supervisor Dr. Aldo Vezzoni before moving to UK. He worked at Eastcott Referral Veterinary Hospital (UK) for three years and, in 2020 he received the European Diploma in Small Animal Surgery. In the same year, Filippo achieved the Italian qualification of Assistant Professor in Small Animal Surgery (ASN). He is a member of the ECVS Small Animal Credentials Committee. Filippo has specific interest in soft tissue surgery, minimally invasive surgery, and neurosurgery.

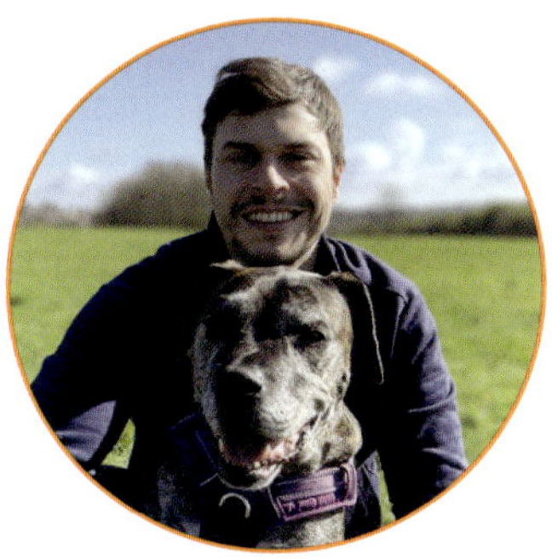

Matteo Rossanese

DVM, CertAVP, SPSA, MSc, DECVS, PGCertVeTEd, FHEA, MRCVS,
EBVS® and RCVS Specialist in Small Animal Surgery

Matteo is a lecturer in Small Animal Surgery, and he is the co-head of Soft Tissue Surgery at the Department of Clinical Science and Services at the Royal Veterinary College. Matteo graduated from the University of Bologna, Italy, in 2009. In 2011, he embarked on a postgraduate research project and internship in surgery and neurosurgery at North Downs Specialist Referrals, followed by a general internship at the Animal

Health Trust. In 2013, Matteo gained the certificate of Specialist in Animal Health from the University of Padua, and, in 2015, completed the RCVS Certificate in Advanced Veterinary Practice. In 2015, Matteo joined the Small Animal Teaching Hospital at the University of Liverpool, where he completed an ECVS-approved residency in Small Animal Surgery. In 2018, he gained a Master in Veterinary Professional Studies and in 2021 he received the European Diploma in Small Animal Surgery. In 2022, he achieved the Postgraduate certificate in Veterinary Education and the Fellowship of the Higher Education Academy. Matteo's primary clinical interests include cardiothoracic surgery and minimally invasive surgery.

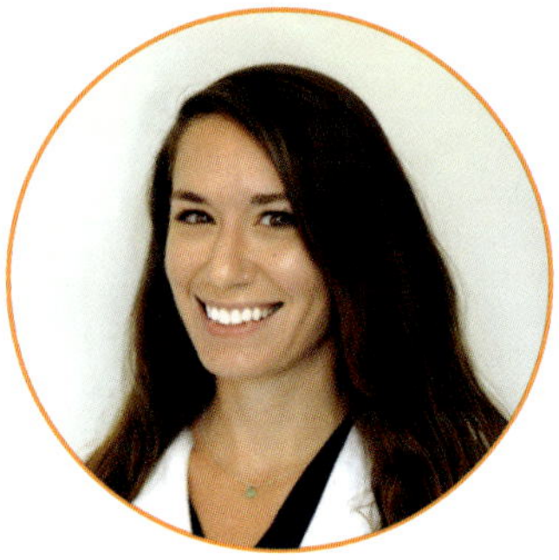

Marie Burneko

VMD, DACVS (Small Animal)

Marie Burneko is an Assistant Professor of Small Animal Surgery at the University of Pennsylvania School of Veterinary Medicine, with a focus on minimally invasive surgery. Marie received her VMD from the University of Pennsylvania in 2016 and completed a small animal rotating internship at the Tufts University Cummings School of Veterinary Medicine following graduation. She then completed a one-year surgical internship at Gulf Coast Veterinary Specialists in Houston, Texas, and a three-year surgical residency at the University of Pennsylvania in 2021. Marie has a specific interest in minimally invasive soft tissue and orthopedic surgery, as well as in the development of surgical educational tools to improve the quality and efficiency of intraoperative and extraoperative resident education.

Contributors

Adrien Aertsens
DVM, MRCVS, DECVS
College of Veterinary Medicine
University of Minnesota
Saint-Paul, MN, USA

Lillian R. Aronson
VMD, DACVS
Department of Clinical Sciences & Advanced Medicine, School of Veterinary Medicine
University of Pennsylvania
Philadelphia, PA, USA

Boaz Arzi
DVM, DAVDC, DEVDC, FF-AVDC-OMFS
Department of Surgical and Radiological Sciences, School of Veterinary Medicine
University of California
Davis, CA, USA

Daniel J. Brockman
BVSc, CVR, CSAO, DACVS, DECVS, FHEA, MRCVS
Royal Veterinary College
Hawkshead, UK

Paolo Buracco
DVM, DECVS, former Professor
Department of Veterinary Sciences
University of Torino
Grugliasco, TO, Italy

Benito de la Puerta
DVM, CertSAS, DECVS, MRCVS
North Downs Specialist Referrals
Bletchingley, London, UK

Ricardo De Sousa
DVM, DECVS, MRCVS
Department of Veterinary Medicine
University of Cambridge
Cambridge, UK

Christiana Fischer
VMD, DACVECC
Metropolitan Veterinary Associates
Norristown, PA, USA

Maria-Christine Fischer
DVM, DECVO, FHEA, MRCVS
Royal Veterinary College
Hawkshead, UK

Dario A. Floriano
DVM, DACVAA
Department of Clinical Sciences & Advanced Medicine, School of Veterinary Medicine
University of Pennsylvania
Philadelphia, PA, USA

Anna Frykfors von Hekkel
BVetMed(Hons), PGDipVCP, MVetMed, PGCertVetEd, DECVS, FHEA, MRCVS
Royal Veterinary College
Hawkshead, UK

Erin Gibson
DVM, DACVS
Department of Clinical Sciences & Advanced Medicine, School of Veterinary Medicine
University of Pennsylvania
Philadelphia, PA, USA

Contributors

David E. Holt
BVSc, DACVS
Department of Clinical Sciences & Advanced Medicine, School of Veterinary Medicine
University of Pennsylvania
Philadelphia, PA, USA

Sara D. S. Janssens
DVM, DECVS
Department of Clinical Sciences of Companion Animals, Faculty of Veterinary Medicine
Utrecht University
Utrecht, The Netherlands

Benjamin Kaye
BVSc, MANZCVS (ECC), MVetMed, DECVS
Southpaws Speciality and Referral Hospital
Melbourne, Australia

Natalie Kovak
DVM, DACVECC
Eastern Pennsylvania Veterinary Medical Center
Allentown, PA, USA

Anne Kummeling
DVM, DECVS
Department of Clinical Sciences of Companion Animals, Faculty of Veterinary Medicine
Utrecht University
Utrecht, The Nederlands

Karla Lee
MA, VetMB, PhD, MBA, CertSAS, DECVS, PGCAP, FHEA, MRCVS
Hamilton Specialist Referrals
Buckinghamshire, UK

Mark Longley
BVM&S, MSc, GPCertSAS, DECVS, MRCVS
Pride Veterinary Referrals
Derby, UK

Stephen Martin
MVB, BSc(Hons), DVMS, DECVS MRCVS
CityU Veterinary Medical Centre
Hong Kong, China

Anna M. Massie
DVM, DACVS-SA
Department of Clinical Sciences & Advanced Medicine, School of Veterinary Medicine
University of Pennsylvania
Philadelphia, PA, USA

Benjamin Mielke
BVSc(Hons), MVetMed, MANZCVS (SAS), DECVS, MRCVS
Melbourne Animal Referral Services
Melbourne, Australia

Alison Moores
BVSc(Hons), CertSAS, DECVS, FRCVS
Moores Soft Tissue
Winchester, UK

Sarah van Rijn
DVM, PhD, DECVS
Department of Clinical Sciences of Companion Animals, Faculty of Veterinary Medicine
Utrecht University
Utrecht, The Nederlands

Tommaso Rosati
DVM, DACVECC, DECVECC
Department for Small Animal Emergency and Intensive Care, Vetsuisse Faculty
University of Zurich
Zurich, Switzerland

Lynda Rutherford
BVM&S, MVetMed, DECVS, PGCertVetEd, FHEA, MRCVS
Royal Veterinary College
Hawkshead, UK

Thaleia Stathopoulou
DVM, MVetMed, DECVAA, PGCertVetEd, FHEA, MRCVS
Royal Veterinary College
Hawkshead, UK

Rhiannon Strickland
BVetMed, MVetMed, PGCertVetEd, DECVS, FHEA, MRCVS
Royal Veterinary College
Hawkshead, UK

Roberta Troia
DVM, PhD, DECVECC, EBVS
Department of Veterinary Medicine
University of Bologna
Bologna, BO, Italy

Ingrid Tundo
DVM, DEVDC, MRCVS, EBVS
IVC Evidensia, Haddington
Haddington, Scotland, UK

Rosario Vallefuoco
DVM, DESV, DECVS, MRCVS
Pride Veterinary Referrals
Derby, UK

Simona Vincenti
DVM, PhD, DECVS, MRCVS
Department of Clinical Veterinary Science
University of Bern
Bern, Switzerland

Rachel Williams
DVM, DACVS-SA
Small Animal Clinical Sciences
University of Florida
Gainesville, FL, USA

Foreword

This book is specifically designed to address the urgent and intricate world of small animal surgical emergencies. This volume emerges from a profound understanding of the challenges, exigencies, and high-stakes decisions veterinary professionals face when confronted with urgent surgical needs for our beloved patients. It is with a sense of profound responsibility and a commitment to the advancement of veterinary care that we, the editors, have curated this book and brought together this collection of knowledge and expertise.

The conception of this book was motivated by a clear and persistent need within the veterinary community for an authoritative, yet swiftly accessible resource that could demystify the complex decision-making and procedural intricacies of emergency surgeries in cats and dogs. Recognizing the high-pressure scenarios that veterinarians, veterinary technicians, and students frequently encounter, our aim was to distill the essence of surgical emergency care into a format that is not only informative but also immensely practical and immediate in its utility.

This book is structured to provide the reader with an intuitive and logical progression through the myriad of surgical emergencies that a practitioner might face. Each section is meticulously organized to address a specific category of emergencies, from trauma-related injuries to acute abdominal crises, ensuring that readers can quickly find the guidance they need. Within these sections, individual chapters delve into specific conditions, offering a concise overview of the emergency at hand, followed by a detailed, bullet-pointed walkthrough of the recommended surgical intervention. This format is designed to facilitate and promote rapid comprehension and retention of critical steps, enabling effective communication with the patients' owners and the rest of the team and confident action in the operating room.

The features that distinguish this book are manifold. Foremost among these is the emphasis on clarity and accessibility, achieved through bullet-pointed procedural guides, complemented by high-resolution photographs and videos that provide visual clarity to the textual descriptions guiding the reader through each surgical step. Additionally, each chapter includes 'Pro Tips' from experienced surgeons, which offer invaluable insights and distilled wisdom. Furthermore, 'Pitfall Alerts' are strategically placed to forewarn surgeons of common mistakes and complications, fostering a proactive approach to surgical planning and execution.

This book is intended to serve a wide audience within the veterinary community. It represents an essential tool for practicing veterinarians who face the unpredictability of emergency cases, offering a quick-reference reliable guide that supports decisive and effective surgical intervention. Veterinary students will find this volume an invaluable companion during their clinical rotations, providing a clear roadmap through the complexities of surgical emergencies. Veterinary technicians and nurses will also benefit from the detailed procedural guides, enhancing their ability to assist in surgeries and manage postoperative care effectively. Moreover, for residents in small animal surgery or surgeons in training, this book serves as a critical stepping stone in their journey towards specialization, offering depth and insight that will contribute significantly to their growth and development as specialist surgeons.

In essence, this book is more than just a reference; it is a guide and mentor for those moments when the stakes are high and the need for precise, confident surgical intervention is paramount. It embodies our collective aspiration to empower veterinary professionals with knowledge, confidence, and the ability to make a tangible difference in the lives of their patients. As you turn these pages and explore the book, we hope you will find not only the information you seek but also inspiration and a renewed sense of commitment to provide the highest level of care in any emergency surgical situation. This book stands as our commitment to our shared dedication to improving the quality of life for our patients through excellence in surgical care.

We would like to extend our deepest gratitude to all the authors and contributors who have worked along with us and enriched this book with chapters, videos, and pictures. Thank you for the time you invested to share your knowledge, dedication, and passion ensuring that this book is a valuable resource for the veterinary community. We also want to express our gratitude to Edra Publishing, who made the production of this book possible.

Filippo, Matteo, Marie

Acknowledgments

This book is dedicated to all veterinary colleagues, residents and students.
May this text help readers update their knowledge and improve the surgical management of their patients.
To my family for always supporting and believing in me.
To my wife Marta, and our kids Edoardo and Margherita for their love and for making every day of my life extraordinary.

Filippo Cinti

"If I have seen further, it is by standing on the shoulders of giants." Isaac Newton.
To my family and Bettie.

Matteo Rossanese

I would like to thank my colleagues and all contributors to this textbook for the insight and specialized clinical expertise provided in these chapters. I would also like to thank the faculty, house officers, students, and staff at the University of Pennsylvania for their support and the motivation they provided for the development of this textbook. Drs. Holt and Aronson have been instrumental in my development as a surgeon, and this book would not be possible without them. Finally, I would like to acknowledge my family and friends for their continued support and guidance—thank you for all you do!

Marie Burneko

Table of Contents

Chapter 4

THORACIC APPROACHES

Matteo Rossanese, Simona Vincenti

SECTION 3 • TUBE PLACEMENT AND STAPLING/SEALING DEVICES

Chapter 5

TUBE PLACEMENT

Anna Frykfors von Hekkel, Rhiannon Strickland

Chapter 6

STAPLERS AND VESSEL-SEALING DEVICES

Rhiannon Strickland, Anna Frykfors von Hekkel

SECTION 4 • SURGICAL WOUND MANAGEMENT

Chapter 7

BITE WOUNDS

Alison Moores

Chapter 13

BILIARY DISEASE

Karla Lee

Chapter 14

HEPATIC SURGICAL EMERGENCIES

Sara D. S. Janssens, Anne Kummeling

SECTION 6 • ABDOMINAL CAVITY SURGICAL EMERGENCIES

Chapter 15

ABDOMINAL HERNIAS

Filippo Cinti, Paolo Buracco

Chapter 16

PERITONITIS

Rosario Vallefuoco, Mark Longley

SECTION 7 • URINARY SURGICAL EMERGENCIES

Chapter 17

UROABDOMEN

Natalie Kovak, Christiana Fischer

Chapter 18

TRAUMA OR PROLAPSE OF THE URINARY TRACT

Marie Burneko, Lillian R. Aronson

Chapter 19

URINARY TRACT OBSTRUCTION

Lillian R. Aronson, Marie Burneko

SECTION 8 • REPRODUCTIVE SURGICAL EMERGENCIES

Chapter 20

GENITAL EMERGENCIES

Erin Gibson, Rachel Williams

SECTION 9 • RESPIRATORY SURGICAL EMERGENCIES

SECTION 10 • CARDIAC AND VASCULAR SURGICAL EMERGENCIES

SECTION 13 • OPHTHALMIC SURGICAL EMERGENCIES

Chapter 31

EYELID LACERATIONS

Maria-Christine Fischer

Chapter 32

GLOBE PROPTOSIS

Maria-Christine Fischer

Chapter 33

ENUCLEATION

Maria-Christine Fischer

Chapter 1

Triage of the emergency patient

Tommaso Rosati, Roberta Troia

Triage is a systematic and dynamic process employed in the context of small animal emergency medicine that involves the rapid assessment, prioritization, and categorization of patients based on the severity of their medical conditions and the availability of healthcare resources. The primary objective of small animal triage is to ensure that the most critically ill patients receive immediate and appropriate care, while also addressing the needs of less urgent cases. A structured systematic triage technique optimizes resource allocation and timing of medical interventions, thus contributing to maximize the chances of positive clinical outcomes for all small animal patients. This chapter aims to provide a comprehensive guide to small animal triage in the context of emergency surgery, covering the principles, protocols, and practical considerations involved.

Principles of triage

Triage, derived from the French word *trier* (to sort or select), refers to the process of prioritizing and categorizing patients based on their urgency. Small animal triage revolves around a systematic approach that encompasses the essential elements of targeted clinical history collection, clinical assessment, and judicious use of supportive point-of-care diagnostics. These fundamental principles guide veterinary professionals in categorizing the level of care required for each patient, ensuring a prioritized response based on urgency. Subsequently, a problem-directed stabilization approach is employed, tailoring interventions to address immediate concerns and optimize time and resources management.

Targeted clinical history collection

During triage, the emphasis in clinical history collection lies in discerning the primary reason for the current visit and understanding the nature of the observed clinical signs. Strategically posed questions, including "What happened?" and "How long ago did it happen / these signs started?", are aimed at extracting information directly related to the immediate concerns at hand. This focused approach allows for prompt decision-making and interventions to ensure patient stability.

It is paramount to recognize that, at this initial stage, the goal is to grasp the essential details that directly contribute to the current condition. A more comprehensive and detailed clinical history will be pursued at a subsequent stage, once the patient's stability has been assured and emergency issues have been addressed. This targeted strategy ensures that crucial information is promptly gathered, facilitating a timely and effective response during the essential moments of small animal triage.

Clinical assessment

The cornerstone of small animal triage is a rapid and comprehensive clinical assessment. This involves a systematic evaluation of the patient's respiratory, circulatory, and nervous systems.

Triage effectiveness begins before hands-on patient contact. Initial observation with visual and auditory assessment of the respiratory rate, effort, and pattern allows for swift evaluation and helps localize the anatomic origin of respiratory distress. Increased respiratory noises can signal the presence of an upper airway problem. Stertor sounds are associated with the vibration of tissues due to the turbulent airflow caused by narrowed air passages. Stertor can be indicative of conditions such as soft palate abnormalities, laryngeal collapse, or other causes of upper respiratory tract obstruction. Stridor is typically a high-pitched, harsh sound that occurs during inspiration, and it often indicates that there is resistance to the flow of air (obstruction or narrowing) in the upper airway, specifically in the larynx. Conditions such as laryngeal paralysis, laryngeal edema, and foreign body obstruction can lead to the development of stridor. Both stertor and stridor sounds serve as clear indicators that immediate attention is warranted.

Increased respiratory rate and effort, presence of abdominal breathing, and specific body postures (e.g., extended head and neck with abducted elbows—i.e., orthopneic posture) may be indicative of respiratory distress. Thoracic auscultation via a stethoscope might provide additional information, such as the presence of abnormal respiratory sounds (e.g., diffuse vs. localized fine crackles) or muffled respiratory noises (e.g., pneumothorax, thoracic effusion). However, the impact of pain, stress, and anxiety on the respiratory rate and effort should not be underestimated. Cyanosis, characterized by a grey to bluish tint to the mucous membranes, suggests a high level of circulating deoxygenated hemoglobin, although its absence does not rule out hypoxemia. Pulse oximetry could be a simple noninvasive method to assess the blood oxygen content in animals showing an abnormal breathing pattern.

Effective evaluation of perfusion parameters is an integral part of the primary assessment during small animal triage. Perfusion refers to the delivery of oxygen and nutrients to the tissues and the removal of waste products, and it is a critical component of a patient's overall stability. Proper perfusion assessment can help identify and determine the severity of shock and guide the consecutive treatment decisions. Key perfusion parameters to evaluate include mentation, mucous membrane color, capillary refill time, heart rate, pulse quality, and extremities temperature. Specifically, pale mucous membranes, tachycardia (or bradycardia, especially in cats), abnormal capillary refill time, poor or absent pulse, hypothermia, and dull mentation are all indicators of systemic hypoperfusion (Table 1.1).

Following physical examination, emergency diagnostic tools that can aid cardiovascular triage can be used, including indirect blood pressure and electrocardiography. In the early stages of shock (i.e., well compensated shock), patients may only show mild signs of hypoperfusion with normal blood pressure, such that shock may not be appropriately recognized until it progresses into a more advanced stage. On recognition, it is imperative to promptly initiate emergency treatment interventions to rectify compromised tissue oxygenation and ensure the adequacy of overall perfusion.

During small animal triage, the assessment of neurological parameters precedes any physical contact. This initial evaluation is focused on assessing the level of consciousness, gauging the animal's responsiveness to stimuli and awareness. Decreased mentation may be determined by various causes, including intracranial factors, such as neoplasia or traumatic hemorrhage, as well as extracranial or metabolic issues like severe hypoperfusion due to sepsis, hypoglycemia, or sodium derangements. Animals presenting with ongoing or recent seizures necessitate immediate admission to the treatment area for prompt stabilization based on their current status. Additionally, particular attention should be dedicated to assessing ambulation status,

TABLE 1.1 - KEY CLINICAL PARAMETERS WARRANTING PRIORITIZATION DURING SMALL ANIMAL TRIAGE

Parameter	Potential abnormalities
RESPIRATORY	
Respiratory rate	Apnea, >40 rpm
Breathing pattern	Increased respiratory noises, increased respiratory effort, open-mouth breathing (cats)
PERFUSION	
Mentation	Decreased mentation
Mucous membrane color	White, pale-pink, hyperemic, cyanotic
Capillary refill time	<1 s, >2 s
Heart rate	Small-breed dogs <50 bpm, >160 bpm Large-breed dogs <50 bpm, >100 bpm Cats <160 bpm, >220 bpm
Pulse quality	Absent, weak, bounding, nonrhythmic
Extremity temperature	Cold, warm
NEUROLOGICAL	
Mentation	Obtundation, stupor, coma, sudden change in mentation, hyperexcitability
Ambulation	Nonambulatory status (absent or decreased motor function)
OTHERS	
Body temperature	>39.5°C
Abdominal palpation	Severe abdominal pain
Urinary bladder	Enlarged, firm, painful, absent

discerning whether the patient exhibits normal motor function or if there are indications of impaired mobility. Patients with a history of trauma could report spinal instability and, consequently, should be handled with extreme care until any spinal instability is fully ruled out.

Once respiratory, cardiovascular, and neurologic assessments have been completed, and urgent conditions have been addressed, attention can shift to evaluating the abdominal cavity and the urinary tract. Suspicion for urinary tract dysfunction may arise from reported changes in urine production, stranguria, pigmenturia, or recent trauma. It is crucial to perform urinary bladder palpation in all patients to identify potential urethral obstruction, characterized by a large, firm, and painful bladder that cannot be expressed. In trauma cases, the presence of a palpable bladder does not rule out organ injury and leakage. Conversely, the absence of a palpable bladder could indicate rupture or may be observed in cases of severe dehydration (relative oliguria) or intrinsic renal failure with reduced or absent urinary output.

Following the initial triage assessment, a more comprehensive and focused evaluation of the patient's physical status becomes imperative once clinical stability has been ensured and a thorough clinical history has been gathered.

Supporting point-of-care diagnostics

Alongside the physical examination performed during the primary survey, a minimum database including evaluation of packed cell volume (PCV), total protein (TP), blood smear, acid–base status, electrolytes, blood glucose and lactate, and laboratory markers of organ dysfunction (serum creatinine, urea, and bilirubin) can provide useful diagnostic information about the patient and may help guide emergency therapeutic interventions. A small amount of blood drawn during placement of the intravenous catheter could be used for this purpose. The PCV can be measured to assess for the presence of severe anemia or hemorrhage. Blood glucose measurement can be critical in indicating whether to supplement glucose or not in collapsed or critical patients; in addition, both hypo- and hyperglycemia in association with a deteriorating clinical status can be markers of severe metabolic impairment or occurrence of sepsis (e.g., surgical site infection, or intestinal suture dehiscence after major gastrointestinal surgery). Measuring electrolytes can be lifesaving in many critical conditions requiring medical stabilization prior to surgery (e.g., hyperkalemia in a patient with uroabdomen). In addition to point-of-care blood testing, a complete blood count, biochemistry screen, urinalysis, and coagulation testing should be performed depending on the clinical situation.

Point-of-care ultrasound (POCUS) can provide relevant information otherwise unattainable on physical examination alone, and it should be intended as complementary to triage and other point-of-care diagnostics. A key approach to the use of POCUS is to perform a focused assessment of the abdomen and the thorax guided by the initial findings of the triage (e.g., presence of pulsus paradoxus, shock, respiratory distress, muffled lung or heart sounds) and through clinically driven binary questions (e.g., in a dyspneic patient, is there pleural effusion? Yes/no). Keeping this in mind, POCUS is performed to search for free abdominal fluid, basic lung and heart pathologies (e.g., pleural effusion, diaphragmatic hernia, pneumothorax, interstitial lung disease, pericardial effusion), and selected abdominal diseases (e.g., pyometra, free abdominal gas) (Fig. 1.1). POCUS can also be used to perform ultrasound-guided procedures for diagnostic and therapeutic purposes (e.g., therapeutic thoracentesis in the presence of pleural effusion or pneumothorax, abdominocentesis) within minutes of patient triage.

Table 1.2 summarizes the supporting point-of-care diagnostics for the triage of small animal patients and lists potential causes for the most common abnormalities.

Categorization

Following clinical assessment, patients are categorized into distinct priority levels. Classification often includes the following levels:

- Emergent—immediate care required.
- Urgent—care must be started within the first hour from presentation.
- Nonurgent—care can be delayed.

Categorizations serve as a structured approach to facilitate decision-making and to adequately allocate staff and equipment resources. There is currently no standardized triage system in veterinary medicine, and, to this day, patient conditions are often assessed intuitively. A recent veterinary study tested the use of triage list categories based on a human five-point scoring system that links clinical complaints to urgency and target waiting times. According to this veterinary triage list, animals were categorized into four urgency color-coded categories with target waiting times: red, immediate; orange, 15 minutes; yellow, 30–60 minutes; green, 120 minutes. This system was more effective at categorizing emergency cases with target waiting times compared with intuitive triage performed by nurses. However, it should be taken into account that employing overly complex triage systems with numerous color codes may counteract the intended purpose of rapid and intuitive patient categorization. Therefore, readers are encouraged to adopt systems with a limited range, ideally consisting of two or three levels.

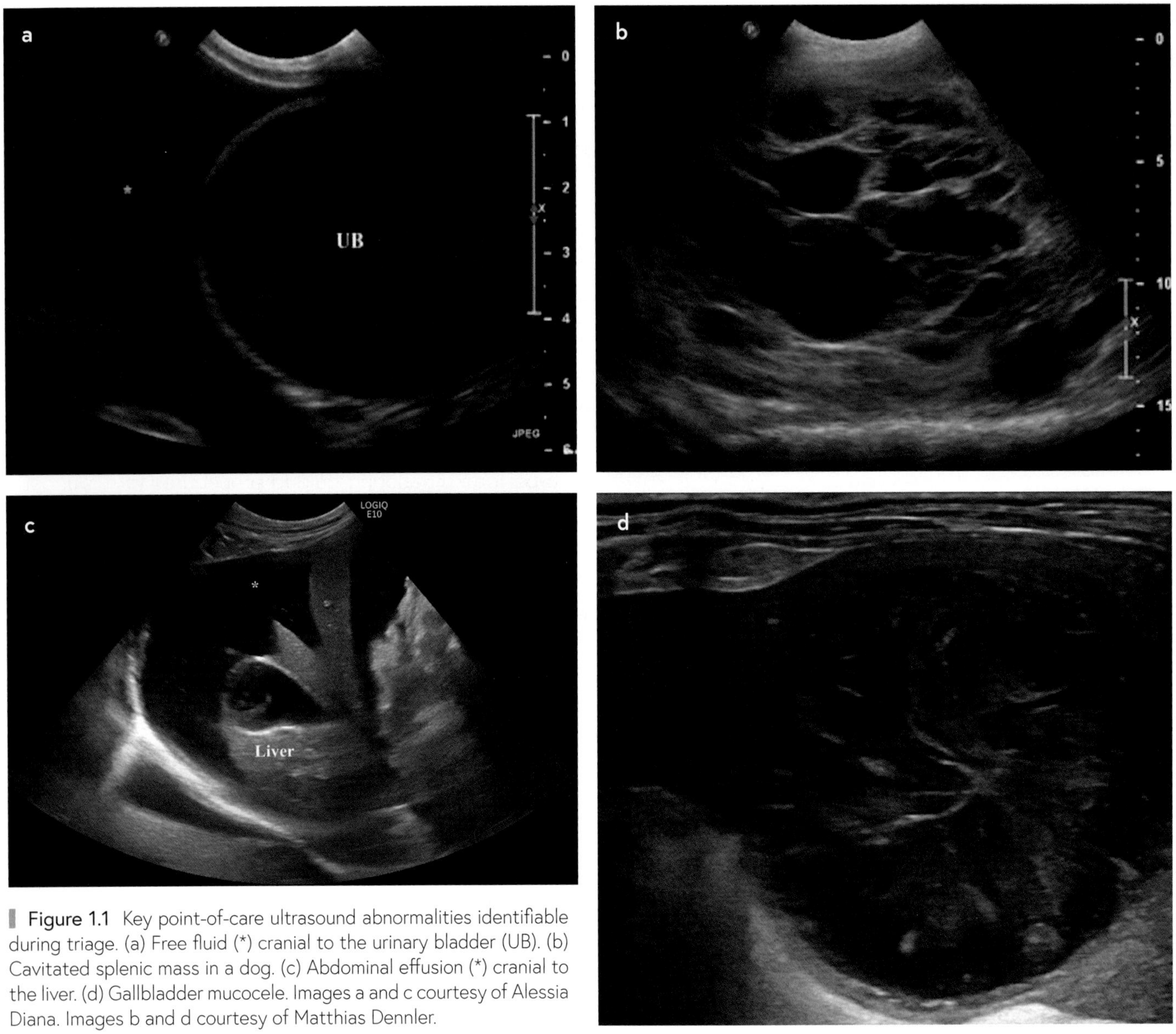

Figure 1.1 Key point-of-care ultrasound abnormalities identifiable during triage. (a) Free fluid (*) cranial to the urinary bladder (UB). (b) Cavitated splenic mass in a dog. (c) Abdominal effusion (*) cranial to the liver. (d) Gallbladder mucocele. Images a and c courtesy of Alessia Diana. Images b and d courtesy of Matthias Dennler.

Level allocation should be determined by the initial clinical assessment (see Table 1.1) and nature of the presenting complaint (Fig. 1.2). Furthermore, it is worth noting that, although it is crucial to recognize that inaccurate categorization might undermine the effectiveness of the overall triage effort, it remains imperative to approach patient assessment with a heightened diligence, as delayed care could significantly compromise the overall status of patients.

Initial stabilization

All patients triaged as requiring immediate care should be promptly transported to the treatment area for stabilization of major organ systems. If the animal has patent airways but exhibits an abnormal respiratory rate and/or effort, supplemental oxygen therapy should be initiated, initially using flow-by or a mask while concurrently conducting the remainder of the clinical and diagnostic assessment. If airway patency is compromised (e.g., abnormal airways conformation, laryngeal dysfunction, obstructive foreign body) or if the patient is not breathing, prompt endotracheal intubation should be performed and positive-pressure ventilation initiated.

Any critically ill animal should have vascular access established for the administration of emergency and/or lifesaving treatments. When intravenous access proves difficult or delayed due to cardiovascular collapse, a cutdown approach or intraosseous catheterization may be considered. In patients displaying signs of poor tissue perfusion, efforts to identify the

TABLE 1.2 - SUPPORTING POINT-OF-CARE DIAGNOSTICS FOR THE TRIAGE OF SMALL ANIMAL PATIENTS

Parameter	Significant variation	Potential causes
INSTRUMENTAL		
PCV/TP	Diminished (both)	Hemorrhage
	PCV diminished, TP normal within normal limits	Hemolysis (e.g., IMHA, infectious)
	Increased (both)	Hemoconcentration (e.g., dehydration)
Blood glucose	<60 mg/dL	Sepsis, starvation, xylitol ingestion, paraneoplastic, liver dysfunction
	>180 mg/dL	Diabetes mellitus, sepsis
Potassium	>6 mmol/L	Urinary tract obstruction, uroabdomen, AKI with oliguria/anuria
Sodium	<130 mmol/L	Chronic hypovolemia, excessive water ingestion, secondary to hypoglycemia
	>160 mmol/L	Excessive free water loss (e.g., gastrointestinal vs. renal), water deprivation
Ionized calcium	<0.8 mmol/L	Pancreatitis, AKI, hypoparathyroidism, citrate toxicosis
Lactate	>2.5 mmol/L	Hypoperfusion, liver dysfunction
Blood pressure	Systolic <90 mmHg	Systemic hypotension, hypoperfusion
	Systolic >140 mmHg, Mean >100 mmHg	Pain, Cushing's reflex (combined with bradycardia), systemic hypertension
SpO_2	<95%	Hypoventilation (e.g., airway obstruction), pulmonary disease (e.g., CHF, pneumonia)
Effusion/serum potassium ratio	Dogs: >1.4; Cats: >1.9	Uroabdomen
Effusion/serum creatinine ratio	Dogs & Cats: >2	
Effusion: serum bilirubin ratio	>2	Bile peritonitis
Blood glucose minus effusion glucose	>20 mg/dL	Septic peritonitis
POCUS		
Abdominal cavity		
Free fluid	Present	Septic abdomen, uroabdomen, hemorrhage, hypoalbuminemia, right-sided CHF, physiologic (mild, in puppies)
Discrete lesions	Present	Liver, splenic, gastrointestinal, and lymphatic neoplasia, abscess
Gallbladder	Kiwi-like structure	Gallbladder mucocele
Thoracic cavity		
Free fluid	Present	Pyothorax, hemothorax, chylothorax, neoplastic effusion, left-sided CHF (cats)
B-lines	Present (numerous)	Left-sided CHF, pneumonia, atelectasis, neoplasia
Glide signs	Absent	Pneumothorax
Heart		
Left atrium:aorta ratio	Dogs >1.6 Cats >1.8	Increased left atrium size secondary to MMVD (dogs), cardiomyopathy Potential risk for left-sided CHF
Left ventricle volume (subjective)	Diminished	Hypovolemia, hypertrophic cardiomyopathy
Pericardial effusion	Present	Neoplasia, coagulopathies, idiopathic

AKI, acute kidney injury; CHF, congestive heart failure; IMHA, immune-mediated hemolytic anemia; MMVD, myxomatous mitral valve disease; PCV, packed cell volume; POCUS, point-of-care ultrasound; TP, total protein.

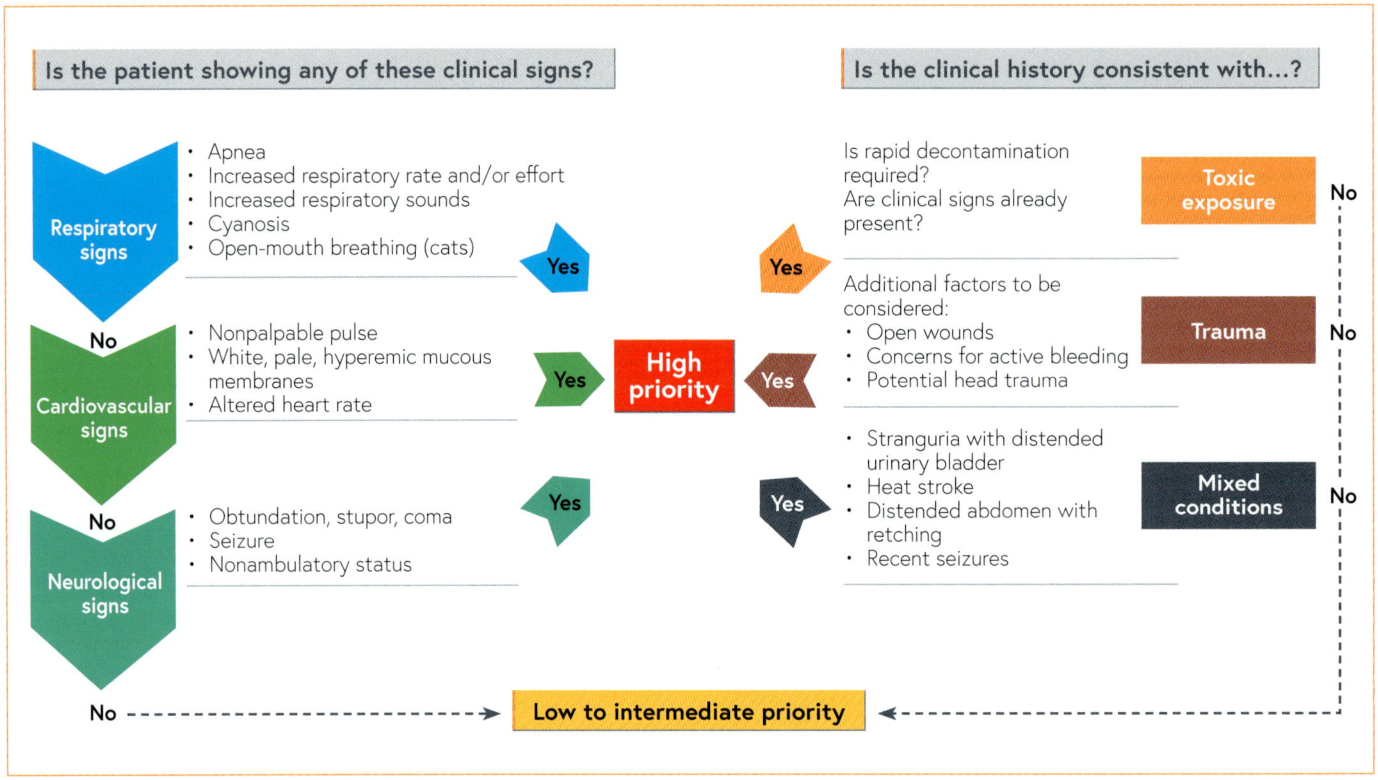

Figure 1.2 Flowchart illustrating a suggested triage strategy for prioritizing emergency veterinary patients.

underlying cause of the shock state (hypovolemic, cardiogenic, distributive, obstructive, hypoxic, metabolic) should be undertaken through historical data (e.g., fluid losses, trauma), clinical assessment, and point-of-care diagnostics.

The primary treatment for circulatory shock, except for cardiogenic shock, involves the rapid administration of intravenous fluids to restore an effective circulating volume. The crystalloid "shock dose" (60 mL/kg in cats, 90 mL/kg in dogs) represents the total amount that could theoretically be administered to patients during stabilization. Shock doses are never administered in full immediately but are divided into aliquots (e.g., 5–15 mL/kg bolus). These aliquots are administered over 10–20 minutes and adjusted based on the patient's clinical response. It is worth noting that the complete shock dose is rarely necessary to stabilize a patient. Once half of the shock dose has been administered, alternative strategies (e.g., colloids, catecholamines) should be considered. In specific situations, the use of 7.5% sodium chloride (hypertonic saline) may be considered for both small volume resuscitation and hyperosmolar treatment, particularly in cases involving increased intracranial pressure, such as head trauma. In persistently hypotensive animals despite appropriate fluid resuscitation, distributive shock should be suspected and vasopressor therapy instituted. Early vasopressor use in septic shock may be beneficial to reduce the risk of volume overload and inadequate achievement of resuscitation goals. A mean arterial blood pressure of 65 mmHg is considered the minimum goal.

Neurological problems requiring immediate stabilization include seizures, altered mentation, and acute paralysis. Seizure activities should be immediately terminated by the rapid administration of a benzodiazepine (e.g., midazolam, diazepam) as first-line rescue therapy to prevent further brain injury, cerebral edema, and progressive hyperthermia, irrespective of the underlying cause. Long-term anticonvulsant therapies such as phenobarbital or levetiracetam could then be initiated to prevent further seizure activities. In any patient exhibiting severely altered mental status, such as stupor or coma, an increase in the intracranial pressure should be suspected and appropriately treated with hyperosmolar therapy (mannitol or hypertonic saline); hypertonic saline should be the preferred choice in case of concurrent hypovolemia or hypotension (e.g., in animals with polytrauma). Elevating the head at a 15–30-degree angle helps enhance venous outflow from the brain. Caution must be exercised to avoid jugular vein compression and any maneuver leading to a potential increase in intracranial pressure. Patients with suspected traumatic spinal cord injury should be immobilized on a backboard, and any movement should be minimized to prevent further injury.

TABLE 1.3 - SELECTED KEY INTERVENTIONS FOR THE INITIAL STABILIZATION OF CRITICALLY ILL SMALL ANIMAL PATIENTS			
Intervention	**Indications**	**Dose**	**Comments**
OXYGEN THERAPY			
Flow-by **Oxygen mask**	Hypoxemia, hypoventilation	2–5 L/min or 50–200 mL/kg/min	
Oxygen cage	Hypoxemia, hypoventilation	21%–60%	Control temperature
FLUID THERAPY			
Ringer's lactate **Plasma-Lyte**	Hypovolemia	5–10 mL/kg bolus over 10–15 min, then reassess perfusion parameters	Consider alternative strategies once 40 mL/kg is reached
Hypertonic saline 7.5%	Hypovolemia, increased intracranial pressure	2–4 mL/kg over 10–15 min	Sodium derangements
ANALGESIA, SEDATION			
Methadone	Analgesia	0.1–0.4 mg/kg IV, IM	
Butorphanol	Sedation, weak analgesia	0.1–0.4 mg/kg, IV, IM	Variable analgesia
INDUCTION AGENTS			
Propofol	Urgent intubation	2–4 mg/kg titrated to effect 0.1–0.4 mg/kg/min CRI	Adverse effects: Hypotension, apnea
Ketamine+Midazolam	Cardiovascularly compromised patients	5–10 mg/kg (ket)+0.5 mg/kg (mid) IV, titrated to effect	Adverse effects: Hyperexcitability during recovery
ANTI-SEIZURE MEDICATIONS			
Midazolam	Seizure control	0.1–0.5 mg/kg IV, IN, IM 0.1–0.5 mg/kg/h CRI	
Diazepam	Seizure control	0.1–0.5 mg/kg IV, R	
CATECHOLAMINES			
Norepinephrine	α_1 and α_2 activity (+++) β_1 activity (+)	0.1–1 µg/kg/min	First-line vasopressor in sepsis
Dobutamine	β_1 and β_2 activity (+++) α_1 and α_2 activity (+)	5–15 µg/kg/min	High doses and prolonged infusions can cause seizures in cats
OTHERS			
Glucose 50%	Hypoglycemia	0.25–0.5 mL/kg, equivalent to 0.5–1 g/kg IV	Dilute 1:4
Calcium gluconate 10%	Hyperkalemia, hypocalcemic crisis	0.5–1.5 mL/kg IV over 15 min	ECG monitoring during administration (bradyarrhythmia)
Lidocaine 20%	Ventricular tachycardia	2 mg/kg IV	Cardio- and neurotoxicity in cats

CRI, constant-rate infusion; ECG, electrocardiogram; IM, intramuscular; IN, intranasal; IV, intravenous; R, rectal.

Table 1.3 summarizes the key interventions, indications, and dosages for the initial stabilization of critically ill small animal patients.

Spaces dedicated to triage and initial stabilization play a pivotal role in ensuring prompt and effective care of critically ill patients. These areas should be meticulously equipped with essential instruments and monitoring devices to facilitate seamless interventions.

Crucial equipment such as electrocardiography monitors ensures continuous cardiac monitoring, while the provision of oxygen and fluid pumps allows for immediate respiratory support and fluid administration. The inclusion of emergency drugs and an anesthesia machine further enhances the capability to address emergency situations swiftly.

These well-equipped spaces not only enable the rapid assessment of patients but also lay the foundation for timely and precise interventions, fostering an environment conducive to the delivery of optimal emergency care.

KEEP IN MIND

- Triage is a crucial technique in small animal practice that involves rapid assessment and prioritization of patients based on the severity of their condition and the availability of resources.
- The goal of triage is to ensure that the most critical patients receive immediate care while also addressing the needs of less urgent cases.
- During clinical evaluation in triage, a systematic assessment of the respiratory, circulatory, and nervous systems is conducted. To further understand the cause of clinical deterioration, based on the clinical history reported, point-of-care ultrasound techniques and blood testing are routinely performed.
- Patients are categorized into priority levels as immediate, delayed, or minor based on the severity of their condition. These levels guide the allocation of resources and the timing of interventions. Immediate cases require prompt attention, delayed cases can be managed after initial stabilization, and minor cases have less critical needs.
- Triage areas should be well equipped with essential supplies, such as oxygen, monitoring equipment, fluids, and medications. Having these resources readily available expedites the care of critically ill patients.

References

1. Ruys LJ et al. Evaluation of a veterinary triage list modified from a human five-point triage system in 485 dogs and cats. *J Vet Emerg Crit Care (San Antonio)*. 2012; 22(3):303–312.
2. Lisciandro GR. Abdominal and thoracic focused assessment with sonography for trauma, triage, and monitoring in small animals. *J Vet Emerg Crit Care (San Antonio)*. 2011; 21(2):104–122.
3. DeFrancesco TC, Ward JL. Focused canine cardiac ultrasound. *Vet Clin North Am Small Anim Pract*. 2021; 51(6):1203–1216.
4. Cole L, Humm K, Dirrig H. Focused ultrasound examination of canine and feline emergency urinary tract disorders. *Vet Clin North Am Small Anim Pract*. 2021; 51(6):1233–1248.
5. Boysen SR. Lung ultrasonography for pneumothorax in dogs and cats. *Vet Clin North Am Small Anim Pract*. 2021; 51(6):1153–1167.
6. Boag AK, Hughes D. Assessment and treatment of perfusion abnormalities in the emergency patient. *Vet Clin North Am Small Anim Pract*. 2005; 35(2):319–342.
7. Reineke EL, Rees C, Drobatz KJ. Association of blood lactate concentration with physical perfusion variables, blood pressure, and outcome for cats treated at an emergency service. *J Am Vet Med Assoc*. 2015; 247(1):79–84.
8. Cortellini S, Seth M, Kellett-Gregory LM. Plasma lactate concentrations in septic peritonitis: A retrospective study of 83 dogs (2007–2012). *J Vet Emerg Crit Care (San Antonio)*. 2015; 25(3):388–395.

Chapter 2

Analgesia and anesthesia for critically ill patients

Thaleia Stathopoulou, Dario A. Floriano

The term *emergency anesthesia* applies to patients that need to be anesthetized either immediately (within minutes of decision to operate) or urgently (within hours of decision to operate).[1] Following the initial triage and before anesthesia, the patient should be as hemodynamically stable as possible. Addressing any fluid and electrolyte imbalances, acute hemorrhage, or underlying causes of respiratory compromise, such as pneumothorax or pleural effusion, is crucial.

The above is essential because the stress response triggered by anesthesia and surgery includes physiological and pathophysiological mechanisms that, especially in compromised animals undergoing emergency surgery, can lead to systemic inflammatory response syndrome (SIRS), hypermetabolism and hypercatabolism, and immune system impairment.[2] Additionally, most anesthetic agents are associated with vasodilation, hypoventilation, hypothermia, and other effects that can further compromise the critically ill animal.[2]

Providing emergency anesthesia differs significantly from utilizing anesthesia in elective cases in several ways:

- 24/7 staff availability, often during odd hours.
- Limited or minimal patient's clinical history is common.
- Time pressure can impact adherence to guidelines in clinical practice; therefore, accurate anesthesia recordkeeping is crucial.
- Preoperative assessment should be brief and concise, focusing on identifying relevant risks and recognizing the appropriate responses.

Points for a successful anesthesia for emergency surgery are:

- Ensure adequate and trained personnel.
- Emphasize teamwork and communication.
- Implement structured handover (if applicable) for continuity of care with clear standardized documentation.
- Maintain equipment for emergency anesthesia, including portable induction carts, anesthetic machines and monitors, and crash carts.
- Have readily available medications for immediate use and dosing charts.
- Regularly conduct audits to improve outcomes.

Analgesia

Pain is a complex experience that has a sensory, a cognitive, and an emotional dimension. The vast majority of animals presenting for emergency surgery experience different intensities of acute pain depending on the condition. Untreated pain can impair respiratory function, immune response, and wound healing. It also affects coagulation, decreases gastrointestinal motility, and increases sodium and water retention and infection rate. Additionally, pain can elevate metabolic and oxygen demands and sympathetic stimulation, further complicating patient outcomes.[3] In the critically ill patient that will undergo emergency surgery, pain needs to be recognized, assessed, and treated as soon as it is safe to do so, normally following the initial triage. Beyond the physiological consequences, untreated pain prolongs unnecessary suffering and can be linked with further distress and prolonged recovery.[3]

Pain recognition and assessment

Pain recognition and assessment are based on behavioral features and can differ between dogs and cats. Several validated pain scales are available to aid recognition and assess the efficacy of pain management in small animals. In cats, the feline grimace scale (FGS), the UNESP–Botucatu feline pain scale (UFEPS-SF), and the Glasgow feline composite measure pain scale (CMPS-Feline) have been validated and are used for pre- and postoperative assessment of acute pain.[4] In dogs, examples of validated tools to assess acute pain include the short form of the Glasgow composite measure pain scale (CMPS-SF) and the University of Melbourne pain scale (UMPS).[4]

Intraoperatively, conscious pain perception is absent, and the term *nociception* is used instead. Nociception refers to the unconscious conduction and processing of noxious stimuli by the central nervous system. It is associated with physiological responses that include tachycardia, hypertension, tachypnea or apnea, and decreased anesthetic depth or even body movement.[5] Objective quantification of nociception during surgery is challenging, but over the past years, various monitoring systems have been developed to assess nociception and antinociception balance in patients under anesthesia. Some monitors measure the parasympathetic tone activity (analgesia nociception index, ANI), others the sympathetic nervous system activity like the pupillometry and the surgical plethysmographic indexes, and there are also monitors utilizing electroencephalography and electromyography.[5] Despite the limited data available in veterinary species and the various limitations, this is a promising area for accomplishing objective nociception assessment under anesthesia and aid optimal analgesia.[5]

Pain management

The nociceptive pain pathway consists of five phases: transduction, conduction, transmission, modulation, and perception. To improve pain management, multimodal analgesia and preventive analgesia are employed. Multimodal analgesia refers to the use of different pharmacological and nonpharmacological modalities to target different receptors in the pain pathway,[4] and to achieve better pain relief by taking into account the complexity of pain physiology. The aim is to reduce the dosage and the side effects following monotherapy, especially of opioid agents. It is important to distinguish appropriate multimodal analgesia from polypharmacy, where different agents are administered concurrently without rationale or assessment, risking drug interactions and side effects.[4]

Preventive analgesia refers to the administration of analgesics to minimize sensitization throughout the perioperative period (i.e., pre-, intra-, and postoperative). This approach is wider in scope than preemptive analgesia, which necessitates pain relief before the onset of nociceptive stimuli, often not feasible in critically ill patients experiencing ongoing pain. Current evidence supports the practice of preventive analgesia, rather than preemptive analgesia, in both human and veterinary medicine.[6]

Perioperative analgesia in emergency surgery can involve different classes of pharmacological agents (Table 2.1). Opioids continue to be the cornerstone of perioperative analgesia in veterinary medicine. However, considering their side effects, particularly in critically ill animals, the often problematic access to controlled substances, and the availability of alternative agents and adjuvant analgesics, opioid-sparing or opioid-free anesthesia can be achieved by minimizing or eliminating the use of opioids.[4]

Analgesic agents encompass alpha-2 agonists, nonsteroidal anti-inflammatory drugs, acetaminophen (paracetamol), NMDA antagonists, tramadol, anticonvulsant agents, antidepressant agents, local anesthetics, and cannabinoids. Depending on the pharmacological class, analgesics can be administered as a single dose or as a continuous infusion (Table 2.1).

Regional anesthesia plays a significant role as an adjuvant in perioperative analgesia. By integrating new technology, the accuracy of nerve location has improved, and the side effects decreased, compared to previously practiced blind techniques.[7] In critically ill and possibly hemodynamically compromised animals undergoing emergency surgery, regional anesthesia can be beneficial in reducing the requirement for inhalation anesthesia, minimizing the side effects of systemic opioids, and promoting a faster recovery. In addition to epidural analgesia, which is a well-established technique in veterinary medicine, there is a plethora of locoregional techniques available that can provide analgesia for surgeries involving the abdomen and thorax.[7,8] Following an initial learning curve, these techniques can be safe, time-efficient, and cost-effective, ultimately improving patient outcomes by minimizing side effects and expediting recovery.[4]

Postoperative analgesia is crucial for promoting recovery and wound healing. Pain relief is a dynamic process that varies among individuals and must be regularly assessed and modified as needed. Continuous infusion of analgesic agents and opioid transdermal patches as well as epidural catheters (Fig. 2.1), wound soaker catheters, and peripheral nerve catheters can be used postoperatively to achieve optimal analgesia over an extended period, with minimal side effects. Nonpharmacological modalities, including nursing care, supportive therapy,

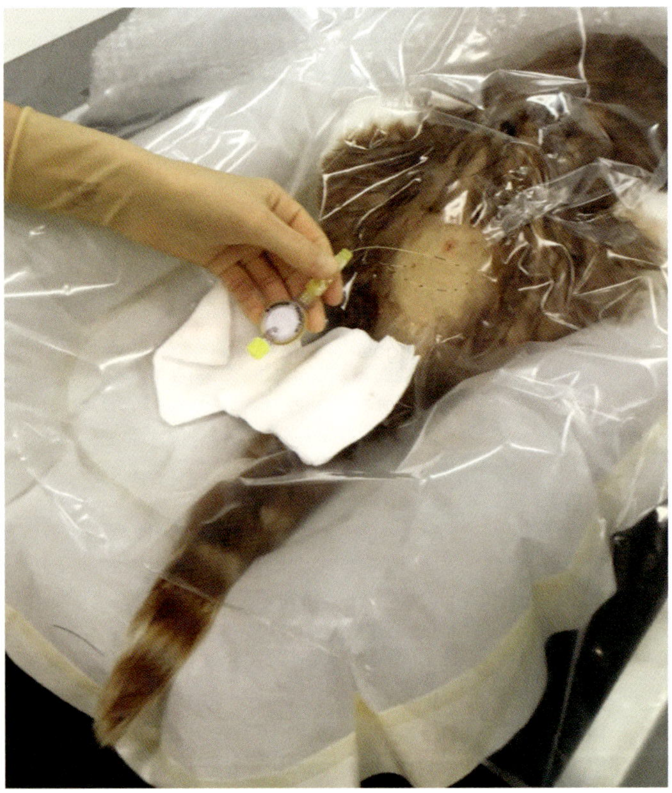

Figure 2.1 Epidural catheter placement for postoperative analgesia in a cat.

TABLE 2.1 - MOST COMMON SYSTEMIC ANALGESICS AND SEDATIVES USED IN EMERGENCY SURGERY

Drug	Classification	Dosage	Duration	Comments
ANALGESICS				
Methadone	Opioid, synthetic, pure mu agonist NMDA antagonist	0.1–0.3 mg/kg IV, IM, or SC	3–4 h Wide references in literature	• Racemic mixture, lipophilic • Similar analgesic potency to morphine • Minimal sedation • Emesis (rare) • Hemodynamic changes like other opioids
Morphine	Opioid, pure mu agonist	0.1–0.3 mg/kg IV, IM, or SC	2–6 h	• Hydrophilic, suitable for epidural route • Emesis (common) • Possible histamine release (especially after rapid IV injection)
Pethidine	Opioid, synthetic, pure mu agonist	3–5 mg/kg IM	60–90 min	• Synthesized originally as an anticholinergic agent, maintains HR antispasmodic effect • Mild sedation • Low incidence of vomiting • Metabolite norpethidine can cause seizures
Fentanyl	Opioid, synthetic, pure mu agonist	Bolus: 2–10 μg/kg IV CRI: • Intraoperative: 0.1–0.4 μg/kg/min • Postoperative: 0.05–0.1 μg/kg/min Transdermal: 4 μg/kg/h	20–30 min	• High potency, rapid onset • In high doses: mild sedation in dogs, euphoria/dysphoria in cats • Respiratory depression • Coinduction with benzodiazepines
Remifentanil	Opioid, synthetic, pure mu agonist	CRI: • Intraoperative: 0.1–0.4 μg/kg/min	3–6 min	• High potency, rapid onset, short latency to peak effect • No bolus due to the very short effect • Does not prolong recovery • Unique: metabolism by nonspecific esterases, no hepatic involvement • Limited postoperative use due to ultrashort action in case of infusion disruption
Buprenorphine	Opioid, high-affinity partial mu agonist Weak kappa antagonist	0.01–0.04 μg/kg IV, IM, or oral transmucosal in cats Transdermal patch in cats	4–12 h 36 h (transdermal)	• Bell-shaped dose-response curve • More appropriate for postoperative analgesia • Minimal respiratory depression
Butorphanol	Opioid, kappa receptor agonist Mu antagonist	0.1–0.4 mg/kg IV, IM, or SC	1.5–2 h	• Good sedation, but limited analgesia • Premedication in nonpainful procedures/ diagnostics • Antitussive
Hydromorphone	Opioid, semisynthetic, pure mu agonist	0.05–0.1 mg/kg IV, IM, or SC	4 h	• Ten times more potent than morphine • Popular due to reduced cost • Hyperthermia has been reported in cats
Ketamine	Noncompetitive NMDA antagonist	Bolus: 0.2–0.5 mg/kg IV CRI: • Intraoperative: 5–10 μg/kg/min • Postoperative: 2–5 μg/kg/min	20–40 min	• Antihyperalgesic • Interaction with opioid receptors • Activation of noradrenergic and serotonergic receptors • Sympathomimetic • Dysphoria in high infusion rates
Lidocaine	Local anesthetic Blocks voltage-gated Na^+ channels	Dogs: Bolus: 2 mg/kg IV CRI: 20–80 μg/kg/min	30–90 min	• Antiarrhythmic • Anesthetic-sparing effect • Appropriate for neuropathic/visceral pain • Antinociceptive, immune modulating, prokinetic, and anti-inflammatory properties described • Monitor for signs of possible toxicity • Avoid in cats

Dosages are based on the authors' practice at the Royal Veterinary College, UK, and on the published literature.
CRI, constant rate infusion, IM, intramuscular; IV, intravascular; SC, subcutaneous.

TABLE 2.1 - (CONTINUED) MOST COMMON SYSTEMIC ANALGESICS AND SEDATIVES USED IN EMERGENCY SURGERY

Drug	Classification	Dosage	Duration	Comments
ANALGESICS				
Acetaminophen (paracetamol)	NSAID Weak inhibitor of prostaglandin synthesis	Dogs: licensed product Pardale-V (only in UK) 15 mg/kg IV 30 mg/kg PO every 8 h	8 h	• No anti-inflammatory properties • Avoid in dehydrated, hypovolemic, or hypotensive animals • Licensed for 5 days • Contraindicated in cats
Medetomidine Dexmedetomidine	Alpha-2 agonists Dose-dependent decrease in release and turnover of noradrenaline, dopamine, and serotonin in CNS	Medetomidine: 1–5 µg/kg IV or IM CRI: 1–5 µg/kg/h Dexmedetomidine: 0.5–2.5 µg/kg IV or IM CRI: 0.5–2.5 µg/kg/h	30–180 min, depending on the dose	• Can be used as sedatives, part of the premedication, or analgesics • Synergistic action with opioids • Anesthetic-sparing effect • Avoid in cardiovascularly unstable animals • Vasoconstriction, bradycardia
Meloxicam	NSAID Inhibition of cyclooxygenase enzyme (COX)	Dogs: 0.2 mg/kg IV or SC on day 1 and 0.1 mg/kg subsequently Cats: 0.2-0.3 mg/kg SC once	24 h	Do not use in animals with: • Gastrointestinal disorders such as irritation and hemorrhage • Impaired hepatic, cardiac, or renal function • Hemorrhagic disorders
SEDATIVES				
Acepromazine	Phenothiazine tranquilizer Blocks dopamine receptors and alpha-1 receptors	0.005–0.01 mg/kg IV 0.01–0.02 IM	6–8 h	• Anxiolytic, sedative • Can be part of premedication • Causes vasodilation • Avoid in hypovolemic or hypotensive patients • Avoid in patients with hepatic/renal insufficiency • Useful in brachycephalic breeds that could develop upper airway obstruction due to stress
Medetomidine + vatinoxan hydrochloride	Combination of alpha-2 agonist and peripherally acting alpha-2 antagonist	1 mg medetomidine/m^2 BSA, or according to dosing table provided Half dose when coadministered with opioids	45 min	• Analgesic and sedative effect of alpha-2 agonist without the cardiovascular side effects of peripheral alpha-2 receptors (vasoconstriction, bradycardia) • Can be used only as a sedative, not as premedication • Not licensed in cats • Risk of developing hypoglycemia

Dosages are based on the authors' practice at the Royal Veterinary College, UK, and on the published literature.
BSA, body surface area; CNS, central nervous system; CRI, constant rate infusion, IM, intramuscular; IV, intravascular; NSAID, nonsteroidal anti-inflammatory drug; PO, by mouth; SC, subcutaneous.

physiotherapy techniques (e.g., low-level laser therapy, cold therapy, massage, acupuncture), and appropriate nutritional support, can be utilized to promote positive outcomes and aid in recovery.[4]

Sedation/anxiolysis

It is not uncommon for small animals requiring emergency surgery to need sedation. Sedation can facilitate diagnostic imaging or be necessary for behavioral reasons. Critically ill dogs and cats can suffer from distress, anxiety, aggression, and sleep deprivation, which can lead to increased sympathetic stimulation and oxygen consumption, potentially worsening their condition.[3] Appropriate analgesia should always be administered first, as pain management can often alleviate these behaviors and aid in further diagnosis. Additionally, once adequate pain relief is achieved, the use of anxiolytics and sedatives can improve the health-related quality of life of critically ill dogs and cats, promoting rest and a near-normal sleep–wake cycle, particularly in a stressful hospital environment. A list of agents that can be used as sedatives is provided in Table 2.1.

General anesthesia

Critically ill patients may require general anesthesia for various emergency surgical procedures. Depending on the invasiveness or painfulness of the procedure and the presence of concomitant diseases (e.g., regurgitation), sedation may not always be safer than general anesthesia. Inducing unconsciousness through general anesthesia allows for orotracheal intubation, thereby protecting the airways from aspiration of foreign or gastrointestinal material. Moreover, general anesthesia enables adequate ventilation and provides comprehensive monitoring of the cardiovascular and respiratory systems.

In addition to achieving unconsciousness, general anesthesia should also provide analgesia, immobility, and muscle relaxation. Unfortunately, no single anesthetic agent encompasses all these properties in concentrations that are safe for critically ill patients, as they may lead to severe cardiovascular and respiratory depression. For this reason, multimodal, balanced anesthesia employs multiple drugs in an attempt to decrease the dose of each drug, lowering the likelihood of potential side effects, and taking advantage of synergistic and summative effects between different drugs. The choice of which anesthetic protocol to administer in an emergency should be based on the underlying cause of the disease. Common anesthetic protocol examples are illustrated in Table 2.2.

Critically ill patients are at increased risk of complications, as they are less tolerant to the cardiopulmonary depression induced by anesthesia. All emergency patients undergoing anesthesia should be intubated and connected to an anesthetic machine to deliver 100% oxygen, regardless of whether an inhalation anesthetic is delivered.

The administration of preanesthetic drugs can help to reduce the dosage of potentially more dangerous drugs used to produce general anesthesia, facilitate induction, and enhance perioperative analgesia.[9]

Premedication

Premedication is an important component of a well-balanced anesthetic protocol, typically involving a combination of an analgesic and a sedative agent. Premedication offers several benefits, including reducing the

TABLE 2.2 - ANESTHETIC PROTOCOLS FOR COMMON EMERGENCIES

Premedication	Induction	Maintenance	Postoperative
Opioid: • Nonpainful procedures: Butorphanol 0.1–0.4 mg/kg IV or IM • Painful procedures: Fentanyl 3–5 μg/kg, hydromorphone 0.2–0.5 mg/kg, methadone 0.2–0.5 mg, IM or IV Otherwise healthy: • Acepromazine: 10–30 μg/kg IV or IM • Dexmedetomidine: 1–5 μg/kg IV or IM Sick/debilitated: • Benzodiazepine: Midazolam 0.1–0.3 mg/kg IV or IM, or diazepam 0.1–0.3 mg/kg IV	Propofol: 2–4 mg/kg IV to effect: • Alfaxalone: 2–4 mg/kg IV to effect • Ketamine: 2–5 mg/kg IV (with diazepam or midazolam: 0.2–0.3 mg/kg IV to effect) • Etomidate: 2 mg/kg IV (with diazepam or midazolam: 0.2–0.3 mg/kg IV) Recumbent/debilitated: • Fentanyl: 2–10 μg/kg IV (with diazepam or midazolam: 0.3 mg/kg IV)	Isoflurane or sevoflurane + O_2 or Propofol: 70–400 μg/kg/min CRI or Alfaxalone: 100–400 μg/kg/min CRI with/without: • Fentanyl: 0.1–0.5 μg/kg/min CRI • Lidocaine: 50 μg/kg/min CRI, dogs only • Ketamine: 0.6 mg/kg/h CRI • Dexmedetomidine: 0.5–3 μg/kg/h CRI	For painful procedures, continue pure mu agonist opioid intermittently or fentanyl (1–3 μg/kg/h IV CRI) Consider reversal of benzodiazepines and alpha-2 agonists during prolonged recoveries. Consider loco-regional analgesic techniques whenever is possible.

REVERSALS

Drug	Antagonism	Dose	Special considerations
Atipamezole	Alpha-2 adrenergic agents	Equal volume of dexmedetomidine, administered IM or 0.1 mg/kg Can be given IV during CPR	• May reverse effects rapidly; caution in aggressive patients • Given IM because IV can cause profound vasodilation and hypotension
Flumazenil	Benzodiazepines	0.01 mg/kg IV or IM	• May need to repeat due to short half-life (1 h) • Do not administer in patients predisposed to seizures
Naloxone	Opioids	0.02–0.04 mg/kg IV or IM	• May need to repeat due to short half-life (1 h) • Titration is essential to preserve analgesia

Doses reflect those commonly used at the University of Pennsylvania, School of Veterinary Medicine.
CPR, cardiopulmonary resuscitation; CRI, constant rate infusion; IM, intramuscular; IV, intravenous.

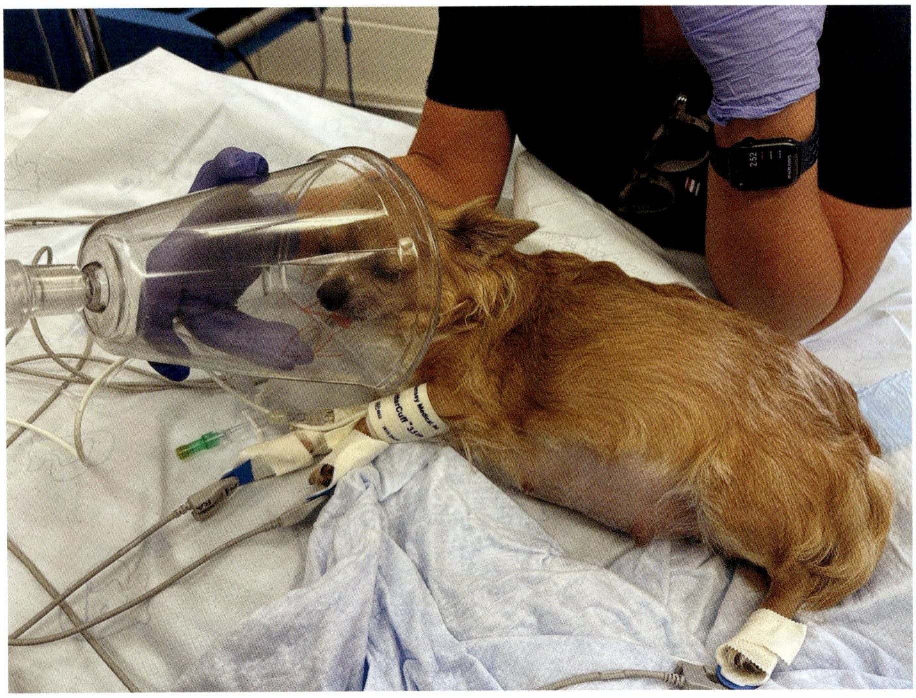

Figure 2.2 Preoxygenation with a mask.

required dosage of induction and maintenance agents, facilitating smooth induction and recovery, and providing analgesia.[10] The choice of premedication agents depends on factors such as pain intensity, duration of the surgical procedure, temperament of the animal, and the American Society of Anesthesiologists classification (ASA I–V). Critically ill patients usually fall into ASA grades III and above, and depending on their condition, premedication may consist solely of an opioid agent, with the omission of an additional sedative or anxiolytic agent. In severely compromised and obtunded patients that have received appropriate analgesia, premedication may be omitted altogether.
It is important to provide supplemental oxygen via a mask, if tolerated, following premedication and before induction (Fig. 2.2). The aim is to increase the body's oxygen store and delay the onset of arterial hemoglobin desaturation.

Induction

After preoxygenation with a mask, titration of drugs with the goal of maintaining spontaneous ventilation while attempting to establish a patent airway and avoiding cardiovascular collapse is of critical importance.[11] In circumstances where the risk of regurgitation is high (e.g., esophageal/gastric foreign bodies, pregnancy, gastrointestinal disturbances), rapid sequence intubation may be necessary, and drugs should be administered more quickly. It is important to note that in emergency situations patients are often not fasted, and regardless of the specific disease process, the risk of regurgitation and aspiration of gastric content during induction is higher than in scheduled elective procedures.[12]
Injectable anesthetics are typically the preferred method of inducing general anesthesia due to their fast onset, which results in smooth induction and rapid metabolism and excretion.

- **Propofol** is a short-acting intravenous anesthetic agent that allows very rapid and smooth anesthesia induction and recovery. An increase in heart rate may occur as a reflex response to the temporary drop in arterial blood pressure, which is due to vasodilation and reduced myocardial contractility. Respiratory depression and apnea are dose and rate dependent; therefore, propofol should be titrated slowly to effect. Preanesthetic medication significantly reduces the amount of propofol required for anesthesia induction, thus lowering the risk of blood pressure decline.[13] In cats, multiple exposures (consecutive days) to propofol can result in oxidative injury to red blood cells.[14]
- **Alfaxalone** is a synthetic neuroactive steroid solubilized in a cyclodextrin. It provides anesthesia and muscle relaxation, and, similarly to propofol, it can also cause cardiovascular and respiratory depression, although these effects may be less pronounced than with propofol, especially in cats.[15] In unstable patients, the dose should be minimized through concurrent use of cardiovascular-sparing premedications such as benzodiazepines and opioids. Potential side effects include opisthotonos, paddling activity,

and rough recovery when higher doses are used, especially if administered without premedication. Alfaxalone may also be administered via the intramuscular route.[16]

- **Etomidate** is a carboxylated imidazole derivative with hypnotic effects and a short duration of action. Induction with etomidate is characterized by a very rapid induction and smooth recovery when associated with sedatives such as benzodiazepines, acepromazine, or alpha-2 agonists. In contrast, excitement, myoclonus, pain on injection, vomiting, and apnea can be observed if etomidate is administered alone without preanesthetic medication.[17] Its minimal cardiovascular and respiratory depression makes etomidate an ideal intravenous induction agent for patients with advanced heart disease or cardiovascular instability/disease. However, since etomidate suppresses adrenal function and cortisol synthesis, it should not be administered to septic patients, Addisonian patients, or severely debilitated patients in which adrenocortical function is already suppressed.[18] Supplementation with a short-acting glucocorticoid may be indicated in these patients. Etomidate is prepared in a propylene glycol base and has a high osmolality; therefore, dilution is recommended prior to administration to avoid pain on injection.
- **Ketamine**, a dissociative anesthetic acting as a competitive antagonist for NMDA receptors, is used as a short-acting general anesthetic. When administered in low doses, it can serve as an adjunct analgesic during general anesthesia and for conscious patients. Ketamine has minimal effects on respiration, although apnea has been reported. It also stimulates the cardiovascular system by causing an increase in central catecholamine levels, mainly by inhibiting their reuptake. However, in critically ill patients, ketamine can cause direct inhibition of myocardial contractility, mitigating the advantageous indirect sympathetic effects. Potential side effects include myoclonus activity and rough recovery. To decrease the adverse effects of rigidity, it is advisable to always coadminister ketamine with diazepam or midazolam.

In patients with severe cardiovascular compromise, the coadministration of a potent opioid, such as fentanyl, and a benzodiazepine can help to achieve a level of unconsciousness adequate to tolerate endotracheal intubation, avoiding the detrimental effects of induction agents.

Typically, it is not recommended to induce anesthesia using volatile anesthetics, as the substantial dosage required could result in significant hypotension and hypoventilation.

Maintenance

Inhalational volatile anesthetics are typically used for maintenance of general anesthesia because they are administered and eliminated through the respiratory system. They do not accumulate in tissues and do not require hepatic metabolism, ensuring a rapid and predictable recovery, even after prolonged anesthetic events. The most commonly used inhalational anesthetics in veterinary medicine are isoflurane and sevoflurane. Both agents cause severe dose-dependent cardiovascular and respiratory depression and have no analgesic properties. Peripheral vasodilation is the primary mechanism of hypotension and, as a general principle, the lowest effective concentration of isoflurane or sevoflurane that guarantees an appropriate surgical depth of anesthesia should be delivered. Because of their potent respiratory depressant activity, mechanical ventilation may be necessary to prevent hypoxemia and hypercapnia. These conditions could trigger pulmonary vasoconstriction and exacerbate or trigger arrhythmias. Therefore, expired carbon dioxide should be monitored with a capnometer. High concentrations of inhalant anesthetics impair autoregulation of cerebral blood flow and should be avoided in patients with increased intracranial pressure. The use of preanesthetic medications and intravenous induction significantly reduces the amount of inhalants necessary to maintain an appropriate anesthetic plane and is strongly recommended to decrease the likelihood of adverse effects.

Propofol and alfaxalone can also be administered as intravenous boluses or as a constant rate infusion for maintenance of anesthesia. Due to the cumulative effects after prolonged anesthesia, especially in more critically ill animals, maintenance with injectable anesthetics is typically used for shorter procedures or procedures where inhalants cannot be used (e.g., when there is potential for room contamination, such as airway or pulmonary surgery), as they can lead to delayed recovery.

Cardiovascular support

Cardiovascular function should be monitored in every patient under general anesthesia, using ECG, pulse oximeters for oxygen saturation, invasive (gold standard) or noninvasive blood pressure, capnometry, and capnography. Despite aggressive fluid resuscitation, cardiac function may be poor and systemic vasodilation may occur as a result of both the disease process and the effect of administered anesthetic agents with vagotonic, vasodilatory, and negative inotropic properties. Parasympatholytic and sympathomimetic agents are typically used perioperatively to support

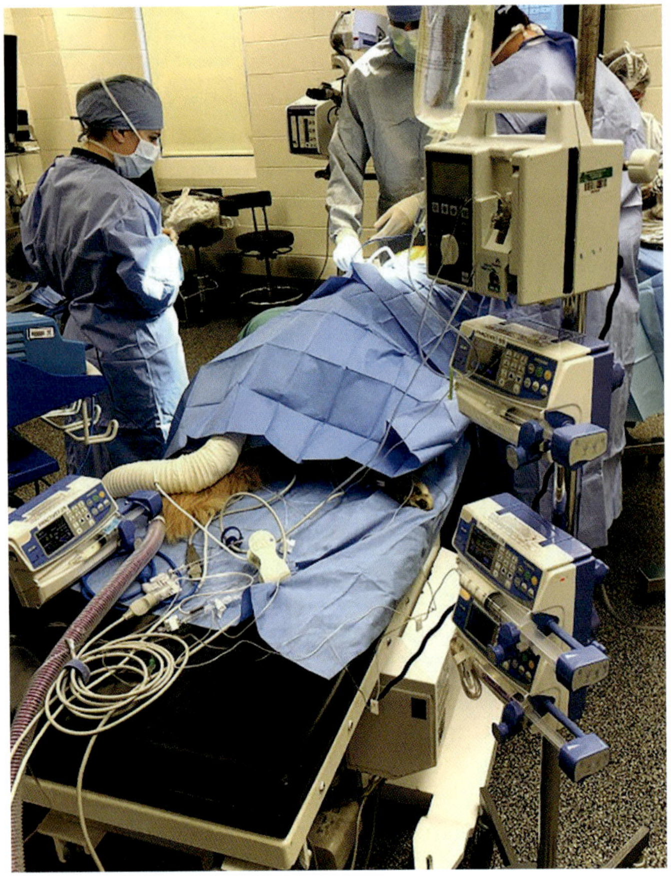

Figure 2.3 Multiple infusion pumps should be available to administer analgesics, blood pressure support medications, fluids, antimicrobials, and other perioperative medications.

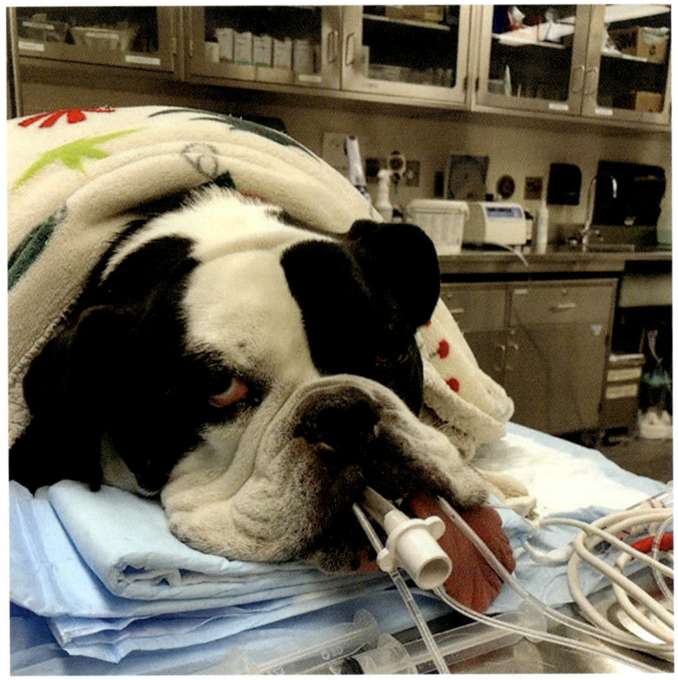

Figure 2.4 In some circumstances, extubation can be delayed until the patient is able to maintain patent airway. Patients with brachycephalic syndrome often tolerate the endotracheal tube for longer periods of time during the recovery phase.

blood pressure and counteract the cardiovascular effects of many sedatives and anesthetics, and often multiple medications have to be infused to maintain acceptable blood pressure levels (Fig. 2.3). Parasympatholytics or anticholinergics, such as atropine, block the binding of acetylcholine to cardiac muscarinic receptors and are mainly used to treat bradyarrhythmias and to increase heart rate. Sympathomimetics, mainly belonging to the class of catecholamines, act on specific adrenergic receptors, causing, within other effects, an increase in cardiac contractility and peripheral vasoconstriction (Table 2.3).[19]

Recovery

Recovery from anesthesia carries many potential complications, and patients should never be left to recover unobserved. Dogs and cats should be extubated as soon as the swallowing reflex is detected. In brachycephalic patients or patients predisposed to airway obstruction and regurgitation, however, it is recommended to delay extubation until they are more awake or able to lift their head or until they do not tolerate the tube (Fig. 2.4).[20] Hypothermia, hypotension, hypoglycemia, hypoxemia, and hypercapnia can all be the cause of prolonged recoveries, and intra- and postoperative interventions should be implemented to avoid such complications. Active and passive warming should be continued until the patient can spontaneously maintain normal body temperature. Respiratory and cardiovascular function should be monitored and oxygen administered to maintain adequate hemoglobin oxygen saturation. ECG cables should be left connected to identify arrhythmias that may develop during the recovery phase. If the patient has received considerable doses of opioids and benzodiazepines, administration of the proper antagonist agent should be considered. In some situations, emergence delirium can be caused by dysphoria and/or pain, and it is important to distinguish between them as early as possible and administer the most appropriate sedative or analgesic.

TABLE 2.3 - DOSES AND EFFECTS OF COMMONLY USED BLOOD PRESSURE SUPPORT DRUGS

Drug	Dose	Effects
ANTICHOLINERGICS		
Atropine	0.01–0.04 mg/kg IV or IM	• Fast onset, short duration • Preferred during CPR • Transient bradycardia or 2nd-degree AV blocks can be seen
Glycopyrrolate	0.005–0.01 mg/kg IV or IM	• Longer onset, longer duration • Transient bradycardia or 2nd-degree AV blocks can be seen with low doses or soon after administration
SYMPATHOMIMETICS		
Dopamine	Low: 1–4 μg/kg/min IV Medium: 5–10 μg/kg/min High: >10 μg/kg/min	• Both α and β receptors, depending on the dose • Low dose: Renal vasodilation • Medium dose: Increased cardiac contractility (β effect) • High dose: Vasoconstriction (α_1 effect)
Dobutamine	1–5 μg/kg/min IV	• β receptors • Increase in cardiac contractility (β_1 effect), but because of some vasodilatory effect (β_2 effect), BP does not always increase • HR increases with higher doses
Ephedrine	0.05–0.2 mg/kg IV	• Both α and β receptors • Increase in BP and CO through inhibition of reuptake of endogenous norepinephrine; tachyphylaxis and ineffective with repeated doses • Causes CNS stimulation
Norepinephrine	0.1–1.0 μg/kg/min IV	• Both α and β receptors • Increase in BP mainly through vasoconstriction (α_1 effect); some positive inotropic effect present • Often combined with dopamine or dobutamine to increase CO
Epinephrine	10 μg/kg or 100 μg/kg IV	• Both α and β receptors • Typically administered as IV boluses during CPR to cause potent vasoconstriction and increase cardiac contractility
Phenylephrine	0.1–0.5 μg/kg/min IV	• α receptors • Potent vasopressor; increases BP through intense vasoconstriction • HR can severely decrease due to baroreceptor reflex

AV, atrioventricular; BP, blood pressure; CNS, central nervous system; CO, cardiac output; CPR, cardiopulmonary resuscitation; HR, heart rate.

KEEP IN MIND

- Pain needs to be assessed and treated as a priority in the pre-, intra-, and postoperative periods.
- Anesthesia for emergency procedures requires preparation and trained staff.
- Sedation is not always safer than general anesthesia.
- Emergency cases are more likely to experience perioperative complications.
- Multimodal balanced anesthesia aims to use multiple drugs with lower doses, thereby decreasing potential side effects.

References

1. Bahlmann UB, Morris C, Kakokdar P. *Chapter 5: Guidelines for the Provision of Emergency Anaesthesia Services 2023*. Royal College of Anaesthetists, published July 2, 2023. Available at https://www.rcoa.ac.uk/gpas/chapter-5.
2. Layton R et al. The impact of stress and anesthesia on animal models of infectious disease. *Front Vet Sci*. 2023; 10:1086003.
3. Hansen BD. Analgesia and sedation in the critically ill. *J Vet Emerg Crit Care*. 2005; 15(4):285–294.
4. Monteiro BP et al. 2022 WSAVA guidelines for the recognition, assessment and treatment of pain. *J Small Anim Pract*. 2023; 64(4):177–254.
5. Ruíz-López P, Domínguez JM, Granados MDM. Intraoperative nociception-antinociception monitors: A review from the veterinary perspective. *Vet Anaesth Analg*. 2020; 47(2):152–159.
6. Clark L. Pre-emptive or preventive analgesia—lessons from the human literature? *Vet Anaesth Analg*. 2014; 41(2): 109–112.
7. Portela DA, Verdier N, Otero PE. Regional anesthetic techniques for the thoracic limb and thorax in small animals: A review of the literature and technique description. *Vet J*. 2018; 241:8–19.
8. Portela DA, Verdier N, Otero PE. Regional anesthetic techniques for the pelvic limb and abdominal wall in small animals: A review of the literature and technique description. *Vet J*. 2018; 238:27–40.
9. Bednarski R et al. AAHA anesthesia guidelines for dogs and cats. *J Am Anim Hosp Assoc*. 2011; 47(6):377–385.
10. Murrell J. Premedicants in cats and dogs: Which one should you choose and when? *In Practice*. 2022; 44(4):205–213.
11. McNally EM, Robertson SA, Pablo LS. Comparison of time to desaturation between preoxygenated and nonpreoxygenated dogs following sedation with acepromazine maleate and morphine and induction of anesthesia with propofol. *Am J Vet Res*. 2009; 70(11):1333–1338.
12. Davies JA et al. Incidence of and risk factors for postoperative regurgitation and vomiting in dogs: 244 cases (2000–2012). *J Am Vet Med Assoc*. 2015; 246(3):327–335.
13. Robinson R, Borer-Weir K. A dose titration study into the effects of diazepam or midazolam on the propofol dose requirements for induction of general anaesthesia in client owned dogs, premedicated with methadone and acepromazine. *Vet Anaesth Analg*. 2013; 40(5):455–463.
14. Andress JL, Day TK, Day D. The effects of consecutive day propofol anesthesia on feline red blood cells. *Vet Surg*. 1995; 24(3):277–282.
15. Campagna I et al. Comparison of the effects of propofol or alfaxalone for anaesthesia induction and maintenance on respiration in cats. *Vet Anaesth Analg*. 2015; 42(5):484–492.
16. Suarez MA, Dzikiti BT, Stegmann FG, Hartman M. Comparison of alfaxalone and propofol administered as total intravenous anaesthesia for ovariohysterectomy in dogs. *Vet Anaesth Analg*. 2012; 39(3):236–244.
17. Muir WW 3rd, Mason DE. Side effects of etomidate in dogs. *J Am Vet Med Assoc*. 1989; 194(10):1430–1434.
18. Qin B, Hu H, Cao B, Zhu Z. Effects of continuous infusion of etomidate at various dose rates on adrenal function in dogs. *BMC Anesthesiol*. 2016; 16:2.
19. Skelding AM, Valverde A. Sympathomimetics in veterinary species under anesthesia. *Vet J*. 2020; 258:105455.
20. Gruenheid M et al. Risk of anesthesia-related complications in brachycephalic dogs. *J Am Vet Med Assoc*. 2018; 253(3): 301–306.

Chapter 3

Abdominal approaches

Simona Vincenti, Matteo Rossanese

Midline celiotomy

Midline celiotomy is the preferable approach for the majority of abdominal surgeries in dogs and cats. Reported complications include seroma, incisional infection, ventral edema, excessive wound inflammation, wound discharge, wound dehiscence, and abdominal hernia.

Surgical technique (Video 3.1)

1. The patient is positioned in dorsal recumbency.
2. The ventral abdomen is clipped and prepped from cranial to the xiphoid process to caudal to the pubis.
3. A skin incision is made along the ventral midline, from the xiphoid process to the pubis, using a number 10 scalpel blade. Based on the procedure, the incision can be made only in the cranial, middle, or caudal abdomen. In male dogs, the incision should be deflected along the penis (i.e., parapreputial incision—between prepuce and nipple) (Fig. 3.1).
4. The subcutaneous tissue is dissected using a combination of sharp and blunt dissection to expose the linea alba.
5. In male dogs, the branches of the caudal superficial epigastric artery to the prepuce are ligated and transected. The preputial muscle is transected with scissors or electrocautery.
6. The penis is retracted to the side opposite to the surgeon, and further exposure of the linea alba is performed.
7. The linea alba is elevated with a pair of forceps (preferably Adson or Adson–Brown forceps), and a reverse or stab incision is made at the level of the umbilicus using a scalpel blade (most commonly a number 10 or 15 scalpel blade) (Fig. 3.2).
8. The peritoneal surface is checked cranially and caudally for the presence of adhesions using the fingers or closed blunt forceps to avoid damage to any abdominal organs.
9. The incision is then extended along the linea alba, cranially up to the xiphoid process and/or caudally as needed based on the surgical procedure, using scissors or a scalpel blade.

Video 3.1. Midline celiotomy in a female dog. Hemostasis is achieved with electrocautery. Note the excision of the falciform fat to improve exposure.

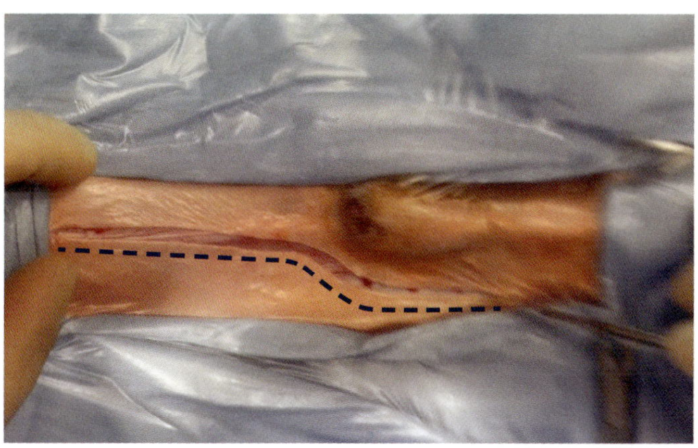

Figure 3.1 Parapreputial skin incision performed in male dogs. Note how the incision is deflected along the penis. The dashed line indicates the shape of the incision.

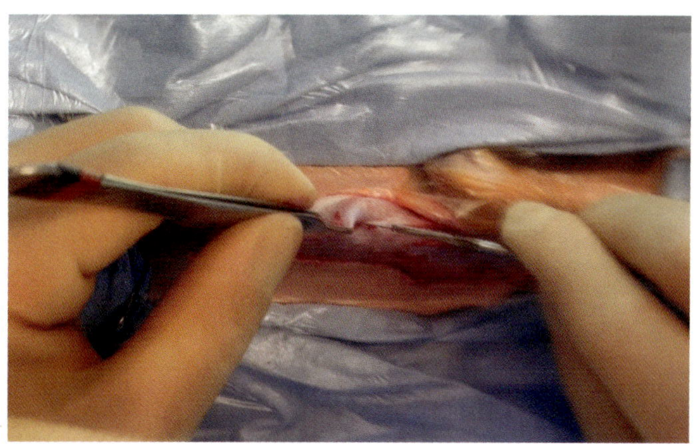

Figure 3.2 The linea alba is elevated with a pair of Adson forceps to avoid damaging the abdominal organs and a reverse or stab incision is made with a number 10 scalpel blade.

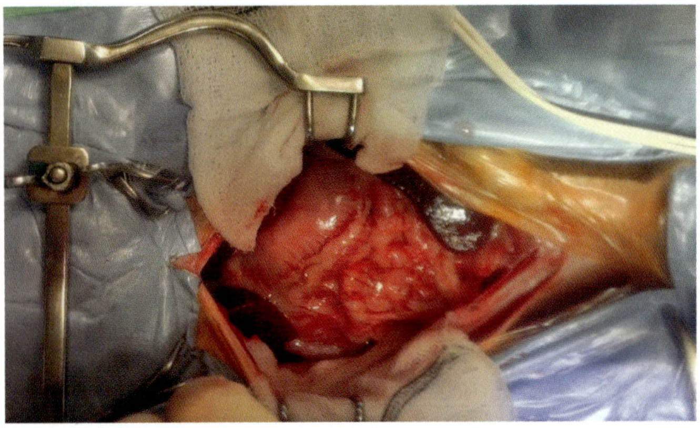

Figure 3.3 Midline celiotomy is completed. Moist laparotomy sponges and an abdominal retractor have been placed.

10. The falciform fat is resected along the incision edges and on the xiphoid process using electrocautery to increase exposure and improve visualization of the abdominal organs.
11. Moist laparotomy sponges are placed around the incision edges, and an abdominal retractor (Balfour retractor or ring retractor) is inserted (Fig. 3.3).

Closure

1. An appropriate suture size (2-0/1) should be selected based on the patient's size and weight. Absorbable monofilament suture material (e.g., polydioxanone) should be used in a simple interrupted or continuous pattern.
2. The abdomen is closed taking deep bites (>5 mm) of the fascia and the linea alba, avoiding full-thickness bites that might include muscle and/or peritoneum.
3. An assistant can maintain tension on the suture material to help with the closure.
4. The subcutaneous layer is closed in a simple continuous pattern using absorbable monofilament suture material. Incorporating the fascial layer in the bites can minimize dead space.
5. Obese animals may require closure of an additional deep layer of subcutaneous tissue to reduce dead space and to appose the skin edges.
6. The skin edges should be apposed with no tension. Absorbable monofilament in an intradermal pattern, nonabsorbable monofilament in a simple interrupted or cruciate mattress pattern, or skin staples can be used for skin closure.

Parapreputial caudal celiotomy

This approach can be used alone or as the caudal component of the standard midline celiotomy in male dogs, as described above. Parapreputial caudal celiotomy alone allows for a limited approach to the caudal abdomen and can be used to access the urinary bladder, the intra-abdominal urethra, the prostate gland, and, in general, to explore the structures in the caudal abdomen. The surgical procedure is the same as described for midline celiotomy, with the difference that the incision is focused only at the parapreputial portion of the ventral abdomen (Video 3.2).

Video 3.2. Midline celiotomy with a parapreputial approach in a 3-year-old Chihuahua (3.4 kg). Note the use of electrocautery for hemostasis and the placement of an abdominal retractor to improve abdominal exposure.

Paracostal/lateral abdominal approach

Although this approach is less commonly used, it can be helpful for some specific conditions. Indications include access to the mesenteric lymph nodes for lymphangiography; to the cisterna chyli, ipsilateral adrenal gland, kidney, or ovary; and to the stomach for gastrostomy tube placement or prophylactic gastropexy. It can also be combined with a transdiaphragmatic approach for ligation of the thoracic duct. The location of the incision should be determined based on the target organ. In case of a cranial incision near the last rib, care should be taken to leave enough muscle tissue cranially for suturing. If needed the ribs can be incorporated into the closure.

There are two main surgical techniques described to perform a lateral abdominal approach: the grid incision and the through-and-through incision. In both cases the incision is carried through three muscular layers: the external abdominal oblique muscle, the internal abdominal oblique muscle, and the transversus abdominis muscle.

Surgical technique: Grid incision

The grid approach is a minilaparotomy incision aimed at reducing as much as possible the muscle trauma caused by a standard through-and-through paracostal abdominal incision. Each muscle is bluntly separated following the direction of its fibers, which is different in each muscular layer of the abdominal wall.[1–5]

1. The patient is positioned in lateral recumbency with the side to be approached uppermost.
2. The lateral abdomen and caudal thorax are clipped and prepped from the spinous processes to beyond the ventral midline.

3. A sandbag or a rolled towel can be placed beneath the cranial abdomen or caudal thorax to improve the exposure and elevate the abdominal organs.
4. A skin incision is made from the ventral edge of the epaxial muscles toward the ventral midline, approximately 2 cm caudal to the last rib.
5. The subcutaneous tissue is dissected from the fascia of the external abdominal oblique muscle.
6. The external abdominal oblique muscle is split along its fibers with scissors or electrocautery. Gelpi retractors or a ring retractor are placed to retract the muscle.
7. The internal abdominal oblique muscle is exposed, split along its fibers with scissors or electrocautery, and retracted.
8. The transversus abdominis muscle is exposed, split along its fibers with scissors or electrocautery, and retracted, exposing the abdominal cavity (Fig. 3.4).
9. Stay sutures can be placed in the muscles to help recognize the different layers for closure.
10. Moist laparotomy sponges are placed around the incision edges, and a retractor is inserted.

Surgical technique: Through-and-through incision

1. Following the skin and subcutaneous incision, the abdominal wall muscles are incised from dorsal to ventral.
2. The external and internal abdominal oblique muscles are incised in the same direction, almost perpendicular and crosswise to the direction of the muscles.
3. An incision is then made in the transversus abdominis muscle. Depending on the location of the approach, this last incision will be performed in the muscular or tendinous portion (transverse fascia) of the muscle.
4. Stay sutures can be placed in the muscles to help recognize the different layers for closure.
5. Moist laparotomy sponges are placed around the incision edges, and a retractor is inserted.

Closure

1. Each muscle of the body wall previously incised should be apposed individually. Absorbable monofilament suture material (2-0/3-0 polydioxanone) should be used in a simple continuous pattern.
2. The subcutaneous layer is closed using absorbable monofilament suture material in a simple continuous pattern.
3. The skin is then apposed using monofilament suture material in an intradermal pattern (absorbable suture material) or in a simple interrupted or cruciate mattress pattern (absorbable or nonabsorbable suture material). Skin staples can be used for closure.

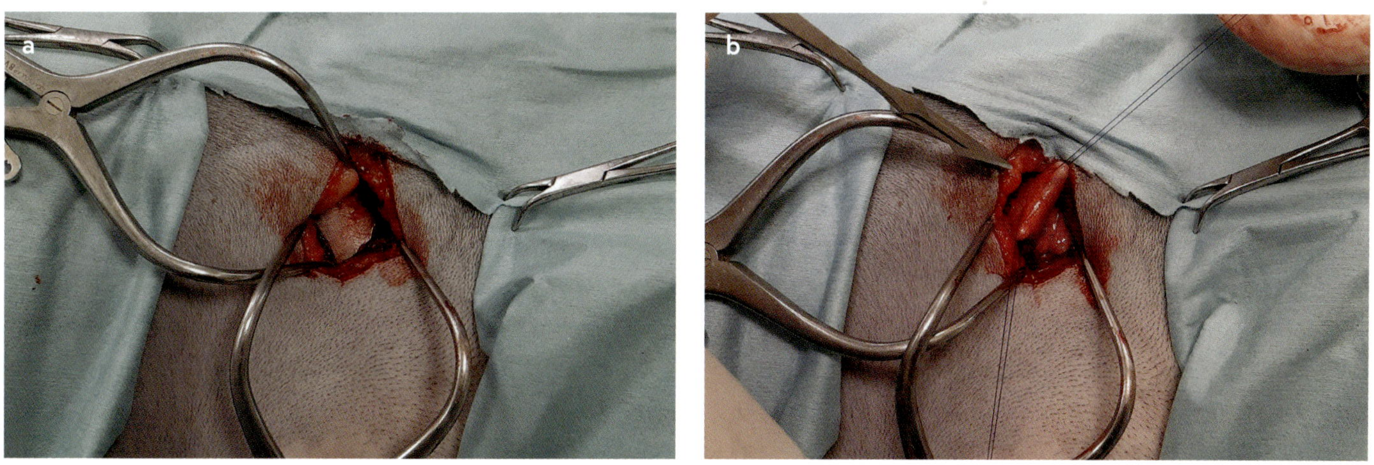

Figure 3.4 Grid approach on the right lateral abdominal wall in a dog for a routine gastropexy. After splitting the abdominal wall muscles along their fibers, two Gelpi retractors are placed to improve visualization. (a) Note the peritoneum as the last layer before entering the abdominal cavity. (b) The abdominal cavity is exposed and stay sutures are placed on the gastric wall. Images courtesy of Filippo Cinti.

KEEP IN MIND

- Parapreputial caudal celiotomy is a limited approach that allows exploration of the structures in the caudal abdomen.
- Paracostal approaches are not commonly used; however, they can be helpful for some specific conditions. The location of the incision should be determined based on the target organ.

References

1. van Sluijs F, L'Eplattenier H, Jonker J, Ensink J. Abdominal surgery. In: Kirpensteijn J, ter Haar G (eds.). *The Cutting Edge: Basic Veterinary Surgery Techniques*, 3rd ed. Lawrence, KS: Sorry For Saying Sorry Media; 2021.
2. Scavelli TD. Endocrine system. In: Bojrab MJ, Ellison GW, Slocum B (eds.). *Current Techniques in Small Animal Surgery*, 4th ed. Baltimore, MD: Williams & Wilkins; 1998.
3. Cornell K. The stomach. In: Johnston SA, Tobias KM (eds.). *Veterinary Surgery: Small Animal*, 2nd ed. St. Louis, MO: Elsevier; 2018.
4. Knecht CD, Allen A, Williams DJ, Johnson JH. *Fundamental Techniques in Veterinary Surgery*, 3rd ed. Philadelphia, PA: Saunders/Elsevier; 1987.
5. Steelman-Szymeczek SM, Stebbins ME, Hardie EM. Clinical evaluation of a right-sided prophylactic gastropexy via a grid approach. *J Am Anim Hosp Assoc*. 2003; 39(4):397–402.

Chapter 4

Thoracic approaches

Matteo Rossanese, Simona Vincenti

Median sternotomy

Median sternotomy permits access to the entire thoracic cavity, provides better exposure of ventral mediastinal structures, and allows bilateral exploratory surgery. The postoperative complication rate ranges from 17% to 78%; however, recently, closure-related complication rates of 7.7% in cats and 14.1% in dogs have been reported.[1,2] Complications have been associated with sternal instability and lack of adequate fixation leading to postoperative pain and prolonged recovery; therefore, anatomical reduction and rigid stabilization of the sternum is critical to promote sternal healing and to reduce the risk of complications.[1–3] Leaving either the manubrium or the xiphoid process intact facilitates sternal closure and increases its stability. Stainless steel orthopedic wire is commonly used for sternal closure in dogs; however, heavy-gauge suture material and crimped monofilament leader line have been described as suitable closure methods.[4–6] The authors use orthopedic wire or appropriately sized crimped monofilament leader line in dogs over 20 kg, whereas they use absorbable suture material (2-0 to 1 USP polydioxanone) in dogs under 20 kg and cats.

Surgical technique (Video 4.1)[7–10]

1. The patient is positioned in dorsal recumbency with the thoracic limbs extended and secured cranially.
2. The thorax is clipped and prepped from the ventral cervical area to the cranial ventral abdomen. Clipping should extend dorsally enough to allow placement of a thoracostomy tube during the surgical procedure.

Video 4.1. Caudal median sternotomy (manubrium left intact) in a dog diagnosed with pyothorax. Note the use of a sternal saw. This involves an approach to the xiphoid process and sternotomy in a caudal to cranial direction.

3. A skin incision is made on the ventral midline along the length of the sternum, from the manubrium to the xiphoid process, using a number 10 scalpel blade.
4. The subcutaneous tissue is dissected to expose the superficial and deep pectoral muscles.
5. Using a periosteal elevator or electrocautery, the superficial and deep pectoral muscles are separated in the midline to expose the sternebrae.
6. The sternebrae are scored along the midline with a scalpel or electrocautery to guide the osteotomy (Fig. 4.1).
7. Once the sternum is exposed, the osteotomy is performed transecting the sternebrae longitudinally with an oscillating saw. It is important to stay on the midline to avoid inadvertent fracture of the sternebrae and hemorrhages from the internal thoracic arteries (Fig. 4.2).
8. Moderate lavage with saline during the osteotomy helps prevent thermal injuries to the sternebrae and keeps the incision line clear. The oscillating saw is moved along the midline using a back-and-forth motion (Fig. 4.3).
9. The surgeon should inform the anesthetist before entering the thoracic cavity, as intermittent positive-pressure ventilation (IPPV) should be started.

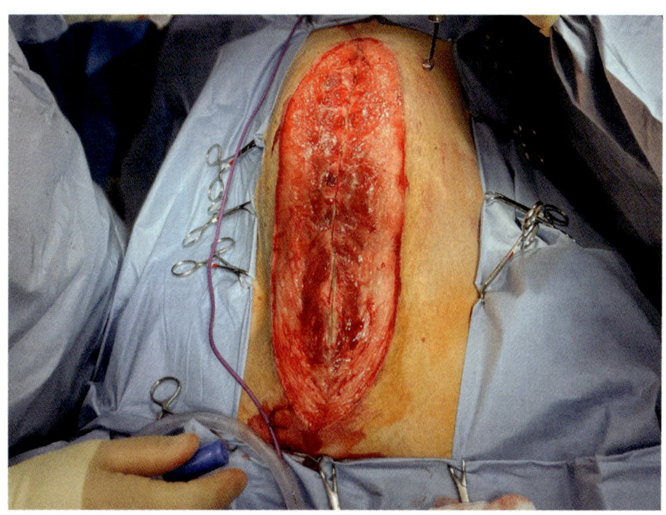

Figure 4.1 The sternebrae have been scored with electrocautery to guide the sternotomy. Cranial is to the bottom of the image.

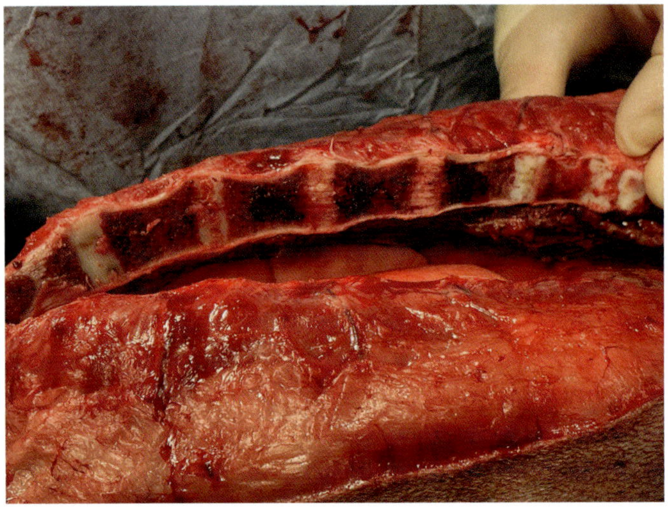

Figure 4.2 The sternebrae have been transected longitudinally in the midline using an oscillating saw. This increases the stability of the sternotomy closure.

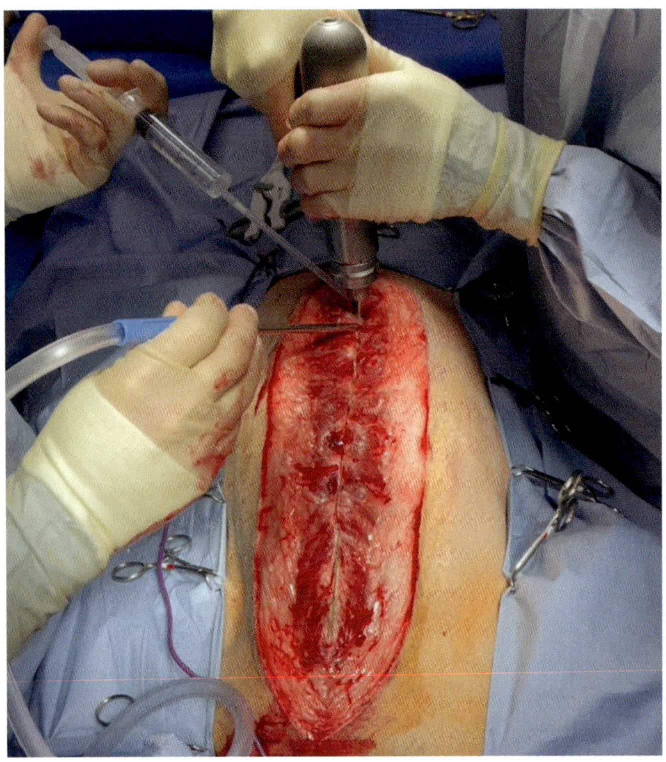

Figure 4.3 Flushing with saline and continuous suction are used during sternotomy to prevent thermal injury and facilitate visualization.

10. Once one or two sternebrae have been sectioned, a Gelpi retractor is placed on the osteotomy edges to retract the sternum.
11. The connective tissue of the ventral thorax should be perforated to establish a pneumothorax, avoiding any damage to intrathoracic structures.
12. An assistant can introduce a long pair of forceps and keep them against the dorsal aspect of the sternum to protect the intrathoracic structures from the oscillating saw.
13. The osteotomy is continued in a cranial to caudal direction. It should be noted that, based on the surgical procedure to be performed, the xiphoid process or the manubrium should be left intact in order to increase the stability of the sternotomy after closure.
    - Cranial sternotomy: The sternotomy should extend from the manubrium to the 6th–7th sternebrae.
    - Caudal sternotomy: The sternotomy should extend from the xiphoid process to the 2nd–3rd sternebrae.
    - Full (complete) sternotomy: The sternotomy should extend from the manubrium to the xiphoid process.
14. Moist laparotomy sponges are placed around the edges of the osteotomized sternum, and a Finochietto retractor is inserted (Fig. 4.4).

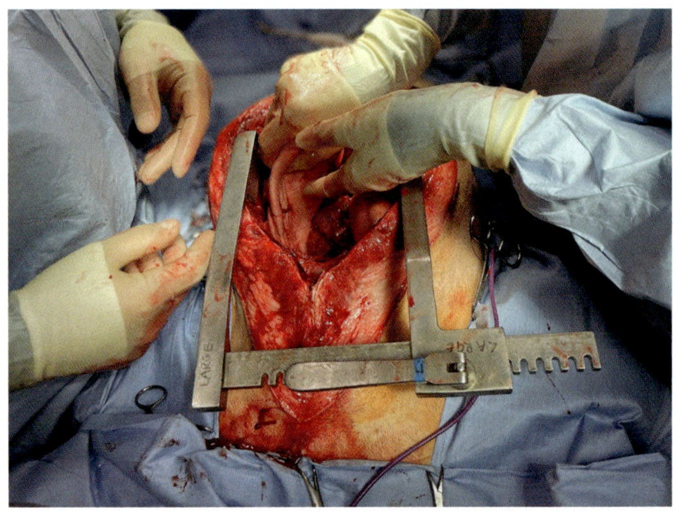

Figure 4.4 Placement of a Finochietto retractor after sternotomy. This allows exposure of ventral mediastinal structures. In the image, the left cranial lung lobe is being examined.

Closure (Video 4.2)

1. Before closure, a thoracostomy tube should be placed as described in Chapter 5.
2. The sternotomy is closed using an alternating figure-of-eight pattern of stainless steel wire or 2-0 to 1 absorbable or nonabsorbable monofilament based on the size of the patient.

Video 4.2. Sternotomy closure in a 36 kg dog using stainless steel wire in an alternating figure-of-eight pattern.

3. Sutures or wires are preplaced at each sternebra incorporating the costal cartilage. The tip of the wire or needle should be passed carefully to avoid injury to the lungs or other soft tissues (e.g., internal thoracic vessels).
4. An assistant should place traction on one or more sutures or wires to reappose the sternebrae while the remaining sutures are tied or the wires twisted.
5. If orthopedic wire is used, the ends are cut short, leaving two or three twists, and bent over to minimize soft tissue injuries and help with soft tissue coverage (Fig. 4.5).
6. The superficial and deep pectoral muscles are reapposed using 3-0 or 2-0 absorbable monofilament suture material in a simple continuous pattern.
7. Residual air (and fluid) should be removed from the thoracic cavity using the thoracostomy tube.
8. The subcutaneous layer and the skin are closed routinely.

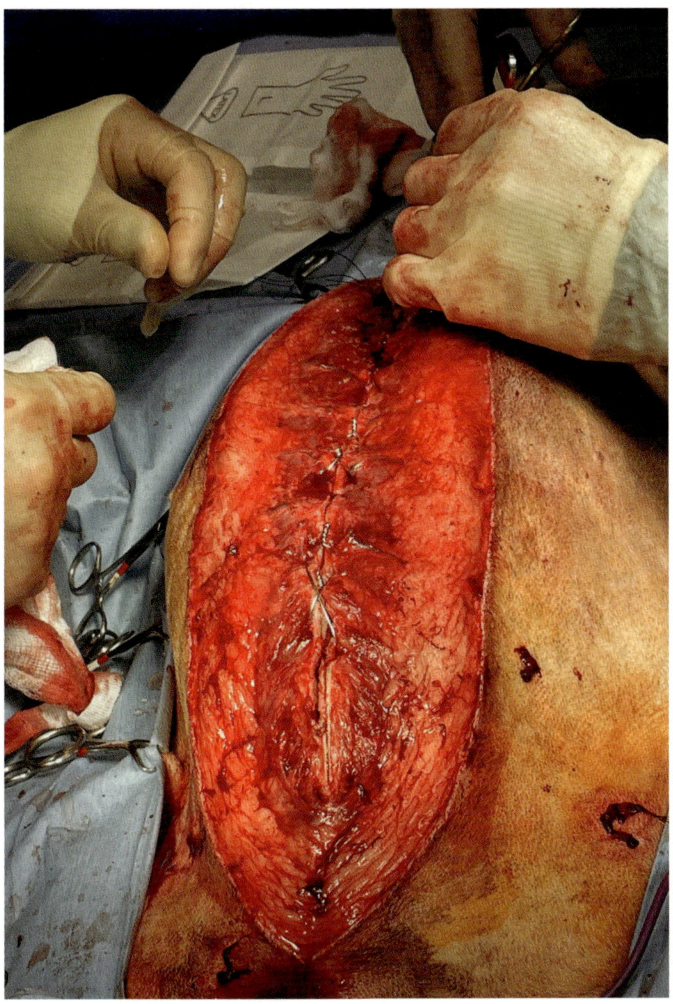

Figure 4.5 Sternotomy closure using orthopedic wire. Note that the wires have been twisted and cut short, leaving two or three twists, and bent over toward the sternum to help with soft tissue coverage.

Intercostal thoracotomy

The decision to use intercostal thoracotomy depends on the exposure needed and underlying disease (Table 4.1). This approach allows access to only one hemithorax, and the exposure of intrathoracic structures is limited; therefore, determining the correct location for the thoracotomy incision is a critical step.[6,8–10] Due to the deep and narrow shape on the thorax in cats and dogs, intercostal thoracotomy overall provides an adequate exposure for the majority of surgical procedures. Dogs and cats have 13 pairs of ribs (12 intercostal spaces), with the first 9 ribs articulating with the sternebrae via the costal cartilage. It is important to remember that due to the natural curvature of the ribs, the ribs cranial to an intercostal incision are more easily retracted than the caudal ribs; therefore, when choosing between two adjacent intercostal spaces, the more caudal one should be preferred.[8–10] Complications associated with intercostal thoracotomy include seroma, ventral edema, excessive wound inflammation, ipsilateral limb lameness, wound discharge, and infection.[3]

Surgical technique (Video 4.3)[7–10]

1. The patient is positioned in lateral recumbency with the side to be approached uppermost.
2. The lateral thorax is clipped and prepped from the axilla to the last rib and from the thoracic spinous processes to the sternum.
3. A sandbag or a rolled towel can be placed beneath the thorax caudal to the scapula to spread the ribs and elevate the intrathoracic structures. The thoracic limb can be secured in an extended position if needed.
4. The incision site should be located by counting the intercostal spaces from the last rib.
5. A skin incision is made using a number 10 scalpel blade, centered over the intercostal space of interest. For thoracotomy in the 4th or 5th intercostal spaces, the incision should be made about 2 cm caudal to the scapula, starting at the caudodorsal angle of the scapula and ending below the costochondral junction.
6. The subcutaneous tissue is incised and the cutaneous trunci muscle is transected to expose the latissimus dorsi muscle.

Video 4.3. Right 5th intercostal thoracotomy using a muscle-sparing technique. Note the dorsal retraction of the latissimus dorsi muscle. Cranial is to the right side.

TABLE 4.1 - RECOMMENDED INTERCOSTAL SPACES FOR THORACOTOMY BASED ON THE STRUCTURE OF INTEREST		
Structure	**Intercostal space**	
	Left	**Right**
Heart/pericardium	4, 5	4, 5
PDA, PRAA	4, (5)	—
Cranial lung lobe	5, (4)	5, (4)
Middle lung lobe	—	5
Accessory lung lobe	—	5, (6)
Caudal lung lobe	5, (6)	5, (6)
Cranial vena cava	(4)	4
Caudal vena cava	(6, 7)	6–9
Thoracic duct		
Dogs	—	8–11
Cats	8–11	—
Thoracic esophagus		
Cranial	3, 4	3–5
Caudal	7–9	7–9

Modified from Tobias KM, Darrow BG, Radlinsky MG. Thoracic cavity. In: Johnston SA, Tobias KM (eds.). *Veterinary Surgery: Small Animal*, 2nd ed. St. Louis, MO: Elsevier; 2018. Numbers in parenthesis indicate alternative surgical sites. PDA, patent ductus arteriosus; PRAA, persistent right aortic arch.

7. The latissimus dorsi muscle can be (Fig. 4.6):
   - elevated dorsally after incising its ventral fascial attachments (muscle-sparing technique)—an Army-Navy retractor can be used;
   - transected vertically along the incision if additional exposure is required.
8. It is important to correctly identify the intercostal space of interest:
   - A finger can be inserted under the latissimus dorsi muscle to locate the first rib and count the ribs or intercostal spaces in a caudal direction (Fig. 4.7).
   - The last rib can be located, and the ribs or intercostal spaces can be counted in a cranial direction.
   - The caudal extent of the muscular portion of the scalenus muscle can be identified inserting on the 5th rib (Fig. 4.8).

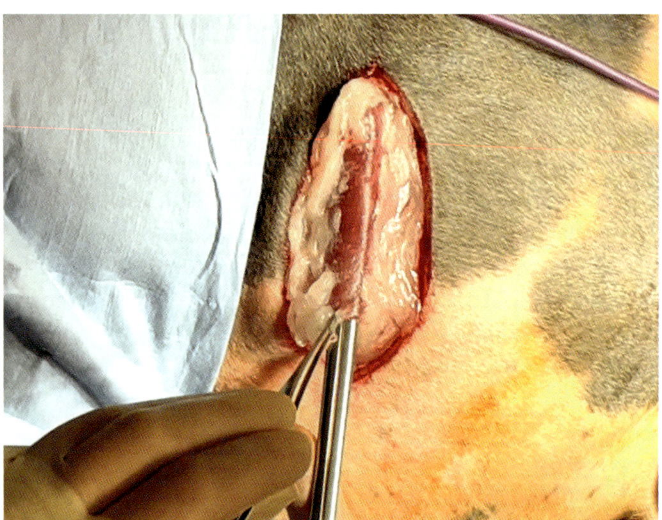

Figure 4.6 Intercostal thoracotomy with isolation of the latissimus dorsi muscle. This muscle can be preserved and retracted dorsally or incised to improve exposure. Cranial is to the left of the image.

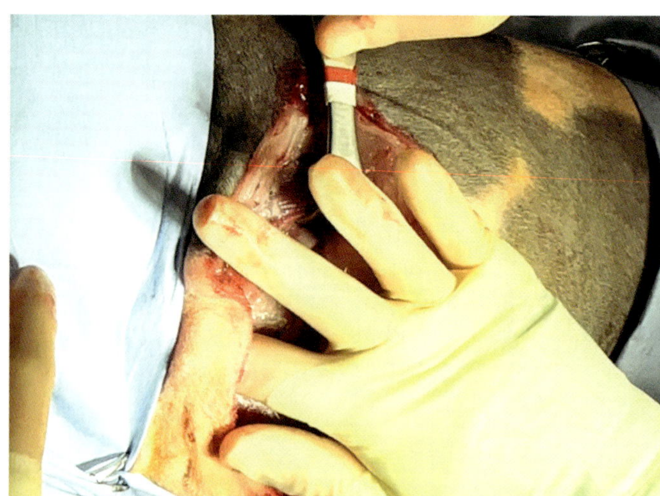

Figure 4.7 A finger is inserted under the latissimus dorsi muscle up to the first rib. The intercostal spaces are then counted from cranial to caudal until the intercostal space of interest is located. Cranial is to the left of the image.

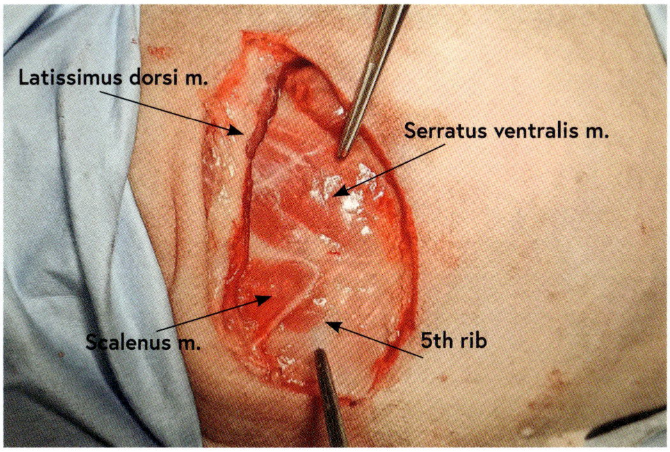

Figure 4.8 Musculature of the lateral thoracic wall after incision of the latissimus dorsi muscle. Note the bellies of the serratus ventralis muscle and the scalenus muscle inserting on the 5th rib. Image courtesy of Filippo Cinti

9. The bellies of the serratus ventralis muscle are divided at the proposed intercostal incision to gain access to the correct intercostal space.
10. The external and internal intercostal muscles are individually elevated and transected in the middle of the intercostal space, preserving the pleura. It should be remembered that the intercostal vessels and nerves lie in the caudal aspect of the intercostal spaces.
11. The surgeon should inform the anesthetist before entering the thoracic cavity, as IPPV should be started.
12. The pleura is punctured with a pair of forceps to avoid damage to the underlying lungs. This allows air to enter the thoracic cavity, causing collapse and retraction of the lungs away from the thoracic wall. Mechanical ventilation can be temporarily suspended just before entering the pleura to allow the lung lobes to deflate and move away from the pleura, avoiding potential damage to the lungs.
13. The pleural incision is extended from the medial angle of the ribs to below the costochondral junction. Attention should be paid dorsally and ventrally to avoid damage to the epaxial muscles and to the internal thoracic artery, respectively (Fig. 4.9).
14. Moist laparotomy sponges are placed on the edges of the incision, and the ribs are gradually spread apart using a Finochietto retractor.

Closure (Video 4.4)

1. Before closure, a thoracostomy tube should be placed as described in Chapter 5.
2. The sandbag or rolled towel should be removed from beneath the patient's thorax to facilitate rib apposition.

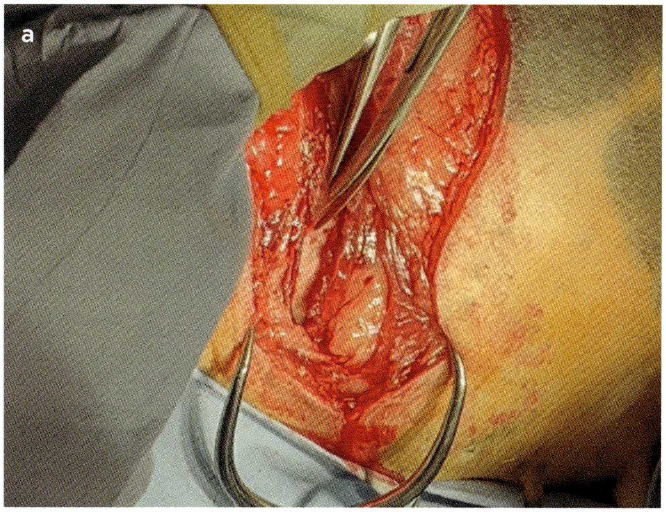

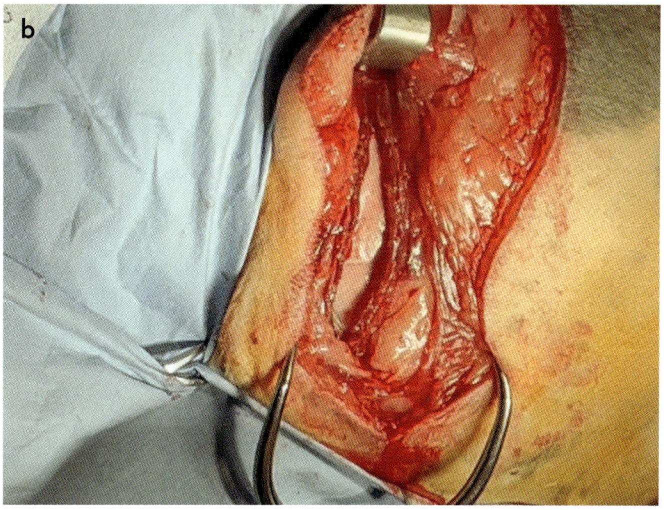

Figure 4.9 (a) Incision of the pleura with Metzenbaum scissors. Note the use of a pair of DeBakey forceps under the pleura to protect the intrathoracic structures during the incision. (b) The pulmonary tissue is exposed after incising the pleura.

3. Circumcostal sutures (2-0 to 1 absorbable or nonabsorbable monofilament) are preplaced around the ribs cranial and caudal to the incision every 1.5–3 cm based on the patient's size.
4. An assistant should place traction crossing two sutures to appose the ribs while the remaining sutures are tied (Fig. 4.10). Overlapping of the ribs should be avoided.

Video 4.4. Closure of a right 5th intercostal thoracotomy. Note the use of 0 polydioxanone circumcostal sutures and how the assistant applies traction to appose the ribs and aid in closure.

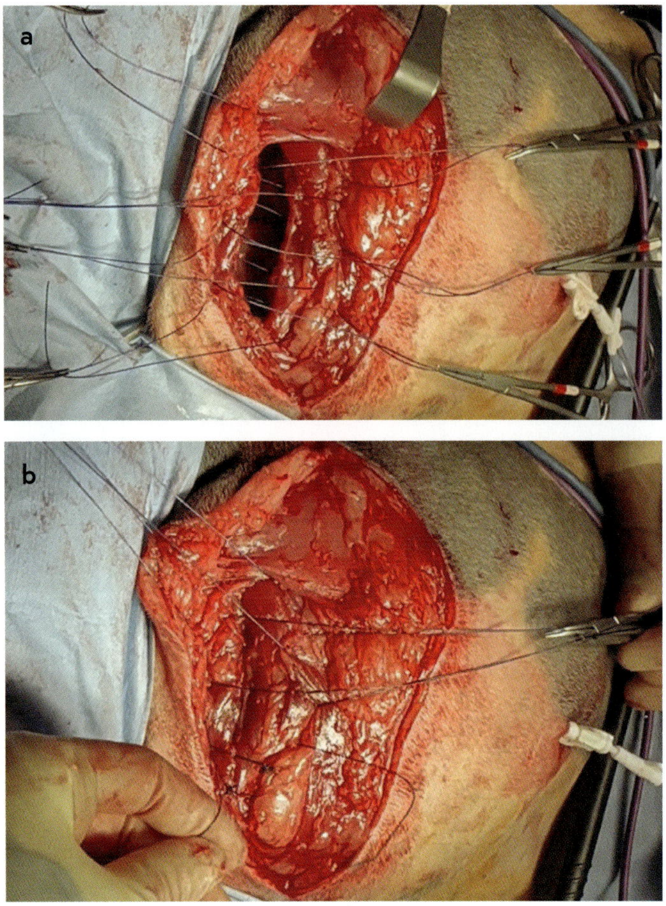

Figure 4.10 (a) Preplacement of circumcostal sutures. (b) An assistant apposes the ribs by applying traction on the sutures to aid closure of the thoracic cavity.

5. In medium- and large-breed dogs, the external and internal intercostal muscles can be reapposed using 2-0 or 3-0 absorbable monofilament in a simple continuous pattern. However this is not necessary and usually not performed.
6. The bellies of the serratus ventralis muscle are reapposed using 2-0 or 3-0 absorbable monofilament in a simple continuous pattern.
7. The scalenus and pectoral muscles should be reapposed (if included in the initial incision) using 2-0 or 3-0 absorbable monofilament in a simple continuous pattern.
8. Residual air (and fluid) should be removed from the thoracic cavity using the thoracostomy tube.
9. The subcutaneous layer and the skin are closed routinely.

Transdiaphragmatic thoracotomy

Transdiaphragmatic thoracotomy provides good access to the caudal thoracic cavity, including the thoracic duct, caudal lung lobes, caudal vena cava, caudal thoracic esophagus, and heart.[11] Cardiopulmonary resuscitation is also possible via this approach.

Surgical technique (Video 4.5)[10]

1. The patient is positioned in dorsal recumbency with the thoracic limbs extended and secured cranially.
2. The ventral abdomen and the caudoventral thorax are clipped and prepped.
3. A skin incision is made on the cranioventral midline using a number 10 scalpel blade.
4. The subcutaneous tissue is dissected to expose the linea alba.
5. The linea alba is elevated with a pair of forceps, and a stab incision is made with a scalpel blade.
6. Using Mayo scissors, the abdominal cavity is opened by incising along the linea alba cranially up to the xiphoid process and caudally as needed.
7. The falciform fat is resected along the incision edges using electrocautery.
8. Moist laparotomy sponges are placed around the incision edges, and an abdominal retractor is inserted.
9. A moist laparotomy sponge is placed to protect and retract the liver caudally and dorsally.
10. Before the diaphragm is incised, the caudal vena cava and esophagus are identified.
11. An incision is made on the ventral portion of the diaphragm and extended in a dorsoventral direction using Metzenbaum scissors. Care should be taken to avoid injury to the nearby hepatic veins and caudal vena cava.
12. Stay sutures (2-0 or 3-0 absorbable or nonabsorbable monofilament) are placed at the edges of the incision to expose the intrathoracic structures (Fig. 4.11).
13. If more exposure is needed, a caudal sternotomy should be considered.

Video 4.5. Transdiaphragmatic thoracotomy in a 3-year-old Chihuahua for placement of an epicardial pacemaker. After performing a midline celiotomy, an incision is made on the ventral aspect of the diaphragm and enlarged in a dorsoventral direction. Note the stay sutures placed on the diaphragmatic and pericardiotomy incision edges to expose the apex of the heart.

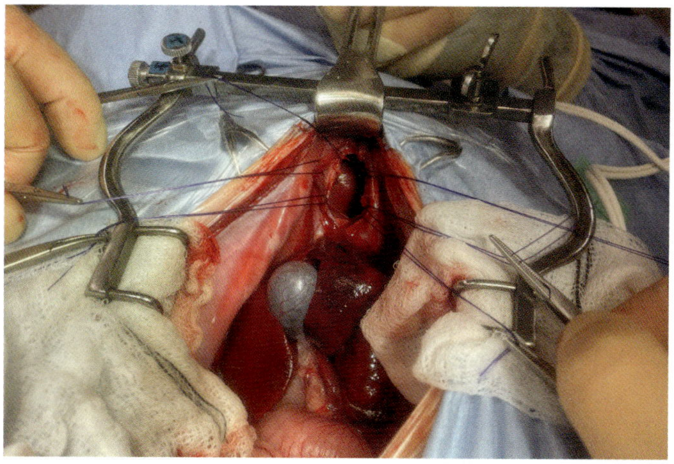

Figure 4.11 Placement of stay sutures at the edges of the diaphragm incision after a transdiaphragmatic thoracotomy to expose the caudal intrathoracic structures. Note the vertical incision on the ventral aspect of the diaphragm and the use of ventrocranial retraction of the sternum.

Closure

1. The diaphragmatic incision is closed using 2-0 or 3-0 absorbable monofilament in a simple continuous or interrupted pattern, starting at the most dorsal part of the incision.
2. The thoracic cavity should be drained before closure to restore negative intrathoracic pressure, using a butterfly catheter or an over-the-needle catheter transdiaphragmatically connected to an extension set, a three-way tap, and a syringe. Placement of a thoracostomy tube can be considered. Return of the concave shape of the diaphragm indicates appropriate thoracic evacuation.
3. The cranial abdominal incision is closed routinely as described in Chapter 3.

KEEP IN MIND

- It's crucial to perform a meticulous count of all swabs and sharps after concluding each surgical intervention.
- Sternotomy allows for better exposure of ventral mediastinal structures and is the preferable approach for bilateral exploratory surgery.
- Intercostal thoracotomy allows access to only one hemithorax. Determining the correct location for the thoracotomy incision is a critical step.
- Transdiaphragmatic thoracotomy provides good access to the caudal thoracic cavity.

References

1. Pilot MA, Lutchman A, Hennet J et al. Comparison of median sternotomy closure-related complication rates using orthopedic wire or suture in dogs: A multi-institutional observational treatment effect analysis. *Vet Surg*. 2022; 51(6):990–1001.
2. Hennet J, Pilot MA, Anderson DM et al. Closure-related complications after median sternotomy in cats: 26 cases (2010–2020). *J Feline Med Surg*. 2022; 24(6):e109–e115.
3. Bleakley S, Phipps K, Petrovsky B, Monnet E. Median sternotomy versus intercostal thoracotomy for lung lobectomy: A comparison of short-term outcome in 134 dogs. *Vet Surg*. 2018; 47(1):104–113.
4. Rossanese M, Tomlinson A. Crimped monofilament nylon leader for median sternotomy closure in 10 dogs. *Vet Surg*. 2021; 50(2):402–409.
5. Pelsue DH, Monnet E, Gaynor JS et al. Closure of median sternotomy in dogs: Suture versus wire. *J Am Anim Hosp Assoc*. 2002; 38(6):569–576.
6. Tillson DM. Thoracic surgery; important considerations and practical steps. *Vet Clin North Am Small Anim Pract*. 2015; 45(3):489–506.
7. Fossum TW. Surgery of the lower respiratory system: Lungs and thoracic wall. In: Fossum TW (ed.). *Small Animal Surgery*, 4th ed. St. Louis, MO: Elsevier; 2013. pp. 958–990.
8. Hunt GB. Thoracic wall. In: Johnston SA, Tobias KM (eds.). *Veterinary Surgery: Small Animal*, 2nd ed. St. Louis, MO: Elsevier; 2018.
9. Tobias KM, Darrow BG, Radlinsky MG. Thoracic cavity. In: Johnston SA, Tobias KM (eds.). *Veterinary Surgery: Small Animal*, 2nd ed. St. Louis, MO: Elsevier; 2018.
10. Risselada M. Thorax. In: *Atlas of Surgical Approaches to Soft Tissue and Oncologic Diseases in the Dog and Cat*. Hoboken, NJ: John Wiley & Sons; 2020.
11. Fox PR, Matthiesen DT, Purse D, Brown NO. Ventral abdominal, transdiaphragmatic approach for implantation of cardiac pacemakers in the dog. *J Am Vet Med Assoc*. 1986; 189(10):1303–1308.

Chapter 5

Tube placement

Anna Frykfors von Hekkel, Rhiannon Strickland

Feeding tubes

Feeding tube placement should be considered in patients where the use of nutritional support is necessary or anticipated. A number of factors should be taken into consideration, including the underlying disease process and associated clinical signs, expected duration of tube feeding, method of tube placement, risk of complications related to the specific procedure performed, and any contraindications. Common types of feeding tubes include nasoesophageal (NE)/nasogastric (NG), esophagostomy, gastrostomy, and enterostomy tubes. After placement, it is important to secure the feeding tube to avoid dislodgment and to confirm appropriate placement to avoid potentially life-threatening complications. Nonabsorbable monofilament suture material (2-0 to 3-0) in a finger-trap pattern is commonly used to secure feeding tubes. A biomechanical study which evaluated several finger-trap patterns utilized to secure an esophagostomy tube concluded that the patterns shown in Figure 5.1 performed best in axial loading and that a minimum of six rows of sutures should be placed.[1] Reported methods of confirming appropriate tube placement include direct laryngeal visualization, capnography, presence of negative pressure during aspiration, direct palpation in the stomach, instillation of sterile saline, and radiography.[2] Misinterpretation of single lateral radiographs has been reported, due to superimposition of the tube over the target region (esophagus/stomach).[3,4] In the absence of direct palpation, the authors recommend performing orthogonal radiographs to confirm appropriate placement.

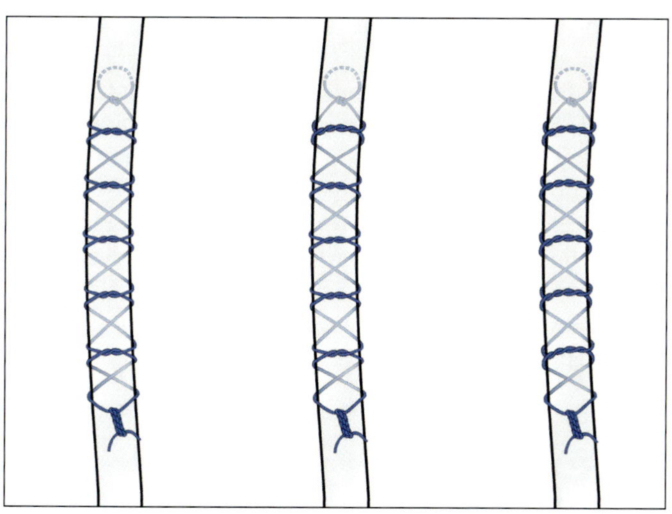

Figure 5.1 Finger-trap suture patterns that performed best in a biomechanical study evaluating esophagostomy tube securement.[1]

Any tube (and drain) needs to be protected from patient interference, which can be achieved with an Elizabethan collar or body stocking. In instances of feeding tube blockage, a small volume (3–5 mL) of a carbonated drink (e.g., cola) can be instilled into the tube and left for 5–10 minutes in an attempt to dissolve the blockage. Following removal of an esophagostomy or gastrostomy tube (also cystostomy tubes and thoracic/abdominal drains), the resultant wound is left open to heal by second intention. A light dressing can be applied to protect the wound from contamination and patient interference, and should be changed daily.

Nasoesophageal/nasogastric tubes

A small-bore (3Fr–8Fr) feeding tube is passed via the nostril into the esophagus (NE tube) or stomach (NG tube). This can typically be performed in a conscious patient, precluding the need for sedation or anesthesia. Reported complication rates of NE and NG tubes are comparable,[5] although NG tubes have the advantage of allowing gastric decompression and measurement of gastric residual volume. The small luminal diameter restricts diet consistency to very liquid formulations only; despite this, tube obstruction is common. The patient can be fed immediately after tube placement, and the tube can be removed at any time. These tubes should be avoided in patients with abnormal gag reflex, esophageal dysfunction, or high risk of aspiration.

Technique

1. A topical local anesthetic agent (e.g., lidocaine) is administered into the nostril and allowed to take effect.
2. The tube is premeasured from the nose to the 7th–8th rib (NE tube) or the 9th–11th rib (NG tube) and marked.

3. The tube is lubricated and inserted into the nostril in a ventromedial direction to allow entry into the ventral nasal meatus (Fig. 5.2).
4. The patient's head is held in a neutral position to allow swallowing as the tube is advanced through the pharynx into the esophagus or stomach up to the level of the mark. Coughing can indicate incorrect placement into the trachea, in which case the tube should be withdrawn and the procedure repeated.
5. The tube is secured to the patient's head, typically using a finger-trap suture (Fig. 5.3) or sutures through tape "butterflies" applied to the tube.

Esophagostomy tubes

Esophagostomy tube placement allows use of a larger-bore tube (10Fr–20Fr) but requires general anesthesia. Patients can be fed via the tube as soon as they have recovered from anesthesia and there is no minimum requisite time until the tube can be removed, unlike gastrostomy tubes. Complications are reported in 36%–44% of cases, although they are usually minor.[6] The most frequently encountered complications are related to stoma site inflammation/infection or tube dislodgement; however, complications such as severe hemorrhage, tracheal laceration, mediastinal or subcutaneous misplacement, and wound infection requiring surgical debridement have also been infrequently reported.[4,6,7] Esophagostomy tube placement should be avoided in patients with persistent vomiting or esophageal disorders/surgery.

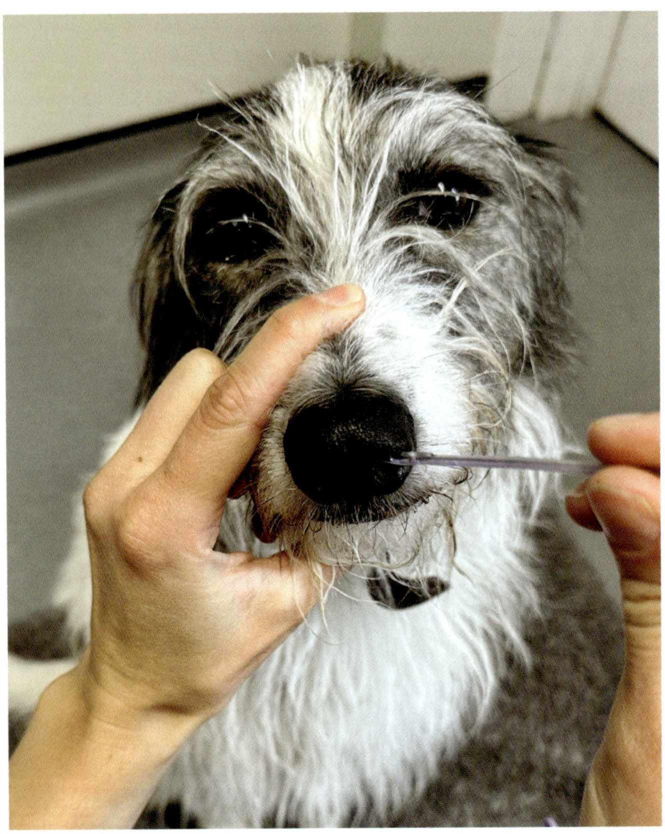

Figure 5.2 Nasogastric feeding tube (8Fr) being inserted into the left nostril of a conscious patient.

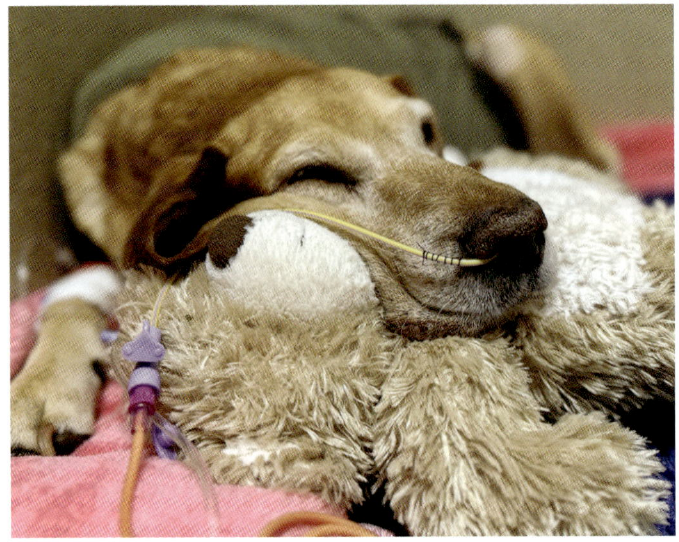

Figure 5.3 Right-sided nasogastric tube in a dog secured with a finger-trap suture, for administration of a constant-rate infusion of the requisite diet.

Technique (Fig. 5.4; Video 5.1)

1. The equipment is prepared and the patient positioned in lateral recumbency (typically right) with a sandbag under the neck.
2. The lateral aspect of the neck is clipped and the skin is aseptically prepared.
3. The tube is premeasured from the midcervical region to the 7th–8th rib and marked.
4. Curved Carmalt or Kelly forceps are advanced from the mouth into the cervical esophagus, distal to the hyoid apparatus. Downward pressure is applied to the forceps handle in order to lift the forceps tips, tenting the tissue overlying them.
5. The area adjacent to the skin tent is palpated to ensure the forceps have not been inadvertently placed into the trachea and that the carotid artery or jugular vein are not appreciable at the intended incision site.

Video 5.1. Placement of a transesophageal esophagostomy tube secured using a finger-trap suture and a butterfly attachment.

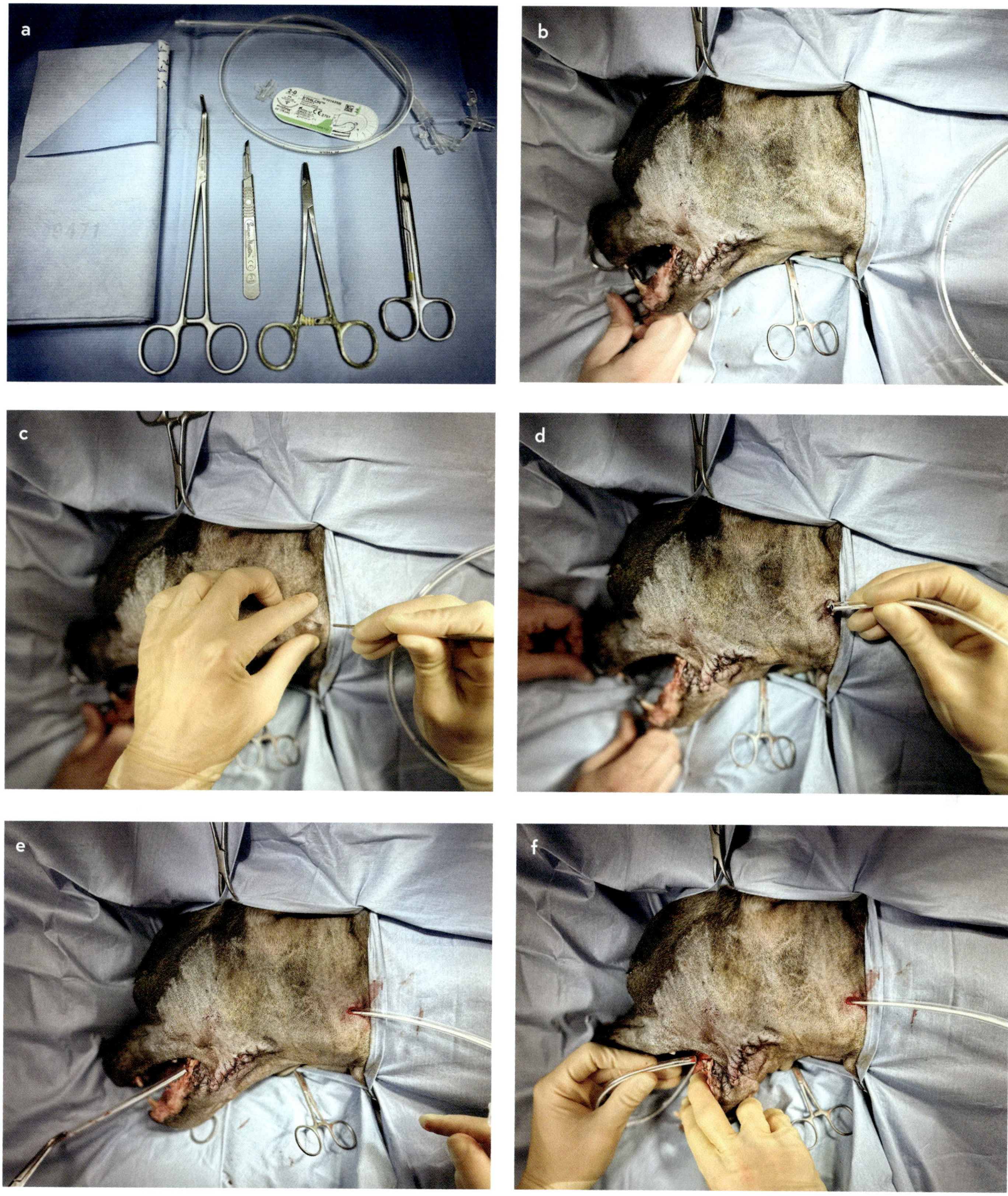

Figure 5.4 Esophagostomy tube placement. (a) Equipment required: (top) esophagostomy tube and suture to secure the tube; (bottom, from left to right) sterile drape, curved forceps, scalpel blade, needle holders, and suture scissors. (b) Curved forceps are advanced from the mouth into the cervical esophagus. Downward pressure on the forceps handle causes the forceps tips to protrude from the lateral neck, tenting the tissue overlying them. Note the jugular vein just ventral to the tented skin. (c) A skin incision is made over the forceps tips. (d) The forceps tips are advanced through the incision and the tip of the tube is grasped. (e) The forceps and tube are withdrawn out of the mouth. (f) The tube tip is redirected back into the mouth.

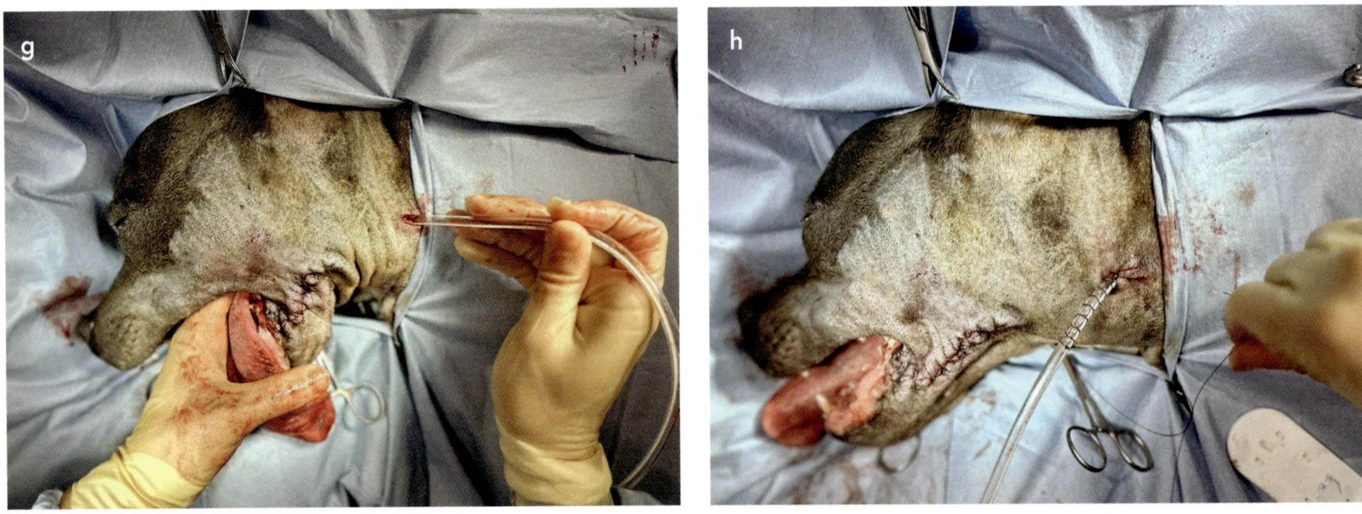

Figure 5.4 Esophagostomy tube placement. (g) The tube tip is advanced into the esophagus by hand while the external portion is simultaneously withdrawn to facilitate tube flipping. (h) The tube is secured to the patient's neck using a finger-trap suture.

6. The forceps tips are forced through the esophageal wall and subcutaneous tissue by applying downward counterforce over the tips.
7. A small skin incision is made over the forceps tips using a scalpel blade.
8. The forceps tips are advanced through the incision and the tip of the esophagostomy tube is firmly grasped.
9. The forceps (and tube tip) are withdrawn out of the mouth.
10. The tube tip is redirected back into the mouth. Care should be taken to ensure that the esophagostomy tube has not become entangled with the anesthetic equipment present in the mouth.
11. The tube tip is advanced into the esophagus by hand or using an instrument—simultaneously withdrawing the cervical portion of the tube can facilitate the tube flipping to lie caudally.
12. The tube is advanced to the level of the premeasured mark.
13. The tube is secured to the patient's neck using a finger-trap suture, and a light dressing is applied.
14. Prior to feeding, appropriate positioning of the tube is confirmed using radiography or fluoroscopy.

Gastrostomy tubes

Gastrostomy tube feeding allows the oral cavity and esophagus to be bypassed as well as placement of large-bore tubes (14Fr–28Fr) and measurement of gastric residual volume. These tubes can be placed surgically (ventral midline or paracostal approach) or endoscopically (percutaneous endoscopic gastrostomy or PEG tube). Complications have been reported to occur in around 42% of cases, most commonly related to peristomal infection/inflammation.[8–10] Major complications such as septic peritonitis or tube removal/dislodgment requiring intervention are reported in approximately 10% of cases, with PEG tubes being associated with a higher rate of complications than surgically placed ones.[10] Gastrostomy tube placement has been reported in the face of preexisting septic peritonitis.[8,9]

Commercially available kits are used for placement of PEG tubes. For surgically placed tubes, Malecot or de Pezzer gastrostomy tubes are preferred to Foley catheters, as gastric contents can lead to degradation and deflation of the Foley balloon bulb.[11] The authors typically use a de Pezzer gastrostomy tube with an XL mushroom tip (Fig. 5.5).

Tube use should be delayed for 24 hours following placement to allow a seal to form between the stomach and body wall. The tube should remain in place at least until a permanent adhesion has formed between the stomach and body wall (typically 8–14 days). Malecot and de Pezzer tubes are removed by cutting the finger-trap suture and applying fast, firm traction to the external portion of the tube (Video 5.2). Gastrostomy tubes should be avoided in animals with primary gastric disease or persistent vomiting.

Video 5.2. Removal of a de Pezzer mushroom-tipped gastrostomy tube (size 16 XL) in a conscious dog.

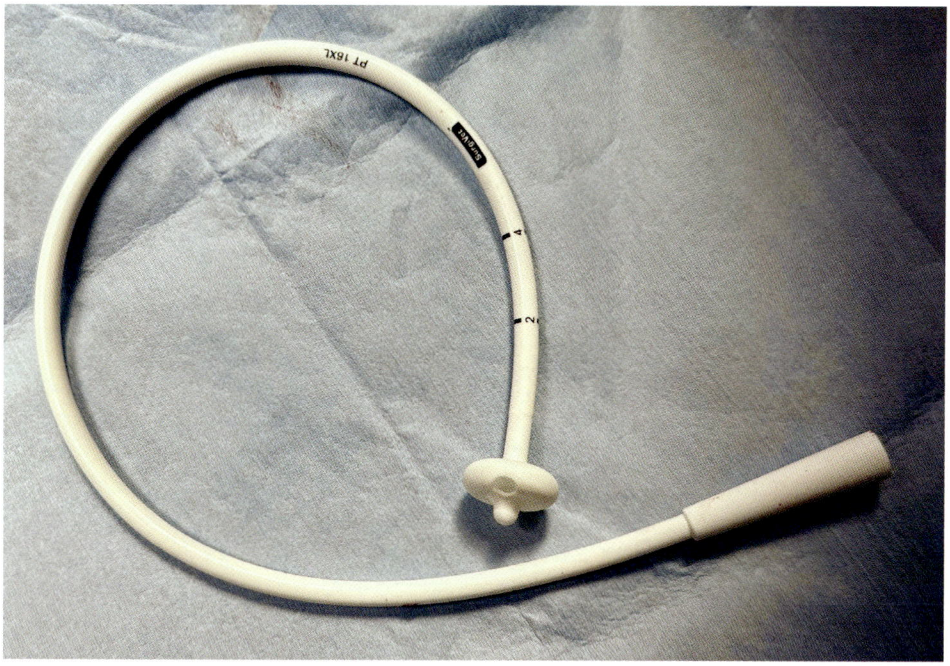

Figure 5.5 De Pezzer gastrostomy tube (size 16 XL).

Technique: Percutaneous endoscopic placement

1. The patient is positioned in right lateral recumbency.
2. A 15 cm^2 area (from the costal arch caudally) on the left lateral flank is aseptically prepared.
3. The endoscope is advanced into the stomach and the stomach is insufflated.
4. The endoscope light is directed toward the left flank and visualized externally. An assistant applies digital pressure to the intended insertion site and the resultant indentation is visualized endoscopically.
5. A small skin incision is made at the level of the intended insertion site with a number 11 scalpel blade.
6. The endoscope is withdrawn to the level of the cardia.
7. The introducer catheter is inserted via the skin incision into the insufflated stomach.
8. Endoscopic grasping forceps are advanced to sit at the tip of the introducer catheter.
9. A guidewire is advanced through the introducer catheter into the stomach and grasped with the endoscopic grasping forceps.
10. The introducer catheter is removed.
11. The grasping forceps with guidewire are withdrawn (along with the endoscope) out of the mouth. Care should be taken to maintain a grasp of the external flank guidewire at all times to avoid fully advancing the wire into the stomach.
12. The guidewire is released from the grasping forceps and the end (external portion) of the PEG tube is attached to the oral end of the guidewire.
13. The external flank guidewire is withdrawn, drawing the gastrostomy tube from the mouth into stomach and out through the body wall.
14. Once the gastrostomy tube can be grasped at the flank, traction is applied until the PEG tube mushroom tip is apposed to the stomach wall and the stomach wall is apposed to the body wall.
15. The endoscope is reinserted to confirm appropriate positioning.
16. The tube is secured by applying the external fixation device.
17. A light protective dressing is applied.

Technique: Surgical placement

1. The patient is placed in dorsal recumbency; the cranial abdomen, caudal thorax, and left paracostal area are clipped and aseptically prepared.
2. A cranial midline celiotomy is performed; a paracostal approach can also be used (see Chapter 3).
3. The cuff of the endotracheal tube should be well inflated to prevent aspiration in case of regurgitation during stomach manipulation.
4. Moistened laparotomy swabs are used to isolate the stomach from the rest of the abdomen, reducing the risk of peritoneal contamination.
5. Stay sutures are placed in the ventral surface of the gastric body to facilitate manipulation.
6. Forceps are used to apply pressure from the abdominal cavity through the left ventrolateral body wall. Care should be taken to ensure this is performed caudal to the costal arch and in a position approximating normal patient anatomy (approximately lev-

el with the left body/fundus of the stomach when the patient is standing).

7. An incision is made in the skin over the forceps tips with a number 11 scalpel blade, and the forceps are advanced through the body wall and skin to grasp the tip of the gastrostomy tube.
8. The tube tip is pulled through the body wall into the abdomen.
9. A full-thickness purse-string suture (2-0 to 0 absorbable monofilament) is placed in the ventral aspect of the left gastric body, midway between the lesser and greater curvatures. The suture is not tied at this stage.
10. Using a number 11 blade, a full-thickness stab incision is made through the center of the purse-string suture into the gastric lumen. Care should be taken not to lacerate the purse-string suture during this process.
11. The gastrostomy tube is advanced through the stab incision into the stomach and the purse-string suture is tightened and tied (Fig. 5.6). A simple interrupted suture can be placed across the stab incision to further close the site.
12. Box sutures are preplaced between the stomach and body walls to enclose the stoma site (see "Box sutures" section below).
13. The gastrostomy site is omentalized.
14. The gastrostomy tube is secured externally using a finger-trap suture (Fig. 5.7).
15. The abdomen is closed routinely.
16. A light protective dressing is applied.

Video 5.3. De Pezzer (size 16 XL) gastrostomy tube placement secured using box sutures between the gastric and abdominal walls (×2 speed).

Box sutures (Video 5.3)

Box sutures are used to enclose a stoma site between the body wall and associated tissue (e.g., stomach, urinary bladder). It consists of four horizontal mattress sutures, each oriented to form one side of a square.

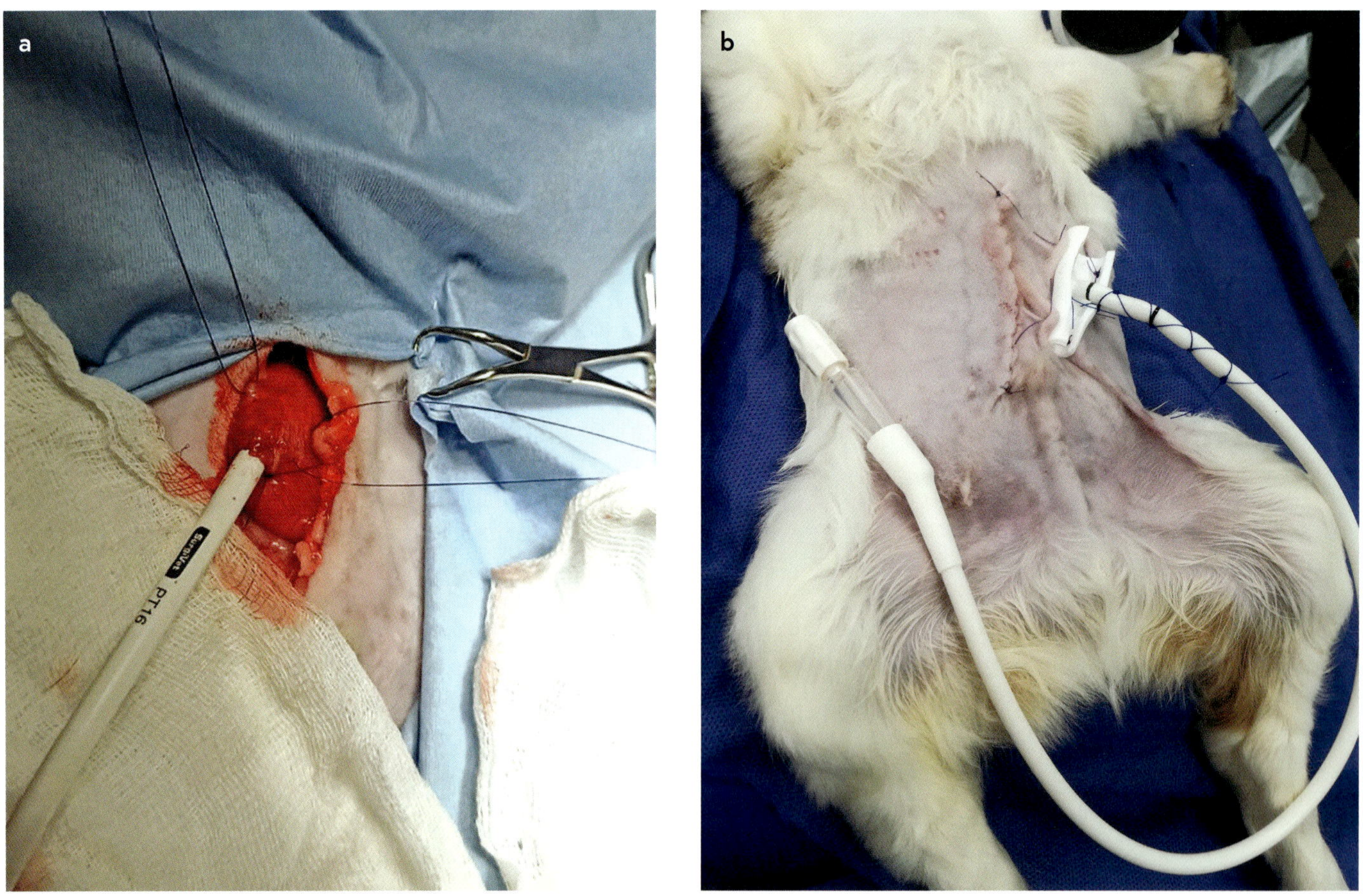

Figure 5.6 (a) After a cranial midline celiotomy and placement of stay sutures in the ventral surface of the gastric body, the gastrostomy tube is advanced through a stab incision into the stomach and the purse-string suture is tightened and tied. Note that in this case the gastrostomy tube is placed in the stomach before advancing it through the abdominal wall. (b) The gastrostomy tube is secured externally using a finger-trap suture. Note that in this case the tube was also secured with a flange. Images courtesy of Filippo Cinti.

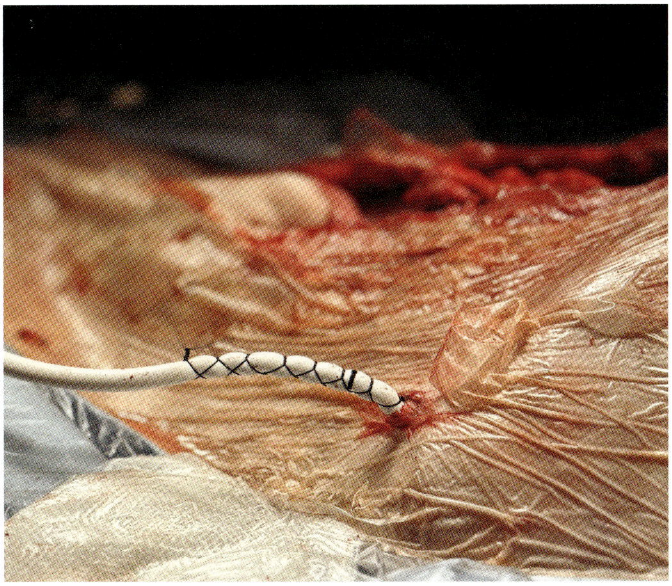

Figure 5.7 Left-sided de Pezzer gastrostomy tube secured externally using a finger-trap suture.

1. A ventrodorsally directed bite of transversus abdominis muscle is taken cranial to the gastrostomy tube.
2. The needle is repositioned in the needle holder and a second dorsoventrally directed bite of gastric wall is taken cranial to the gastrostomy tube.
3. The suture is not tied but left long, with hemostat forceps on the suture ends.
4. This is repeated along the caudal aspect of the tube (suture bites directed along ventrodorsal planes) and the ventral and dorsal aspects of the tube (suture bites directed along craniocaudal planes).
5. Gentle traction is applied to the external portion of the tube to appose the body wall and gastric wall.
6. The box sutures are tied snugly.
7. The site is omentalized.

Enterostomy tubes

Enterostomy tube placement is rarely indicated in the emergency setting, and the reader is directed to alternative resources for further details. It is worth noting that commercially available and homemade gastrojejunostomy tubes can be used to deliver postgastric feeding (Fig. 5.8); these tubes negate some of the concerns related to enterostomy tube placement.[12]

Tube feeding guidelines

Selecting the appropriate diet for tube feeding is crucial and should be determined based on the specific nutritional requirements of the patient, the primary disease, and the size of the tube. Liquid diets are suitable for NE/NG or enterostomy tubes, while blenderized diets are preferred for esophagostomy and gastrostomy tubes. Most oral medications can be crushed and administered through the feeding tube. Feeding methods can vary between bolus feeding and constant-rate infusion. Daily fluid and calorie requirements should be calculated on the individual patient taking into account their current condition:

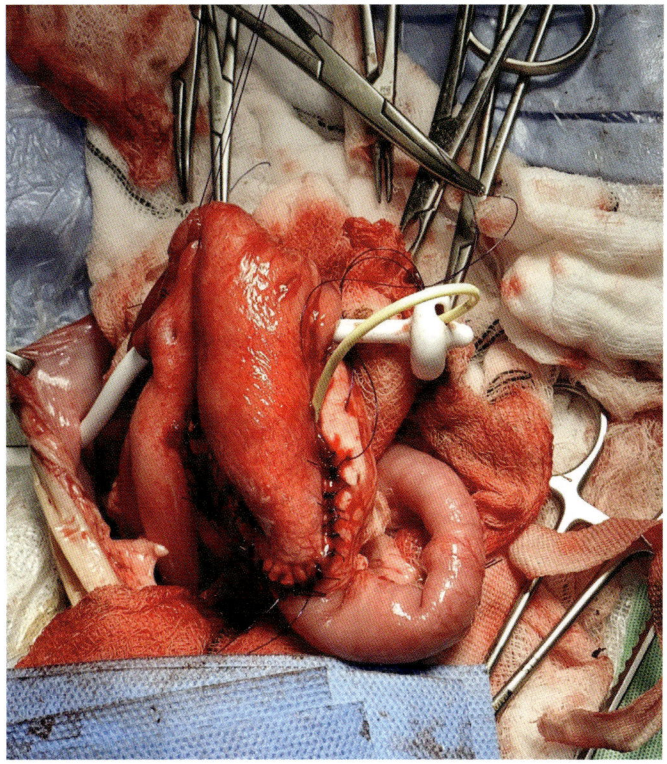

Figure 5.8 Placement of a right-sided gastrojejunostomy tube following a Y-U pyloroplasty for management of pyloric stenosis. Note the small-bore (yellow) tube passing through the mushroom tip of the de Pezzer gastrostomy tube (white).

- Daily fluid requirement: 50–100 mL of water × body weight (kg).
- Daily resting energy requirement (RER) in kcal/day: $70 \times (\text{body weight [kg]})^{0.75}$

The daily RER should be divided into three to five feedings per day. If the patient has been anorexic for several days, it is recommended to begin the feeding with 25% of the RER and, if tolerated, gradually increase it daily with the goal of reaching 100% of the RER within 3–4 days.

Tube feeding procedure

It is important to note that, unless contraindicated, oral food should be offered before resorting to tube feeding.

1. The feeding tube is flushed with 5–10 mL of tepid water.
2. Warm to room temperature food is administered over 15–20 minutes. If the patient exhibits signs of

nausea, vomiting, or other clinical signs, the feeding should be stopped and delayed. If these clinical signs persist, the feeding tube position should be reassessed, the gastric motility evaluated, and/or the feeding volume reduced or switched to a constant-rate infusion.
3. After feeding, the tube is flushed with an additional 5–10 mL of tepid water to ensure tube clearance.

Thoracostomy tubes/drains

Thoracostomy tubes are used when repeated drainage of air or fluid from the pleural space is anticipated, and they can also be utilized for intrapleural delivery of local anesthetics. They can be large bore (16Fr–20Fr) or small bore (12Fr–14Fr). A canine cadaveric study revealed no discernible difference in efficacy between small- and large-bore tubes, irrespective of whether they were tested with air or low- or high-viscosity fluid.[13] Placement of large-bore thoracostomy tubes requires general anesthesia, whereas small-bore tube placement is typically well tolerated with sedation only.[14] Thoracostomy tubes are placed using a strict aseptic technique, typically at the ventral third of the thoracic wall for management of pleural fluid and at the dorsal third for management of pneumothorax. When thoracostomy tubes are placed percutaneously, orthogonal thoracic radiographs should be taken to ensure their correct positioning: along the sternum, with all the fenestrations within the pleural cavity.

Complications associated with thoracostomy tubes include pneumothorax, soft tissue swelling, subcutaneous emphysema, discharge at the tube insertion site, tube kinking, tube displacement, and lung perforation.[15] Thoracic drainage can be intermittent or continuous, with surgical patients typically undergoing intermittent drainage at approximately 4-hour intervals or sooner if clinical signs suggestive of air or fluid accumulation in the pleural cavity manifest. Thoracic fluid production depends on the underlying condition but typically decreases by the second or third day following the thoracic procedure.

The presence of a thoracostomy tube induces pleural fluid production, with progression to septic suppurative fluid frequently noted even under experimental conditions in healthy dogs.[16,17] This should be borne in mind when evaluating cytology or bacteriology results in the presence of a thoracostomy tube, as tube fluid production is unlikely to reach zero. A clinical study in dogs with thoracostomy tubes reported a median fluid production rate of 0.09 mL/kg/h (2.1 mL/kg/day), ranging between 0 and 7.0 mL/kg/h (0–168 mL/kg/day) at the time of tube removal. Fluid production rate was not associated with the presence of pleural fluid 2 weeks later.[18] Due to the potential risk of bacterial infection, tubes should be removed as soon as possible, although this decision should be carefully considered in conjunction with the patient's progress and ongoing fluid production.

Technique: Small-bore tube placement (Fig. 5.9; Videos 5.4 and 5.5)

1. An area over the thorax approximately from the 3rd to the 12th rib is clipped and the skin is aseptically prepared.
2. The patient is positioned in sternal recumbency (unless the tube is placed during intrathoracic surgery).
3. The tube is premeasured by holding it alongside the thorax with the tip aligned with the 2nd rib.
4. A small skin incision is made with a number 11 scalpel blade at the level of the 8th–9th intercostal space, and the introducer catheter is inserted through the skin and advanced subcutaneously to the level of the 7th–8th intercostal space.
5. The introducer catheter is advanced through the intercostal musculature and parietal pleura at the 7th–8th intercostal space. The catheter should be inserted at the cranial aspect of the rib to avoid inadvertent damage to the neurovascular structures that lie along the caudal aspect of the ribs.
6. Once the pleura has been punctured, the catheter stylet is removed and the catheter is advanced into the pleural cavity.
7. A guidewire is advanced through the catheter into the pleural cavity in a cranioventral direction.
8. The catheter is then removed, while the guidewire is left in situ. Care should be taken to maintain a grasp of the guidewire at all times to avoid fully advancing (and losing) the wire into the pleural cavity.

Video 5.4. Percutaneous placement of a small-bore thoracostomy tube using a modified Seldinger technique. Video courtesy of Ben Mielke.

Video 5.5. Intraoperative placement of a small-bore thoracostomy tube using a modified Seldinger technique. Note that the technique is the same without surgical access to the thoracic cavity, but the guidewire/tube cannot be manually positioned within the thoracic cavity.

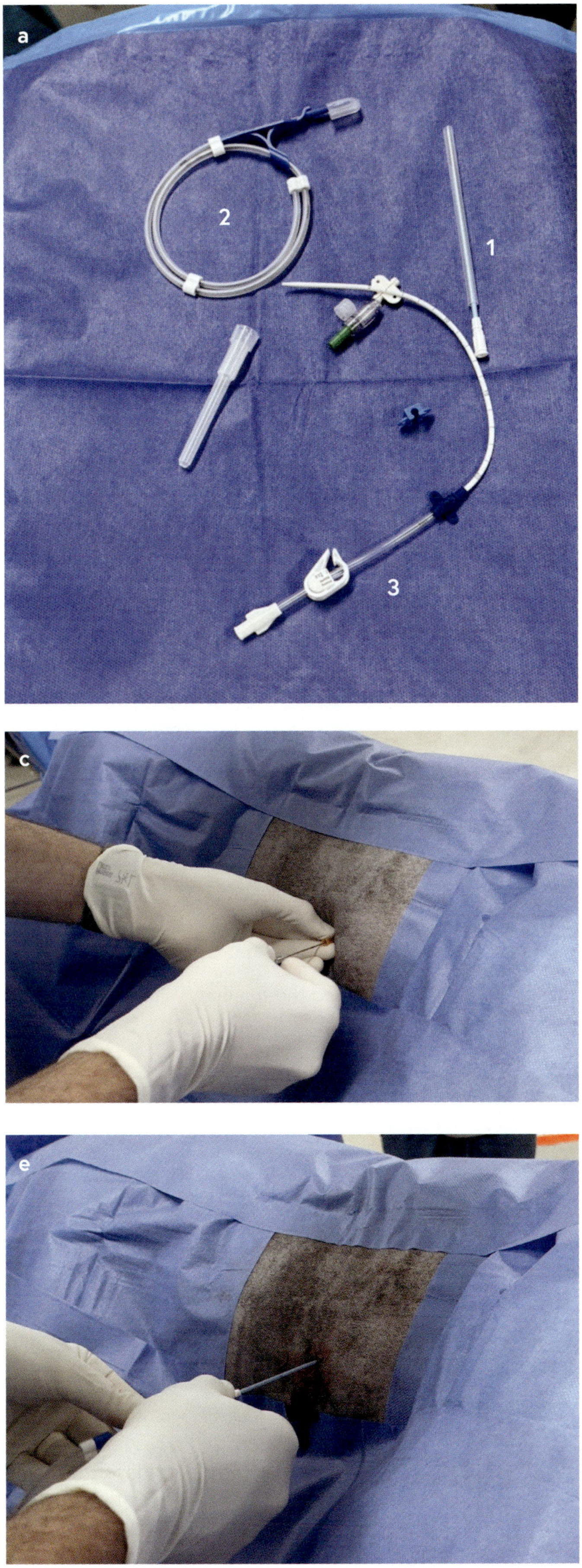

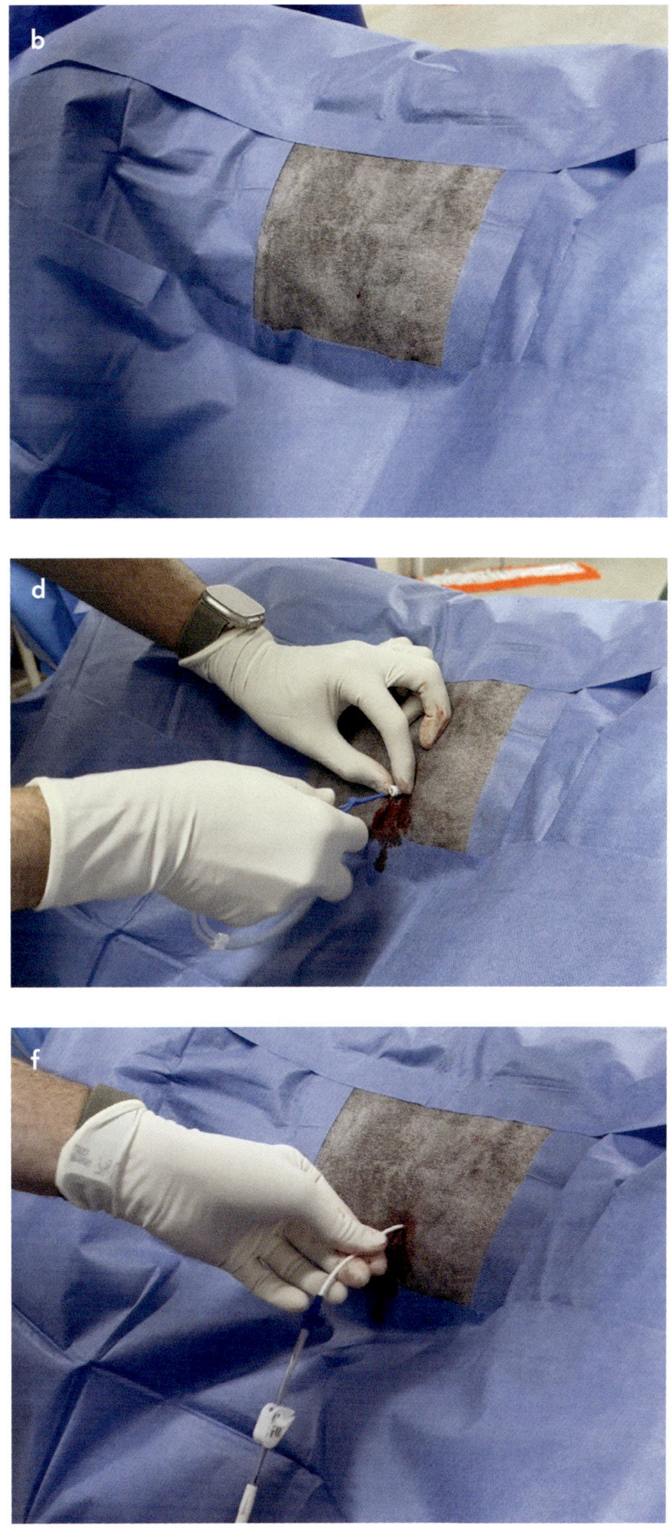

Figure 5.9 Small-bore thoracostomy tube placement. (a) Equipment required, main components: 1, dilator; 2, guidewire; 3, thoracostomy tube. (b) An area of the lateral thorax is aseptically prepared, and the patient is positioned in sternal recumbency. (c) The introducer catheter is inserted through the thoracic wall. (d) The stylet is removed and the guidewire is advanced through the catheter into the pleural cavity. (e) A dilator is advanced over the guidewire. (f) The thoracostomy tube is advanced over the guidewire.

9. A dilator can be inserted over the guidewire to enlarge the insertion point for the thoracostomy tube. Otherwise, a small stab incision with a number 11 scalpel blade can be made in the skin.
10. The thoracostomy tube is advanced over the guidewire into the pleural cavity. Care should be taken to advance the tube far enough so that all the fenestrations are within the thoracic cavity.
11. The tube is aspirated to confirm it is functioning.
12. The tube is secured to the skin using a finger-trap suture or through the suture holes present in the tube.
13. Thoracic radiography should be used to confirm proper tube placement.
14. A light protective dressing is applied.

Technique: Trocar tube placement (Figs. 5.10 and 5.11)

1. An area over the thorax approximately from the 3rd to the 12th rib is clipped and the skin is aseptically prepared.
2. The patient is positioned in lateral recumbency.
3. The tube is premeasured by holding it alongside the thorax with the tip aligned with the 2nd rib. A clamp is preplaced on the tube.
4. The tube is inserted through a skin incision on the dorsal third of the 10th–11th intercostal space and tunneled in a cranioventral direction using the stylet or, if not present, hemostatic forceps.
5. The tube is held vertical at the level of the 7th–8th intercostal space in the midthorax.
6. The anesthetist is asked to pause ventilation in

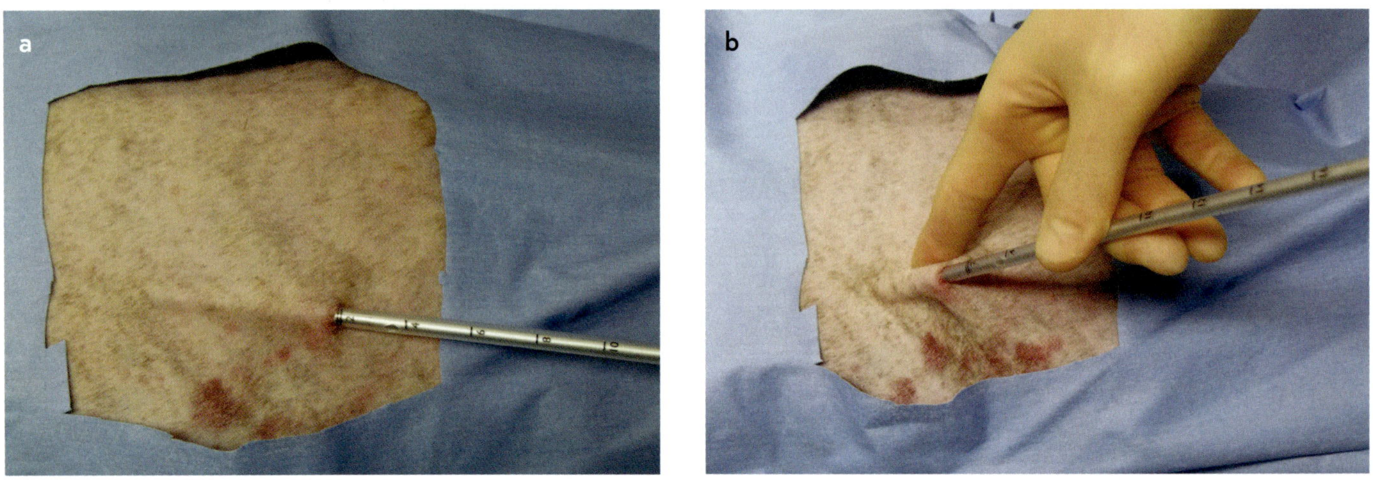

Figure 5.10 Trocar thoracostomy tube placement. (a) The tube is inserted through a skin incision and tunneled under the skin up to the desired point of insertion into the thoracic wall. (b) The tube is elevated and held vertically to the thoracic wall before forcing it through the intercostal space and into the pleural cavity. Images courtesy of Rosario Vallefuoco.

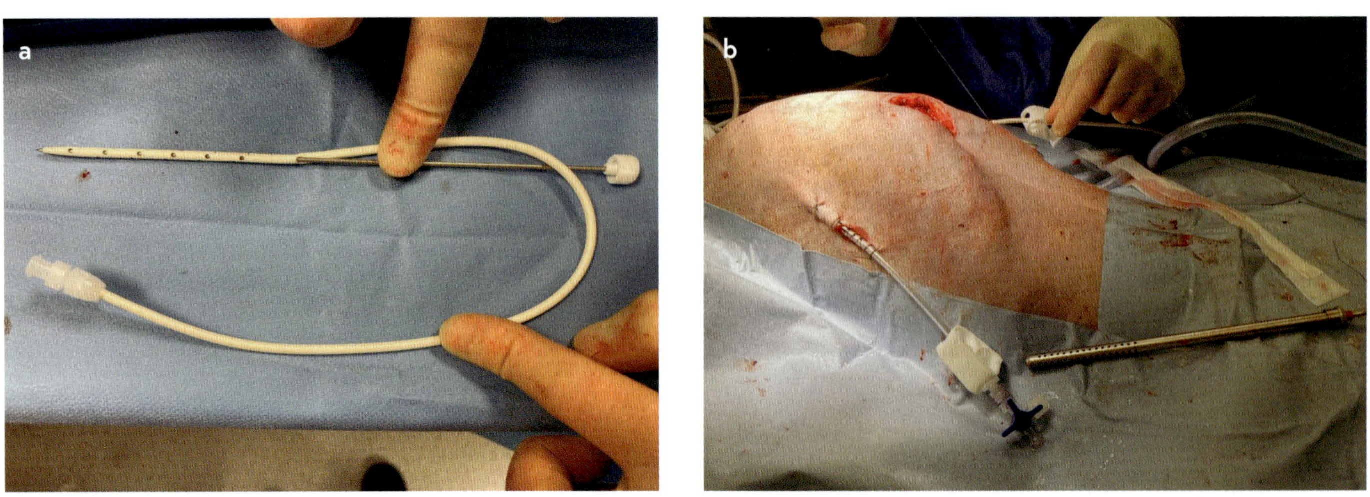

Figure 5.11 Intraoperative bilateral trocar thoracostomy tube placement. (a) One of the tubes before implantation. (b) The tubes are secured to the skin using a finger-trap suture. Images courtesy of Rosario Vallefuoco.

order to minimize the risk of lung injury. The tube is forced through the intercostal space with firm, abrupt pressure on the stylet or hemostatic forceps. Once the pleura is penetrated, ventilation is reestablished.

7. The stylet is aimed at the contralateral elbow and the tube is advanced cranially into the thorax. It is essential that all the fenestrations are within the thoracic cavity.
8. The stylet is removed and the tube is compressed with the preplaced clamp and capped with a stopcock.
9. The tube is aspirated to confirm it is functioning.
10. The tube is secured to the skin using a finger-trap suture or through the suture holes present in the tube.
11. Thoracic radiography should be used to confirm proper tube placement.
12. A light protective dressing is applied.

Abdominal drains

Abdominal drains are frequently used when repeated abdominal drainage is necessary, such as in cases of uroabdomen or septic peritonitis. They can be placed surgically or percutaneously. Percutaneously placed drains are advantageous in that they do not require general anesthesia.[19] Abdominal drains are typically placed as closed active drains, characterized by a tube connected to a suction device, with a reduced risk of infection compared with open drains. Suction can be continuous (e.g., "grenade" suction bulbs used with Jackson–Pratt drains) or intermittent (e.g., manual aspiration). A number of commercially produced drains are available, which function to generate suction in a variety of ways. Grenade suction bulbs have been found to perform most reliably.[20] The presence of a collection reservoir allows ready visualization and monitoring of the abdominal fluid produced. Similar to thoracostomy tubes, the presence of an abdominal drain induces peritoneal fluid production, and it is unlikely that drain fluid production will reach zero. Complications associated with drains include drain-associated infections, patient interference, tube obstruction, drain breakage, neoplastic seeding along the drain tract, and erosion of underlying structures.

Technique: Percutaneous placement

1. The patient is positioned in dorsal recumbency.
2. A wide area around the umbilicus is clipped and the skin is aseptically prepared.
3. Using a number 11 scalpel blade, a small skin incision is made a few centimeters lateral to the umbilicus.
4. The introducer catheter is advanced through the skin incision and tunneled 1–2 cm caudally before being directed through the abdominal wall musculature.
5. Once the peritoneum has been punctured, the catheter stylet is removed and the catheter is advanced into the abdominal cavity.
6. A guidewire is advanced through the catheter into the abdominal cavity in a caudoventral direction.
7. The catheter is then removed, and the guidewire is left in situ. Care should be taken to maintain a grasp of the guidewire at all times to avoid fully advancing (and losing) the wire into the abdominal cavity.
8. If necessary, a dilator is advanced over the guidewire to enlarge the entry hole and is then removed.
9. The drain is advanced over the guidewire into the abdominal cavity. Care should be taken to advance the tube beyond all fenestrations.
10. The drain is secured to the skin using a finger-trap suture or through the suture holes present in the drain.
11. A closed collection system is connected to the drain.
12. A light protective dressing is applied.

Technique: Surgical placement (Fig. 5.12)

1. A midline celiotomy approach is performed (see Chapter 3).
2. Forceps are used to apply pressure from the caudolateral area of the abdominal cavity through the lateral body wall. The drain should not exit through the original incision. Care should be taken to avoid the caudal superficial epigastric vessels.
3. An incision is made in the skin over the forceps tips with a number 11 scalpel blade, and the forceps are advanced through the body wall. The forceps are opened and used to grasp the tips of a second pair of forceps, which are withdrawn into the abdomen.
4. The end of the abdominal drain is placed into the tips of the intra-abdominal forceps, and both are pulled out through the body wall together.
5. The drain is positioned appropriately within the abdomen, that is to say with the drain tip in the deepest part of the abdomen, typically cranial to the liver.
6. Excess drain length is trimmed from the external portion of the drain.
7. The drain is secured externally using a finger-trap suture.
8. A collection system is attached and activated.
9. A light protective dressing is applied.

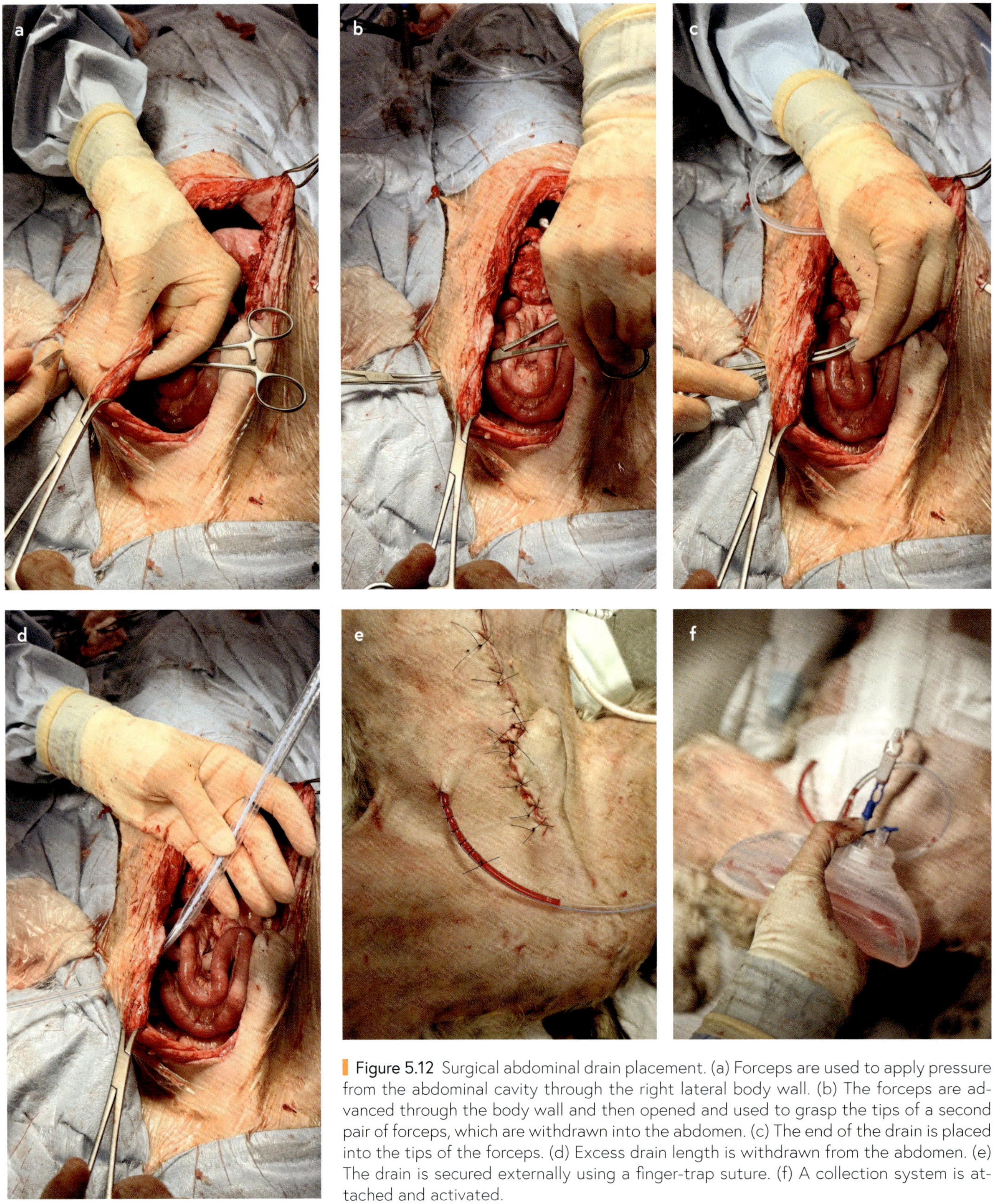

Figure 5.12 Surgical abdominal drain placement. (a) Forceps are used to apply pressure from the abdominal cavity through the right lateral body wall. (b) The forceps are advanced through the body wall and then opened and used to grasp the tips of a second pair of forceps, which are withdrawn into the abdomen. (c) The end of the drain is placed into the tips of the forceps. (d) Excess drain length is withdrawn from the abdomen. (e) The drain is secured externally using a finger-trap suture. (f) A collection system is attached and activated.

Cystostomy tubes

Cystostomy tubes are indicated when urinary diversion is required, commonly in patients with injury to the lower urinary tract, or to avoid bladder overfilling. These tubes are usually temporary, although permanent cystostomy tube placement may be considered for detrusor atony or obstructive neoplasia.

Mushroom-tipped (also known as de Pezzer) catheters and Foley catheters (8Fr–14Fr) are examples of surgically placed cystostomy tubes (Fig. 5.13). Foley catheters may be less traumatic to remove, as the bulb can be deflated; however, clinicians should be mindful that the bulb can be prematurely deflated or damaged, resulting in dislodgement of the cystostomy tube. Although this is less applicable to de Pezzer catheters, they can be traumatic to remove and may require a stiffening stylet to straighten out the mushroom.

The cystostomy tube should be attached to a closed collection system that is emptied every 6–8 hours, with an aseptic technique, and the urine output should be recorded. Alternatively, the tube can be closed with a bung and the bladder drained every 4–8 hours; this can be useful to assess if the patient is able to urinate.

Surgically placed cystostomy tubes may be left in place for a protracted period, with reports of up to 49 days,[21] although they are usually removed when the underlying issue is resolved. Percutaneous pigtail catheters may be more short-lived, with a median of 8 days, although the longest duration in one study was 27 days. The longer a tube is left in place, the more confident the clinician can be that a stoma has formed at the cystopexy site, leading to a reduced risk of uroabdomen on removal. At the authors' institution, a minimum of 10 days is advised to allow time for a secure adhesion between the bladder and the body wall.

Complications occur frequently in patients with cystostomy tubes. In one study up to 49% of cases suffered complications, the most common being inflammation of the stoma site and urine leakage, but also inadvertent tube removal, patient chewing the tube, breakage of the mushroom tip during removal, and fistula formation following tube removal.[22] Complications of percutaneous tube placement have been reported in 2 cats out of 25 and included bladder rupture at placement and dislodgement of the tube resulting in uroabdomen.[23]

Cystostomy tubes predispose the patient to urinary tract infection due to the presence of residual urine in the bladder and the formation of a biofilm on the surface of the cystotomy tube. The requirement for antibiotics should be assessed on an individual basis, but they should be avoided whenever possible while the tube is in place to prevent the development of a multiresistant or nosocomial urinary tract infection. In a retrospective study of 24 animals with a positive urine culture, only 13 had clinical signs.[22] Antibiotics should only be considered if the patient has clinical signs of urinary tract infection that warrant treating (e.g., pyrexia, persistent dysuria, lethargy).

Cystostomy tubes can be placed via a midline celiotomy or a minimally invasive approach.[21] In unstable patients, temporary urinary diversion may be achieved by placement of a percutaneous locking-loop pigtail catheter into the urinary bladder if the bladder is large and palpable.[23]

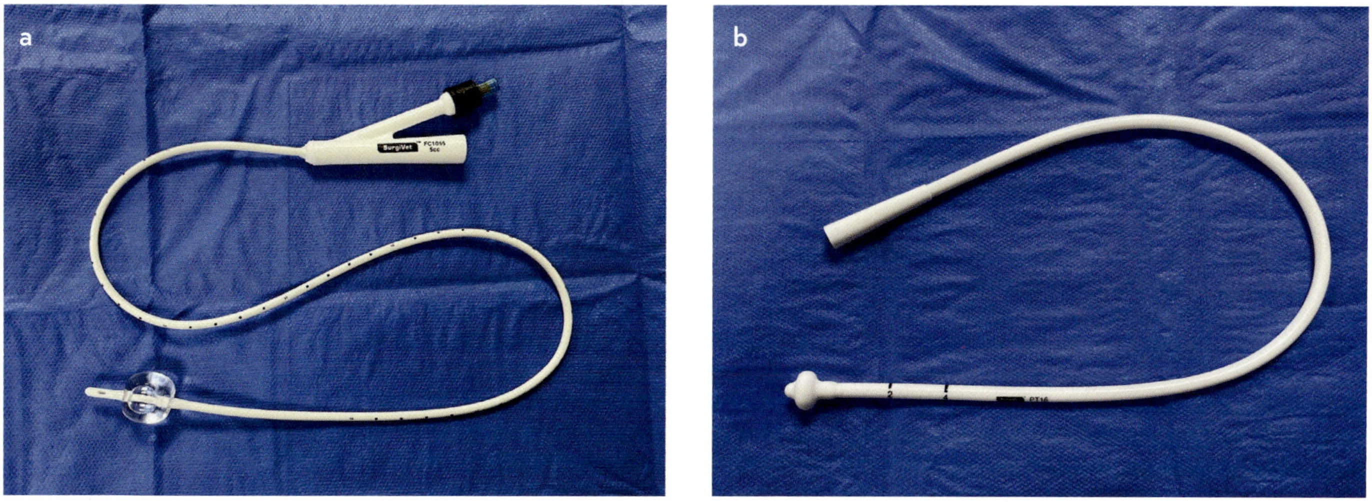

Figure 5.13 (a) Foley catheter with bulb inflated. The bulb of this Foley catheter should be inflated with 5 mL of saline. (b) De Pezzer or mushroom-tipped catheter.

Technique: Ventral midline approach (Fig. 5.14)

1. The patient is placed in dorsal recumbency, and a caudal ventral midline celiotomy is performed (see Chapter 3).
2. A stay suture is placed in the apex of the bladder using a round-bodied needle with monofilament suture such as polydioxanone or polyethylene.
3. The location for the cystostomy is chosen on the ventral surface of the bladder. Generally, cystostomy tubes should be ventral and lateral, away from the bladder trigone to avoid interference with the ureteral openings, avoiding visible vessels on the serosal surface.
4. On the corresponding body wall, in an area that is close to the location of the bladder, forceps are

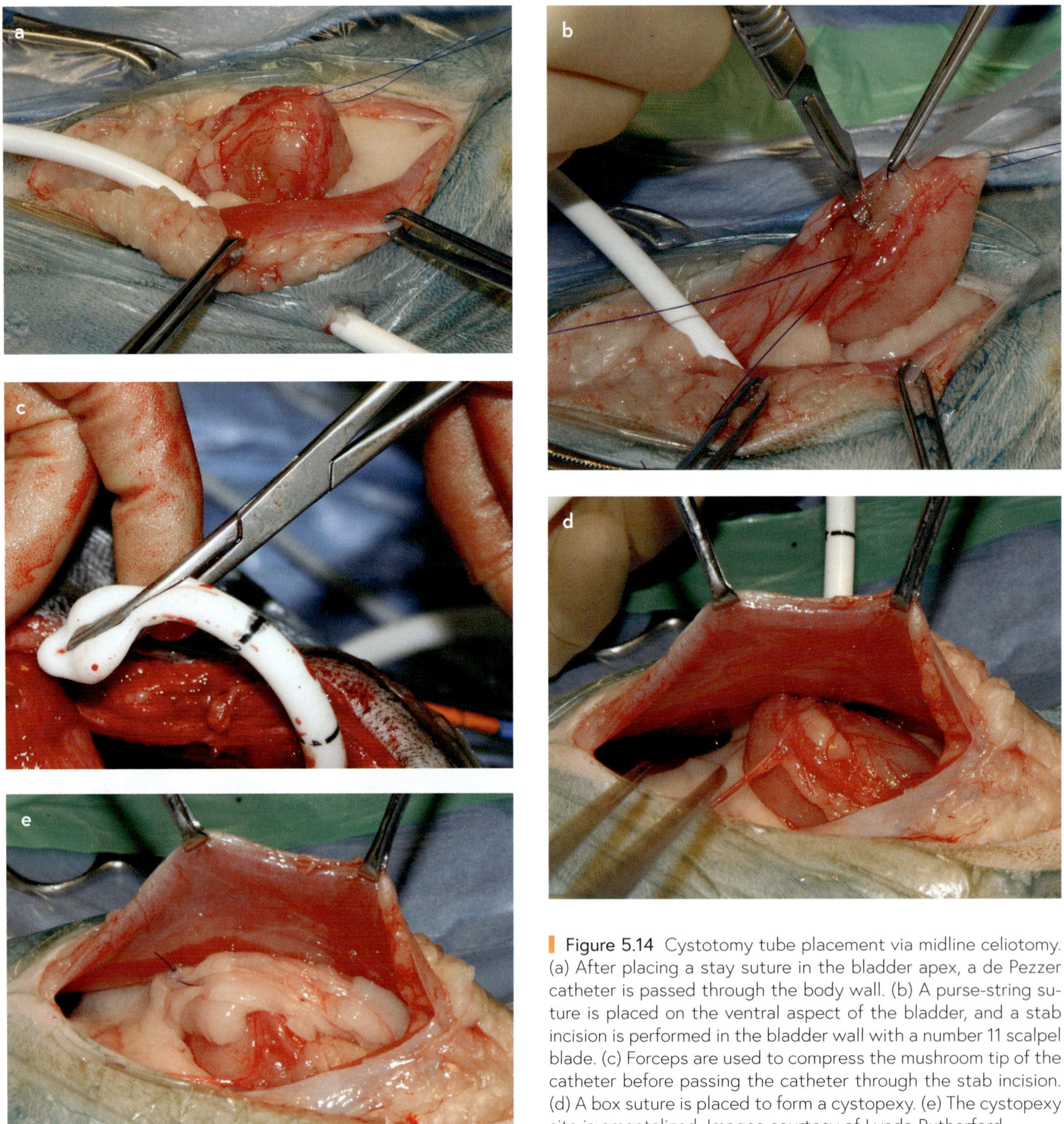

Figure 5.14 Cystotomy tube placement via midline celiotomy. (a) After placing a stay suture in the bladder apex, a de Pezzer catheter is passed through the body wall. (b) A purse-string suture is placed on the ventral aspect of the bladder, and a stab incision is performed in the bladder wall with a number 11 scalpel blade. (c) Forceps are used to compress the mushroom tip of the catheter before passing the catheter through the stab incision. (d) A box suture is placed to form a cystopexy. (e) The cystopexy site is omentalized. Images courtesy of Lynda Rutherford.

used to apply pressure from the abdominal cavity through the right caudolateral body wall.

5. With a number 11 scalpel blade, an incision is made in the skin over the forceps tips, and the forceps are advanced through the body wall and skin to grasp the tip of the cystostomy tube.
6. An appropriate catheter (mushroom-tipped or Foley catheter) is passed through the body wall so that the tip lies in the abdomen.
7. A purse-string suture is placed in the bladder wall at the cystostomy site, with long-acting absorbable monofilament suture (2-0 or 3-0).
8. A full-thickness stab incision is made in the center of the purse-string suture using a number 11 scalpel blade.
9. If using a mushroom-tipped catheter, the mushroom is compressed laterally with hemostat forceps to allow passage into the bladder lumen through the stab incision. Once within the lumen, the tip expands, keeping the catheter in place. If using a Foley catheter, the bulb is inflated with saline, not exceeding the designated volume.
10. The purse-string suture is then tied.
11. A box suture (see above) is placed between the bladder and the transversus abdominis muscle. This consists of four horizontal mattress sutures placed in a "box" around the cystostomy tube, securing the bladder to the body wall and forming a cystopexy. It is easier to place the most dorsal suture first and preplace the sutures before tying.
12. The cystostomy site is omentalized.
13. Gentle traction is placed on the tube to bring the tip to sit against the body wall. At this point, the catheter can be moved within the lumen to ensure a suture has not been placed inadvertently through the tip or tube.
14. The tube is secured to the skin using a finger-trap suture (see Fig. 5.1). Care should be taken not to occlude the lumen when tying.

Technique: Minimally invasive approach

1. The patient is placed in lateral recumbency with the pelvic limbs positioned caudally.
2. A wide area of the ventrolateral abdomen is clipped and aseptically prepared.
3. The bladder is located with palpation (the bladder can be filled with saline using a urethral catheter).
4. An oblique skin incision is made in the inguinal region, directly over the palpable bladder.
5. The subcutaneous and fascial tissue of the external abdominal oblique muscle is sharply dissected.
6. A grid approach (see Chapter 3) is used to access the abdominal cavity. The internal abdominal oblique and transversus abdominis muscles are split along the muscle fibers.
7. The bladder is typically pressed against the abdominal body wall. If the bladder is not full, it may be dilated via a urethral catheter (if possible).
8. The cystostomy tube is passed into the abdominal cavity through a stab incision 2–3 cm cranial to the approach.
9. A purse-string suture is placed (but not tied) in the exposed bladder wall at the site of the cystostomy with long-acting absorbable monofilament suture (2-0 or 3-0).
10. A full-thickness stab incision is made in the center of the purse-string suture using a number 11 scalpel blade.
11. The catheter tip is inserted into the bladder lumen. If a Foley catheter is used, the bulb is inflated with saline, not exceeding the designated volume.
12. The abdominal muscle layers are apposed either separately or in a single layer; the innermost muscle layer incorporates bites of the bladder wall (including the submucosa) to form a cystopexy. Care should be taken to leave a small gap in the closure to avoid obstructing the tube, and to avoid penetrating the tube or bulb with the suture.
13. The cystostomy tube is secured to the skin with a finger-trap suture (see Fig. 5.1).

Technique: Percutaneous placement (pigtail)[23]

1. The patient is appropriately sedated and placed in lateral recumbency.
2. A wide area of the ventrolateral abdomen is clipped and aseptically prepared.
3. The bladder is located by palpation and/or ultrasound.
4. A superficial skin incision is made overlying the bladder with a number 11 scalpel blade.
5. The entire device is advanced through a stab incision until seated in the urinary bladder.
6. The stylet is removed and placement confirmed by withdrawing urine.
7. The locking-loop mechanism is activated by pulling and securing the locking suture (may vary between manufacturers).
8. The cystostomy tube is secured to the body wall with a finger-trap suture (see Fig. 5.1).
9. The tube is attached to a closed collection system.
10. Radiographs are taken to confirm the presence of the tube within the urinary bladder.

KEEP IN MIND

- All tubes and drains must be protected from patient interference with the use of an Elizabethan collar or body stocking as necessary.
- It is essential that all the fenestrations of a thoracostomy tube are within the thoracic cavity.
- Nasoesophageal/nasogastric tubes, esophagostomy tubes, and thoracic and abdominal drains can be removed at any time, while gastrostomy and cystostomy tubes must remain in place at least until a mature adhesion has formed between organ and body wall (7–14 days).
- A small volume of a carbonated drink (e.g., cola) can be instilled in a feeding tube and left for 5–10 minutes to dissolve tube blockages.
- Once the tube/drain has been removed, the site is left open to heal by second intention.
- Radiographs are recommended after tube placement to confirm location.

Bibliography

1. Earley NF et al. Mechanical properties of 6 finger-trap suture techniques. *Vet Surg.* 2017; 46(6):765–772.
2. Aronson LR (ed.). *Small Animal Surgical Emergencies*, 2nd ed. Wiley Blackwell; 2022.
3. Rodriguez-Diaz J, Sumner JP, Miller M. Fatal complications of nasogastric tube misplacement in two dogs. *J Am Anim Hosp Assoc.* 2021; 57(5):242–246.
4. Kelly S, Bandt C. Inadvertent placement of an esophagostomy tube into the mediastinum of a cat. *Can Vet J.* 2022; 63(11):1124–1128.
5. Yu MK et al. Comparison of complication rates in dogs with nasoesophageal versus nasogastric feeding tubes. *J Vet Emerg Crit Care (San Antonio).* 2013; 23(3):300–304.
6. Breheny CR et al. Esophageal feeding tube placement and the associated complications in 248 cats. *J Vet Intern Med.* 2019; 33(3):1306–1314.
7. Nathanson O et al. Esophagostomy tube complications in dogs and cats: Retrospective review of 225 cases. *J Vet Intern Med.* 2019; 33(5):2014–2019.
8. Elmenhorst K, Pérez López P, Belch A, Demetriou JL. Retrospective study of complications associated with surgically-placed gastrostomy tubes in 43 dogs with septic peritonitis. *J Small Anim Pract.* 2020; 61(2):116–120.
9. Hansen SC, Hlusko KC, Matz BM, Bacek LM. Retrospective evaluation of 24 cases of gastrostomy tube usage in dogs with septic peritonitis (2009–2016). *J Vet Emerg Crit Care (San Antonio).* 2019; 29(5):514–520.
10. Salinardi BJ, Harkin KR, Bulmer BJ, Roush JK. Comparison of complications of percutaneous endoscopic versus surgically placed gastrostomy tubes in 42 dogs and 52 cats. *J Am Anim Hosp Assoc.* 2006; 42(1):51–56.
11. Davidson JR. Feeding tubes. In: Johnston SA, Tobias KM (eds.). *Veterinary Surgery: Small Animal*, vol. 2. Elsevier. p. 1907.
12. Risselada M, Griffith E, Kapler M, McDonald-Lynch M. Evaluation of various gastrojejunostomy tube constructs for enteral support of small animal patients. *J Am Vet Med Assoc.* 2018; 252(10):1239–1246.
13. Fetzer TJ, Walker JM, Bach JF. Comparison of the efficacy of small and large-bore thoracostomy tubes for pleural space evacuation in canine cadavers. *J Vet Emerg Crit Care (San Antonio).* 2017; 27(3):301–306.
14. Valtolina C, Adamantos S. Evaluation of small-bore wire-guided chest drains for management of pleural space disease. *J Small Anim Pract.* 2009; 50(6):290–297.
15. Boullhesen Williams T et al. Retrospective evaluation of the use and complications of small-bore wire-guided thoracostomy tubes in dogs and cats: 156 cases (2007–2019). *Front Vet Sci.* 2022; 9:818055.
16. Szabo SD, Jermyn K, Neel J, Mathews KG. Evaluation of postceliotomy peritoneal drain fluid volume, cytology, and blood-to-peritoneal fluid lactate and glucose differences in normal dogs. *Vet Surg.* 2011; 40(4):444–449.
17. Hung GC et al. Quantification and characterization of pleural fluid in healthy dogs with thoracostomy tubes. *Am J Vet Res.* 2016; 77(12):1387–1391.
18. Racette MA et al. Retrospective evaluation of fluid production at the time of thoracostomy tube removal following elective and emergency surgery in dogs (2010–2017): 185 cases. *J Vet Emerg Crit Care (San Antonio).* 2022; 32(1):58–67.
19. Crosby J, Humm K, Cook SD. Retrospective evaluation of the use of small-bore wire-guided catheters for the management of peritoneal effusion in cats and dogs. *J Vet Emerg Crit Care (San Antonio).* 2023; 33(1):91–97.
20. Halfacree ZJ, Wilson AM, Baines SJ. Evaluation of in vitro performance of suction drains. *Am J Vet Res.* 2009; 70(2):283–289.
21. Bray JP, Doyle RS, Burton CA. Minimally invasive inguinal approach for tube cystostomy. *Vet Surg.* 2009; 38(3):411–416.
22. Beck AL et al. Outcome of and complications associated with tube cystostomy in dogs and cats: 76 cases (1995–2006). *J Am Vet Med Assoc.* 2007; 230(8):1184–1189.
23. Nurra G et al. Clinical use and complications of percutaneous cystostomy pigtail catheters in 25 cats. *J Feline Med Surg.* 2022; 24(6):e28–e33.

Chapter 6

Staplers and vessel-sealing devices

Rhiannon Strickland, Anna Frykfors von Hekkel

Stapling devices

Stapling devices are commonly used in small animal surgery for various thoracic and abdominal procedures. They vary in configuration, staple height, and number of staple rows deployed, but each device has a handle and a separate cartridge. Staplers are designed to be single use, with a limited number of cartridge reloads (seven reloads for a total of eight firings); however, in reality they are commonly reused in veterinary surgery to limit waste and costs. Potential benefits of these devices include decreased anesthetic and surgical time, tissue trauma, and intraoperative contamination. The most frequently used devices in veterinary patients are linear stapling devices, including thoracoabdominal (TA) and gastrointestinal anastomosis (GIA) staplers. There are also stapling devices designed for use in minimally invasive surgery, such as the Endo GIA (Covidien–Medtronic), which may also be used in open surgery. All these devices (TA, GIA, and Endo GIA staplers) are available in different lengths, ranging from 30 to 100 mm, and deploy two to three staggered rows of staples. Some may have a cutting device, with staples deployed on either side of a blade that cuts the tissue after staple deployment.

Thoracoabdominal staplers

TA staplers are versatile devices with application in a wide range of surgical interventions, particularly in those involving vascular tissues such as lung and liver lobectomies. They may also be used to complete a functional end-to-end intestinal anastomosis. These devices consist of a handle with a trigger mechanism and a U-shaped end containing a cartridge (Fig. 6.1). Tissues are carefully inserted through the U-shaped end and secured by a retaining pin. By squeezing the handle, the staples are deployed from the cartridge and secured through the tissue (Video 6.1).

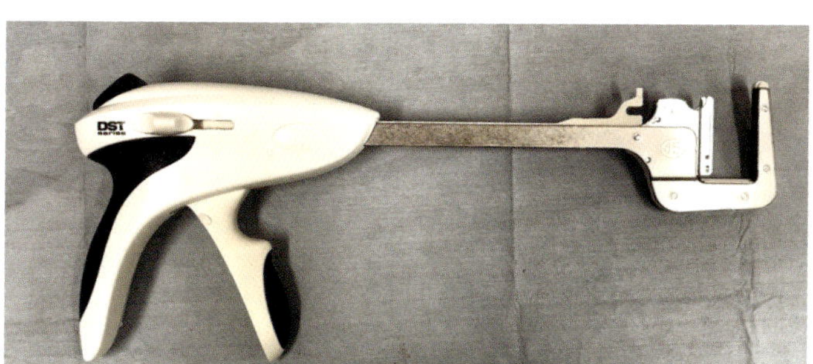

Figure 6.1 Thoracoabdominal stapler without cartridge. Image courtesy of Matteo Rossanese.

Video 6.1. Use of a thoracoabdominal stapler. Note that the retaining pin is in the cartridge and not present in this video. Video courtesy of Matteo Rossanese.

TA staplers and associated cartridges are available in various widths and staple sizes. Cartridges are color-coded according to the closed staple height (Table 6.1). They contain two or more staggered rows of B-shaped titanium staples. Vascular (white) cartridges deploy three rows of staples, with a closed staple height of 1 mm; they are recommended for lung and liver lobectomies, as a closed staple height over 1 mm (blue and green cartridges) is more likely to lead to hemorrhage or air leakage (Figs. 6.2 and 6.3).

Technique (Video 6.2)

The reader is referred to the information provided by the manufacturer, as device characteristics may vary. The following are the instructions for the TA Stapler (Covidien–Medtronic).

1. The correct cartridge is mounted on the U-shaped end of the device.

Video 6.2. Use of a TA 30 Stapler for typhlectomy. The remaining cecum is inserted through the U-shaped end of the device and secured by the retaining pin. The handle is squeezed twice, the first time to compress the tissue, and the second time to deploy the staples from the cartridge. Note that after the second squeeze the system remains locked.

TABLE 6.1 - COMMONLY USED THORACOABDOMINAL STAPLERS AND AVAILABLE CARTRIDGES						
Cartridge color	Devices		Staple rows	Open staple height (mm)	Closed staple height (mm)	Indications
	Covidien–Medtronic	Ethicon				
White (vascular)	TA 30 (V3)	TX 30V	3	2.5	1.0	Liver lobectomy Lung lobectomy
Blue	TA 30, 45, 90	TX 30, 60	2	3.5	1.5	Particularly large vascular pedicles (white cartridge is preferred in most cases) Typhlectomy Functional end-to-end anastomosis closure (transverse end)
Green	TA 30, 45, 90	TX 30, 60	2	4.8	2.0	Partial gastrectomy

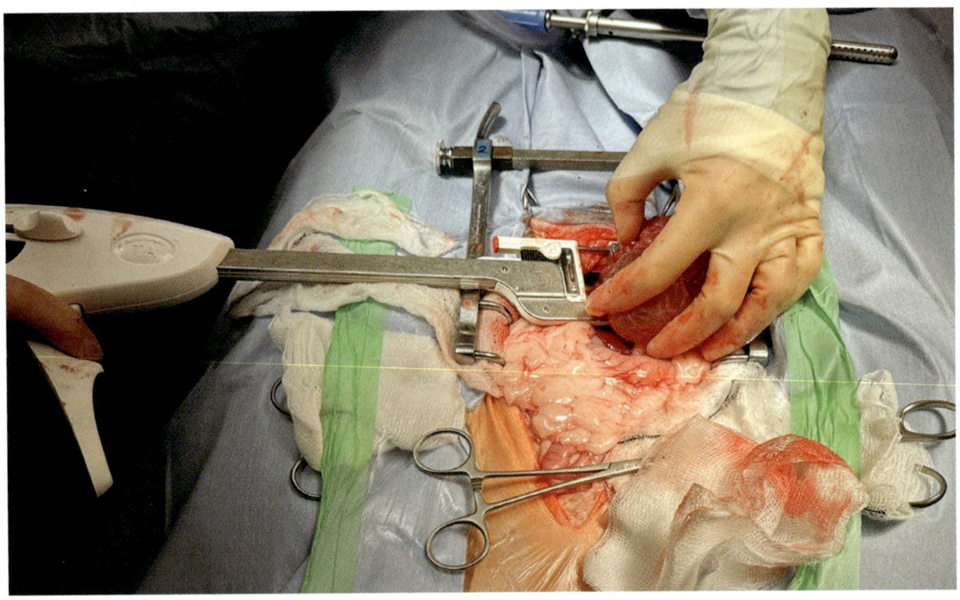

Figure 6.2 Thoracoabdominal stapler with a vascular (white) cartridge passed around the hilus of a liver lobe. The retaining pin has been advanced.

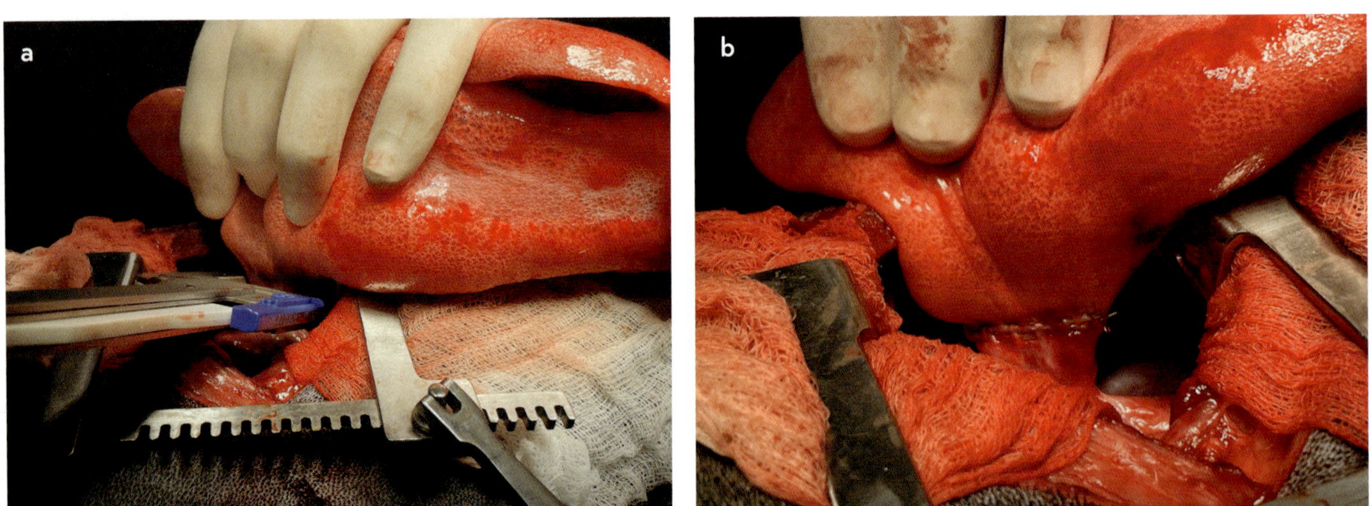

Figure 6.3 (a) Lobectomy of an emphysematous lung lobe performed with two thoracoabdominal blue cartridges (a white cartridge is preferred in most cases). (b) Note the four rows of staggered staples deployed across the large vascular pedicle before resection. Images courtesy of Filippo Cinti.

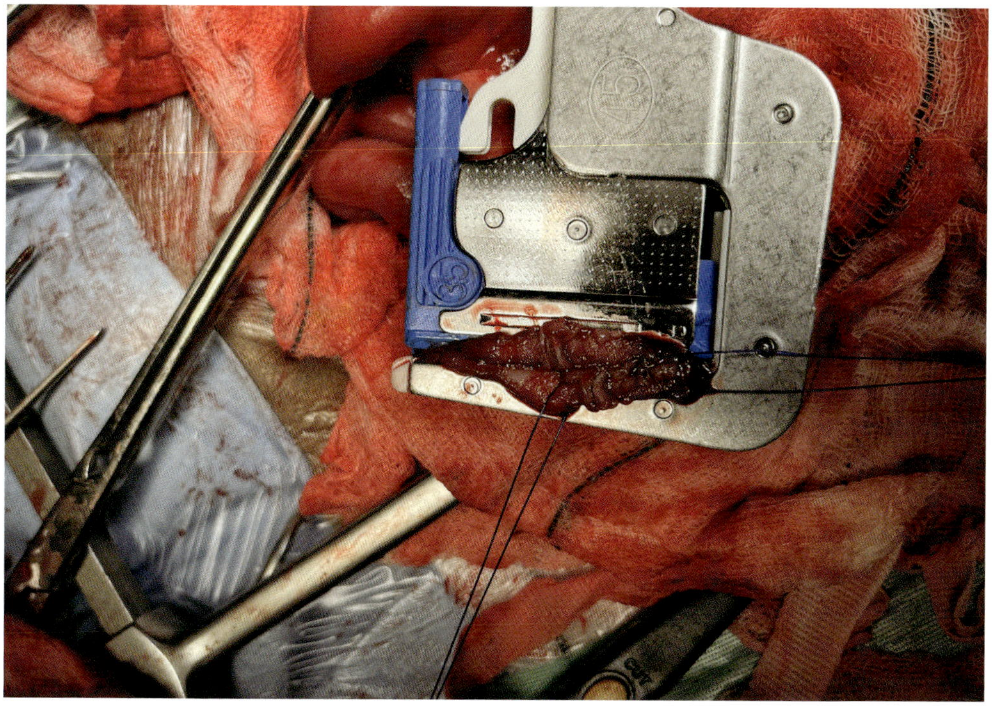

Figure 6.4 A thoracoabdominal stapler with a blue cartridge is used to place a transverse staple line to complete an end-to-end functional intestinal anastomosis.

2. After isolating the tissue to be excised, the open end of the device is passed around the base of the tissue. Only the intended tissue should be included within the device.
3. The retaining pin is driven via manual advancement of the firing knob.
4. The handle is squeezed once to clamp the tissue. Staples are not deployed at this stage. Anesthesia parameters and surrounding tissue should be checked for unintended consequences. This step is reversible, so the device can be altered as necessary.
5. The handle is squeezed a second time; the lever should not fully revert to its previous position, confirming staple deployment (Fig. 6.4).
6. A number 11 scalpel blade is used to resect the tissue distal to the staple line. There is a cutting guide on the anvil to guide the scalpel blade and protect nearby tissues.
7. Vascular clamps are prepared for use in case of hemorrhage, and the device is released.
8. The surgical site is checked for hemorrhage and/or air leakage and treated if necessary.

Gastrointestinal anastomosis staplers

GIA staplers consist of two halves that lock together to form a handle with two "legs" (Fig. 6.5). Unlike TA staplers, they have an integrated cutting device. Four rows of staggered B-shaped titanium staples are deployed, and the device simultaneously cuts between the second and third staple rows. GIA staplers are mostly used in gastrointestinal surgery such as gastrectomy or functional end-to-end stapled anastomosis. However, they have also been used for cardiac, pulmonary, hepatobiliary, or genital surgery. A specific endoscopic stapler is also available.

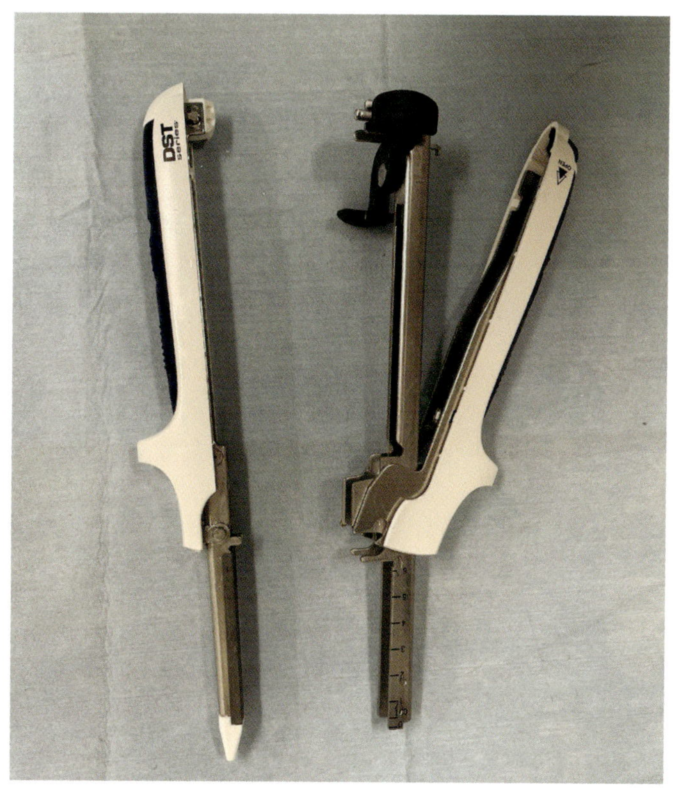

Figure 6.5 Gastrointestinal anastomosis stapler without cartridge. Note the two separate halves, which lock together. Image courtesy of Matteo Rossanese.

The GIA Stapler (Covidien–Medtronic) and the Proximate Linear Cutter (Ethicon) are commonly used examples of this type of device. The GIA Stapler is available in 60 mm, 80 mm, and 100 mm lengths. The Proximate Linear Cutter is available in 55 mm, 75 mm, and 100 mm lengths. Both devices deploy staples with a closed height of 1.0 mm, 1.5 mm, or 2.0 mm.
Cartridge choice is driven by tissue thickness; staples should penetrate the full thickness of the tissue. The authors use a blue cartridge (1.5 mm closed staple height) for gastrointestinal anastomosis. For a partial gastrectomy, where the tissue is thicker, a green cartridge (2 mm closed staple height) might be more appropriate.

Technique

1. The two halves of the stapler are separated.
2. The appropriately sized cartridge is loaded. Care should be taken to select the correct length cartridge for the device.
3. The safety insert covering the cutting blade is removed.
4. Each half of the device is inserted into each bowel lumen (for anastomosis; Fig. 6.6) or placed across the tissue to be resected.
5. The device is aligned and clamped at either the rear or the center of the device.
6. The tissue is inspected to ensure that it lies flat between the handles and that no extra tissues are included.

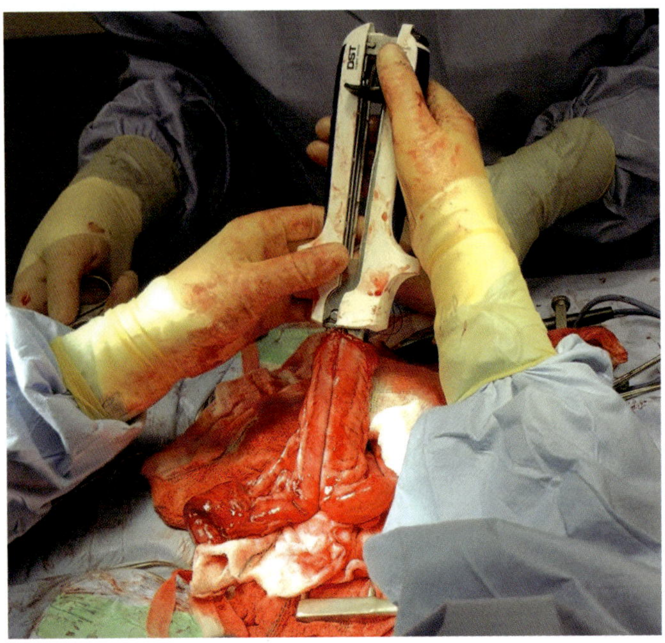

Figure 6.6 Gastrointestinal anastomosis stapler being assembled after inserting each half of the device into each jejunal lumen to perform a functional end-to-end anastomosis. The antimesenteric surface of the jejunum is clamped within the device. The firing knob has not yet been advanced.

7. The firing knob is advanced fully to deploy the staples and cut between them. The cutting device stops short of the staple line.
8. The firing knob is returned all the way back to the original position. The device is released and then removed. The staple line is inspected to ensure the staples have penetrated the full thickness of the tissue.

Endoscopic gastrointestinal anastomosis staplers

Staplers intended for minimally invasive surgery deploy 3 staples rows on each side of an integrated cutting device, and they typically deploy staples also around the distal end of the blade to prevent leakage in the event of incomplete excision. The Endo GIA (Covidien–Medtronic) and the Echelon (Ethicon) are common examples (Fig. 6.7).
Endoscopic cartridge lengths range from 28 mm to 60 mm. The most frequently utilized endoscopic stapling devices are 12 mm in diameter. Cartridge choice is driven by tissue thickness, and different staple sizes are available. The 2.0 mm Endo GIA stapler (grey cartridge) is the smallest cartridge available from Covidien–Medtronic. It fires three rows of 2 mm staples on each side of the blade, and the staples compress to 0.75–1.0 mm. This device has been shown to prevent air leak in canine cadavers up to 27 kg, providing an alternative that may reduce air leakage and hemorrhage.[1] The 2.5 mm (white or vascular) cartridge should be used on tissue that can comfortably compress to 1.0–1.5 mm, and it is specifically designed for vascular tissue to prevent bleeding. The 3.0 mm to 4.0 mm (purple) and 3.5 mm (blue) cartridges are intended for regular tissue stapling. They should be used on tissue that can compress to 1.5–2.0 mm. The 4.8 mm (green) cartridge is used for thick or dense tissues and should be used on tissue that compresses to 2.0 mm.

Technique (Video 6.3)

The reader is referred to the information provided by the manufacturer, as device characteristics may vary. The following are the instructions for the Endo GIA stapler (Covidien–Medtronic).

1. The black return knob on the device is pulled back completely, and the articulating lever is set to the neutral position (0 degrees).
2. The Endo GIA reload cartridge is loaded. The pin located at the distal end of the device shaft is insert-

Video 6.3. Use of an endoscopic stapler (Endo GIA, Covidien–Medtronic). Video courtesy of Filippo Cinti.

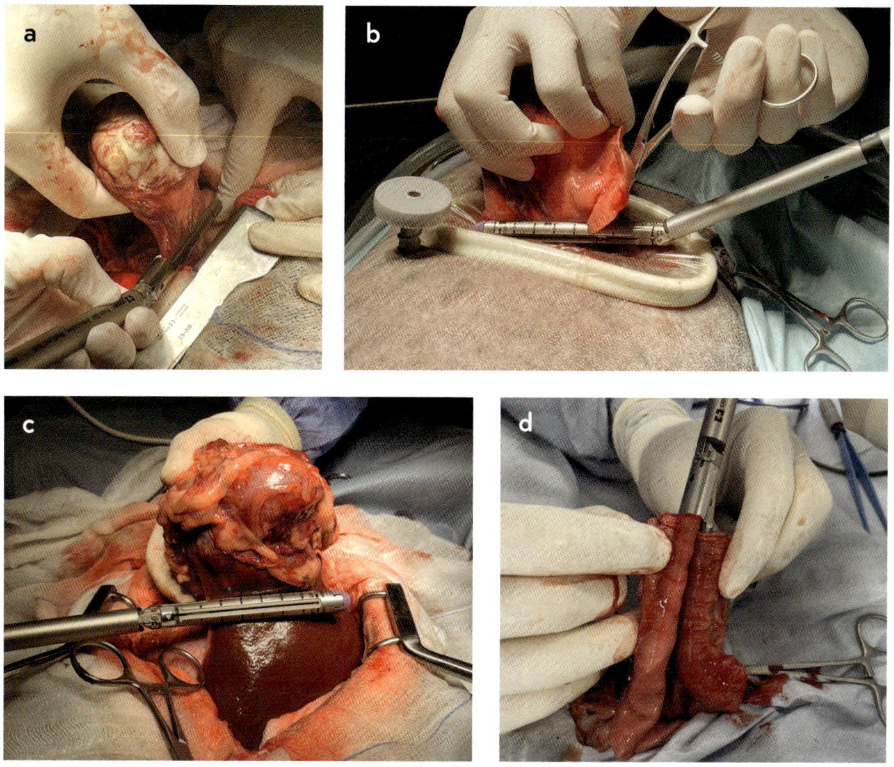

Figure 6.7 Endo GIA (Covidien–Medtronic) endoscopic stapler used for (a,b) lung lobectomy, (c) liver lobectomy, and (d) functional end-to-end gastrointestinal anastomosis. Images courtesy of Filippo Cinti.

ed into the reload. The load alignment indicators on the reload and on the shaft must be aligned. The reload is pushed in and twisted clockwise 45 degrees relative to the device.

3. The "shipping wedge" is removed from the reload. The instrument is checked to confirm proper loading of the reload.
4. In a minimally invasive surgical procedure, the jaw of the reload is closed prior to inserting it into the trocar.
5. The jaw of the reload is opened by pulling back the knob completely.
6. The tissue of interest is atraumatically grasped within the reload jaw by squeezing the handle to close the jaws. The green firing button is pushed down and held (the handle will return to the firing position). The stapler is now ready to be fired.
7. The handle is squeezed sequentially until the lower clamp cover reaches the distal end of the cartridge slot, and the handle locks.
8. Once the device has been completely fired, the jaw is opened by pulling back the black return knob completely. The device is gently removed from the tissue.
9. The staple line is inspected to ensure the staples have penetrated the full thickness of the tissue.

Vessel-sealing devices

Advanced bipolar vessel-sealing devices, such as LigaSure (Covidien–Medtronic) and EnSeal (Ethicon), are versatile and valuable tools widely used in veterinary medicine, significantly contributing to reduce surgical time and minimize intraoperative blood loss.[2] These devices provide hemostasis by a combination of pressure and bipolar energy, effectively denaturing collagen and elastin within the vessel wall. Thermal damage to adjacent tissues is limited to 2 mm (LigaSure) and 1 mm (EnSeal). During use, these devices detect tissue impedance and provide real-time feedback to the surgeon (Video 6.4). Vessels up to 7 mm in diameter can be effectively sealed using LigaSure or EnSeal. Additionally, both devices often incorporate a cutting function, making them invaluable tools in both laparoscopic and open procedures (Fig. 6.8). While these devices are generally not intended for reuse, they are frequently employed multiple times. Studies have shown that they can be used an average of eight times before experiencing fail-

Video 6.4. Use of a vessel-sealing device (LigaSure Small Jaw Open Sealer/Divider, Covidien–Medtronic). Note the sound from the generator giving real-time feedback to the surgeon during vessel sealing. The subsequent two beeps indicate that the seal is complete and the vessel/tissue can be cut (by pulling the gray knob). Video courtesy of Matteo Rossanese.

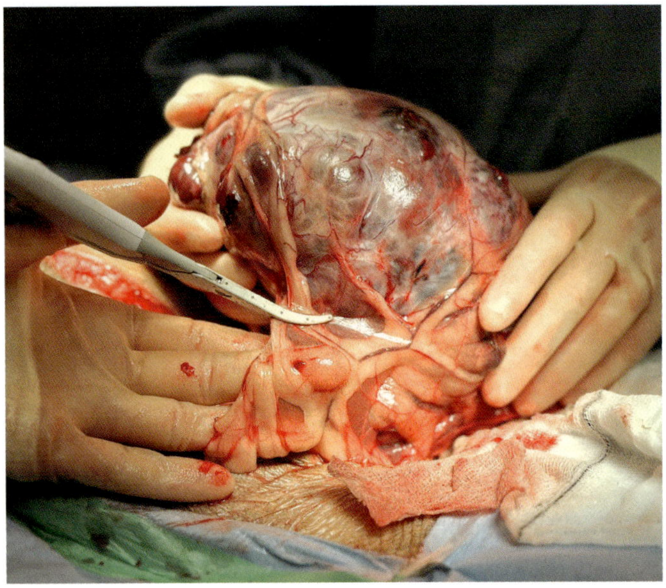

Figure 6.8 Splenectomy using a bipolar vessel-sealing device (LigaSure). The short handpiece is intended for open surgery.

ure,[3] and, in some cases, up to five times while maintaining a bursting pressure equivalent to that of reusable devices.[4]

Harmonic systems are vessel-sealing devices that deliver ultrasound waves at a rate of 55.5 kHz/s, effectively dissecting and coagulating tissues while maintaining a lower temperature range (50°C–100°C) compared to traditional electrosurgery. This system is capable of sealing vessels up to 5 mm in diameter and serves as an efficient tool for tissue dissection, cutting, and coagulation. Its advantages include reduced thermal damage, minimal smoke generation, and the elimination of the risk of electrical current transfer to the patient.

Harmonic devices are available with various handle and tip options, including scalpels, shears, and blades. Their versatility has made them suitable for a wide range of applications in veterinary surgery (Fig. 6.9), including, but not limited to, splenectomy, gonadectomy, liver biopsy, partial lobectomy, adrenalectomy, partial pancreatectomy, and pericardiectomy.

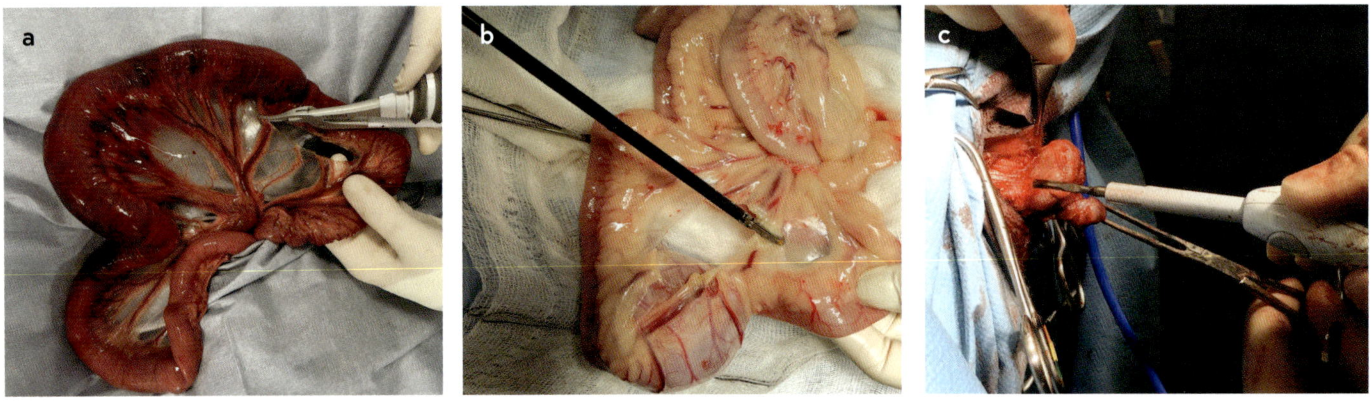

Figure 6.9 Vascular hemostasis during gastrointestinal tract resection achieved using (a) harmonic and (b) EnSeal bipolar vessel-sealing devices. (c) Anal sac tumor resection using a harmonic scalpel. Images courtesy of Filippo Cinti.

KEEP IN MIND

- Every staple must penetrate all layers of the tissue.
- It is preferable to choose a cartridge that is too wide or too long rather than too short. Similarly, if a vascular pedicle is too wide for a 30 mm vascular cartridge, two devices may be used side by side.
- When closing the transverse end of a functional side-to-side anastomosis, care should be taken to offset the staple line of the linear stapler to reduce the risk of dehiscence.
- Vessel-sealing devices can seal vessels up to 7 mm (Ligasure and Enseal) or 5 mm (Harmonic) in diameter.

Bibliography

1. St Blanc AW, Csomos RA. Investigation and validation of a novel Endo GIA stapler for canine lung lobectomies. *Can Vet J*. 2021; 62(11):1207–1210.
2. Sirochman AL, Milovancev M, Townsend K, Grimes JA. Influence of use of a bipolar vessel sealing device on short-term postoperative mortality after splenectomy: 203 dogs (2005–2018). *Vet Surg*. 2020; 49(2):291–303.
3. Valenzano D, Hayes G, Gludish D, Weese S. Performance and microbiological safety testing after multiple use cycles and hydrogen peroxide sterilization of a 5-mm vessel-sealing device. *Vet Surg*. 2019; 48(5):885–889.
4. Gardeweg S, Bockstahler B, Duprè G. Effect of multiple use and sterilization on sealing performance of bipolar vessel sealing devices. *PLoS One*. 2019;14(8):e0221488.

Chapter 7

Bite wounds

Alison Moores

General overview

Bite wounds from dogs are common, representing up to 20% and 26% of feline and canine trauma cases respectively.[1,2] In fact, most thoracic injuries are due to canine bites.

Over 20% of dog owners report aggression of their dog toward other dogs. Sex distribution of canine victims varies between studies, with an equal distribution in cats.[1,3–7] In referral populations, most victims are small (<10 kg), perhaps because they are bitten more frequently, suffer multiple and more severe injuries, or are more likely to be referred.[7,8] In first opinion practice, most victims are medium sized.[1,2,5–10] Injured dogs tend to be young adults, consistent with general hospital populations.[1,2,4,5,7] Feline victims are younger, with speculation that older cats have learnt to avoid dogs.[1,6–8] In low socioeconomic areas, more severe injuries are seen if the attacking dog lives with the victim, whereas in higher socioeconomic areas most bite injuries are from public attacks by unknown dogs. Intrahousehold fights commonly involve at least one female and most involve dogs of the same sex, are usually due to resource guarding, and are usually initiated by the most recent addition to the house, with more severe injuries in same-sex fights and aggression on immediate sight. Terrier breeds are more likely to initiate fights that lead to their own injury than other small breeds.[1,7] Cats are most likely to be attacked at home by a known dog.

In areas where rabies is endemic, transmission of infection can occur from bites from domestic or wild animals.[11]

Bite wounds from cats are considered a separate entity to canine bite wounds, as the clinical effects are related to inoculation of bacteria rather than physical trauma, and they are outside the scope of this book.

Clinical presentation and diagnosis

Bites occur on a single location in 14%–62% of dogs and 29% of cats.[2,6,7,12] Bites to dogs are most commonly to the thorax (18%-35%), head (28%-53%), neck (17%-46%), and limbs and tail (18%-42%).[1,2,7,13] Perineal wounds are uncommon.[11] Since dogs of equal size tend to attack from the front, wounds in larger dogs are commonly to a single area of the head or extremities and are limited to puncture wounds and smaller tearing wounds.[7] Injuries in small dogs and cats are more severe and more commonly occur to the back and thorax, with more thoracic and abdominal injuries than medium or large dogs.[6,7,9] Organized dog fight injuries are usually multiple, involving the head, chest, and forelegs, and there may be older wounds present.

The canine mouth can exert high pressure (150–450 pounds per square inch) and lead to puncture (<1 cm), crushing, laceration (>1 cm), and avulsion injuries, causing immediate cell death, reduced or interrupted tissue blood flow, and decreased defense mechanisms.[1,2,6,7,11,14,15]

Bacteria are inoculated into puncture wounds from the attacker's oral cavity, patient's skin, or environment.[2,15]

Untreated ischemic tissue, compromised blood supply, and dead space provide a medium on which bacteria can grow.[6,7] Due to skin mobility and rib cage elasticity, crushing and shaking can lead to marked deeper tissue injury (muscles, blood vessels, and internal organs) in the absence of superficial puncture wounds, especially in case of attack to small animals.[1,7,16] Failure to recognize and treat injuries can lead to deeper tissue ischemia and necrosis and death of the patient.[3]

Two grading systems have been established to categorize wound severity and depth (Tables 7.1 and 7.2).

Cervical wounds

One-quarter of animals with cervical bite wounds have damage to vital structures. Tracheal or laryngeal trauma is seen in 17% of patients, which clinically presents as inspiratory stridor and subcutaneous or mediastinal emphysema.[8,15] It is possible to have airway laceration without skin penetration; therefore, cervical and thoracic imaging is indicated for all cervical bite wounds.[8] Assessment of laryngeal function under anesthesia should be performed to assess for recurrent laryngeal nerve injury.[8]

Other reported injuries include complete tracheal rupture with pseudotracheal membrane formation, jugular vein damage, nerve damage (left recurrent laryngeal nerve and vagosympathetic trunk), damage to soft tissue structures (mandibular salivary gland, pharynx,

TABLE 7.1 - WOUND SEVERITY GRADING SYSTEM[2,4,5]

Grade	Definition	Incidence (%)*
1	Superficial wounds with partial-thickness dermal laceration	5–12
2	Superficial wounds with full-thickness dermal laceration	10–13
3	Full-thickness puncture wounds with dermal penetration, but without systemic illness	26–38
4	Full-thickness punctures or lacerations with avulsion of underlying tissues and dead space, underlying muscle trauma, possible penetration of a joint, abscess, or systemic illness	40–46
5	Severe injury including penetration into body cavities (abdomen, thorax) and open fractures	0.9–4

* In two large studies involving more than 1,000 dog bite wounds.[4,5]

TABLE 7.2 - WOUND DEPTH GRADING SYSTEM[1,3,6,9]

Grade	Incidence (%)		
	Thoracic wounds in dogs	Thoracic wounds in cats	Wounds (all) in cats
No external wound	11	4–25	4
Superficial (skin only)	35	20–33	33
Deep (involving subcutaneous tissue)	28	15–40	40
Penetrating (communication between skin and peritoneal cavity, thoracic cavity, or retroperitoneum)	30	18–40	18

esophagus, thyroid, and parathyroid gland—with syndromes including trauma-induced primary hypoparathyroidism, inappropriate antidiuretic hormone secretion, and spontaneously resolving atrial fibrillation), and damage to bony structures (mandibular/zygomatic arch synostosis secondary to fracture, occipital condyle, tympanic bulla, hyoid apparatus, and spine).[8]

Thoracic wounds

Over half of dogs and one-quarter of cats with thoracic bite wounds have injuries elsewhere.[3–9] Thoracic bites can cause soft tissue trauma, rib and sternal fractures, pseudoflail chest (paradoxical respiratory movement of part of the chest wall) or true flail chest (≥ two fractures of ≥ two adjacent ribs), pleural effusion, pulmonary contusion or laceration, and diaphragmatic rupture.[9,17] Bite wounds are the most common cause of flail chest, especially in cats, and the second most common cause of rib fractures (after road traffic accidents).[18] Pseudoflail chest is generally palpable in conscious dogs.[9] Respiratory compromise secondary to flail and pseudoflail chest is due to direct pulmonary damage, with pulmonary contusion, subcutaneous emphysema, and pneumothorax being the most prevalent additional radiographic abnormalities.[18] The presence of pseudoflail chest is positively correlated to the depth of thoracic injury in dogs.[9]

Clinical signs in dogs and cats with thoracic bite wounds include tachypnea (22% of dogs, 68% of cats), dyspnea (17% of dogs, 54% of cats), or both (10% of dogs, 40% of cats).[3,9] These clinical signs are not consistently correlated to thoracic injury depth.[3,9]

Thoracic imaging is indicated in patients with thoracic bite wounds, as deeper injuries may be visible on imaging in animals without superficial wounds or breathing abnormalities.[1,3,9] In cats, three or more radiographic lesions are significantly associated with the presence of a penetrating wound and the need for thoracic exploration. Rib fractures are more frequently associated with deep wounds, and cats with sternal fractures are more likely to require thoracic exploration.[3] Pneumothorax, rib fracture, pulmonary contusion, and pleural effusion are all related to an increased length of hospitalization in dogs.[9]

Older studies recommended a conservative approach to thoracic bite wounds due to the high mortality rates reported after thoracotomy, but more recent studies found no association between thoracotomy and mortality, and exploration of all wounds is recommended.[1,7,9,16] While thoracic radiography can help determine if thoracotomy is required, it may underestimate underlying pathology and is not a substitute for wound probing and surgical exploration.[1,3,9] The absence of skin penetration may not reflect deeper injury, and in one study half of dogs requiring lung lobectomy had no skin wounds.[16] In most studies, exploratory thoracotomy and lung lobectomy was more commonly performed in dogs with pseudoflail chest, rib fractures, or pneumothorax and in animals with penetrating thoracic injury.[1,9,16] Most cats with pseudoflail chest have deeper injuries.[3]

Wounds to other areas

Although abdominal penetration and presence of pneumomediastinum is uncommon, bite wounds are the most common cause of traumatic body wall herniation, with a survival rate of 71% in dogs and 80% in cats.[11]

Perineal wounds are rare but require assessment of colorectal and urinary structures. Perineal evisceration has been reported.[11]

Bite wounds rarely cause vertebral fracture but, if present, can lead to paresis and paralysis. External coaptation has been successfully reported.[22]

Limb viability can be assessed by the color and temperature of the extremity, bleeding from clipped nails (in presence of normal blood pressure), peripheral pulse oximetry or Doppler ultrasound, or selective angiography.[11,15]

There are reports[23-29] of other injuries caused from bite wounds, including skull fracture and deep brain laceration managed surgically with good outcome, global brain ischemia treated medically, chronic skull osteomyelitis, discospondylitis, atlanto-occipital instability treated with tension bands, feline penile urethral injury treated with a buccal mucosal graft, cervical vertebral fractures managed with fiberglass casts and lumbar vertebral fractures managed with cage rest, and lung lobe herniation treated by pneumonectomy.

Wound contamination

As the volume of bacteria in a bite wound cannot be quantified over time, these wounds should be considered potentially infected, even if they occurred less than 6 hours previously and whether they are open or closed.[11] In dogs, only 17%–20% of bite wounds are clinically infected at presentation.[12,13] There is an association between infection and longer time between the attack and presentation to hospital, and higher wound grade, but no association with bite location.[2,10,13] Injuries restricted to the dermis are less likely to become clinically infected.[13]

Culture and sensitivity testing of nonpurulent bite wounds is not routinely performed because its validity has been questioned, as infection incidence is low and there is no correlation between initial wound culture results and subsequent development of infection.[2,4–6,11] If wounds are cultured, swabs should be taken after debridement and lavage to best reflect bacteria that could lead to infection rather than surface contaminants.[9,11] Cytology may be an alternative method to assess for infection rather than contamination but will not be relevant in acute bite wounds.[2,4]

Aerobic and/or anaerobic bacterial bite wound cultures are positive in 44%–100% of dogs and 37% of cats.[2,3,9,10,12,13,19] Isolates reflect the florae of the attacking dog's oral cavity, victim's skin, and environment.[11] Most isolates are aerobes, and all wounds that contain anaerobic bacteria will also contain aerobic bacteria.[2,13] The most common bacterial isolates in dogs and cats are *Pasteurella canis* and *Pasteurella multocida*, *Streptococcus* spp., *Staphylococcus* spp. (including *S. intermedius* and *S. pseudintermedius*), *Enterococcus* spp., *Escherichia coli*, and other coliforms.[2,13,20] *Pasteurella multocida* is found more often in cats than in dogs.[20] The most frequently isolated strict anaerobe is *Clostridium perfringens*.[13] Polymicrobial populations are common (50% of wounds).[9] Multidrug-resistant bacteria are reported in 6%–39% of dogs.[9,20]

Treatment of bite wounds

Triage and immediate treatment

Prior to wound treatment, patients are triaged (e.g., using the animal trauma triage scale) for cardiovascular and respiratory abnormalities, the latter being the most common site for organ dysfunction.[14,15] The nervous and urogenital systems are assessed after initial stabilization, followed by orthopedic assessment if there is limb trauma, with radiographs taken as required to rule out fractures or luxations.[10,11] Airway and esophageal endoscopy and neck imaging may be indicated to rule out injury after neck bite wounds. Evaluation of clinicopathological abnormalities can be used to recognize more severe injury.

Immediate treatment includes resuscitation, if necessary, oxygenation, especially if there is thoracic injury, and intravenous fluid therapy.[17] Open wounds should be covered with a sterile dressing to decrease contamination and avoid further injury, but definitive treatment is delayed until the patient is stable.[14,17]

Fluid therapy is used conservatively in the face of marked hemorrhage, while the early use of blood products and antifibrinolytic drugs reduces bleeding from trauma-induced coagulopathy. Life-threatening hemorrhage can be controlled by direct pressure, hemostatic products, wound packing, tourniquets, tamponade of deep hemorrhage by balloon catheter, or direct clamping of vessels.

Thoracic drainage via thoracocentesis or thoracostomy drain may be required if there is tension pneumothorax secondary to lung or airway laceration or penetrating wounds. Tracheostomy may be required in case of upper airway trauma.[11]

Analgesia is provided before patient manipulation. Parenteral analgesia can be augmented with local anesthetic techniques, including intercostal nerve blocks. Interpleural bupivacaine for thoracic bite wounds may have reduced efficacy in the presence of pleural fluid.[17]

Antibiotics

The British Small Animal Veterinary Association (BSAVA) PROTECT ME guidelines recommend antibiotic use only in animals that are systemically unwell, have diffuse tissue involvement, potential joint involvement, or are immunocompromised.[21] There is no indication for antibiotic therapy in uncomplicated low-risk bite wounds.[11,13] Despite this, antibiotics have continued to be widely utilized in dogs with bite wounds; therefore, outcomes based on antibiotic use are not available.[3,5,7,9]

If used, antibiotics are administered intravenously, preferably within an hour of injury.[11] There is no single antibiotic or combination effective against all potential pathogens.[2] Amoxicillin and clavulanic acid is the recommended first-line treatment, with 85%–100% bacterial susceptibility.[19,21] There is no benefit to fluoroquinolones at first presentation.[2,19] The clinician should be prepared to reculture, and institute or change antibiotics, based on clinical indicators of developing or worsening infection.[11]

Surgery and surgical technique

In a study of bite wounds in first opinion practice, surgery was performed in 25% of cases (in 0% of grade 1 and 2, 13% of grade 3, and 40% of grade 4 and 5 wounds).[5] Conservative management was based on veterinary recommendation.[5] Most animals at referral centers are treated surgically, even if there are no open wounds, with the emphasis on surgical debridement.[3,7,9] Thoracic or abdominal exploratory surgery was required in 19% and 6% of dogs with thoracic and abdominal bite wounds, respectively, and lung lobectomy was required in 9%.[9] Of dogs undergoing surgical exploration of thoracic and abdominal bite wounds, 31% and 79%, respectively, had penetrating skin injury.[7]

Initial wound treatment consists of clipping, skin preparation, debridement, lavage, visual exploration, use of a probe to assess wound depth, and surgical exploration as deep as is necessary, including thoracotomy or celiotomy if required.[14,15]

Surgery allows debridement of necrotic tissue and bacterial contamination, reduction of bacterial numbers, and identification and treatment of deeper traumatic lesions.[11,15]

1. Sedation or general anesthesia is required, especially for deeper wounds, but should only be performed when the patient is clinically stable.
2. Sterile, water-soluble gel or moistened surgical swabs are placed over or into the wounds before clipping.[14,15]
3. The hair is widely clipped to reduce wound contamination and to assess for bruising, further puncture wounds, or body wall disruption. Clipping should allow for full surgical exploration of the neck or thoracic or abdominal cavities, depending upon the area of injury.[9,11,14,15]
4. Hair and lubricant are rinsed away, and the skin is cleansed as for aseptic surgery.[2,11,12,14,15] Bacterial resistance to chlorhexidine has been reported, but chlorhexidine is more effective than povidone iodine.[11]
5. Each wound is lavaged with at least 500 mL of an isotonic crystalloid or 2%–4% chlorhexidine to reduce bacterial numbers, but lavage will not remove necrotic debris or foreign particles.[2,14,15,21]
   - Optimum lavage pressure is unknown, but an 18- or 19-gauge needle attached to a 20 or 30 mL syringe, respectively, applied at an oblique angle, is recommended.[14,15] The pressure obtained depends upon the distance from the wound and the force of fluid delivery.[14]
   - Higher pressures should be avoided, as they can drive contaminants into the wound.[14]
   - Intrathoracic lavage is required if there is deep thoracic wall involvement.[17]
6. After draping for aseptic surgery, superficial skin puncture wounds are probed to check for underlying damage.
7. Incision or excision of the puncture wounds is performed to allow assessment of the underlying hypodermis, fascia, and muscle.[11] Hair and foreign debris are physically removed with instruments or a wound debridement pad (e.g., Debrisoft, L&R Medical UK).
8. Contaminated, damaged, nonviable, or necrotic muscle, fat, and fascia are excised from the wound and wound edges (Fig. 7.1).[2,11,14,15] Wounds over the body are debrided more aggressively than extremity wounds to allow primary wound closure in a single surgery.[11,15] Loss of function after removal of large amounts of muscle is rare.[11,15]
9. Drains can be used to manage dead space (Fig. 7.2).
10. Fractures can be fixed at the time of wound exploration or delayed, depending on the extent of initial wound contamination and tissue damage.[11]
11. Reconstructive surgery options for large skin defects include advancement flaps, axial pattern flaps, skin fold flaps, pedicle grafts, skin grafts, and microvascular free flaps.
12. Serial debridement over several days may be necessary if it is difficult to predict the amount of nonviable tissue or if there is high infectious bioburden.[11,14]
13. In the majority of bite wounds, due to the severity of contamination and possibility of infection, delayed primary closure or secondary closure are preferred to primary wound closure (Fig. 7.3).

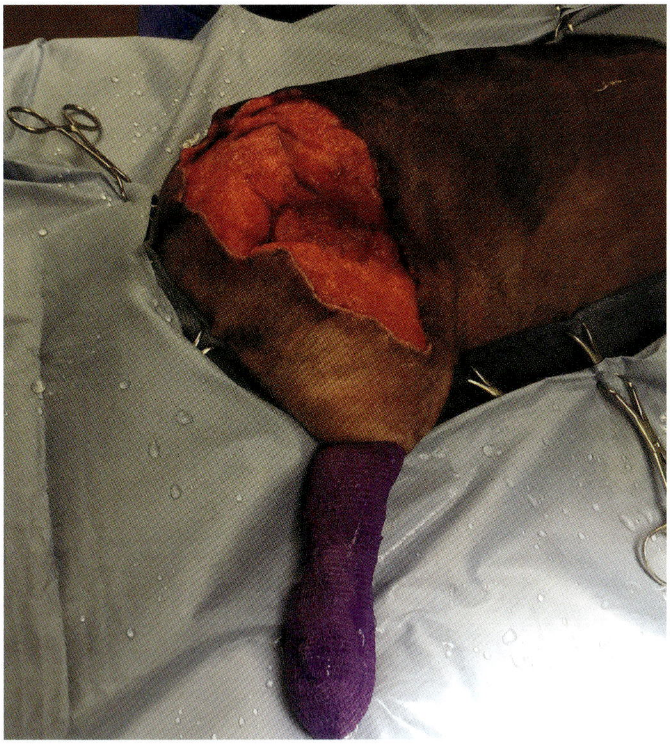

Figure 7.1 Appearance of a bite wound on the right hind limb of a dog following extensive serial debridement and open wound management. Image courtesy of Marie Burneko.

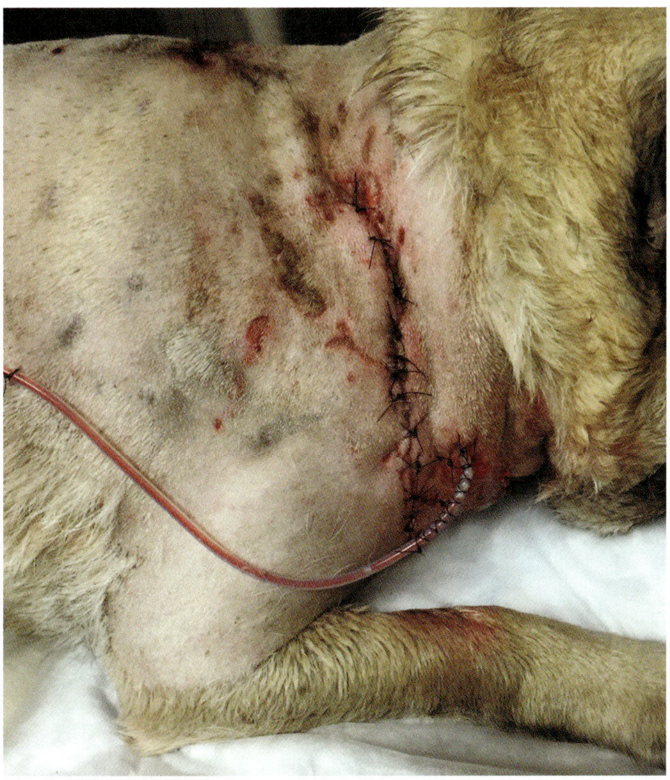

Figure 7.2 Appearance of a bite wound in a 10-year-old dog following immediate debridement and closure. A closed-suction drain was placed to decrease dead space. Image courtesy of Marie Burneko.

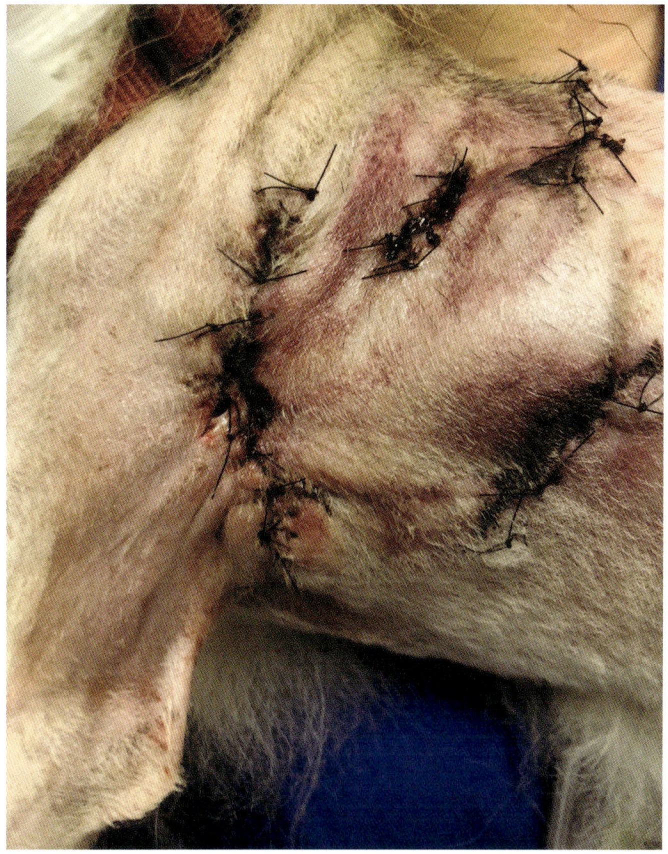

Figure 7.3 Incisional dehiscence and progressive bruising in a 3-year-old Pomeranian with multiple bite wounds to the lateral thorax. The wounds had been immediately debrided and closed following injury; however, ongoing tissue necrosis likely contributed to dehiscence of the debrided wound 5 days after the initial surgery. Image courtesy of Marie Burneko.

- Wound dressings are applied to bite wounds not closed surgically. The choice of contact dressing depends upon wound depth, location, contamination, and degree of exudation (Table 7.3).[14]
- Delayed closure is performed when infection is under control but before granulation tissue formation, typically after 3–5 days.[11]
- Negative-pressure wound therapy can be applied to bite wounds (for 3–5 days) to improve granulation tissue formation and wound healing before final wound reconstruction (Fig. 7.4).
- Alternatively, wounds can be left to heal by second intention.[7]

Head and cervical wounds (Fig. 7.5)

Ventral cervical exploration is indicated for suspected airway injuries, most of which heal after primary repair.[8] Temporary tracheostomy may be required if there is laryngeal injury or marked cervical inflammation.[8] Vascular injuries are managed by ligation. Half of lip avulsion injuries in dogs are caused by bites, and most are as-

TABLE 7.3 - TYPES AND USE OF TOPICAL WOUND DRESSINGS[2,4,5]

Wound dressing	Wound staging	Action of dressing
Hypertonic saline dressing 20% saline	Early phase of healing Inflammatory	Antimicrobial (hypertonicity) 20% saline Autolytic debridement Infected wound
Honey	Early phase of healing Inflammatory Infected wound	Antibacterial Autolytic debridement Reduces inflammation and edema Promotes granulation tissue formation and epithelization
Sugar	Early phase of healing Inflammatory Infected wound	Hyperosmotic Potential nutrient source of the wound
Enzymatic agent	Early phase of healing Inflammatory Debridement	Superficial debridement Debridement of chronic wounds
Maggots	Early phase of healing Inflammatory Debridement	Selective debridement of necrotic tissue Useful when surgical debridement is not an option
Topical antibiotic ointment	Inflammatory Infected wound	Reduces superficial microbial burden
Silver	Early phase of healing Inflammatory Infected wound	Release ionic silver into gel that forms at wound surface to reduce bacterial, yeast, and fungal organisms
Hydrogel	Inflammatory Repair	Keeps wound surface moist and promotes epithelization Wounds with minimal to no exudate (abrasion)
Hydrocolloid	Inflammatory Repair	Absorbs exudate, keeps wound surface moist, and promotes autolytic debridement and granulation tissue formation Wounds with moderate or copious exudate
Alginate	Inflammatory Repair	Absorbs exudate, keeps wound surface moist, and promotes autolytic debridement and granulation tissue formation Wounds with moderate or copious exudate

sociated with other injuries, including facial fractures.[30] They require appositional repair after wound debridement and lavage.

Thoracic wounds

The veterinarian must be prepared to encounter an open thorax after skin incision, as trauma to all soft tissues between the skin and pleural space may be present. Traumatized soft tissues, including muscle, are debrided as described above. Ribs are less likely than long bones to form sequestra after fracture and loss of associated soft tissues; therefore, they rarely need to be excised.[17]

Flail chest injuries are often surgically stabilized, possibly because the anatomical field is already being surgically explored, but this has no impact on survival.[18] Ribs are stabilized with encircling large-gauge sutures around adjacent fractured and intact ribs to create a scaffold for overlying soft tissues (see Chapter 23).[17]

If primary thoracic closure is difficult, options for reconstruction include muscle and myocutaneous flaps (e.g., latissimus dorsi, pectoralis major, and rectus abdominis) and omental advancement, if there is not too much damage to donor tissues.[17] While there will often be complete devitalization of thoracic wall musculature over fractured ribs, the skin is usually intact, and closure has been achieved with only skin and no interposed muscles over the ribs.[17]

Synthetic meshes should be used with care if there is contamination.[17]

Exudate from soft tissues and pleural space can be drained together with a thoracostomy tube or a subcutaneous closed drain, but passive open drains are contraindicated because they compromise the negative pressure of the pleural space.[17] Negative-pressure wound therapy can be applied to thoracic and abdominal bite wounds if primary closure is not possible, but lower pressures are required to avoid decrease in lung compliance.

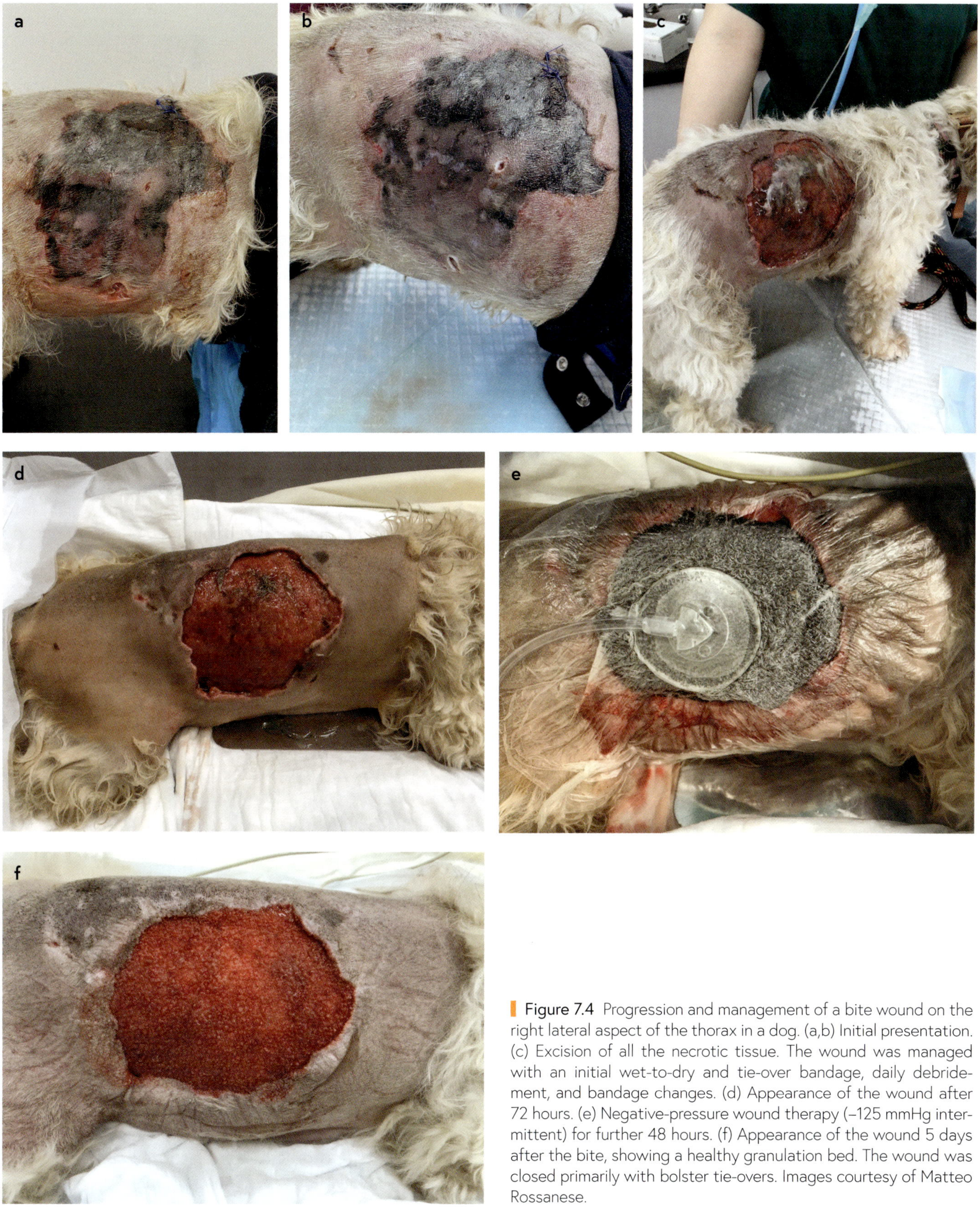

Figure 7.4 Progression and management of a bite wound on the right lateral aspect of the thorax in a dog. (a,b) Initial presentation. (c) Excision of all the necrotic tissue. The wound was managed with an initial wet-to-dry and tie-over bandage, daily debridement, and bandage changes. (d) Appearance of the wound after 72 hours. (e) Negative-pressure wound therapy (–125 mmHg intermittent) for further 48 hours. (f) Appearance of the wound 5 days after the bite, showing a healthy granulation bed. The wound was closed primarily with bolster tie-overs. Images courtesy of Matteo Rossanese.

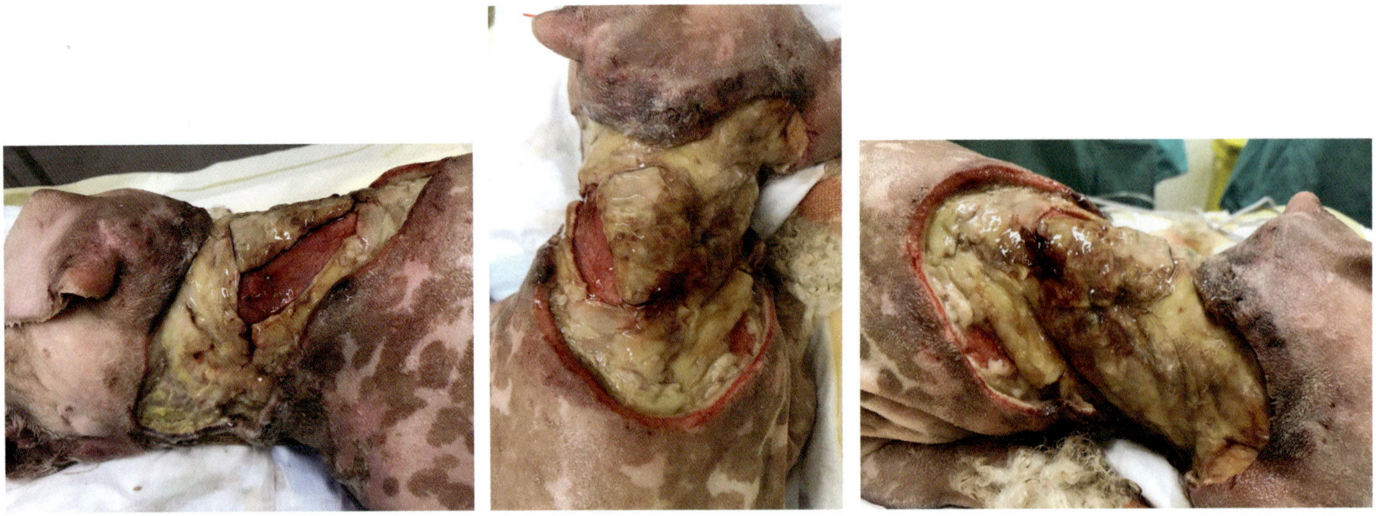

Figure 7.5 Severe cervical bite wound in a dog. Note the involvement of deep tissues and necrosis of the subcutaneous tissue. The patient was septic at presentation. The wound was extensively debrided and a wet-to-dry tie-over bandage was placed. Images courtesy of Matteo Rossanese.

Abdominal and perineal wounds

Celiotomy is indicated if there is concern about damage to abdominal organs (seen in 65% of dogs with abdominal bite wounds), the body wall, or the diaphragm.[7,11] Closure options for large defects include local muscle flaps (e.g., cranial sartorius), surgical mesh, and omental pedicle flaps.[11,15] Skin bite wounds should be explored separately if not accessible via the midline.

Postoperative management of bite wounds

Postoperative care depends on the extent of injury, the surgery undertaken, whether a wound is open or closed, and whether the patient is critically ill (e.g., systemic inflammatory response syndrome). Analgesia and fluid therapy are continued as needed. Postoperative antibiotics are used only in previously indicated cases and are instituted if late clinical wound infection is seen, which occurs in up to 20% of dogs.[4,5,14] Long-term complications are uncommon. Thoracostomy and wound drain care is required if drains are used, and these patients should have constant supervision.

Outcome of bite wounds

Most of the veterinary literature describes cats and small dogs bitten by larger dogs that were referred to specialist hospitals. Populations and outcomes may differ between studies of dog bite wounds in the general population.[5]

Mortality in dogs and cats with bite wounds is 1.7%–20% and 12%–53%, respectively, mostly from sepsis or systemic inflammatory response syndrome when the cause of death was given.[1–10,16] The lowest mortality rate in dogs was in a large first opinion population, and no dogs with grade 1 or 2 wounds died or were euthanized.[5] It is likely that many bite wounds occurring between dogs of matched size are treated in first opinion practice, and most of these will not be referred. It is speculated that the higher mortality rates in cats, compared to dogs, are due to their smaller size, although this could also reflect differences in anatomy and body tissue characteristics.[3] In some studies, small dogs were more likely to die than large dogs.[3,7] Smaller dogs with thoracic bite wounds are more likely to require thoracotomy or lung lobectomy than larger dogs.[9]

Higher mortality rates in dogs have been associated with delayed presentation, thoracic and abdominal injury, pleural effusion, positive bacterial culture, higher animal trauma triage scores, higher wound grade scores, presence of systemic inflammatory response syndrome, lower postoperative white blood cell counts, and the need for fresh frozen plasma administration.[1,7,9,10] Systemic inflammatory response syndrome is exacerbated by the presence of necrotic tissue, highlighting the importance of wound exploration and tissue debridement.[11] Most dogs without thoracic or abdominal injury survive.[7] Higher mortality rates in cats have been associated with increased number of injured areas, category of wound depth, trauma to the thoracic spine, thorax, or abdomen, abdominal wall defects, higher animal trauma triage score and severity of injuries score, and the need for more aggressive treatment or administration of blood and plasma products.[3,6]

KEEP IN MIND

- All bite wounds should be surgically probed or explored to evaluate for deeper injury.
- Severe deeper tissue injury, such as pulmonary trauma, can be present in bite wounds without skin penetration and in animals with no evidence of dyspnea.
- Antibiotics are not always indicated in bite wounds and are not a substitute for lavage and debridement.
- Debridement of damaged or necrotic tissue is required to remove a medium for bacterial growth and potentially allow wound closure at the time of debridement.
- Survival is related to the severity of injury, and most dogs with superficial wounds and/or wounds that do not involve the thoracic or abdominal cavities survive.

References

1. Cabon Q et al. Thoracic bite trauma in dogs and cats: A retrospective study of 65 cases. *Vet Comp Orthop Traumatol.* 2015; 28(6):448–454.
2. Griffin GM, Holt DE. Dog-bite wounds: Bacteriology and treatment outcome in 37 cases. *J Am Anim Hosp Assoc.* 2001; 37(5):453–460.
3. Frykfors von Hekkel AK, Halfacree ZJ. Thoracic dog bite wounds in cats: A retrospective study of 22 cases (2005–2015). *J Feline Med Surg.* 2020; 22(2):146–152.
4. Kalnins NJ et al. A VetCompass Australia study of antimicrobial use in dog-to-dog bite wounds (1998–2018). *Antibiotics (Basel).* 2022; 11(1):55.
5. Kalnins NJ et al. Antimicrobials in dog-to-dog bite wounds: A retrospective study of 1526 dog bite events (1999–2019). *J Vet Intern Med.* 2022; 36(6):2028–2041.
6. Klainbart S et al. Dog bite wounds in cats: A retrospective study of 72 cases. *J Feline Med Surg.* 2022; 24(2):107–115.
7. Shamir MH et al. Dog bite wounds in dogs and cats: A retrospective study of 196 cases. *J Vet Med A Physiol Pathol Clin Med.* 2002; 49(2):107–112.
8. Jordan CJ, Halfacree ZJ, Tivers MS. Airway injury associated with cervical bite wounds in dogs and cats: 56 cases. *Vet Comp Orthop Traumatol.* 2013; 26(2):89–93.
9. Frykfors von Hekkel AK, Pegram C, Halfacree ZJ. Thoracic dog bite wounds in dogs: A retrospective study of 123 cases (2003–2016). *Vet Surg.* 2020; 49(4):694–703.
10. Ateca LB, Drobatz KJ, King LG. Organ dysfunction and mortality risk factors in severe canine bite wound trauma. *J Vet Emerg Crit Care (San Antonio).* 2014; 24(6):705–714.
11. Pavletic MM, Trout NJ. Bullet, bite, and burn wounds in dogs and cats. *Vet Clin North Am Small Anim Pract.* 2006; 36(4):873–893.
12. Meyers B, Schoeman JP, Goddard A, Picard J. The bacteriology and antimicrobial susceptibility of infected and non-infected dog bite wounds: Fifty cases. *Vet Microbiol.* 2008; 127(3–4):360–368.
13. Mouro S, Vilela CL, Niza MM. Clinical and bacteriological assessment of dog-to-dog bite wounds. *Vet Microbiol.* 2010; 144(1–2):127–132.
14. Devriendt N, de Rooster H. Initial management of traumatic wounds. *Vet Clin North Am Small Anim Pract.* 2017; 47(6):1123–1134.
15. Holt DE, Griffin G. Bite wounds in dogs and cats. *Vet Clin North Am Small Anim Pract.* 2000; 30(3):669–679.
16. Scheepens ET, Peeters ME, L'eplattenier HF, Kirpensteijn J. Thoracic bite trauma in dogs: A comparison of clinical and radiological parameters with surgical results. *J Small Anim Pract.* 2006; 47(12):721–726.
17. Shahar R, Shamir M, Johnston DE. A technique for management of bite wounds of the thoracic wall in small dogs. *Vet Surg.* 1997; 26(1):45–50.
18. Olsen D et al. Clinical management of flail chest in dogs and cats: A retrospective study of 24 cases (1989–1999). *J Am Anim Hosp Assoc.* 2002; 38(4):315–320.
19. Kalnins NJ et al. Treatment of moderate grade dog bite wounds using amoxicillin-clavulanic acid with and without enrofloxacin: A randomised non-inferiority trial. *Aust Vet J.* 2021; 99(9):369–377.
20. Nolff MC et al. Assessment of wound bio-burden and prevalence of multi-drug resistant bacteria during open wound management. *J Small Anim Pract.* 2016; 57(5):255–259.
21. British Small Animal Veterinary Association. Antibacterial use in our practice. Guide to Responsible Use of Antibacterials: PROTECT ME. Gloucester, UK: BSAVA; 2018 [accessed June 2019]. Available at https://www.bsavalibrary.com/content/chapter/10.22233/9781910443644.chap6_1#html_fulltext.
22. Chai O, Johnston DE, Shamir MH. Bite wounds involving the spine: characteristics, therapy and outcome in seven cases. *Vet J.* 2008;175(2):259-65.
23. Hodgson N, Walters A, Lawson C, Hague D, Joslyn S, McMichael M. Acute surgical intervention for a depressed skull fracture causing a laceration to the brain parenchyma from a bite wound in a dog. *Can Vet J.* 2018; 59(1):31-35.
24. Lee GW, Park HM, Kang MH. Global brain ischemia in a dog with concurrent multiorgan dysfunction syndrome after bite wound trauma. *Acta Vet Scand.* 2019; 6;61(1):22.
25. Seiler G, Rossi F, Vignoli M, Cianciolo R, Scanlon T, Giger U. Computed tomographic features of skull osteomyelitis in four young dogs. *Vet Radiol Ultrasound.* 2007;48(6):544-9.
26. Kirberger RM. Early diagnostic imaging findings in juvenile dogs with presumed diskospondylitis: 10 cases (2008-2014). *J Am Vet Med Assoc.* 2016;249(5):539-46.
27. Vedrine B, Maurin MP. Dorsal surgical stabilisation using tension bands for treatment of traumatic atlanto-occipital instability in a cat. *Aust Vet J.* 2017;95(12):469-473.
28. Yala W, Suranunt P, Fujisawa Y, Yippaditr W. Application of buccal mucosal graft to establish a new urination passage in male cats with penile traumatic injury. *J Vet Med Sci.* 2022;7;84(10):1442-1446.
29. Ferrell CL, Essman SC. What Is Your Diagnosis? Herniation of the left caudal lung lobe through the left seventh intercostal space. *J Am Vet Med Assoc.* 2016;248(7):759-61.
30. Saverino KM, Reiter AM. Clinical Presentation, Causes, Treatment, and Outcome of Lip Avulsion Injuries in Dogs and Cats: 24 Cases (2001-2017). *Front Vet Sci.* 2018; 5:144.

Chapter 8

Burn injuries

Rachel Williams

Burn wounds, although relatively rare in veterinary medicine, can have significant metabolic and biochemical consequences.

There are multiple ways to classify burn wounds. One common approach is by describing the **mechanism of injury**, and thereby burns can be categorized into four basic types: thermal, chemical, electrical, and radiation.[1] In general, thermal burns are more frequently observed than chemical burns.[2] Thermal burns occur when tissues are exposed to extreme temperatures, whether hot or cold, leading to cellular damage (Fig. 8.1). The most common causes of thermal burns include boiling liquids, electric heating pads, animal-drying cages, and heated metal.[3] It is important to note that frostbite is considered a thermal burn, despite the term *thermal burn* colloquially being used to refer only to hyperthermic injuries.

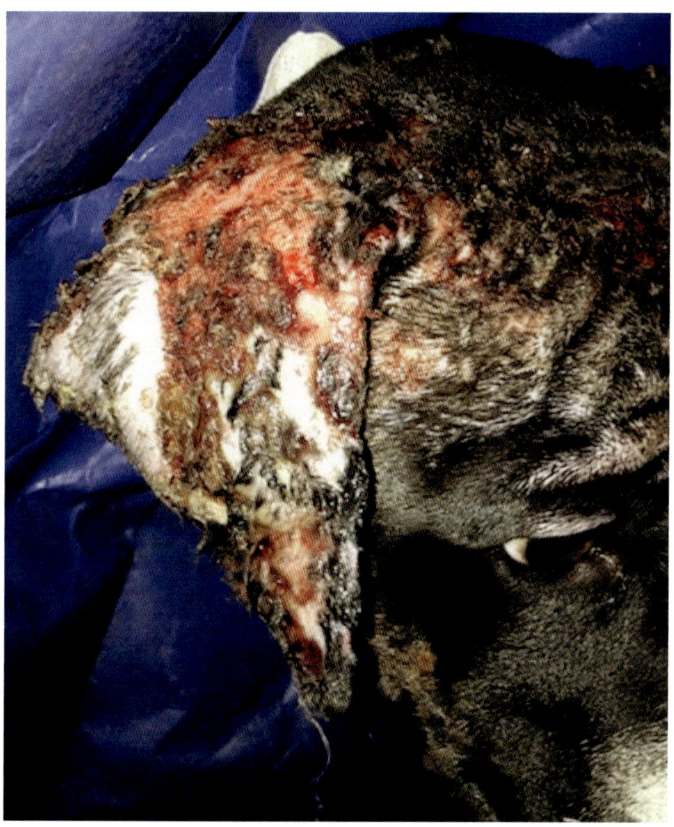

Figure 8.1 Thermal burn caused by a car fire. Image courtesy of Brittany Abrams.

Chemical burns can result either directly from a chemical reaction leading to cellular damage or indirectly through thermal damage secondary to a chemical reaction. Electrical burns occur when an electrical current passes through a patient, either directly or indirectly, resulting in cellular damage and necrosis. Radiation burns occur when ionizing radiation is delivered to an area at levels that result in cell death. This is most commonly seen with exposure to solar radiation or with the use of radiation therapy for treatment of neoplasia (Fig. 8.2).

Other ways to characterize burn wounds are based on the depth of injury and on the total body surface area affected. The **depth of a burn injury** is determined by various factors, including the temperature of the agent, the duration of contact, the thickness of the epidermis and dermis, and the blood supply to the affected area.[3,4] Historically, burns were classified as first- to fifth-degree burns. However, this system does not always accurately reflect the depth of these injuries.[5] A more modern classification utilizes the terms superficial burn (confined to the epidermis), partial-thickness burn (involving the epidermis and superficial dermis), full-thickness burn (involving the epidermis and dermis), and subdermal burn (involving the epidermis, dermis, and subcutaneous tissue) (Fig. 8.3).[3,5,6] Correctly classifying a burn wound based on its depth can aid in prognosis and treatment planning for a patient (Table 8.1). For example, most superficial burn wounds will heal without assistance within 3–5 days, while full-thickness burns will have delayed healing and can lead to more significant scarring and worse cosmesis.[7]

With respect to characterizing burns based on the **total body surface area affected**, a common method is the Wallace rule of nines. This tool is used to estimate the percentage of total body skin area affected by burns in human adults. In children, the Lund–Browder chart is used. When using the rule of nines, each body part is assigned a specific percentage of total body area. The entire head is 9%; the entire trunk is 36%, which can be divided into anterior and posterior and then subdivided into chest and abdomen; each upper extremity is 9%, while the lower extremities are 18% each and can also

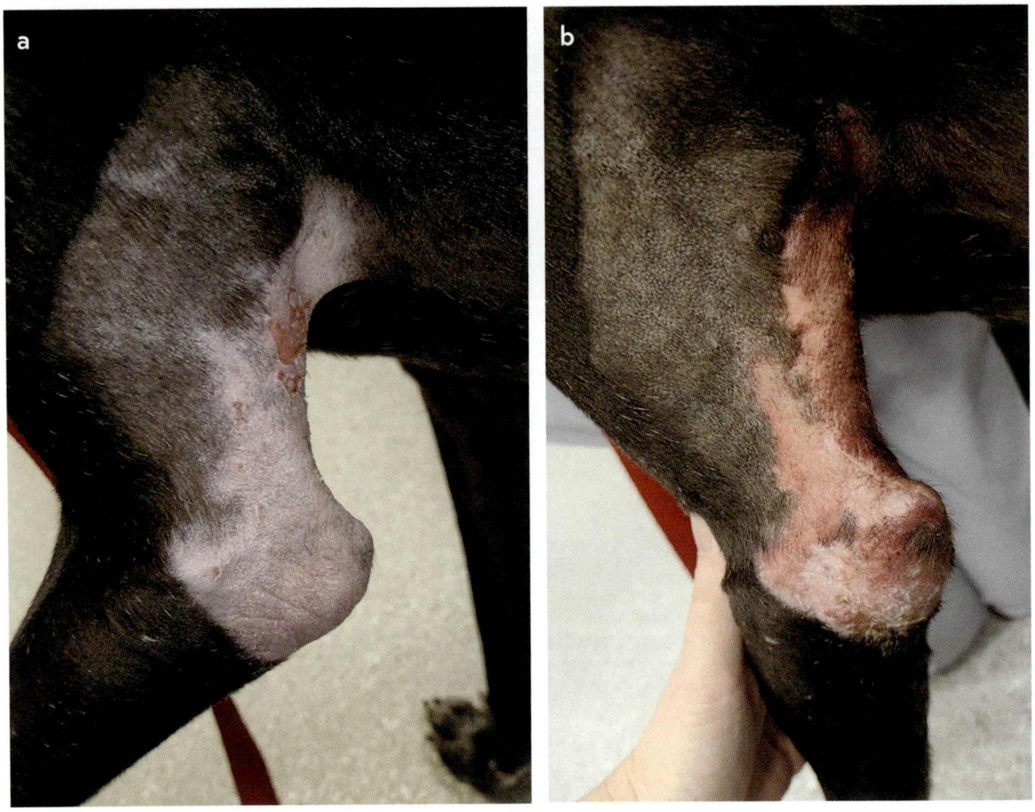

Figure 8.2 Radiation burn (a) 1 week and (b) 2 weeks following definitive radiation therapy for a soft tissue sarcoma. Images courtesy of Sam Yeh.

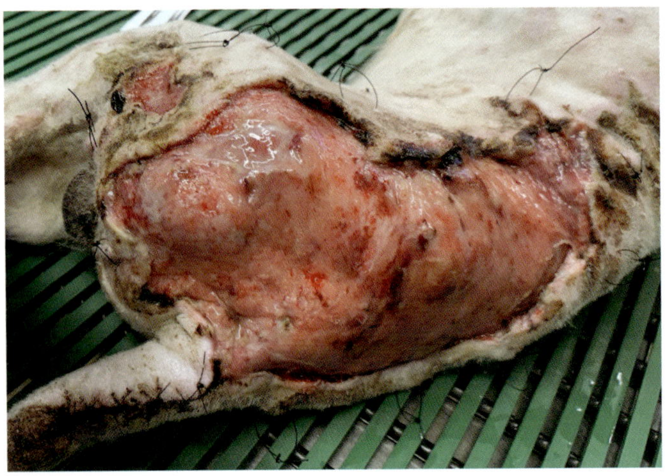

Figure 8.3 Subdermal burn caused by a house fire.

be subdivided into anterior and posterior portions.[6,8] Categorizing a burn using this methodology is important because patients with severe burn injuries (>20%–30% of total body surface area) are known to have more significant systemic and metabolic derangements that require advanced care and intense resuscitation. It is known that there are limitations when applying this classification scheme in human medicine, particularly to very obese or very small patients. Similar limitations may apply to the veterinary population, given the vast differences in size across breeds and species.

There have been attempts to create a veterinary equivalent of the rule of nines. Moderate differences have been found between humans and mesocephalic dogs when comparing the contribution of various body parts to the overall body surface area.[9] While the head and neck represent 9% of the body surface area in the human Wallace rule of nines, in this study the head alone was assigned a value of 14%, with 9% for the neck alone. This system has not yet been validated for clinical use in dogs; however, it demonstrates the limitations of adapting a classification scheme designed for humans to veterinary use.

Another methodology to characterize burns is the burn card system, which makes use of the worldwide standardized dimensions of a plastic credit card: 8.5 cm × 5.3 cm resulting in a 45 cm^2 surface area.[10] In humans, this corresponds to 0.25% of the body surface area of a 70 kg man.[10] Utilizing something that mimics the dimensions and weight of a plastic credit card facilitates ease of carriage and use, particularly in an emergency setting. This method of burn classification has been found to improve assessment of burn wound size, particularly in areas of irregular size and shape.[10] The Veterinary Burn Card has the same dimensions and purpose. In order to determine the percentage of body surface area affected, the number of cards that are needed to cover the wound is calculated, multiplied by 0.45, and divided by the surface area of the patient using a standard weight-to-surface area conversion table.[11]

TABLE 8.1 - CLASSIFICATION OF BURN INJURIES ACCORDING TO THEIR DEPTH

Burn depth	Tissue involvement	Wound characteristics	Pain	Healing capability
Superficial	Epidermis	• Pink to light red • Dry	Minimally painful	Heals in 5–7 days
Superficial partial-thickness	Epidermis, superficial dermis	• Bright red to mottled • Intact hair follicles • Exudative wound surface • Eschar may form	Very painful	Heals in 10–21 days Minimal scarring
Deep partial-thickness	Epidermis, dermis	• Dark red or yellow to white • Some hair follicles remain • Moist wound surface • Eschar may form	Reduced pain sensation	Prolonged duration of healing Increased risk of wound complications and contracture Surgical intervention strongly encouraged
Full-thickness	Epidermis, dermis, subcutaneous tissue ± muscle	• Charred or white • Dry wound surface • Hair epilates easily	Nonpainful	Delayed healing expected Surgical intervention mandatory

Source: Bishop JF. Burn wound assessment and surgical management. *Crit Care Nurs Clin North Am.* 2004; 16(1):145–177; Pavletic MM, Trout NJ. Bullet, bite, and burn wounds in dogs and cats. *Vet Clin North Am Small Anim Pract.* 2006; 36(4):873–893.

Although every burn classification system has its limitations, whether it centers around assessing the depth of injury or the surface area affected, it is important to be as accurate as possible in estimating surface area due to its direct relationship with fluid resuscitation in these cases.

Clinical presentation and diagnosis

The clinical presentation of a burn wound should, in most cases, be relatively straightforward. However, the lack of direct visualization of the inciting cause or the presence of ill-natured intent can complicate an accurate diagnosis. A dark and dense hair coat can also hinder diagnosis by concealing the damage until it becomes significant enough to result in either epilation or an odor.[3,12,13] A recent history of significant sun exposure or of an anesthetic event with exposure to external heating sources, hair dryers, or caustic chemicals can aid in diagnosis.[3] If there is little clinical history to rely on, a burn wound can be easily misdiagnosed as other dermatological disorders, such as toxic epidermal necrolysis, pemphigus vulgaris, erythema multiforme, or other immune-mediated diseases.[2] In these cases, differentiation between an immune-mediated disease and a burn wound relies on accurately assessing wound progression. If there is no progression after the first 5 days of observation, it is more likely to be a burn wound.[2,3]

The clinical signs observed in cases of a burn wound directly correlate with the severity of the insult and can be helpful in establishing a prognosis, in conjunction with the aforementioned classification schemes.

Integument

As a generalization, veterinary patients do not develop blistering as human patients do in the case of a burn wound.[14] In superficial burns, the skin can appear reddened and edematous. In more severe burns (partial or full thickness), varying amounts of exudate can be present over the surface and there can be variable exposure or involvement of subcutaneous fat and muscle. In many cases, the involved skin takes on a dark and thickened appearance, similar to leather. This is called an eschar and is indicative of skin necrosis (Fig. 8.4). Eschars are especially common in the event of a latent wound, such as when a homemade warming element is utilized during surgery or other anesthetic events. Eventually, the eschar will separate from the underlying tissues and surrounding skin. At this point, discharge may be evident or there can be coverage of granulation tissue and early epithelialization, depending on the health of the wound.

In some cases, patients will develop a smoky odor to their fur, and the tips of their fur may be singed. It is important to thoroughly evaluate these patients to monitor for progression of wounds that may not be immediately evident.

Respiratory system

Not all clinical signs secondary to a thermal or chemical injury will be confined to the skin. Perhaps the most obvious body system to be injured in association with thermal burns is the respiratory system. Injuries to the lungs can also trigger a cascade of responses in other

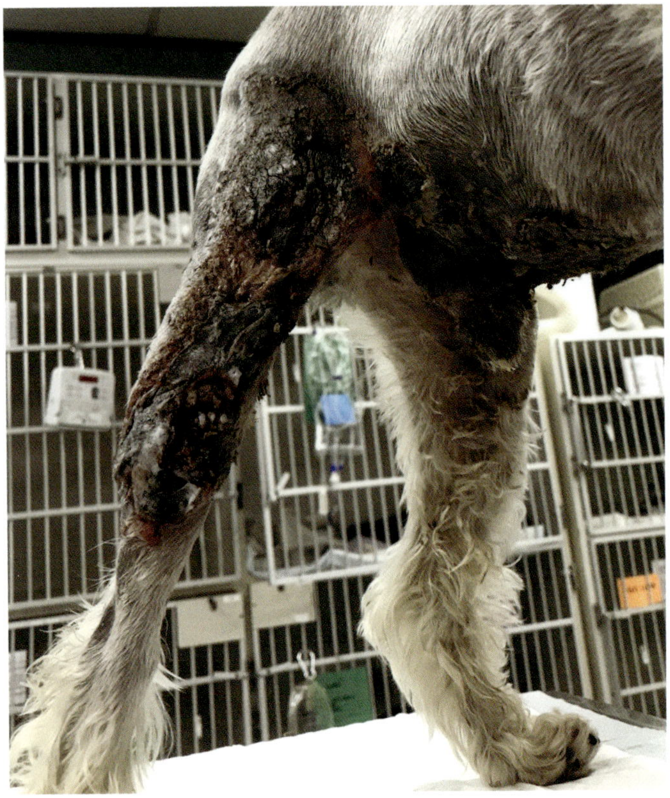

Figure 8.4 Burn wound caused by a house fire. Note the dark, leathery appearance of the tissue overlying the wound (i.e., eschar). Image courtesy of Brittany Abrams.

systems due to a systemic inflammatory response syndrome as well as interference with oxygen delivery secondary to toxic metabolites associated with smoke. Expected clinical signs include tachypnea, hypothermia, and tachycardia.

While pathophysiological changes in the lungs, such as pulmonary edema due to increased pulmonary vascular permeability, can be demonstrated radiographically, it is important to note that the presence of carbon monoxide can be insidious but have profound effects. Carbon monoxide binds to hemoglobin at the same location where oxygen typically binds, displacing oxygen and decreasing the oxygen-carrying capacity of blood.[15,16] In fact, carbon monoxide binds to hemoglobin with approximately 250 times greater affinity than oxygen, resulting in a shift of the oxygen-dissociation curve to the left.[15,16] Despite a significant reduction in the oxygen content of the blood in case of carbon monoxide poisoning, the partial pressure of oxygen in the blood may remain normal, and clinical signs of hypoxemia, such as cyanosis, may be absent.[16] In addition to this, the lack of change in partial pressure of oxygen results in a lack of stimulus to increase ventilation despite the developing hypoxia.[15] This theory has been supported in the veterinary literature by a lack of relationship between respiratory rate and carboxyhemoglobin concentrations.[15,17,18] Thermal injury to the airways and mechanical irritation due to toxicants in smoke can also result in a change in respiratory rate. Although there are few published reference ranges in small animal patients, carboxyhemoglobin can be measured if there is concern for carbon monoxide poisoning. Carbon monoxide poisoning can also result in other clinical signs such as neurological abnormalities, including paresis, change in mentation, and seizures.

Other systems

Other clinical signs that may be observed in a patient with a burn injury can be associated with various body systems. Corneal ulcers can occur in case of thermal or chemical burns. Dehydration and hypovolemia can result from evaporation of fluid from the surface of a burn and fluid migration from the vascular to the interstitial space, secondary to increased vascular permeability.[11] Severe burns can trigger a systemic inflammatory response, leading to myocardial damage, gastrointestinal translocation, and acute kidney injury.[5,7,11,14] It is important to thoroughly evaluate the entire patient in the event of a burn wound and to be aware that some clinical signs can have a delayed presentation.

Treatment

Treatment of burn wounds can be divided into medical and surgical management. Medical management includes initial topical wound therapy, antimicrobial therapy, analgesics, and management of the nonsurgical consequences of burn injuries such as dehydration and alteration of the metabolic state. Surgical management involves initial debridement and wound management as well as both simple and advanced methods to achieve wound closure.

Medical management

Immediate wound care

In the acute setting, initial medical management of burn patients should consist of cooling of the burn wounds and fluid resuscitation. While previously recommended for both burn wounds and heat stroke, ice water is currently not indicated due to the risk of hypothermia[7] and limited healing benefit.[19] The current recommendation is to use cool running water over the burn wound. The optimal temperature is approximately 15°C for 20 minutes, which results in not only a quicker return to baseline temperatures but also a reduction in tissue inflammation and improved scar cosmesis.[19] Cool running water can also provide analgesia, which is crucial in managing pain in burn patients.[20]

Fluid therapy

Fluid resuscitation is the most important factor in the management of burn patients in an acute setting. Initially, patients can experience fluid shifts due to increased vascular permeability, resulting in depletion of the intravascular space. Fluid losses and a hypodynamic state can persist for days to a week after the initial injury due to a loss of protein-rich fluid via the wound surface and via the gastrointestinal tract due to systemic inflammatory response. The loss of fluid through the wound can be difficult to quantify, thereby making treatment more complex.

Since the fluid shifts and inflammatory phase following a burn injury can result in serious morbidity and mortality, appropriate treatment and maintenance of normovolemia are imperative.[11,21] Several formulas for fluid resuscitation have been developed for humans and adapted for veterinary patients. The Parkland formula is currently the most commonly used in human patients.[21] It relies on crystalloids only and requires calculation of the percentage of body surface area affected by the burn. This formula recommends lactated Ringer's solution at 4 × weight of patient in kg × (% burned body surface area × 100) to be given over 24 hours, with the first half given in 8 hours.[21] However, it has been demonstrated in human medicine that patients frequently receive far more fluid than this formula estimates, a term coined *fluid creep*.[21,22] In the initial development of this formula, a fourth 8-hour phase was included in which a dose of plasma was given to provide colloidal support. It is thought that abandoning this phase and switching to a sole crystalloid formula has contributed to fluid creep.[22] Given the relative inaccuracies of measuring the percentage of burned surface area in a wide variety of breeds and species, as well as the risk for fluid creep when limited to only crystalloids, using more objective monitoring parameters (e.g., blood pressure, heart rate, urine output) is recommended when determining the volume and type of fluid resuscitation.

Analgesia

Burn patients frequently have pain levels that are challenging to control without multimodal analgesia and that seem at discordance with the injuries that can be grossly examined. Part of the difficulty in managing pain associated with burn wounds is the multiple sources of pain arising from the wound itself or the surrounding tissues. It is important to remember that burn depth can be variable across the wound; therefore, while a full-thickness burn is classically considered to be painless because of complete destruction of nerve endings, some regions of the burn may be more superficial and can thus be hypersensitized. Pain can also arise as a result of the procedures being performed to treat the wound and also due to tissue regeneration and the formation of new nerve endings as the healing process progresses.[23]

Commonly used analgesics in burn patients include opioids, benzodiazepines, alpha-2 agonists, NMDA antagonists such as ketamine, and local anesthetics such as lidocaine. Nonsteroidal anti-inflammatory drugs may also be beneficial, assuming there are no comorbidities that would preclude their use. Appropriate sedation for bandage changes and debridement can also be considered a component of an analgesic plan in these patients, to reduce the anxiety and anticipation associated with handling.

Antimicrobial therapy

Systemic antibiotics are generally not indicated prophylactically in burn patients, unless there is a concern for sepsis or wound infection.[3,14] Topical antimicrobials are frequently sufficient and provide a moist wound environment to support healing. Silver sulfadiazine is a common topical treatment for burn wounds in veterinary medicine and can be applied even over an eschar if the patient is not stable enough for debridement or if the eschar is healthy enough to remain in place. It has a broad spectrum of antimicrobial coverage, including methicillin-resistant *Staphylococcus aureus* (MRSA), and has been reported to have a soothing effect when applied.[3,24] Mafenide acetate is a less frequently used topical antimicrobial; however, it is known to have much better eschar penetration compared with silver sulfadiazine.[6,24] Other topical antimicrobials include triple antibiotic ointment and medicinal honey.

Following establishment of a robust granulation bed, typical open wound healing strategies can be employed and a variety of dressings utilized. Depending on the stage of healing, hydrocolloid bandages, calcium alginate, or Vaseline-impregnated gauze may be appropriate.

Other medical management

Other affected body systems should be addressed. Treatment of corneal ulcers with appropriate antimicrobials, pain relief, and other therapies should be considered if ocular injury is present. Irritation to the airways and respiratory distress can be treated with bronchodilators, mucolytics, sedatives, and supplemental oxygen.[25] Neurological abnormalities secondary to carbon monoxide poisoning are generally treated supportively, with the focus on the underlying cause. In theory, carbon monoxide poisoning is ideally treated with hyperbaric oxygen, although this is not frequently available in a veterinary setting, and some controversy surrounds its efficacy;[15,25] therefore, intubation with oxygen supplementation is used instead in severe cases.[18]

Nutritional management

Nutrition is a vital component of treatment for burn patients. These patients typically enter a hypermetabolic state leading to increased muscle metabolism and loss of lean body mass.[5] Adequate caloric, and especially protein, intake is crucial to reduce the systemic effects of hypermetabolism. The recommended protein intake is 4–6 g per 100 kcal for dogs and 6 g per 100 kcal for cats.[11] Enteral nutrition is generally preferred over parenteral nutrition, as it can maintain gut motility and decrease the risk of gastrointestinal translocation. This has been shown to result in quicker clinical improvement in patients with gastrointestinal disturbances.[7,25] Feeding tubes may be used if the patient is reluctant to eat. In some cases, strategic planning for tube placement must be considered based on the location and extent of the wounds. However, if enteral nutrition is not possible, parenteral nutrition may need to be used.

Surgical management

Burn wound debridement, although not needed to be done immediately, is eventually necessary in most cases. Debridement can be performed by multiple methods: surgical, ultrasonic, and/or autolytic. Sharp surgical debridement is often pursued due to the relative ease in acquisition of required surgical instrumentation and speed with which a response to therapy is observed. Following debridement, a variety of methods to achieve wound closure are available. Open wound management is a cheap and cost-effective method for treatment of the wound bed (Fig. 8.5); however, it can be time-consuming and is frequently more expensive than anticipated due to the duration of therapy and frequency of bandage changes. Alternatively, secondary wound closure or any number of reconstructive efforts such as flaps or grafts can be performed. While these efforts may reduce the overall timeline of required therapy, they can be costly, and complications can occur that result in persistence of a wound bed and the requirement for ongoing bandage changes or additional surgery.

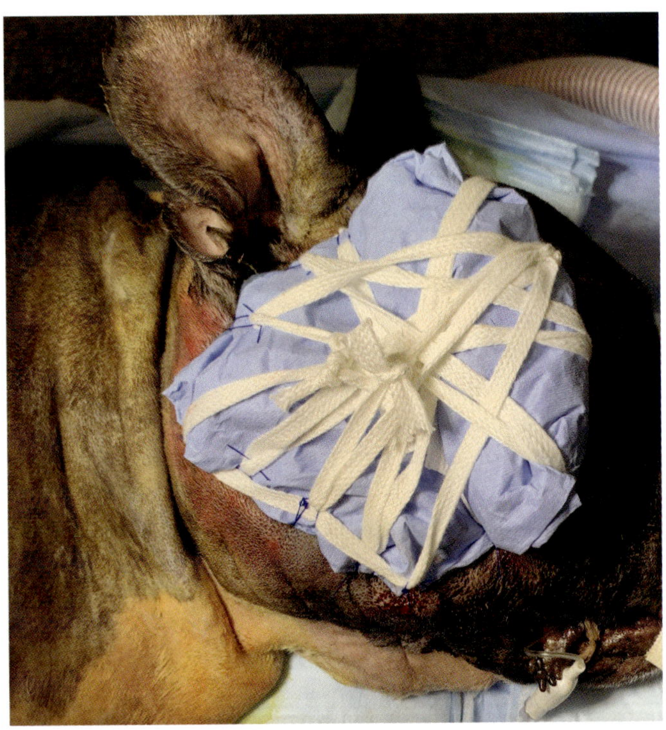

Figure 8.5 Tie-over bandage in place over a chemical wound on the face. These bandages are helpful to provide open wound management in a variety of challenging to bandage locations.

Surgical technique

1. Two forms of debridement are commonly utilized: tangential and layered debridement.
   - Tangential debridement is the preferred choice for addressing partial- or full-thickness burns that do not extend beyond the subcutaneous tissue. This technique involves the use of sharp instruments, such as a scalpel blade or scissors, to incise the interface between the wound and unharmed skin, which creates a natural boundary for resection. Dissection is carried out parallel or tangentially to the wound, resulting in the resection of thin layers of tissue.
   - Layered debridement is more commonly used for deeper wounds that may extend through muscle and even reach the bone. Debridement begins at the periphery of the wound, where it interfaces with healthy skin, and should initially be limited to the outer, superficial zone of hyperemia.[25] As debridement progresses toward the center of the wound (through the zone of stasis and the zone of coagulation), it should reach the deeper regions, as this is where the damage is greatest.
2. Just as with any wound debridement, thorough irrigation of the area throughout the procedure and upon completion is recommended.
3. Due to the known phenomenon of delayed healing associated with burn wounds,[11] immediate wound closure is not recommended. In many cases, the wound can continue to declare itself over the following days, often necessitating further debridement.

Postoperative management

Following debridement of burn injuries, open wound management is commonly employed. This is performed either until the wound is completely healed or until the wound bed is healthy enough to tolerate closure, flap surgery, or grafting (Fig. 8.6).

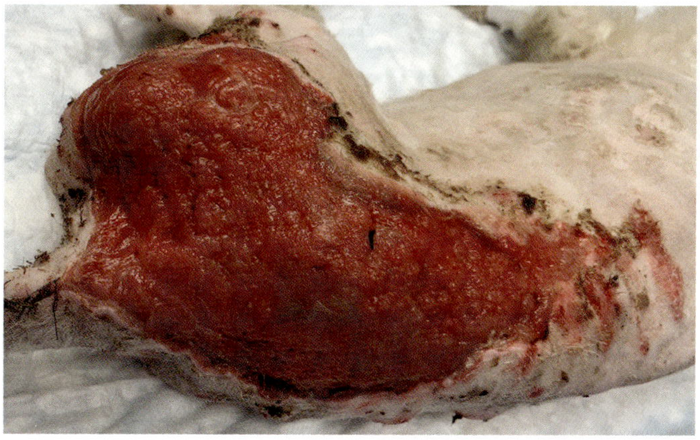

Figure 8.6 Same burn wound from Figure 8.3, with healthy granulation tissue covering the surface. This wound is ready to undergo closure if desired.

The frequency of bandage changes is dictated by the wound bed. Various factors such as exudate volume, progression of healing, and presence of infection can alter the frequency of the changes and may also indicate the need to use a different type of primary dressing. If the animal is treated on an outpatient basis, owners should be instructed to monitor for strikethrough or any change in odor of the bandage.

Injectable analgesics should be continued for at least 12–24 hours postoperatively, although it is common to need a prolonged course, particularly if multiple episodes of debridement are required. A constant-rate infusion of analgesics such as fentanyl, ketamine, or dexmedetomidine can prove beneficial in providing multimodal analgesia. When transitioning to oral pain medications, nonsteroidal anti-inflammatory drugs can be considered, provided there are no contraindications. Gabapentin and codeine have also been used in veterinary patients, although their efficacy is controversial. Exercise should be restricted until healing of the wound has been confirmed.

Outcome

In the event of hypertrophic scar formation and contracture, the outcome may be considered suboptimal. Fortunately, this can be addressed electively once the patient has otherwise fully recovered. Contracture can be problematic, particularly in the extremities, as it can restrict the range of motion and lead to chronic pain during movement. If this occurs, resection of the contracted region can be performed and the surgical wound corrected via primary closure or with the use of skin flaps or grafts.[14] Physical therapy can also be beneficial in preventing this complication.[14]

In general, the prognosis following a burn wound is favorable, provided the patient receives appropriate resuscitation and systemic management. The vast majority of burn wounds will heal completely (Fig. 8.7), although it is important to note that these injuries tend to exhibit delayed healing compared to wounds of other etiologies.[26]

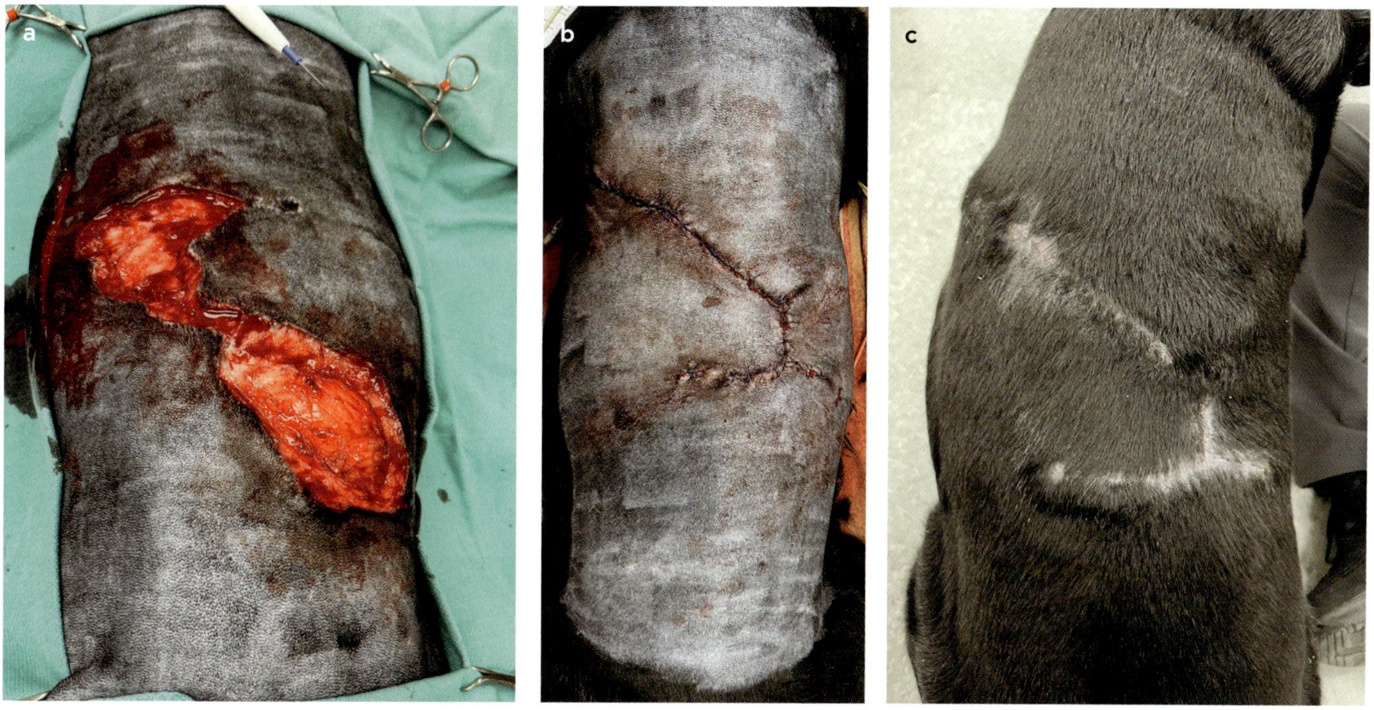

Figure 8.7 Burn wound caused by a heated operating table, (a) immediately after escharotomy, (b) following three-layer closure and use of walking sutures, (c) and 3 weeks after closure.

KEEP IN MIND

- It is important to assess the whole patient. More pressing pathologies (e.g., dyspnea, hypovolemia, burn shock) should not be overlooked for the sake of wound management.
- Burn wounds may not be evident at the time of initial evaluation and may continue to declare themselves for up to a week after injury. In some cases, subsequent episodes of debridement or prolonged therapy duration may be required.
- Multiple sources of pain are present in patients suffering from burn wounds, and all of them should be considered so as to provide appropriate analgesia.
- Systemic antimicrobials are frequently not indicated in these patients, unless there is a concern for sepsis or infection of the wound bed.
- As the wound progresses over time, the requirements for bandage change frequency and type of primary dressing will also evolve. It is important to continually assess the wound and remain dynamic in order to treat the patient appropriately.

References

1. Friedstat J, Brown DA, Levi B. Chemical, electrical, and radiation injuries. *Clin Plast Surg*. 2017; 44(3):657–669.
2. Gross TL, Ihrke PJ, Walder EJ, Affolter VK (eds.). Necrotizing diseases of the epidermis. In: *Skin Diseases of the Dog and Cat*, 2nd ed. John Wiley & Sons; 2005. pp. 75–104.
3. Miller WH, Griffin CE, Campbell KL (eds.). Environmental skin disease. In: *Muller and Kirk's Small Animal Dermatology*, 7th ed. Philadelphia, PA: Saunders; 2012. pp. 659–685.
4. American Burn Association. *Advanced Burn Life Support Course, Provider Manual 2018 Update*. 2018. Available at https://ameriburn.org/wp-content/uploads/2019/08/2018-abls-providermanual.pdf.
5. Vaughn L, Beckel N. Severe burn injury, burn shock, and smoke inhalation injury in small animals. Part 1: Burn classification and pathophysiology. *J Vet Emerg Crit Care (San Antonio)*. 2012; 22(2):179–186.
6. Johnson RM, Richard R. Partial-thickness burns: Identification and management. *Adv Skin Wound Care*. 2003; 16(4): 178–187.
7. Vaughn L, Beckel N, Walters P. Severe burn injury, burn shock, and smoke inhalation injury in small animals. Part 2: Diagnosis, therapy, complications, and prognosis. *J Vet Emerg Crit Care (San Antonio)*. 2012; 22(2):187–200.
8. Moore RA, Waheed A, Burns B. Rule of nines. 2022. In: *StatPearls* [Internet]. Treasure Island, FL: StatPearls Publishing; 2023.
9. Henriksson A et al. Body mapping chart for estimation of percentage of body surface area in mesocephalic dogs. *J Vet Emerg Crit Care (San Antonio)*. 2022; 32(3):350–355.
10. Malic CC, Karoo RO, Austin O, Phipps A. Resuscitation burn card—A useful tool for burn injury assessment. *Burns*. 2007; 33(2):195–199.
11. Bohling MW. Burns. In: Johnston SA, Tobias KM (eds.). *Veterinary Surgery: Small Animal Expert Consult*, 2nd ed. Philadelphia, PA: Saunders; 2017. pp. 1495–1507.
12. Hargis AM, Lewis TP. Full-thickness cutaneous burn in black-haired skin on the dorsum of the body of a Dalmatian puppy. *Vet Dermatol*. 1999; 10(1):39–42.
13. Sumner JP, Pucheu-Haston CM, Fowlkes N, Merchant S. Dorsal skin necrosis secondary to a solar-induced thermal burn in a brown-coated dachshund. *Can Vet J*. 2016; 57(3):305–308.
14. Pavletic MM, Trout NJ. Bullet, bite, and burn wounds in dogs and cats. *Vet Clin North Am Small Anim Pract*. 2006; 36(4):873–893.
15. Ashbaugh EA, Mazzaferro EM, McKiernan BC, Drobatz KJ. The association of physical examination abnormalities and carboxyhemoglobin concentrations in 21 dogs trapped in a kennel fire. *J Vet Emerg Crit Care (San Antonio)*. 2012; 22(3): 361–367.
16. Hall JE. Transport of oxygen and carbon dioxide in blood and tissue fluids. In: *Guyton and Hall Textbook of Medical Physiology*, 13th ed. Amsterdam: Elsevier; 2015. pp. 527–537.
17. Drobatz KJ, Walker LM, Hendricks JC. Smoke exposure in dogs: 27 cases (1988–1997). *J Am Vet Med Assoc*. 1999; 215(9):1306–1311.
18. Berent AC, Todd J, Sergeeff J, Powell LL. Carbon monoxide toxicity: A case series. *J Vet Emerg Crit Care*. 2005; 15(2): 128–135.
19. Cuttle L et al. The optimal temperature of first aid treatment for partial thickness burn injuries. *Wound Repair Regen*. 2008; 16(5):626–634.
20. Cuttle L, Pearn J, McMillan JR, Kimble RM. A review of first aid treatments for burn injuries. *Burns*. 2009; 35(6):768–775.
21. Tricklebank S. Modern trends in fluid therapy for burns. *Burns*. 2009; 35(6):757–767.
22. Saffle JI. The phenomenon of "fluid creep" in acute burn resuscitation. *J Burn Care Res*. 2007; 28(3):382–395.
23. Montgomery RK. Pain management in burn injury. *Crit Care Nurs Clin North Am*. 2004; 16(1):39–49.
24. Honari S. Topical therapies and antimicrobials in the management of burn wounds. *Crit Care Nurs Clin North Am*. 2004; 16(1):1–11.
25. Vigani A, Culler CA. Systemic and local management of burn wounds. *Vet Clin North Am Small Anim Pract*. 2017; 47(6):1149–1163.
26. Nissen NN, Gamelli RL, Polverini PJ, DiPietro LA. Differential angiogenic and proliferative activity of surgical and burn wound fluids. *J Trauma*. 2003; 54(6):1205–1210.

Chapter 9

Penetrating injuries

Marie Burneko, David E. Holt

Penetrating injuries caused by projectiles (e.g., bullets, arrows), knives, and sticks can cause immediate, life-threatening injuries. Other penetrating injuries, such as those caused by porcupine quills and grass seeds, can have more insidious clinical presentations but are no less challenging to manage successfully.

In patients with this type of injury, many body systems may be affected. The initial evaluation of acute cases focuses on the management of the central nervous, respiratory, and cardiovascular systems and on the elimination of immediate threats to life. This may involve intubation and assisted ventilation if the patient is stuporous or comatose, restoring negative intrapleural pressure in cases of pneumo- or hemothorax, and appropriate intravenous resuscitation in cases of severe hemorrhage. The goal of initial treatment is maintaining oxygen delivery to the tissues. Careful reevaluation and imaging, often using several modalities, are required for an accurate diagnosis and appropriate surgical treatment planning. The surgical approach and procedure are dictated by the body systems affected and the nature and severity of the injuries. Careful, often intensive, postoperative monitoring is required in cases with major injuries.

Gunshot wounds

Clinical presentation

Gunshot wounds are relatively uncommon in veterinary medicine, representing 0.76% of hospital admissions in one study.[1] Male dogs are more commonly affected than female dogs, which may be due to the influence of sex hormones on roaming behaviors.[1,2]

The presentation of a gunshot wound depends on the type of projectile, the velocity of the projectile, and the tissue the projectile encounters.[3] High-velocity projectiles, such as those shot from rifles and shotguns, create cavitation on contact with body tissues. Shock waves are generated that travel ahead of the projectile tract; this can result in damage to tissues that are not directly affected by the projectile.[4]

Many cases of acute gunshot injury have a favorable prognosis, with survival rates ranging from 79% to 86%.[1,2] This prognosis is worse in military working dogs, with a survival rate of 38% in one study; these injuries were mostly caused by high-velocity weapons. Thoracic gunshot wounds may be associated with an increase in mortality rate when compared to wounds in other locations.[5] The abdominal region seems to be the most common location of gunshot injury in both cats and dogs.[1,6]

Fractures can occur secondary to gunshot injury, with reports suggesting that 20%–40% of gunshot wounds are associated with a fracture of any bone.[1,6,7] The most common fractures associated with gunshot injuries are those affecting long bones, followed by maxillofacial and vertebral column fractures. These fractures may carry a poor prognosis, especially if there is extensive soft tissue injury present at the location of the fracture.[7]

Diagnosis and treatment

Many gunshot injuries are incidental diagnoses, with evidence of metallic projectiles seen on radiographs. A small number of animals present with acute traumatic gunshot injuries.[1,2,7] The head, neck, and chest are the most vulnerable regions, with fatality potentially occurring quickly, especially in cases of high-velocity projectiles.[5] Wounds present on both sides of the body may represent entry and exit points and should prompt suspicion of a projectile injury. Thoracic, abdominal, and appendicular skeletal radiographs can be helpful to diagnose acute projectile injury if the projectile is still present. In addition, radiographs or focused ultrasound may be useful to diagnose sequelae of projectile injury, such as hemothorax, pneumothorax, hemoabdomen, and septic abdomen. More advanced imaging, such as computed tomography (CT), may be useful when multiple body cavities and organ systems are affected.

As in most penetrating wounds, treatment of gunshot wounds depends on their location and body systems affected. Incidentally found thoracic or abdominal projectiles should not be removed routinely if there are no clinical signs associated with the projectile, as it may be impossible to know the timing of the injury.[1] However, surgical intervention should be recommended in cases of acute penetrating abdominal wounds, thoracic penetrating wounds, and limb injuries requiring internal fixation.[2,4,7]

Impalement injuries

Clinical presentation

Impalement is defined in the Oxford English Dictionary as "piercing or transfixation with a sharp instrument." In small animal medicine, it usually results from running or falling onto a sharp object. In dogs, impalement injuries usually involve the head, neck, or cranial thorax as a result of running into a stationary object. Most commonly, these injuries involve the oropharynx and thoracic cavity and are caused by wooden objects.[8,9] Running with a stick in the mouth can result in oropharyngeal penetration if the end of the stick hits the ground.[8] Impalement with other objects, such as metal rebar or fencing, can also occur, usually after falling from a height onto the object (Fig. 9.1). This has also been reported in several cats with high-rise syndrome.[10] Both of these types of impalement injuries are categorized as type I impalement injuries, in which the animal is moving and the object is not. A type II impalement injury involves a stationary patient and a moving pointed instrument; for example, a stab wound.[11]

Sticks and other wooden foreign bodies most commonly affect dogs in the head and neck regions, with the oropharyngeal location being the most common in cases of wooden foreign body impalement.[12] These dogs typically have a history of stick chewing or trauma associated with a stick or other wooden objects.[8] The presentation of these animals can be acute or chronic. Chronic cases may show abscessation, nasal or ocular discharge, cellulitis/swelling, and/or draining tracts.[13,14] In one report of 50 dogs with penetrating oropharyngeal foreign bodies, 82% presented with chronic signs.[13] Clinical signs of acute penetrating oropharyngeal foreign bodies include dysphagia, oral pain, drooling, dyspnea, and cervical swelling. The most common site of penetration into the oropharynx is sublingual; in these cases, however, the entry wound may not be visible, especially if it is chronic or if the object has been removed. Esophageal perforation, most often in the dorsal wall of the proximal esophagus, may have a more guarded prognosis based on a limited number of cases.[12,13]

Infection is an important component of impalement injury secondary to wooden objects. These wounds

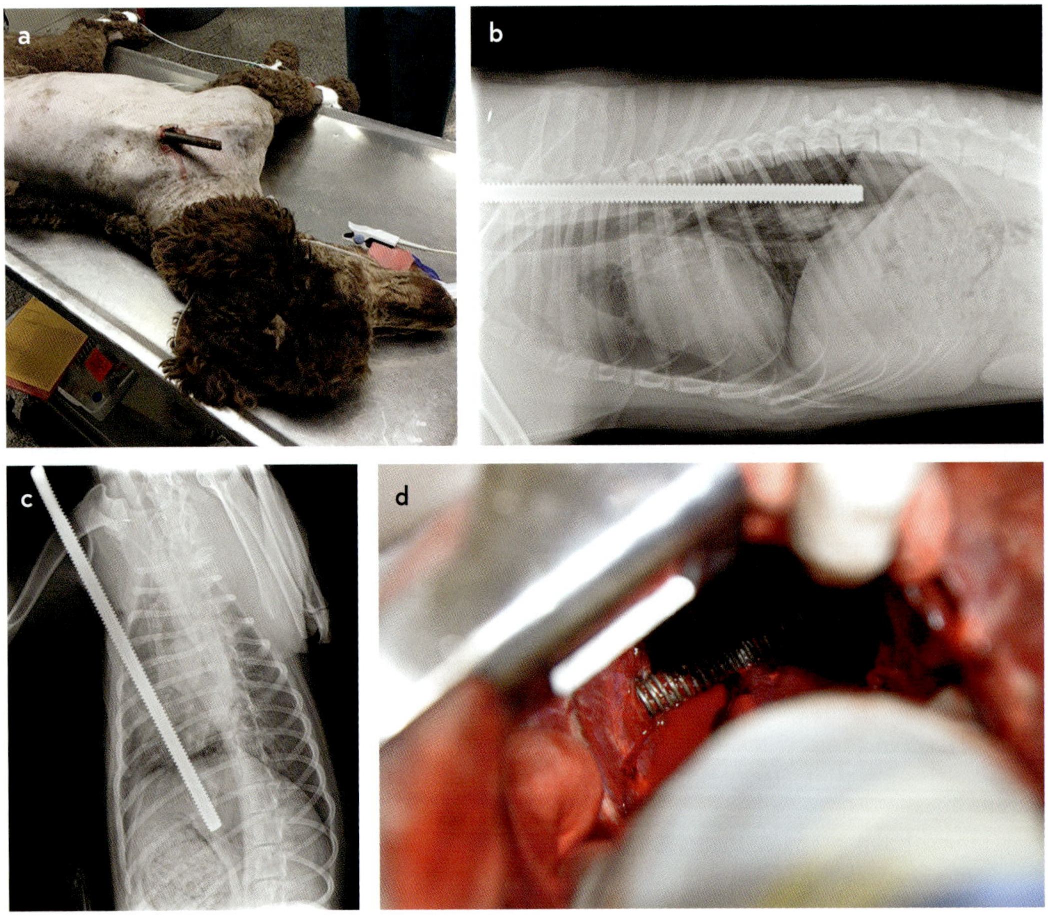

Figure 9.1 (a) Thoracic penetration by a threaded metal rod. (b) Lateral and (c) ventrodorsal thoracic radiographs showing the path of the metal rod. (d) Intraoperative view of the metal rod entering the thorax between the ribs. A median sternotomy was performed to explore the thoracic cavity.

are commonly associated with positive cultures on surgical exploration, with *Escherichia coli* and *Staphylococcus* species being the most frequently cultured organisms.[9]

Diagnosis and treatment

Cervical and thoracic radiography is recommended in all cases of acute oropharyngeal stick injury; performing additional imaging modalities may be prudent to determine the location of the foreign material and the impalement tract. Subcutaneous emphysema, pneumothorax, and pneumomediastinum are common radiographic findings but are not associated with the outcome (Fig. 9.2a).[12]

A thorough oral examination is performed under general anesthesia and intubation is done in cases of suspected oropharyngeal stick injury. Rigid and flexible endoscopy are useful to evaluate the esophagus and the tract created by the impalement.[15]

CT is a very useful diagnostic tool in impalement cases. It has a sensitivity of 64%–79% and a specificity of 88%–93% for detection of penetrating wooden objects in impalement cases.[15,16] CT may also better detect organ damage or inflammation of body cavities secondary to impalement than plain radiographs. Magnetic resonance imaging (MRI) has been reported to be useful in chronic oropharyngeal penetrating injuries, and wooden foreign bodies were visualized in most cases in one report.[17] Cervical ultrasound may also be beneficial in the diagnosis of chronic wooden oropharyngeal foreign bodies.[18] Endoscopy is both a diagnostic and treatment option in dogs with acute oropharyngeal stick injuries. The endoscope is passed through the mouth and penetrating wound, the stick fragments are located and removed, and the tract is evaluated for devitalized tissue and flushed (Fig. 9.2b,c).[15]

Surgery is recommended if there is substantial tissue damage or when endoscopy is not available. The impalement tract is explored and cultured, foreign material removed, damage to deeper structures/organs repaired, and the surgical field lavaged to reduce contamination. The object causing the injury should not be removed until the patient is stable and ideally anesthetized and prepared for surgical exploration.[11] Typically, a ventral midline cervical approach can be used to access the retropharyngeal and cervical tissues and treat most oropharyngeal penetrating wounds. A transoral approach may be necessary if the rostral pharynx is affected. Other approaches, including sternotomy, lateral thoracotomy, and celiotomy can be considered based on the clinical signs, wound appearance, and diagnostic imaging findings. Broad-spectrum antibiotics with coverage against *E. coli* and *Staphylococcus* spp. are administered pending the results of culture and sensitivity testing on specimens obtained during surgery.

Porcupine quills

Porcupines are native to forests in Northern America and Canada, and encounters with dogs often result in quilling.[19] Quills detach on contact, and the backward-facing barbs on their tips anchor the quills in the tissues and facilitate deeper tissue migration.[20] Most dogs are quilled in multiple locations, with the most common sites being the oral cavity, head, and neck. Because of the obvious nature of the injury, most dogs are presented to veterinarians promptly for quill removal. Dogs presented more than 24 hours after quill injury are more

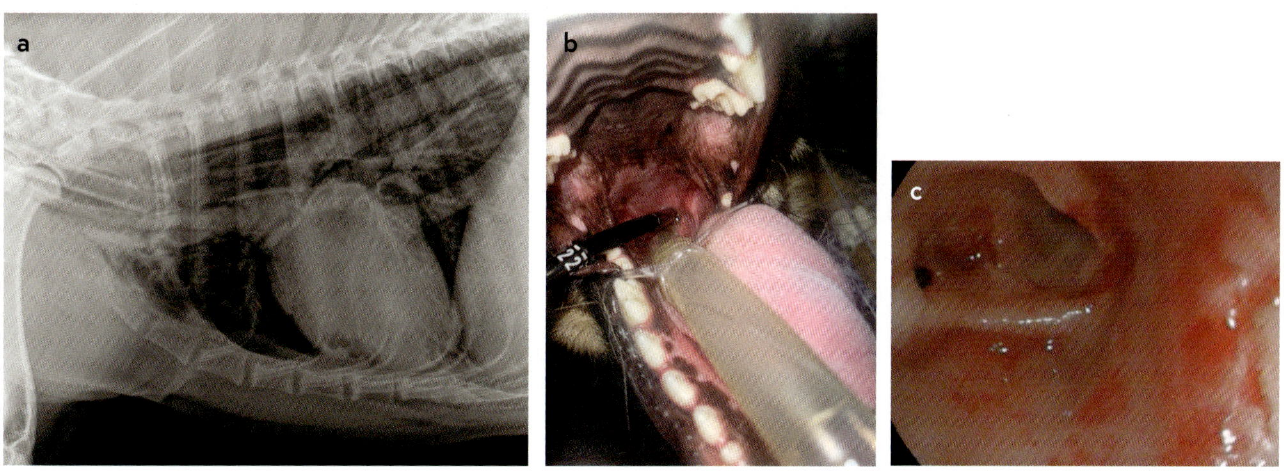

Figure 9.2 (a) Lateral cervical and thoracic radiograph of a dog presented 5 days after oral stick impalement. Note the presence of air in the cervical tissue planes and the pneumomediastinum. (b) Passage of a flexible fiberoptic endoscope into the pharyngeal perforation. (c) Endoscopic view of the tract created by the stick perforation. No residual foreign material was found. The tract was thoroughly flushed with sterile saline.

likely to develop complications, including subcutaneous abscess formation.[19] As such, owners should be advised to have quilled dogs evaluated and treated as soon as possible after injury. Dogs should be monitored carefully after quill removal. Clinical signs of complications, including pneumothorax, develop over a variable period (days to months) after the initial injury.

Clinical presentation

Any quills that break off or are not removed can migrate; reported sites of quill migration include the lungs, mediastinum, heart (Fig. 9.3), eyes, joints, brain, vertebral canal, and soft tissues of the neck and thorax.[21–27] In addition, the authors have seen migration into the abdominal cavity and multiple abdominal organs. Clinical signs will vary depending on the location of the quills. Dogs with thoracic migration and pneumothorax show signs of restlessness, tachypnea, and respiratory distress.[21] Migration into the brain or spinal cord may manifest as depression, weakness, ataxia, changes in cranial nerve reflexes and proprioception, and pain on manipulation of the affected area of the spinal cord.[25,26] Dogs with ocular or periocular quills may exhibit exophthalmos, buphthalmos, periocular swelling, and prolapse of the third eyelid.[27,28] Dogs with migration into or around joints may have intermittent, variable degrees of lameness.

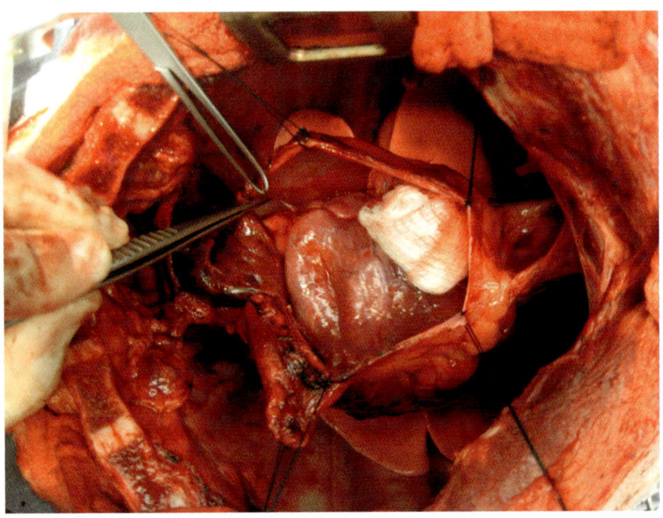

Figure 9.3 Intraoperative view from a median sternotomy showing a porcupine quill at the end of the forceps embedded in the heart.

Diagnosis and treatment

A diagnosis of penetrating porcupine quill migration should be strongly suspected from the history and clinical signs. After initial patient stabilization, imaging is indicated to locate areas of likely quill migration.

A thoracic or abdominal focused assessment with sonography for trauma (TFAST or AFAST) may be used to determine the presence of a pneumothorax or peritoneal fluid, respectively, at initial presentation. Thoracic radiography is a valuable means of diagnosing pneumothorax, but quills will likely not be apparent on radiographs. Ultrasound, CT, MRI, echocardiography, and rhinoscopy have also been used to diagnose quill location.[22–32]

Although advanced imaging may not identify quills, it may indicate areas of tissue damage, determining possible quill location. Even if some quills are visualized with imaging, reports suggest that there are many more that are not, so a complete exploration of the affected area or body cavity must be performed.[21–23] Careful palpation and intraoperative ultrasound may be useful to identify quill location.[31]

Surgical treatment is required, once a diagnosis is made, to prevent further quill migration and organ damage. Although conservative treatment of penetrating quill injury has been reported sporadically, pneumothorax requires complete thoracic exploration, including evaluation of all lung lobes, mediastinum, pericardium, and heart.

Surgical technique

The surgical approach, procedure, and techniques required will depend on the location of the porcupine quills. In cases of pneumothorax, a median sternotomy is performed, allowing complete exploration of each hemithorax, evaluation of all lung lobes, and visualization of the heart and mediastinum.

1. Each lung lobe is carefully evaluated and palpated.
   a. If the quills are protruding from the lung lobes, they can be removed by gentle traction.
   b. The lungs are then leak tested by submerging them in saline during positive-pressure ventilation.
   c. In cases of air leakage, or when the quills are completely within the lung parenchyma, partial or complete lung lobectomy using a surgical stapling device is necessary.
2. The cranial and caudal mediastinum is opened and completely explored.
   a. The pericardium is opened, and stay sutures are placed to create a pericardial basket, allowing for evaluation of the heart.
   a. Quills can be pulled from the myocardium without sutures; however, the use of preplaced mattress sutures with pledgets minimizes the chance of serious hemorrhage.

A similar approach should be taken if clinical signs and diagnostic imaging suggest that quills have penetrated the abdominal cavity, and an exploratory laparotomy should be performed. The authors have removed quills from the liver, pancreas, spleen, and kidney without the need for sutures, but these may be necessary if hemorrhage occurs.

Grass awns

Clinical presentation and diagnosis

Penetrating trauma from grass awns is more insidious than trauma from porcupine quills (see above), as there is often no history to tie the clinical presentation to an underlying cause. Grass awns commonly penetrate the interdigital skin or lodge in the ear canal;[33] however, they can also be inhaled and penetrate the lung, or ingested and penetrate the gastrointestinal tract.[34,35]

Like porcupine quills, grass awns have backward-pointing barbs that promote migration. Grass awn penetration and migration has been associated with pneumothorax, pericarditis, central nervous system (CNS) and soft tissue abscesses, and peritonitis.[34-37] The clinical signs, initial treatment, diagnostic imaging, and surgical techniques in these cases are similar to those described for migrating porcupine quills. The grass awn may or may not be visible on CT scans; however, CT will help identify areas of secondary tissue damage or abscessation and guide surgical planning.[36,38]

A characteristic presentation is associated with grass awns that are inhaled, migrate from the bronchi through the lung and diaphragm, and then lodge in the epaxial muscles. The associated abscess may involve the lumbar vertebrae and often results in a draining tract on the flank. Whilst some more superficial awn-associated abscesses may be amenable to foreign body removal using a clamp through the draining tract under ultrasound guidance, awns located in the hypaxial muscles require an exploratory laparotomy.[39,40] Intraoperative ultrasound is particularly useful for locating the abscess pocket and foreign body.[40]

Penetrating wounds: Treatment, Postoperative management, Outcome

Treatment

In general, the first goal of penetrating wound treatment in small animals is to eliminate immediate threats to life. Penetrating injury to any component of the CNS carries a grave prognosis,[8] and patients with these injuries that present with CNS deficits should be intubated and placed on a ventilator, and given medications to decrease brain swelling, including mannitol or hypertonic saline. Patients may also present with respiratory distress secondary to a thoracic or neck injury. Again, these patients may need to be intubated and ventilated. TFAST can help to quickly diagnose pleural effusion, pneumothorax, and pulmonary contusions. If the respiratory distress is secondary to an intrathoracic injury, thoracocentesis and/or chest tube placement may be necessary. Penetrating thoracic wounds should be covered after evacuation of fluid and/or air from the chest. All potentially penetrating thoracic wounds should be explored to evaluate for deeper tissue and organ damage (Fig. 9.1).

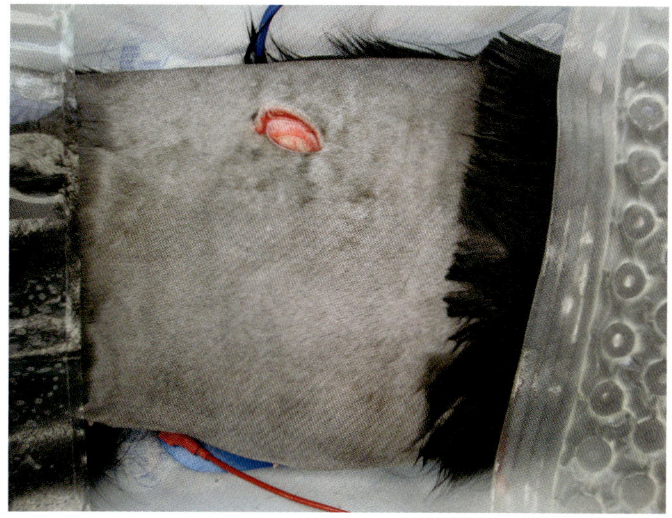

Figure 9.4 Knife wound to the right paracostal area of a cat. Image courtesy Lillian Aronson.

Neck wounds causing respiratory distress should be treated urgently. Ideally, an endotracheal tube should be placed to protect the patient's airway prior to further diagnostics. A temporary tracheostomy may be indicated in these patients after the airway is protected. Wounds to the neck can cause significant hemorrhage if the carotid arteries or jugular veins are lacerated, and they can cause upper airway obstruction secondary to swelling, an object lodged in the upper airways, or laryngeal paralysis if the recurrent laryngeal nerves are damaged.

Penetrating wounds to the abdomen may require urgent stabilization of the patient. AFAST can be helpful to quickly diagnose abdominal effusion, which should increase the index of suspicion for penetration into the abdominal cavity as well as potential organ involvement. Penetrating abdominal wounds should be surgically explored to treat any underlying organ damage and prevent or treat sepsis and control any major hemorrhage (Fig. 9.4). All open wounds should be covered to protect them from contamination prior to surgical exploration.

Surgical technique

Specific surgical techniques to explore penetrating wounds are dependent on the location of the injury.

1. The affected area should be widely clipped to evaluate all potential areas of penetration.
2. The surgeon should be prepared to isolate and temporarily obstruct major vessels that supply the area if there is significant hemorrhage present or anticipated.

3. The penetrating injury tract should be debrided in most cases, and the wound and/or body cavity should be thoroughly lavaged.
   - A tissue culture should also be obtained.
   - A chest drain is applied to manage pneumothorax (in thoracic injury).
4. The closure of penetrating wounds is highly dependent on their presentation, but delayed primary closure or open wound management should be considered for highly contaminated wounds.

Postoperative management

Postoperative management of patients with penetrating wounds is based on maintaining organ and tissue perfusion and maximizing oxygen delivery to tissues. This may include intravascular volume support, such as the use of blood products, isotonic crystalloids, and/or colloidal support. Chest tube management for ongoing pleural effusion or air accumulation is also important in cases of penetrating thoracic wounds. Broad-spectrum antibiotics may be necessary if sepsis is a concern and should be altered based on culture and sensitivity testing.

Systemic inflammatory response syndrome is possible in any critically injured patient, so frequent cardiovascular system monitoring, blood work, and oxygenation status monitoring are vital.

Outcome

The outcome of patients with penetrating wounds is highly variable but is mostly dependent on the type of injury and the ability of the patient to be stabilized. There is a possibility of recurrence of clinical signs with porcupine quills, remaining grass awns, and retained wooden foreign bodies. If there is residual dead or infected tissue in the area of a penetrating wound after surgical exploration, another surgical procedure may be indicated to remove all gross disease.

KEEP IN MIND

- All body systems should be carefully and thoroughly assessed in any patient with a penetrating injury, especially in cases with migrating porcupine quills and grass awns.
- Recurrence of clinical signs is possible, especially in cases with migrating foreign bodies like porcupine quills.
- Outcome is highly variable and depends on the type of injury and overall patient stability.

References

1. Capak H et al. Review of 166 gunshot injury cases in dogs. *Top Companion Anim Med.* 2016; 31(4):146–151.
2. Fullington RJ, Otto CM. Characteristics and management of gunshot wounds in dogs and cats: 84 cases (1986–1995). *J Am Vet Med Assoc.* 1997; 210(5):658–662.
3. Bonath KH, Vannini R, Koch H, Schnettler R. Gunshot wounds—Ballistics, physiopathology, surgical treatment [in German]. *Tierarztl Prax.* 1996; 24(3):304–315.
4. Pavletic MM. A review of 121 gunshot wounds in the dog and cat. *Vet Surg.* 1985; 14:61–63.
5. Baker JL et al. Gunshot wounds in military working dogs in Operation Enduring Freedom and Operation Iraqi Freedom: 29 cases (2003–2009). *J Vet Emerg Crit Care (San Antonio).* 2013; 23(1):47–52.
6. Vnuk D et al. Metal projectile injuries in cats: Review of 65 cases (2012–2014). *J Feline Med Surg.* 2016; 18(8):626–631.
7. Schrock K, Kerwin SC, Jeffery N. Outcomes and complications associated with acute gunshot fractures in cats and dogs. *Vet Comp Orthop Traumatol.* 2022; 35(3):205–212.
8. Pavletic MM. Management of specific wounds. Impalement injuries. In: *Atlas of Small Animal Wound Management and Reconstructive Surgery*, 4th ed. WB Saunders; 2018. pp. 227–228.
9. Matiasovic M et al. Surgical management of impalement injuries to the trunk of dogs: A multicentre retrospective study. *J Small Anim Pract.* 2018; 59(3):139–146.
10. Pratschke KM, Kirby BM. High rise syndrome with impalement in three cats. *J Small Anim Pract.* 2002; 43(6):261–264.
11. Eachempati SR, Barie PS, Reed RL 2nd. Survival after transabdominal impalement from a construction injury: A review of the management of impalement injuries. *J Trauma.* 1999; 47(5):864–866.
12. Doran IP, Wright CA, Moore AH. Acute oropharyngeal and esophageal stick injury in forty-one dogs. *Vet Surg.* 2008; 37(8):781–785.
13. Griffiths LG, Tiruneh R, Sullivan M, Reid SW. Oropharyngeal penetrating injuries in 50 dogs: A retrospective study. *Vet Surg.* 2000; 29(5):383–388.
14. Nicholson I et al. Computed tomography as an aid to management of chronic oropharyngeal stick injury in the dog. *J Small Anim Pract.* 2008; 49(9):451–457.
15. Robinson W, Shales C, White RN. The use of rigid endoscopy in the management of acute oropharyngeal stick injuries. *J Small Anim Pract.* 2014; 55(12):609–614.
16. Lamb CR, Pope EH, Lee KC. Results of computed tomography in dogs with suspected wooden foreign bodies. *Vet Radiol Ultrasound.* 2017; 58(2):144–150.
17. Dobromylskyj MJ, Dennis R, Ladlow JF, Adams VJ. The use of magnetic resonance imaging in the management of pharyngeal penetration injuries in dogs. *J Small Anim Pract.* 2008; 49(2):74–79.
18. Armbrust LJ, Biller DS, Radlinsky MG, Hoskinson JJ. Ultrasonographic diagnosis of foreign bodies associated with chronic draining tracts and abscesses in dogs. *Vet Radiol Ultrasound.* 2003; 44(1):66–70.
19. Johnson MD, Magnusson KD, Shmon CL, Waldner C. Porcupine quill injuries in dogs: A retrospective of 296 cases (1998–2002). *Can Vet J.* 2006; 47(7):677–682.

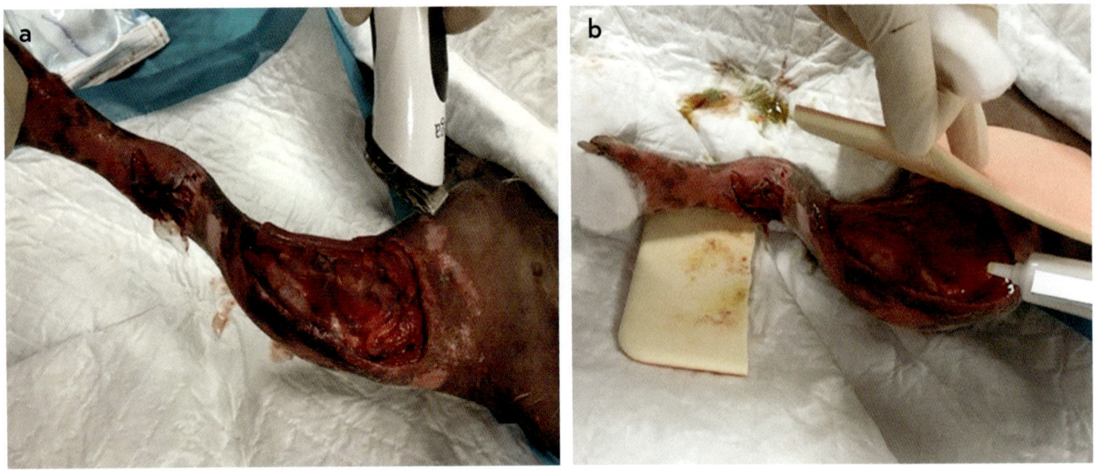

Figure 10.1 (a) Wide clipping of the fur around the wound after protecting the wound bed with a hydrophobic gel. (b) Application of medical-grade honey on the wound and covering with an absorbent, nonadhesive hydrocellular foam dressing.

cuff maintained under 300 mmHg (Fig. 10.2). Pressure must be constant and is independent of needle size.[10]

6. All the necrotic tissue is debrided and removed using a number 11 scalpel blade and/or Metzenbaum scissors. If tissue viability is questionable, reassessment should be performed on the following day (necrosis appears 1–8 days after trauma).
7. At this point samples can be taken for bacterial culture and sensitivity testing.
8. Several debridement interventions may be required to achieve a clean/healthy wound bed in patients with highly contaminated wounds.
9. In case of bone exposure, forage into the medullary canal can be considered to improve the vascular supply to the wound bed. The appropriate Kirschner wire or drill bit size should be selected to prevent inadvertent bone fractures.[11]
10. If there is excessive skin tension, sutures should not be placed. In these cases the wound is left open and wound reconstruction should be considered at a later stage, once infection subsides.
11. The correct selection and use of topical agents are essential for wound healing; using an inappropriate agent or duration can be detrimental.
    - Enzymatic options: collagenase, trypsin (rarely used in veterinary medicine).

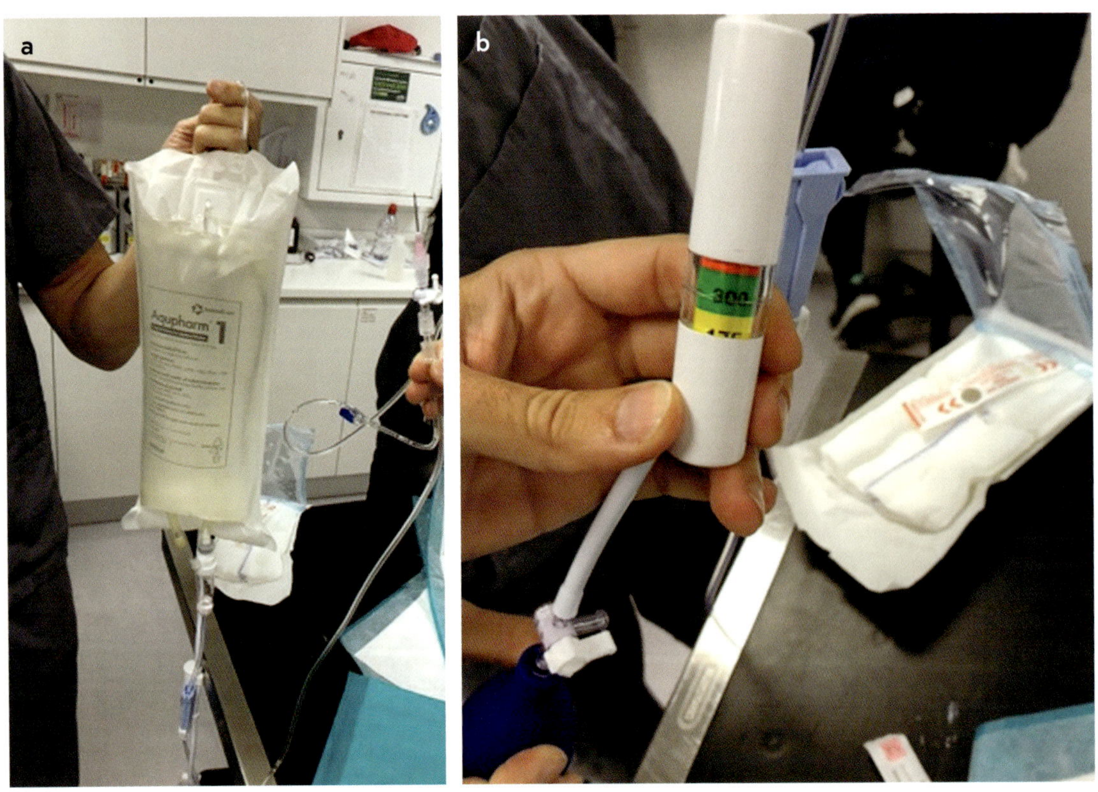

Figure 10.2 Fluid system set up to achieve an irrigation pressure of 7–8 psi. (a) Note the 1 L fluid bag, (b) with a pressure cuff set at 300 mmHg.

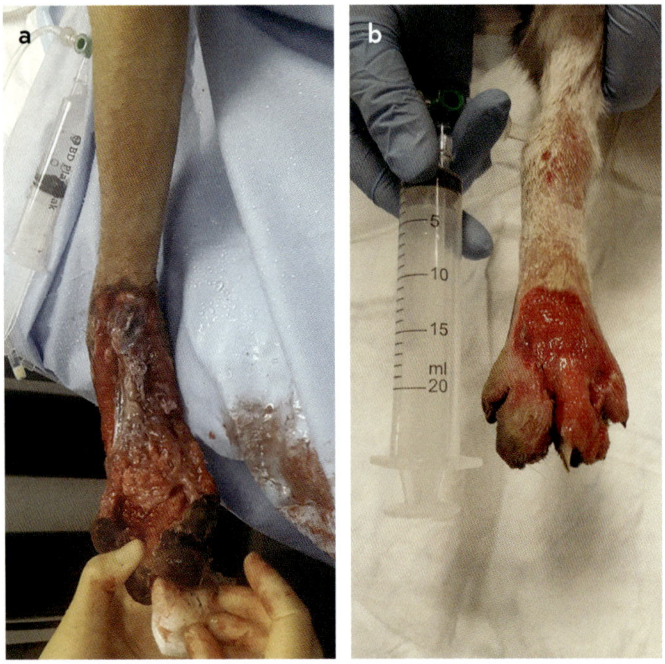

Figure 10.5 Distal degloving/shearing injuries.

Video 10.1. Treatment of a distal hind limb shearing injury in a cat.

Postoperative management

After initial wound care, protecting the wound is indicated to prevent further contamination and reduce damage to healthy tissue. Wound healing comprises three main overlapping phases: the inflammatory phase, the proliferative phase, and the maturation phase.[4] A comprehensive understanding of wound healing physiology is fundamental to adapt the treatment plan accordingly. During the inflammatory phase, the wound should be monitored on a daily basis or every other day depending on the amount of exudate and tissue damage present. As the proliferative phase takes over, the frequency of bandage changes can be decreased. Broad-spectrum antibiotics, such as cephalosporins, effective against potential contaminants (e.g., coagulase-positive staphylococci, *Escherichia coli*, and *Pasteurella* species) should be initiated while awaiting bacterial culture and sensitivity results.[1] During the proliferative phase, angiogenesis occurs, and fibroblasts migrate into the wound so that granulation tissue starts to form. When the wound bed is fully covered with granulation tissue, antibiotic administration can be discontinued. The decision to allow the wound to heal by second intention or opt for surgical reconstruction depends on owner (e.g., commitment, finances), patient (e.g., behavior, concurrent illness), and surgeon (e.g., experience, facilities) factors. Orthopedic injuries requiring internal fixation can be addressed once the soft tissues have healed enough to cover the implants, mitigating the risk of infection.

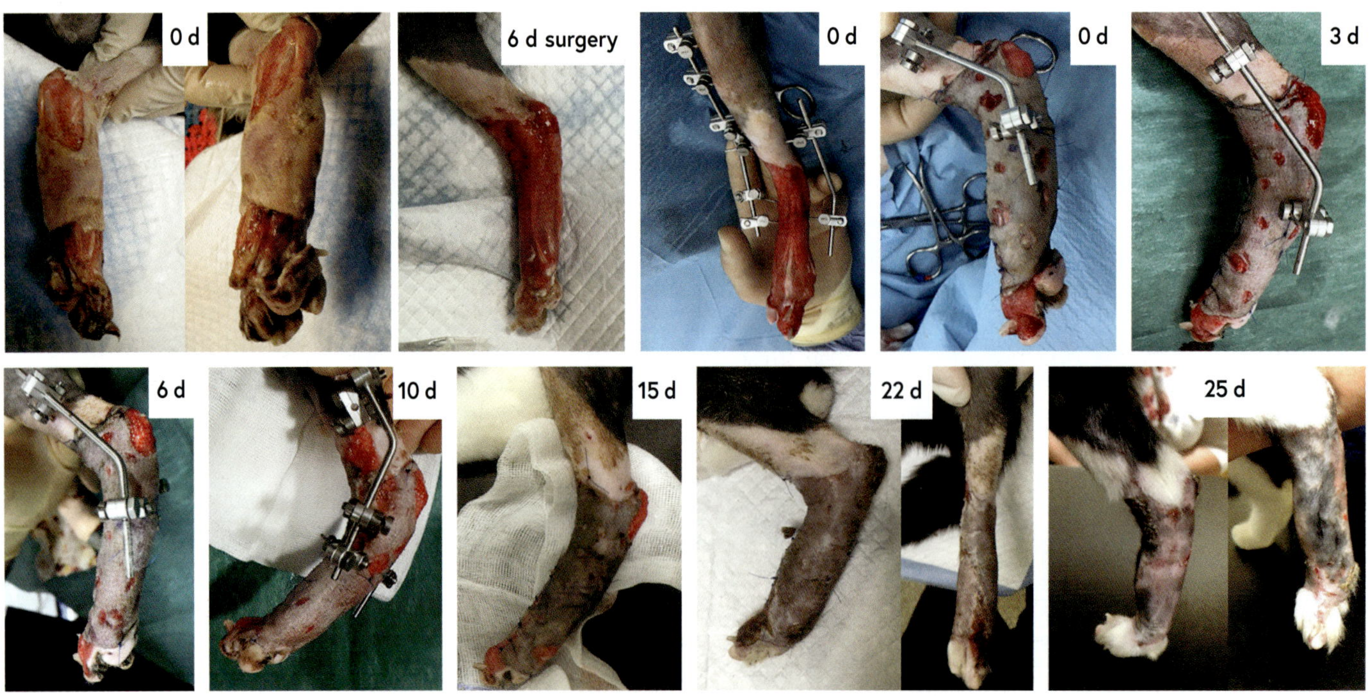

Figure 10.6 Treatment of a distal hind limb degloving injury 6 days after trauma using a free skin mesh graft and transarticular external skeletal fixation.

References

1. Corr S. Intensive, extensive, expensive. Management of distal limb shearing injuries in cats. *J Feline Med Surg.* 2009; 11(9):747–757.
2. Benson JA, Boudrieau RJ. Severe carpal and tarsal shearing injuries treated with an immediate arthrodesis in seven dogs. *J Am Anim Hosp Assoc.* 2002; 38(4):370–380.
3. Diviti S et al. Morel-Lavallee lesions—Review of pathophysiology, clinical findings, imaging findings and management. *J Clin Diagn Res.* 2017; 11(4):TE01–TE04.
4. Hosgood G. Open wounds. In: Tobias K, Johnston S. *Veterinary Surgery: Small Animal.* St. Louis, MO: Elsevier; 2017. pp. 1410–1421.
5. Beardsley SL, Schrader SC. Treatment of dogs with wounds of the limbs caused by shearing forces: 98 cases (1975–1993). *J Am Vet Med Assoc.* 1995; 207(8):1071–1075.
6. Diamond DW, Besso J, Boudrieau RJ. Evaluation of joint stabilization for treatment of shearing injuries of the tarsus in 20 dogs. *J Am Anim Hosp Assoc.* 1999; 35(2):147–153.
7. Harasen GL. Tarsal shearing injuries in the dog. *Can Vet J.* 2000; 41(12):940–943.
8. Moscati RM et al. A multicenter comparison of tap water versus sterile saline for wound irrigation. *Acad Emerg Med.* 2007; 14(5):404–409.
9. Williams JM. Open wound management. In: Fowler D, Williams J (eds.). *BSAVA Manual of Canine and Feline Wound Management and Reconstruction.* Gloucester, UK: BSAVA; 1999. pp. 37–46.
10. Gall TT, Monnet E. Evaluation of fluid pressures of common wound-flushing techniques. *Am J Vet Res.* 2010; 71(11):1384–1386.
11. Clark GN. Bone perforation to enhance wound healing over exposed bone in dogs with shearing injuries. *J Am Anim Hosp Assoc.* 2001; 37(3):215–217.

- Grasping the sialocele with Allis tissue forceps and incising/excising it with Metzenbaum scissors (Video 11.2).

2. Emergency temporary tracheostomy (see Chapter 21).

After stabilization of the patient:

1. Marsupialization:
   a. The sialocele wall is incised and the accumulated fluid removed using suction.
   b. The redundant tissue from the sialocele is resected.
   c. Multiple simple interrupted sutures (3-0 to 4-0 absorbable monofilament) are placed between the remnant wall of the sialocele and the oral mucosa (Fig. 11.2).
2. Sublingual and mandibular sialoadenectomy (ventral approach) (Videos 11.3 and 11.4):
   a. The patient is positioned in dorsal recumbency and a large area is aseptically prepared, from the midcervical region to the most rostral portion of the ventral mandible.

Video 11.2. Patient with respiratory distress. Oral endoscopic examination and identification of an obstructive pharyngeal sialocele. Decompression was performed by excision of the redundant tissue while grasping the sialocele. Video courtesy of Matteo Gobbetti.

Video 11.3. Sublingual and mandibular sialoadenectomy using a tunneling technique. Video courtesy of Matteo Gobbetti.

Video 11.4. Sublingual and mandibular sialoadenectomy using a tunneling technique in a toy-breed dog.

   b. A skin incision is made on the affected side, starting 4–5 cm caudal to the mandibular ramus and extending rostrally toward the mandibular symphysis. Bilateral gland removal requires a midline incision.
   c. The large inflammatory pseudocapsule can be bluntly dissected or incised to provide drainage. It can be partially or totally excised.
   d. After incising the platysma muscle, the external jugular bifurcation should be identified. The mandibular gland is located at or just cranial to this bifurcation.
   e. The capsule of the gland is exposed via blunt dissection and incised. The gland–duct complex (mandibular–sublingual) is then bluntly dissected.

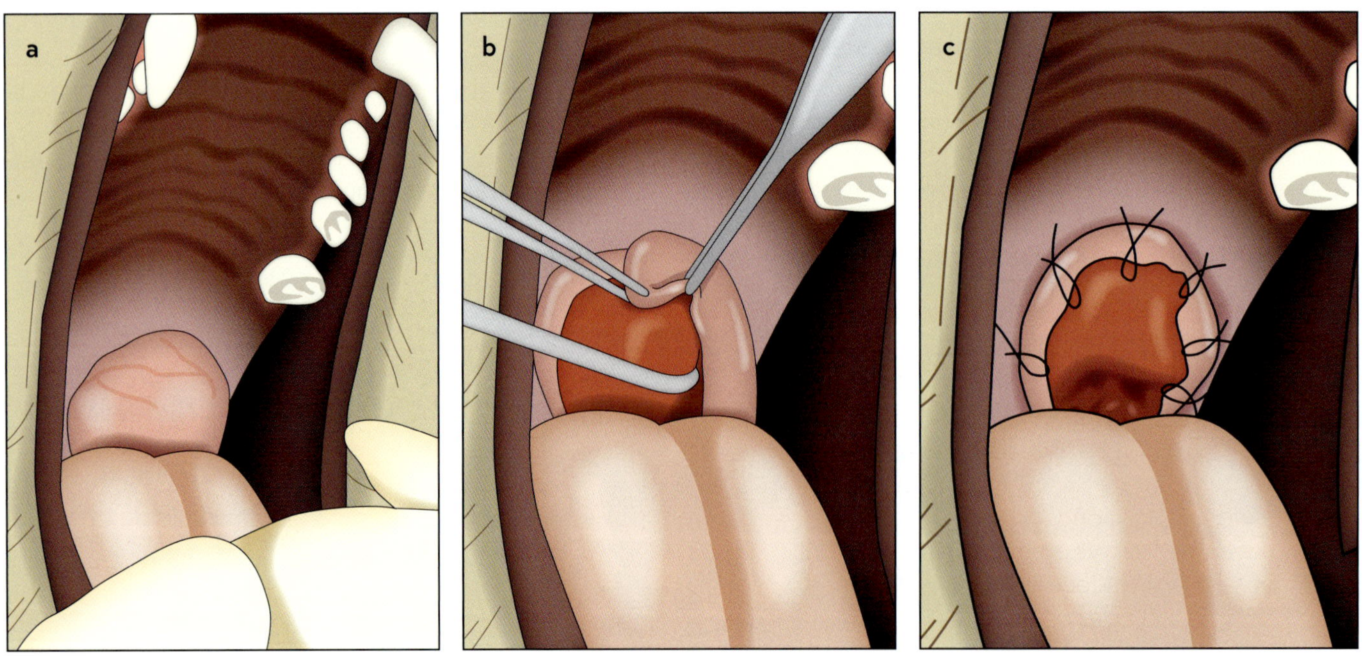

Figure 11.2 Pharyngeal sialocele marsupialization. (a) Airway obstruction due to the pharyngeal sialocele is present on oral examination. (b) Grasping the sialocele with tissue forceps and incising/excising it with Metzenbaum scissors. (c) Multiple simple interrupted sutures are placed between the remnant wall of the sialocele and the oral mucosa.

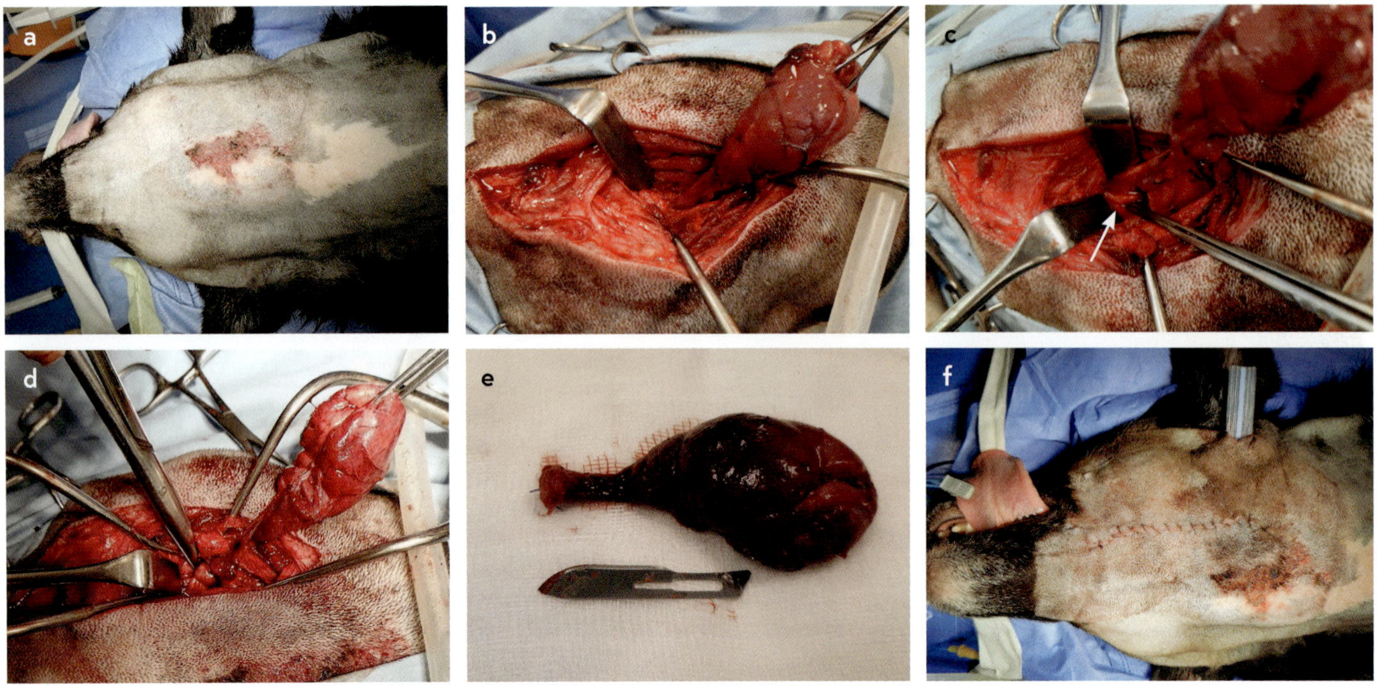

Figure 11.4 Sublingual and mandibular sialoadenectomy without tunneling technique. (a) Ventral approach. (b) Blunt dissection of the gland–duct complex. (c) Using handle retractors, rostral traction is applied to the digastricus muscle for identification of the lingual nerve (white arrow). (d) The salivary duct is ligated as rostral as possible, close to lingual nerve. (e) Sublingual and mandibular gland–duct complex after excision. (f) Skin closure and passive drain placement. Cranial is to the left of the images.

Penetrating injuries to the pharynx

Penetrating oropharyngeal injuries associated with carrying, chewing, or retrieving sticks occur frequently in dogs.[7–9] Although wooden sticks are the main cause, fishhooks, needles, bones, and grass awns have also been reported. Medium- to large-breed dogs appear to be affected most often.[7,8] Affected animals present with either acute (<7 days) or chronic (>7 days) disease, which can result in potentially serious events.[7] In one case series, only 12% of dogs were brought to a veterinarian with acute injury, while 82% of dogs presented with chronic disease (clinical signs for 8 days to 11 months).[8]

Clinical presentation and diagnosis

It is useful to divide the patients into acute (<7 days) and chronic (>7 days) as proposed by White and Lane in 1988,[7] because the clinical approach is different. In case of acute penetrating injury, dogs typically exhibit signs of dysphagia, depression, pain on neck flexion, subcutaneous emphysema, oral pain, and drooling of saliva and blood.[7–9] Chronically affected dogs often present with cervical or facial swelling, abscess formation, and discharging sinus tracts in the head and neck. Common sites of penetration include the lateral and dorsal pharyngeal walls, sublingual region, and esophagus. Esophageal penetration has a guarded prognosis for recovery.[7–9]

Radiography and/or computed tomography of the cervical area and thorax are recommended for the initial diagnostic workup. Ultrasound can also be used, especially helpful to identify small foreign material. After induction of anesthesia, inspection of the oropharynx using a laryngoscope and/or endoscope as well as palpation of the neck can help detect abnormalities. Tracheal and esophageal endoscopy is suggested in cases of cervical swelling or radiographic/computed tomographic signs of gas or tissue reaction within the cervical region.[7–9]

Treatment

The type of treatment depends on the chronicity of the lesion. For acute injuries, oral exploration and retrieval of the foreign body through the entry wound are frequently possible (Fig. 11.5).[9] A recent study described successful retrieval of stick foreign bodies in the oropharynx of dogs using rigid endoscopy, with all animals undergoing endoscopic assessment within 2 days of injury.[10] However, cervical surgical exploration is recommended in acute cases if there is radiographic evidence of tissue emphysema.[9] In chronic cases, the wound may not be obvious on transoral pharyngeal examination, and surgical exploration of the retropharyngeal space is warranted through a ventral midline approach (Fig. 11.6).[8,9]

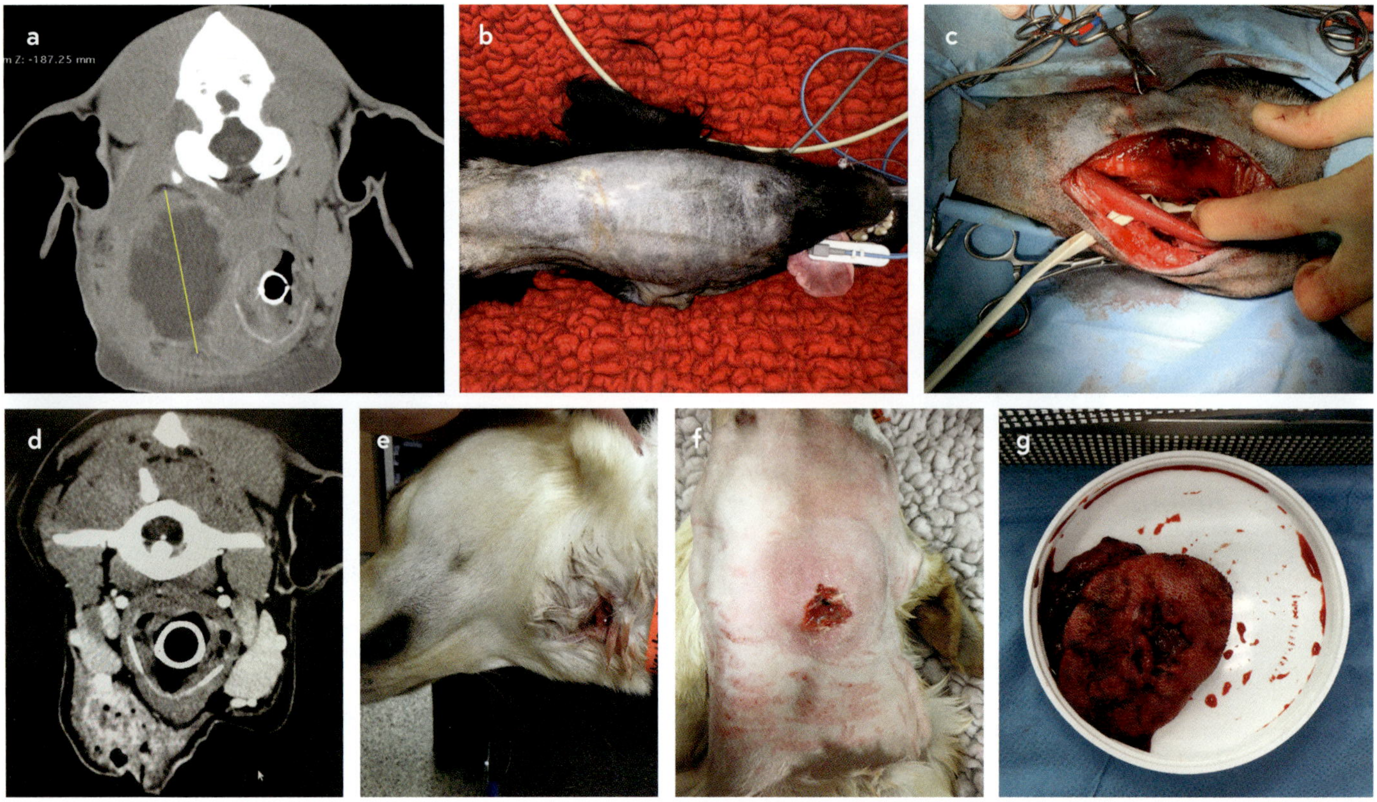

Figure 11.6 Chronic stick injuries. (a–c) First case, with a large, nonmobile, painful swelling on the ventral cervical neck. Computed tomography scan showing a large, chronic, fluid-filled cavity close to the larynx. Ventral approach to the neck, surgical exploration, debridement, and passive drain placement. (d–g) Second case, with a subcutaneous fistula. Computed tomography scan, physical and surgical exploration, and excised tissue after debridement.

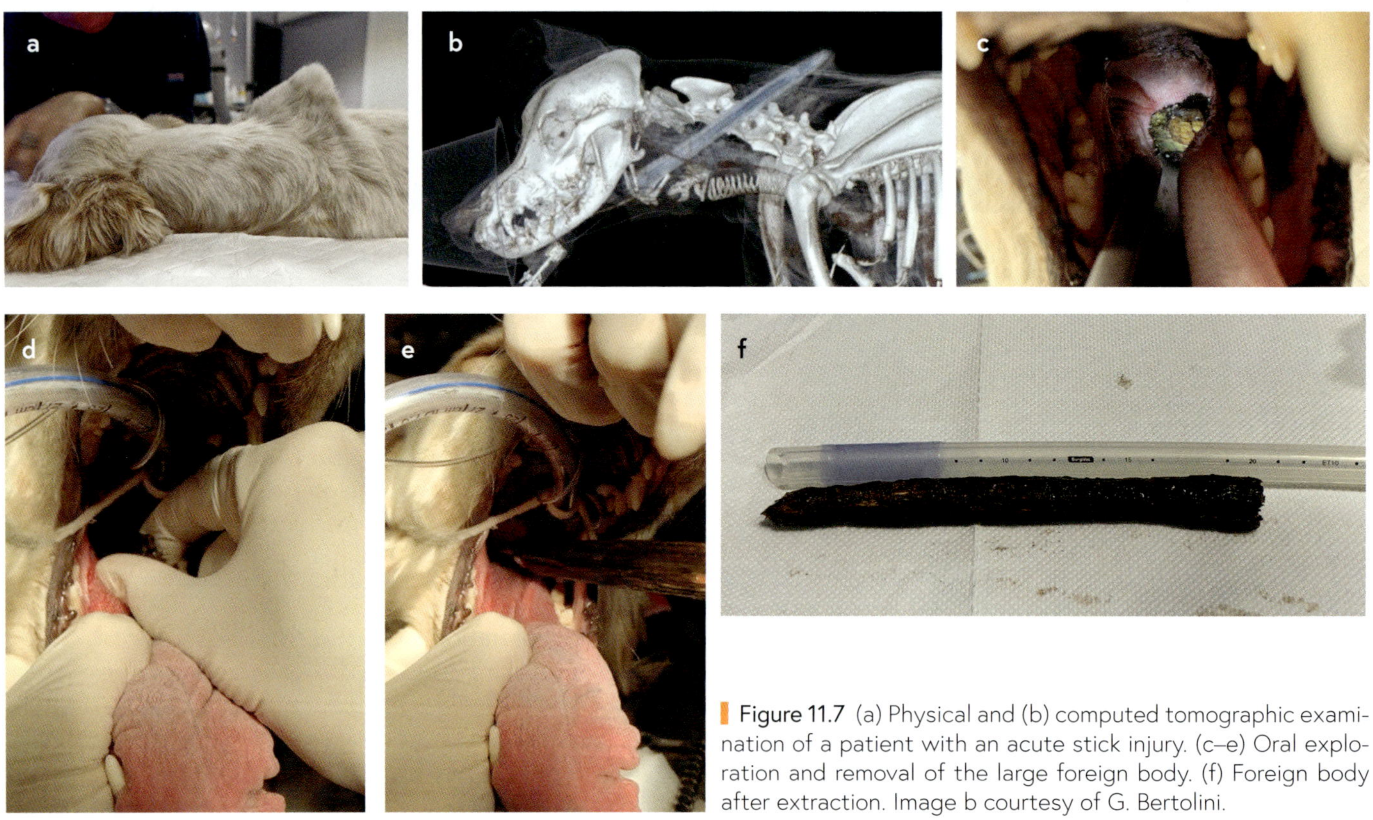

Figure 11.7 (a) Physical and (b) computed tomographic examination of a patient with an acute stick injury. (c–e) Oral exploration and removal of the large foreign body. (f) Foreign body after extraction. Image b courtesy of G. Bertolini.

explored for any foreign body. Tissue and/or fluid should be sampled for cytology and culture.

4. The surgical site is copiously lavaged and a drain (active or passive) is placed.
5. Empirical administration of broad-spectrum antibiotics is recommended until culture and sensitivity testing results are available.
6. In case of penetrating esophageal injury, debridement and esophageal wall reconstruction is necessary (see below).

Postoperative management

Minimal postoperative care is required after uncomplicated surgery. The drain should be kept in place based on the daily fluid production. Standard wound care is delivered, and the sutures are removed after 10–12 days.

Outcome

Acute penetrating injuries of the oropharyngeal region, when treated appropriately, have a better prognosis than acute penetrating esophageal injuries.[9] Aggressive surgical debridement of all sinus tracts and retrieval of foreign material does not eliminate the possibility of recurrence. The recurrence rates in chronic cases are similar regardless of whether foreign material was encountered (45%) or not (43%) during surgery.[8]

Esophageal foreign body or trauma

Obstruction of the esophagus by a foreign body should be considered an emergency because the longer an object remains in the esophagus, the higher the risk of aspiration and esophageal wall injury through pressure necrosis.[11] The most common types of foreign bodies found in the esophagus are bones and plastic items.[12] In dogs and cats, fishhooks account for only 0% to 17% of cases.[11,12] Several techniques have been described to remove esophageal foreign bodies, such as endoscopy, fluoroscopy, and surgery.[12,13] When endoscopic retrieval is unsuccessful, a perforation is present, or if endoscopic removal carries a high risk of perforation, surgery via esophagotomy or gastrotomy is recommended.[12–14]

Clinical presentation and diagnosis

The clinical signs of esophageal foreign body can include gagging, retching, regurgitation, vomiting, dyspnea, pain, lethargy, and inappetence. Terrier breeds, such as the English Bull Terrier and the West Highland White Terrier, are overrepresented among the affected population.[11,15] Esophageal foreign bodies most commonly lodge at the level of the thoracic inlet, the heart base, and the distal esophagus due to extraluminal structures preventing esophageal dilation at these locations.[16]

Cervical and thoracic radiographs can identify most esophageal foreign bodies and may reveal radiographic indicators of esophageal perforation such as pneumomediastinum, pneumothorax, periesophageal fluid collection, and mediastinal widening (Fig. 11.10). Endoscopic examination allows direct visualization of the foreign body and permits assessment of the esophageal mucosa for signs of esophagitis, ulceration, necrosis, or perforation. Computed tomography can be also used to confirm the presence of an esophageal foreign body but has limitation in identifying periesophageal fluid and extraluminal air, which are suggestive of esophageal perforation.[17]

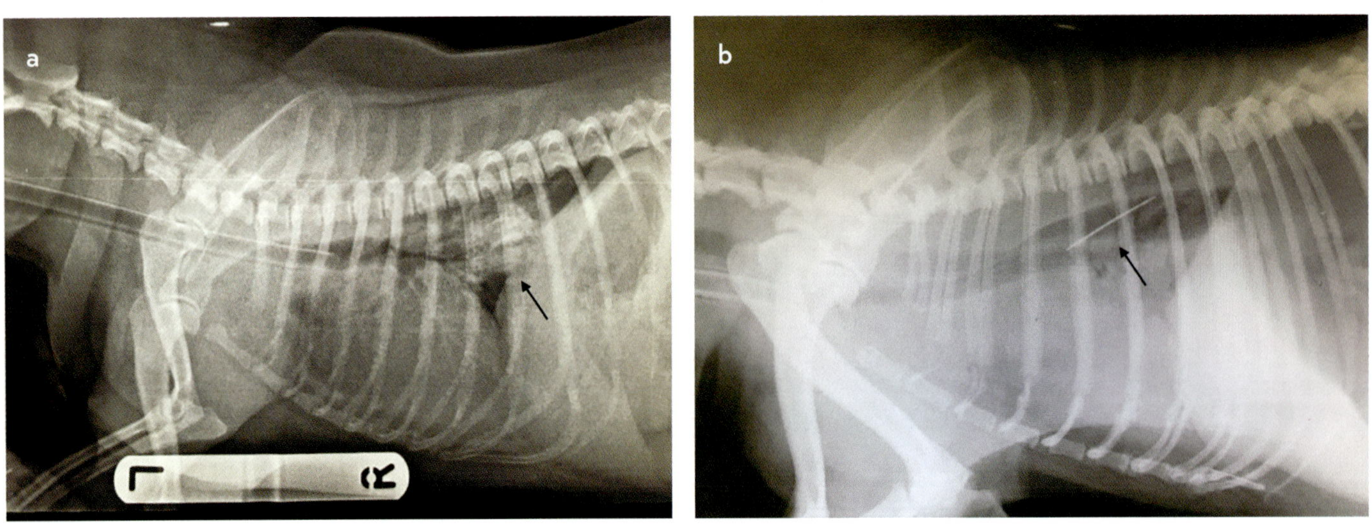

Figure 11.10 Lateral thoracic radiographs of two different esophageal foreign bodies, (a) pork bone and (b) needle, lodged in the caudal thoracic esophagus (black arrow).

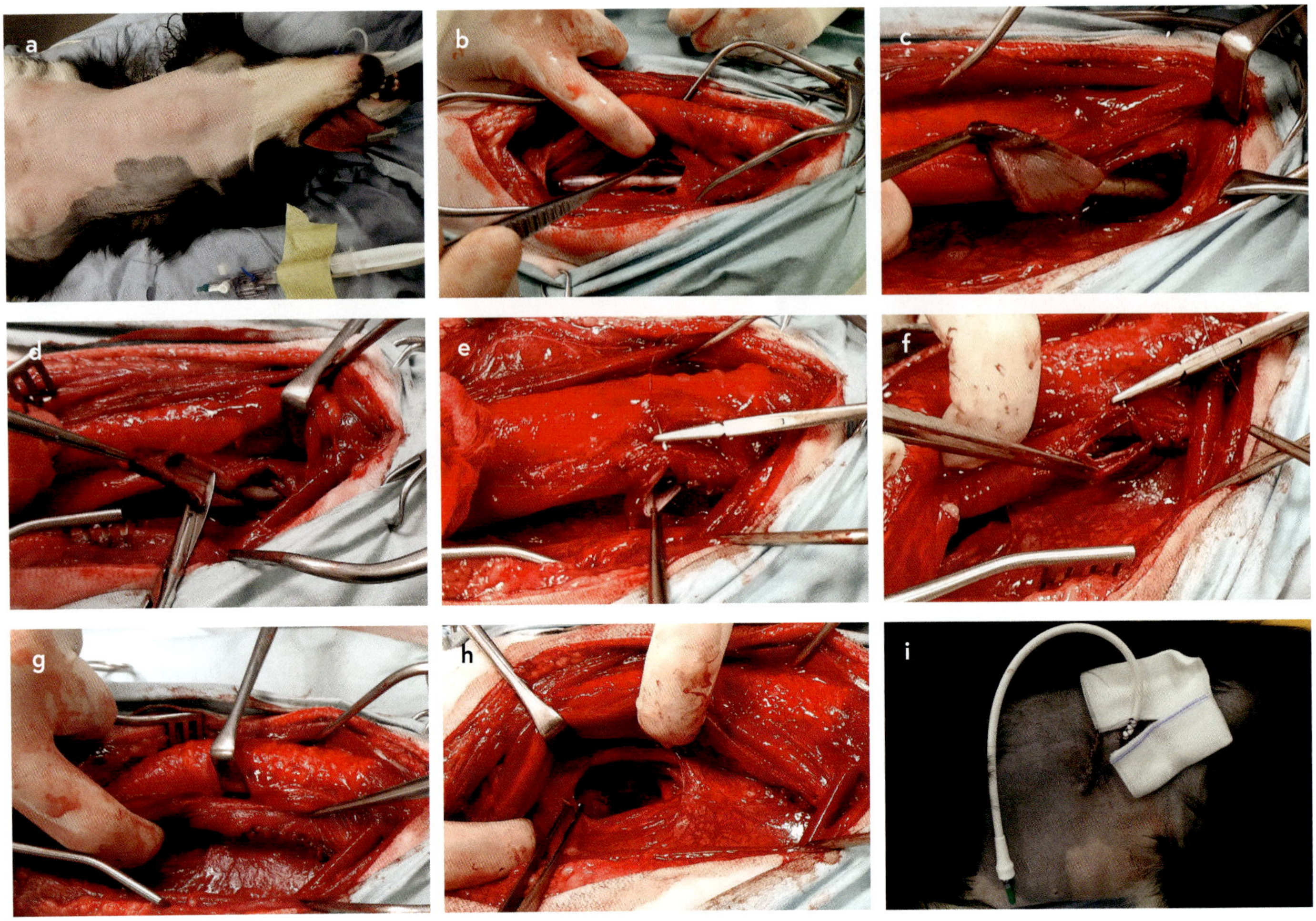

Figure 11.12 Cervical approach in a case of penetrating esophageal injury due to a foreign body (stick) with laceration of the cervical portion of the esophagus. (a–c) Ventral midline approach to the neck and identification of the esophageal laceration. An esophageal probe helps to identify the lesion. (d) Lesion debridement. (e–g) Two-layer closure of the esophageal wall. (h) Exploration, debridement, and closure of the muscular neck wounds. (i) Gastrostomy tube placement.

Transthoracic approach (Video 11.6)

1. A left-sided intercostal thoracotomy (see Chapter 4) is the preferred method to provide access to the esophagus overlying the heart base and caudal thoracic esophagus. The decision of which intercostal space to use is determined by the location of the foreign body on preoperative imaging.
2. Laparotomy sponges are used to isolate the esophagus and retract the lung lobes.

Esophagotomy (Fig. 11.13)

1. The intrathoracic esophagus is elevated using stay sutures or umbilical tape, taking care to avoid damaging the ventral and dorsal vagal trunks.
2. A longitudinal incision is made in the less inflamed area of the esophagus.
3. The foreign body is carefully removed from the esophageal lumen, and the mucosa is carefully inspected for perforations.

Video 11.6. Transthoracic approach for esophageal foreign body removal. Cranial and caudal left-sided intercostal thoracotomy.

4. Any perforation should be debrided before repair. Right-sided intrathoracic perforations can be approached through the esophagotomy incision or by rotating the esophagus with stay sutures.
5. Before repair is started, the mucosal–submucosal limit of the perforation should be visible.
6. Esophageal closure is performed using a simple interrupted suture pattern in two layers. Alternatively, a double-layer technique can be used: the mucosal–submucosal layer is closed with the knots positioned intraluminally, while the muscularis–adventitial layer is closed with extraluminal knots (3-0 or 4-0 slowly

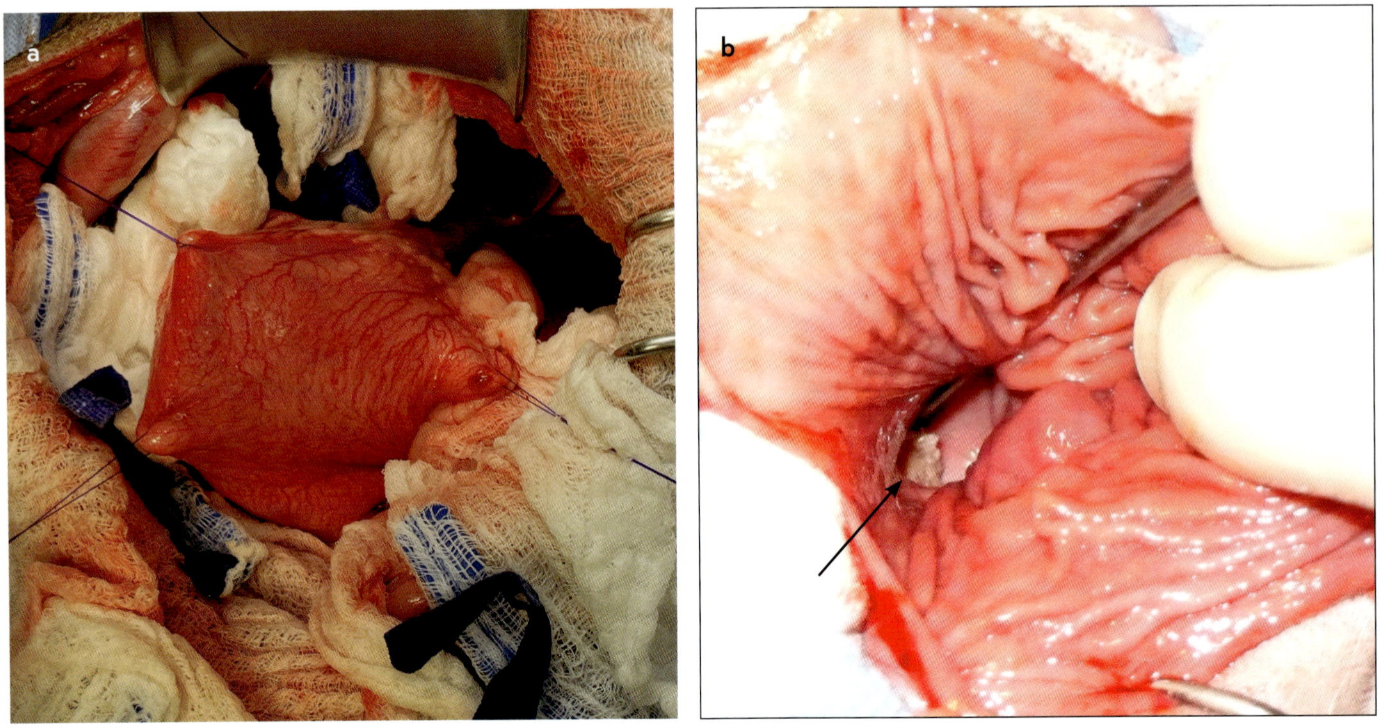

Figure 11.14 Extraction of a caudal esophageal foreign body through a gastrotomy approach. (a) Stomach retraction using stay sutures. (b) Identification of the foreign body (black arrow) in the distal esophagus after gastrotomy. Images courtesy of Adrien Aertsens and *Journal of Small Animal Practice* (2016) 57, 354–359.

reflux, omeprazole and sucralfate are used postoperatively. Broad-spectrum antibiotics (e.g., cefuroxime 15–20 mg/kg every 8–12 h) are indicated due to the high risk of aspiration pneumonia in these patients.

Vital signs including heart rate, blood pressure, respiratory pattern, and temperature should be checked for the first 24–48 hours. Pulse oximetry measurement, blood gas analysis, and thoracic imaging can be performed if indicated. Thoracostomy drains are normally maintained for 12–24 hours. Gastrostomy tubes may be helpful for administration of postoperative nutrition and medications but should be monitored and maintained for a minimum of 10 days. If a nasogastric tube has been placed instead, it should be kept in place for 5–8 days (Fig. 11.15).

Outcome

The prognosis after foreign body removal is generally excellent, except in cases of thoracic esophageal perforation. Early complications may include esophagitis, ischemic necrosis, dehiscence, leakage, and infection. Late complications include esophageal strictures and tracheo- or bronchoesophageal fistulae. The survival-to-discharge rate following surgery for the treatment of esophageal foreign bodies reportedly ranges from 50% to 93%.[12,14,16,23] Recent studies have demonstrated a high survival-to-discharge rate in dogs undergoing surgery for the treatment of esophageal foreign bodies, although esophageal perforation is significantly associated with a lower survival-to-discharge rate. Only 6.1% of esophagotomy incisions dehisced, and most of the dogs that survived had good long-term follow-up with few long-term complications.[18] However, these studies often combined various methods of esophageal foreign body removal, making it difficult to differentiate outcomes following minimally invasive versus surgical removal or to provide detailed information on a significant number of surgical cases.

Gastrointestinal foreign body

In veterinary medicine, the most common indication for a laparotomy is the removal of foreign bodies from the gastrointestinal (GI) tract. GI foreign bodies occur more commonly in dogs compared to cats due to their behavior of ingesting objects. Gastric foreign bodies account for 16% to 50% of all GI foreign bodies. In dogs, the larger esophageal size compared to the intestine or pyloric outflow tract results in the ability to swallow relatively large objects that then lead to obstruction.

Clinical presentation and diagnosis

Gastric foreign body

The clinical signs of gastric foreign bodies include vomiting, regurgitation (secondary to esophagitis caused by

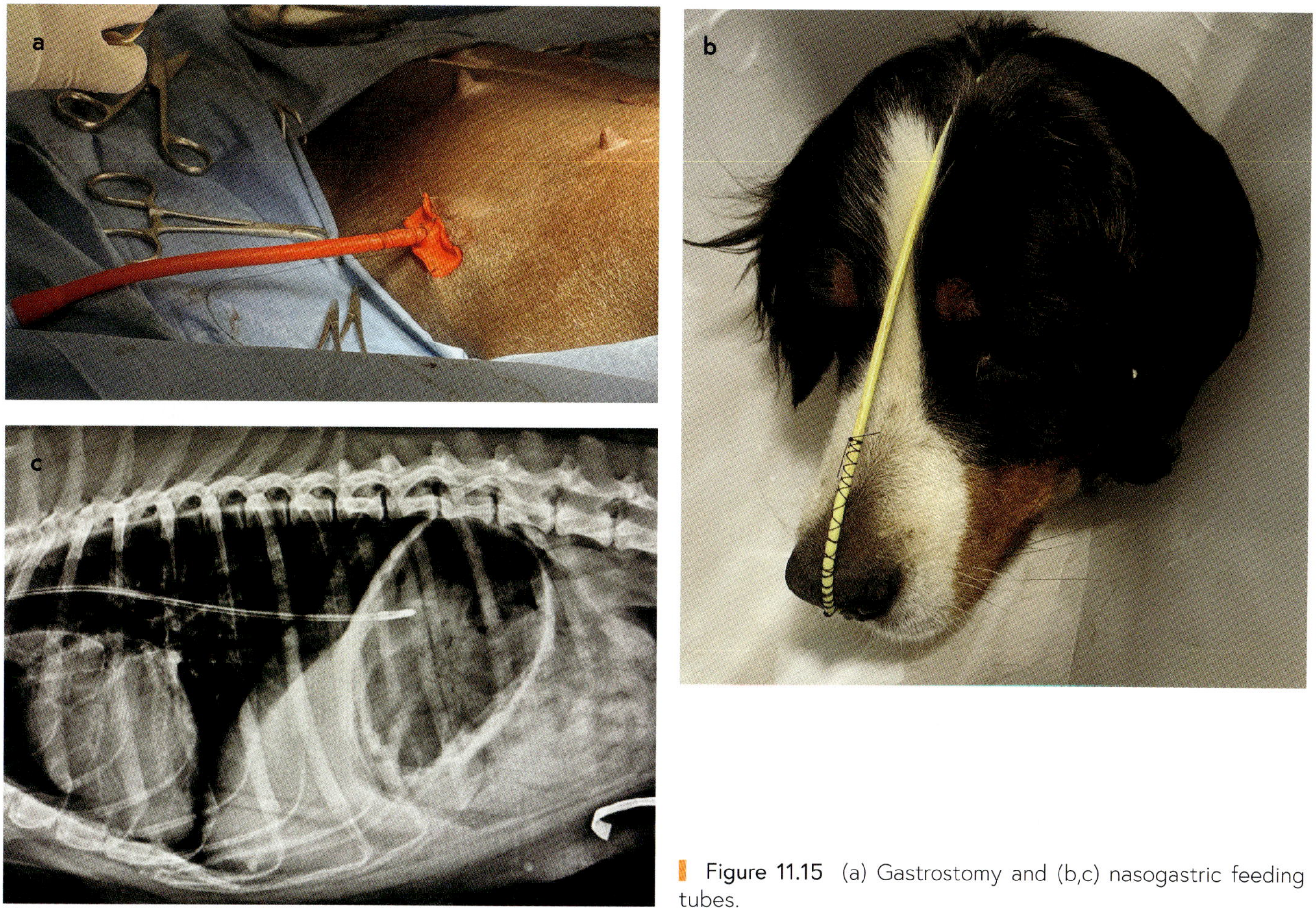

Figure 11.15 (a) Gastrostomy and (b,c) nasogastric feeding tubes.

vomiting), and abdominal pain. Abdominal distension may be noticed in patients that suffer pyloric outflow obstruction. Blood work (hematology, serum biochemistry, electrolytes) may reveal electrolyte and acid–base imbalances, with hypochloremia being the most common abnormality due to vomiting.

The initial diagnostic modality recommended is abdominal radiography. In one study, plain abdominal radiographs (Fig. 11.16) enabled visualization of 95% of gastric foreign bodies; in only two cases the foreign bodies were not observed (a piece of wood and organic material).[24] Contrast radiography can be beneficial in differentiating a foreign body from an intraluminal mass. The use of water-soluble iodinated contrast agents is recommended because they can be easily removed from the abdominal cavity in the presence of a ruptured GI tract. The disadvantage is that they provide poorer contrast compared to barium. The presence of free abdominal air in the abdominal cavity should prompt an emergency exploratory laparotomy due to the presence of a perforated viscus. Ultrasonography can aid in the diagnosis of GI foreign bodies, particularly when there is uncertainty about the presence of GI obstruction on radiography. If free abdominal fluid is visualized, an abdominocentesis with biochemical analysis and cytology of the fluid should be performed to look for signs of septic peritonitis (i.e., intracellular bacteria) (see Chapter 16).

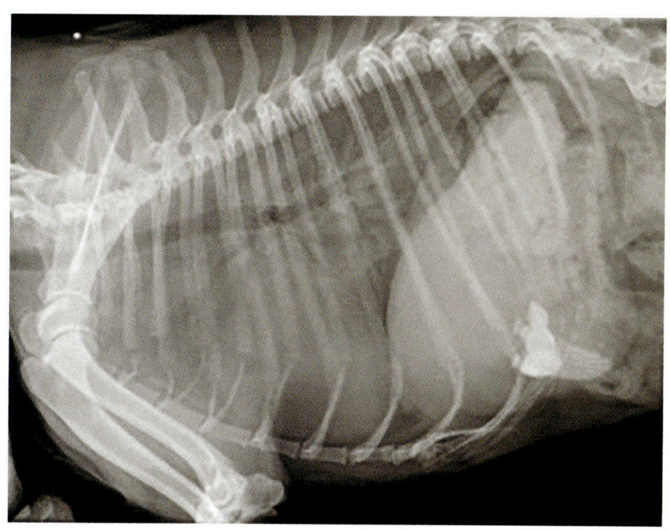

Figure 11.16 Plain lateral abdominal radiograph of a dog revealing the presence of a gastric foreign body.

Intestinal foreign body

The clinical signs of an intestinal obstruction caused by foreign bodies can vary depending on the location, duration, and degree of the obstruction. The most common signs include vomiting, anorexia, lethargy, and abdominal pain. Palpation of the abdomen may reveal the presence of the foreign body. Abdominal radiography can help identify the object, particularly if it is radiopaque. However, more often, signs of mechanical obstruction such as multiple distended, gas- or fluid-filled small intestinal loops are visualized. In case of partial obstruction, these signs may be less severe. Comparing the intestinal diameter to the vertebral height can aid in differentiating between a mechanical/obstructive and functional intestinal ileus. If the ratio between the maximum dilated intestine and the narrowest point of L5 is greater than 2.0, a mechanical obstruction is highly likely and further diagnostics or exploratory laparotomy may be indicated.[25] Contrast radiography can be used but can be time-consuming. Ultrasonography is quicker but operator dependent, and the presence of gas in the intestines may limit the visualization of structures. In a study comparing ultrasound and radiography for identifying GI foreign bodies in 11 dogs and 5 cats, ultrasound identified all 16 foreign bodies, while radiography only identified 9.[26] Comparing the ability of ultrasound and radiography to identify GI foreign bodies, ultrasound revealed a bright interference associated with strong distal acoustic shadowing for all the foreign bodies.

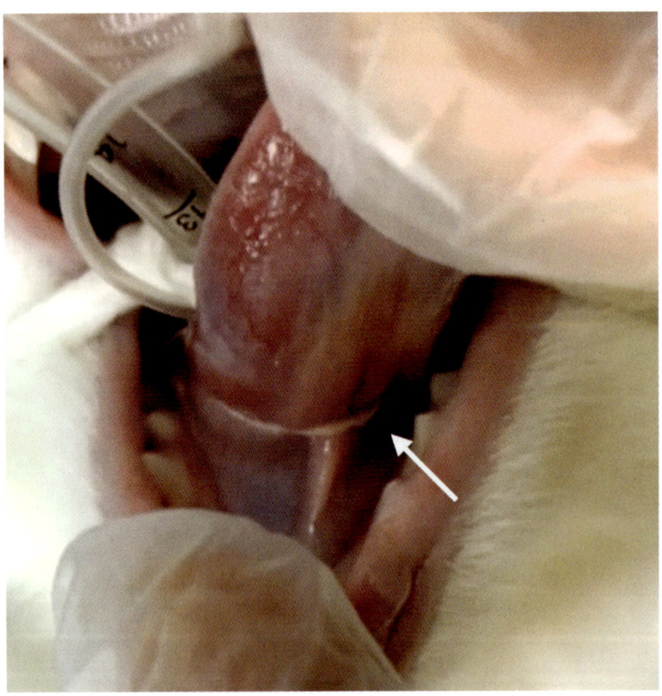

Figure 11.17 Oral examination in a cat showing a linear foreign body trapped around the base of the tongue (white arrow).

Linear foreign body

Linear foreign bodies are more common in cats compared to dogs and include threads, stockings, strings, and carpet. They can cause a specific form of intestinal obstruction. Typically, the linear foreign body becomes anchored in a particular part of the GI tract, most commonly the base of the tongue (cats) or the pylorus (dogs). The peristaltic movements of the intestine cause the linear material to move aborally, resulting in the small intestine bunching up like an accordion. Continued peristaltic movements can lead to the linear material perforating the mesenteric side of the intestine, leading to septic peritonitis. The most common clinical signs are vomiting, anorexia, and lethargy. Linear foreign bodies usually cause partial obstruction; therefore, the clinical signs may not be as severe as with complete obstruction. In approximately 50% of cats, the linear foreign body can be identified attached to the tongue during clinical examination (Fig. 11.17). Abdominal palpation may reveal clumping of the intestines and abdominal pain.

Diagnosis can be aided by plain abdominal radiography, which shows a plicated small intestine in the cranial midabdomen. Gas pockets may be seen instead of the normal curvilinear columns. The use of contrast radiography can reveal more clearly the pleating of the intestines and, in some cases, the foreign material may appear radiolucent. On ultrasound, linear foreign bodies present as bright linear interfaces associated with shadowing, and the affected bowel segment appears plicated. Intestinal distension is normally less pronounced than with larger foreign bodies.

Treatment

Gastric foreign body

When dealing with gastric foreign bodies, it is important to consider their size and duration. This can help in decision-making, such as attempting endoscopy for retrieval. If the foreign body is too large for endoscopic removal or if it has been present for an extended period, surgical intervention should be considered. Prompt removal of the foreign body is crucial to prevent migration into the small intestine, which can lead to obstruction and devitalization of the intestine. The preferred surgical treatment for gastric foreign bodies is gastrotomy.

Surgical technique: Gastrotomy (Figs. 11.18–11.23)

1. A midline celiotomy approach is made (see Chapter 3).
2. Moistened laparotomy swabs are used to isolate the stomach from the rest of the abdomen, reducing the risk of peritoneal contamination.
3. Thorough palpation of the stomach is important to locate and assess the foreign body.

4. To provide retraction and decrease the risk of contamination, two stay sutures are placed in the stomach at either side of the gastrotomy incision, passing the needle through the submucosa to prevent tearing of the tissues (Fig. 11.18).

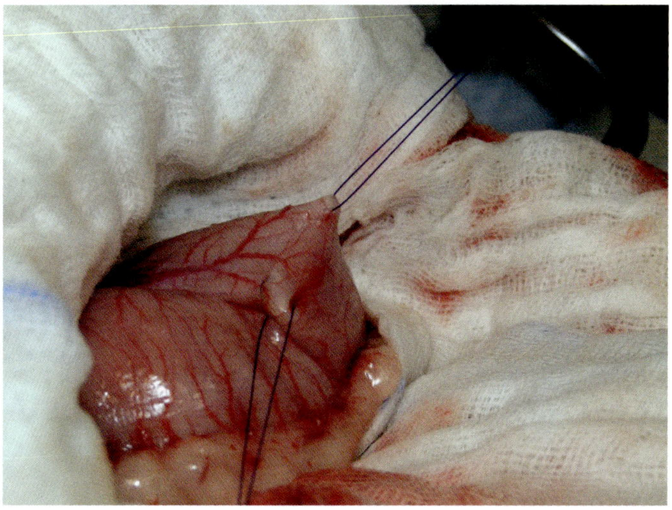

Figure 11.18 Isolation of the stomach from the abdominal cavity using moistened laparotomy swabs. Placement of two stay sutures on either side of the incision to minimize gastric fluid spillage.

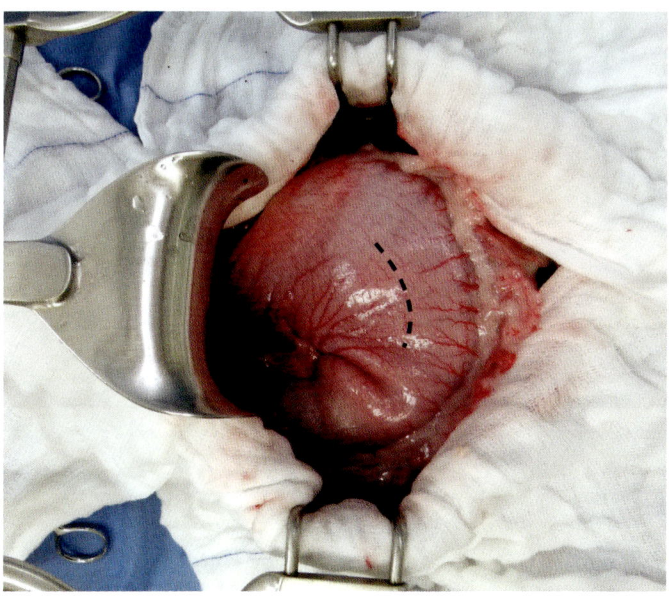

Figure 11.19 Ventral incision of the gastric body.

Video 11.7. Gastrotomy for gastric foreign body removal. After isolating the stomach and placing two stay sutures, the ventral aspect of the gastric body is incised to extract the foreign bodies.

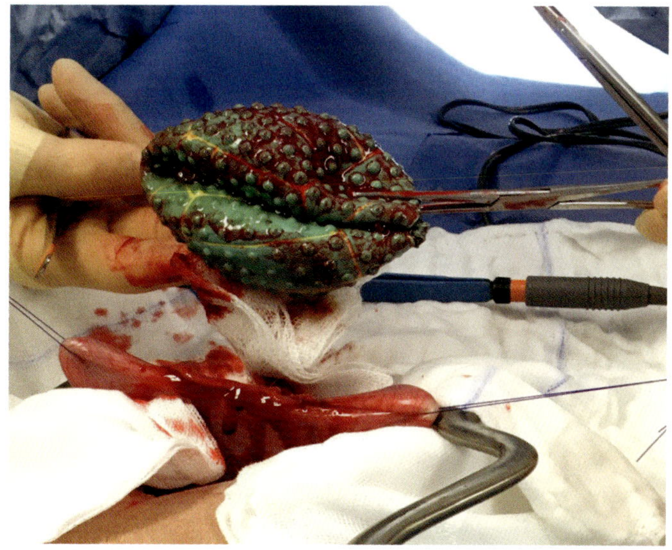

Figure 11.20 Retrieval of a plastic ball from the stomach.

5. An incision is performed with a number 11 scalpel blade in the ventral aspect of the gastric body, parallel to the long axis of the stomach and midway between the greater and lesser curvatures, in an area without mayor blood supply (Fig. 11.19; Video 11.7). In case of a linear foreign body, the incision may be made over the pyloric region.
6. The length of the incision depends on the size of the foreign material, but it should be kept as small as possible.
7. The foreign material is removed using instruments such as DeBakey forceps or Allis tissue forceps (Fig. 11.20).
8. The suture pattern for stomach closure varies depending on the surgeon's preference. Typically, a two-layer closure is performed, with a simple continuous pattern involving all layers (Fig. 11.21) followed by a simple continuous pattern or inverting pattern (Connell or Cushing) incorporating the serosa and muscularis layers (4-0 or 3-0 slowly absorbable monofilament suture) (Fig. 11.22; Video 11.8).
9. Once the stomach is closed, a segment of omentum is placed over the suture site (Video 11.9).
10. In case of contamination of the abdomen, copious abdominal lavage is indicated.
11. The abdominal wall is closed routinely.

Intestinal foreign body

Intestinal foreign bodies require careful evaluation and surgical intervention. An exploratory laparotomy should be performed, with special attention to examining the entire GI tract, as there may be multiple foreign bodies or a perforated segment of intestine oral to the foreign material. Once identified, the segment is assessed for viability. Enterotomy is performed on a viable intestinal

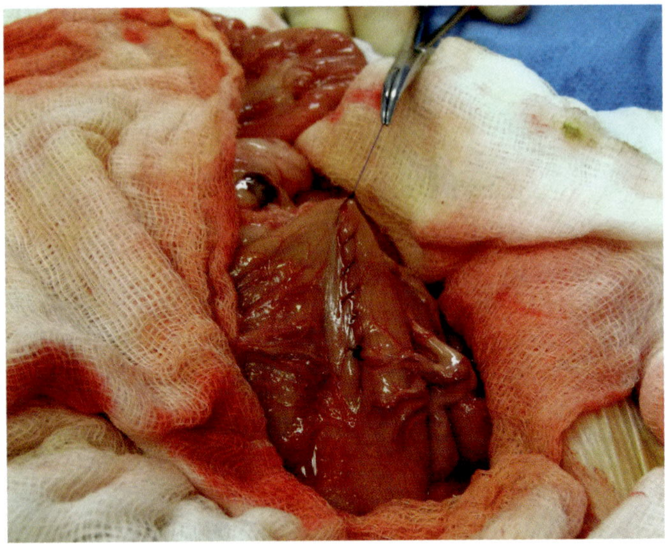

Figure 11.21 Simple continuous suture pattern incorporating all stomach layers.

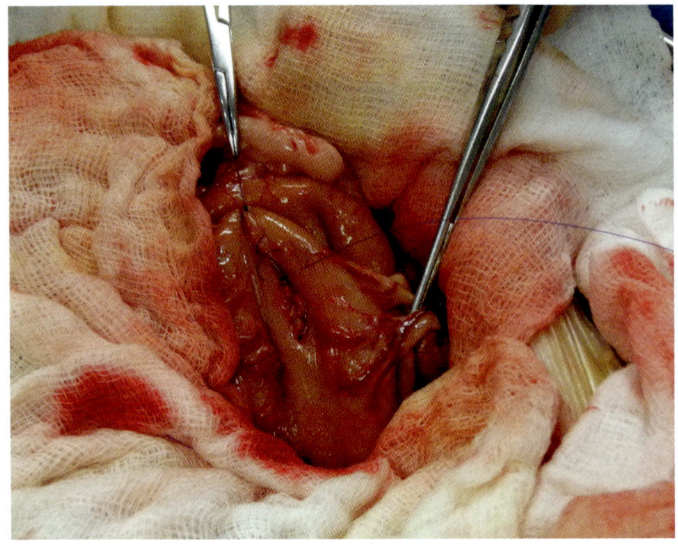

Figure 11.22 Inverting continuous suture pattern incorporating the gastric serosa and muscularis layers.

Video 11.8. Stomach closure via simple continuous suture in two layers: the first layer incorporates the mucosa and submucosa, while the second incorporates the muscularis and serosa.

Video 11.9. Use of omentum to cover the gastric incision.

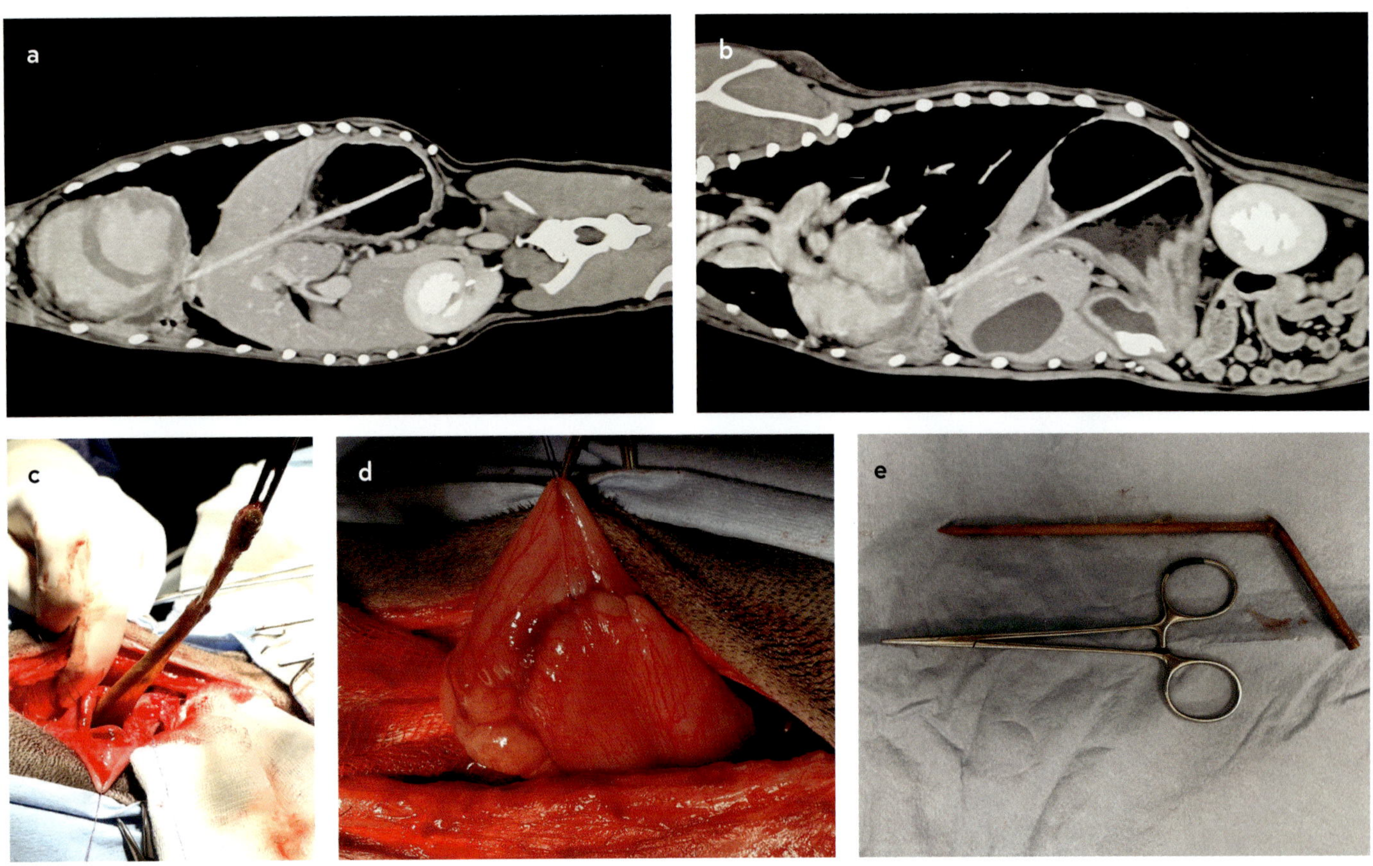

Figure 11.23 (a,b) Computed tomography scans showing a kebab skewer in the stomach. (c) Gastrotomy surgery for foreign body removal. (d) Closure of the stomach in two layers. (e) Foreign body after extraction.

portion aboral to the foreign body, while enterectomy should be performed on nonviable segments. In case of doubt, it may be worthwhile to remove the foreign material and assess the intestinal segment for a few minutes. In some cases, the intestine can appear nonviable due to the pressure from the foreign body; however, once the foreign body is removed and blood flow is restored, the appearance of the intestinal segment starts improving. If this is not the case, then an enterectomy should be performed.

Surgical technique: Enterotomy

1. A midline celiotomy approach is made (see Chapter 3).
2. The digestive tract is thoroughly examined, from the abdominal portion of the esophagus to the colon.
3. The foreign body or bodies are identified, and the presence of necrosis or perforation of the affected intestinal segment is assessed (Fig. 11.24).
4. The segment of intestine is isolated by placing moistened laparotomy swabs around it (Fig. 11.25).
5. A longitudinal incision is made on the antimesenteric border of the intestine, slightly aboral to the foreign body, as this area of the intestine has not been damaged by the passage of the object (Fig. 11.26; Video 11.10). The length of the incision should be sufficient to extract the foreign body without damaging the intestinal wall (Fig. 11.27; Video 11.11).
6. After foreign body removal, the incision is closed using a single-layer simple interrupted or continuous appositional suture pattern (3-0 or 4-0 absorbable monofilament; e.g., polydioxanone). Suture bites should be about 3–4 mm wide and are placed 3–4 mm apart, depending on intestinal thickness and diameter. It is very important to include the submucosal layer, as it provides the greatest strength to the closure (Fig. 11.28; Videos 11.12 and 11.13).
7. Omentum is wrapped around the enterotomy site (Fig. 11.29; Video 11.14).

Surgical technique: Enterectomy

1. A midline celiotomy approach is made (see Chapter 3).
2. The segment of intestine to be resected is identified and evaluated to determine its viability. Subjective criteria for evaluating intestinal viability include intestinal wall thickness, intestinal color, and the presence of peristalsis (pinch test) and vascular pulsation (see "Intussusception" section below).

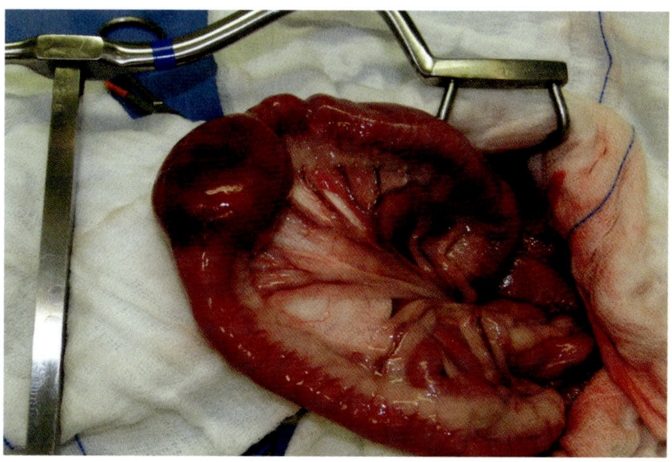

Figure 11.24 Identification of an intestinal foreign body.

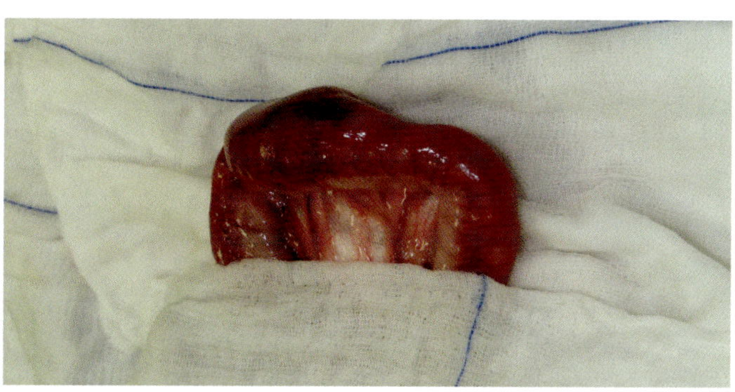

Figure 11.25 Isolation of the affected intestinal loop from the abdominal cavity using moistened laparotomy swabs.

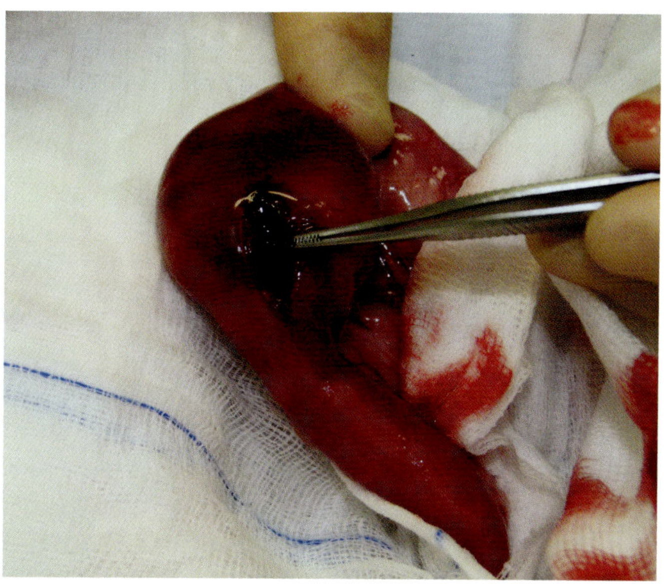

Figure 11.26 Antimesenteric incision made aboral to the foreign body.

Video 11.10. Enterotomy. An incision is made on the antimesenteric border, aboral to the foreign material.

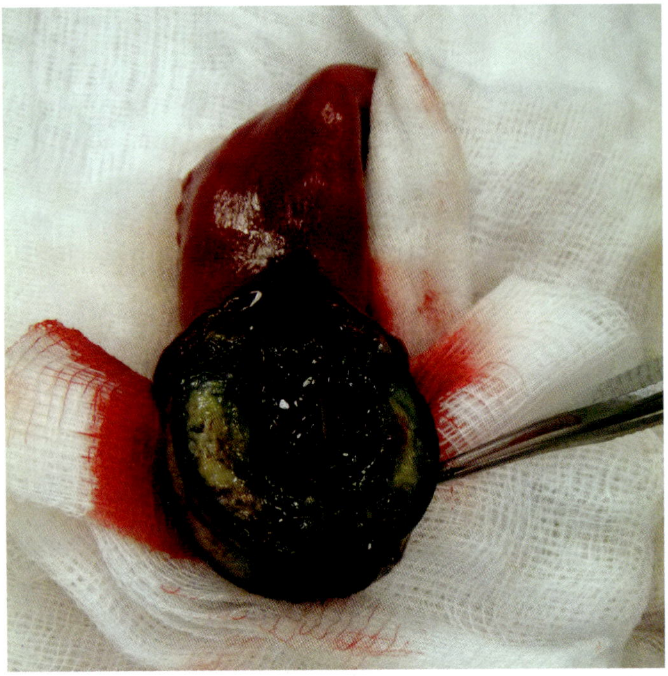

Figure 11.27 Retrieval of the foreign body.

Video 11.11. Intestinal foreign body removal.

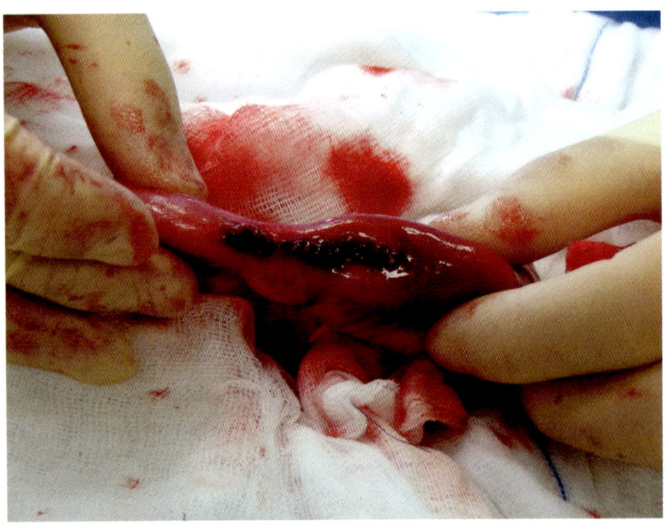

Figure 11.28 Closure of the enterotomy using simple interrupted appositional sutures.

Video 11.12. Enterotomy closure using simple interrupted appositional sutures.

Video 11.13. Examination of the enterotomy closure with DeBakey forceps to assess if more sutures are required.

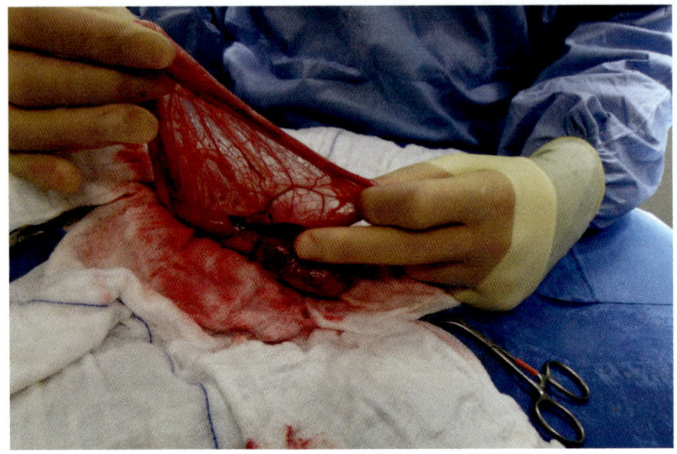

Figure 11.29 Omentalization of the enterotomy.

Video 11.14. Placement of omentum covering the enterotomy site.

3. Moistened laparotomy swabs are used to isolate the segment.
4. If the segment has sufficient mobility, it should be brought out from the abdominal cavity to reduce possible contamination.
5. The length of intestine to be resected is determined:
   - Necrotic tissue: A minimum margin of 1–2 cm of healthy tissue (Video 11.15).
   - Intestinal tumors: Margin of 5–7 cm oral and aboral (Fig. 11.30).
   - Once decided on the margins to remove, the incision of the intestine to be sutured should be close to the main vessel irrigating the section of intestine; this will improve perfusion to the anastomosis.
6. The vessels supplying the bowel segment to be removed are double ligated with a 2-0 to 3-0 monofilament suture and resected, including the con-

Video 11.15. Assessment of multiple intestinal perforations in a dog shot with a pellet gun.

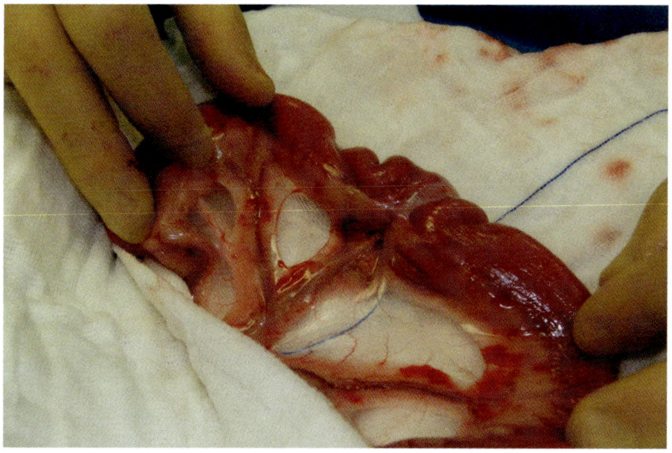

Figure 11.30 Resection of a segment of intestine with a 5 cm margin oral and aboral due to an intestinal carcinoma.

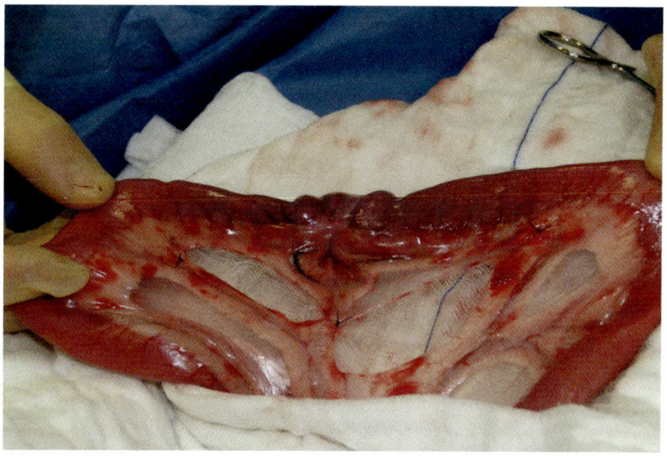

Figure 11.32 Ligation of the arcuate vessels.

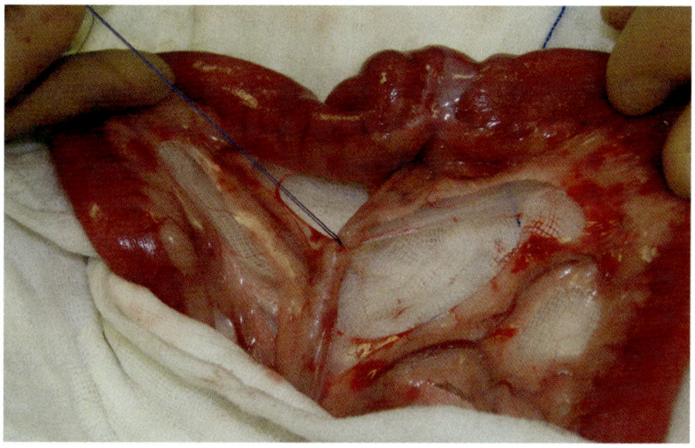

Figure 11.31 Double ligation and resection of the vessels supplying the bowel segment.

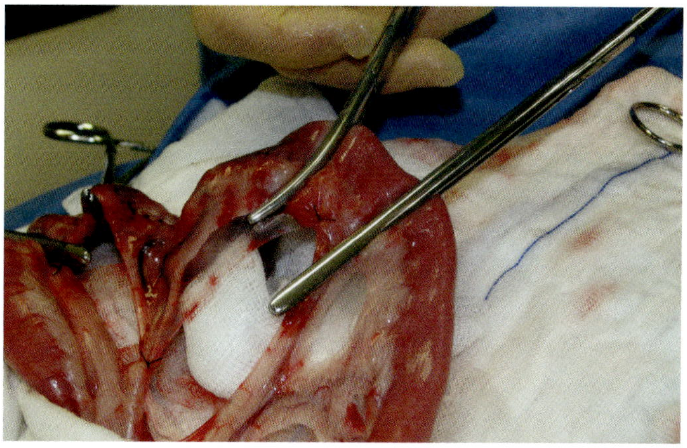

Figure 11.33 Placement of an atraumatic and a traumatic clamp on the edges of the intestine to be sutured and resected, respectively.

necting arcades in the mesenteric border of the intestine (Fig. 11.31). It is important to ligate the arcuate vessels located at the mesenteric border (Fig. 11.32).

7. Atraumatic clamps (e.g., Doyen forceps) or the assistant's fingers are placed on the edge of the intestine to be sutured and traumatic or atraumatic clamps on the edges to be resected (Fig. 11.33).
8. The bowel segment is cut at the level of the atraumatic forceps with a number 11 scalpel blade, leaving at least a 1 cm margin to facilitate suturing (Fig. 11.34; Video 11.16).

Video 11.16. Intestinal resection, ensuring no contamination and leaving enough bowel edge for suturing.

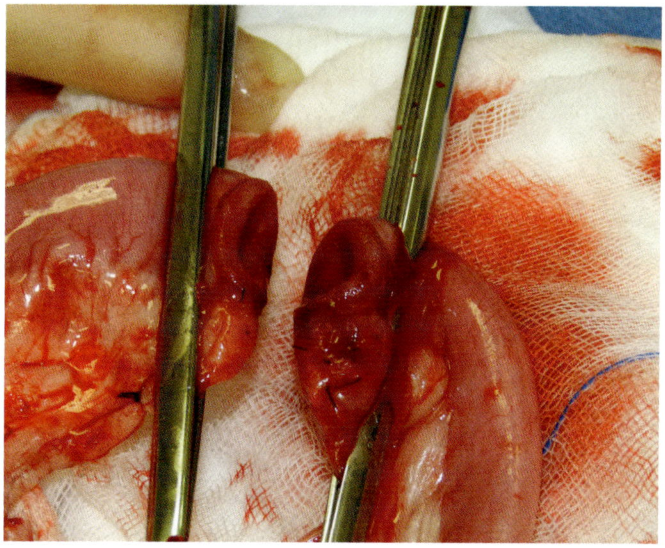

Figure 11.34 Transection of the intestinal segment at the level of the atraumatic forceps, leaving a minimum of 1 cm margin for suture placement.

Suture end-to-end anastomosis:

1. Suturing begins at the mesenteric edge to ensure correct placement of the sutures, as this area has a higher risk of dehiscence due to the presence of mesenteric fat (Fig. 11.35; Video 11.17).
2. Once the first sutures have been placed, anastomosis is continued toward the antimesenteric edge, especially if there is disparity between lumen sizes (Box 11.1). If there is no disparity, a suture can be placed at the antimesenteric edge, followed by the remaining sutures (Figs. 11.36 and 11.37).
3. A simple interrupted appositional suture pattern, with 3-0 or 4-0 long-lasting absorbable monofilament, is used. It is important to include the submucosal layer of the intestine, as it provides the greatest strength. A single layer of interrupted sutures decreases the risk of stricture and leakage of intestinal contents and results in faster wound healing. The needle is inserted about 3–5 mm from the edge of the incision, and sutures are placed every 3–5 mm, depending on intestinal thickness and diameter. The chosen suture should have a good tensile strength for at least 2 weeks, which is when anastomotic strength is close to normal. Examples of suture materials include glycomer 631, polyglyconate, and polydioxanone.
4. Other techniques, such as anastomosis using a continuous suture pattern or a modified Gambee technique, have been described.
5. After suturing, the anastomosis site can be checked:
   - Pushing DeBakey forceps between each suture (Video 11.18).
   - Saline leak test: Injecting saline into the intestine to see if there is any fluid leakage. The application of leak testing in surgery does not predict the likelihood of incisional dehiscence or failure; however, appropriate use of this technique may benefit novice surgeons in intestinal suturing techniques, such as suture number and spacing.[27]

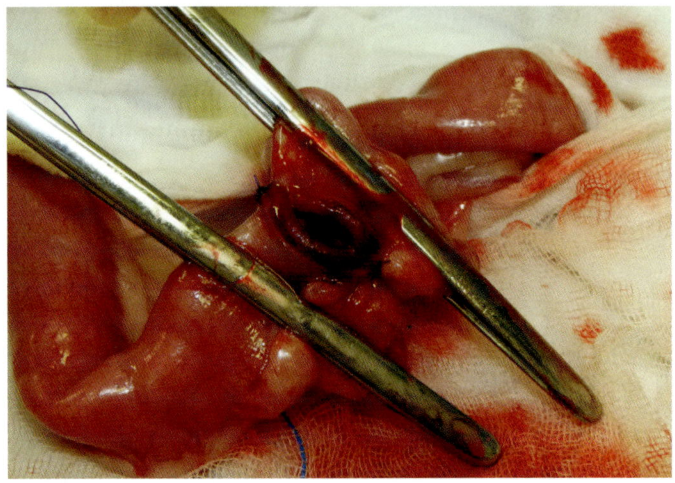

Figure 11.36 Placement of sutures at the antimesenteric border if no disparity exists between the bowel lumen sizes.

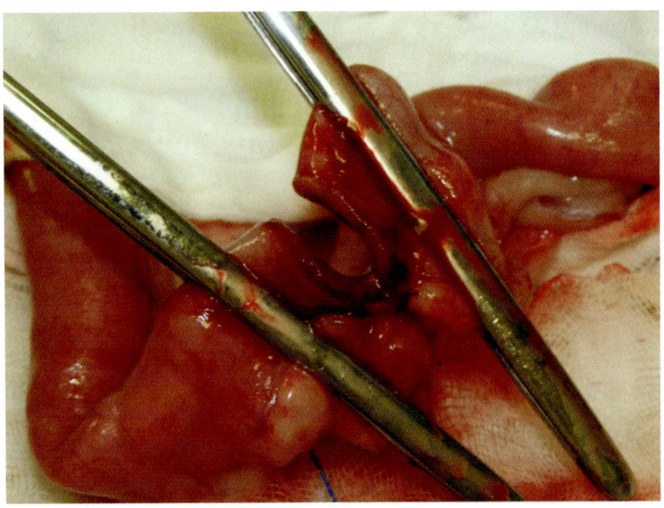

Figure 11.35 Initial sutures placed at the mesenteric side to reduce the risk of dehiscence.

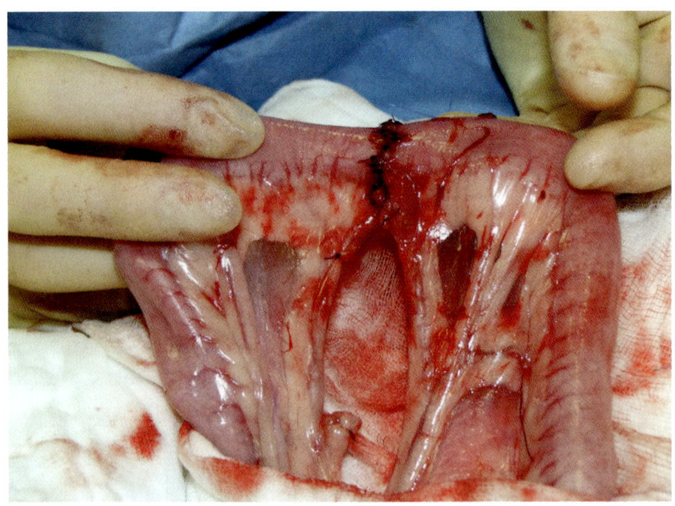

Figure 11.37 Suture placement is continued until a technically correct anastomosis is achieved.

Video 11.17. Placement of the first 2-3 sutures at the mesenteric side of the intestine.

Video 11.18. Assessment of enterectomy closure with DeBakey forceps.

a. The bowel is atraumatically clamped 1–2 cm proximal and distal to the surgical site.
b. Sterile saline is injected into the lumen with a needle (e.g., 22 gauge) and syringe (e.g., 10 mL) to gently distend the bowel.
c. Additional sutures are placed to close any defect detected.

6. Finally, the mesentery is sutured using 3-0 or 4-0 absorbable monofilament (e.g., polydioxanone or poliglecaprone) in a simple continuous or interrupted pattern (Fig. 11.38; Video 11.19).
7. Prior to closing the abdominal cavity, omentum is placed over the anastomosis (Video 11.20).

Box 11.1. Techniques in case of disparity between bowel lumen sizes

- The sutures in the wider lumen may be spaced further apart than those in the narrower lumen.
- The edge of the bowel segment with the narrower lumen can be cut at an angle from the mesenteric border toward the antimesenteric side to increase its surface area (Fig. 11.39).
- The antimesenteric border of the narrower lumen can be spatulated (Fig. 11.40).
- The wider lumen can be partially sutured to reduce its diameter.
- A stapling technique can be used (Fig. 11.41).

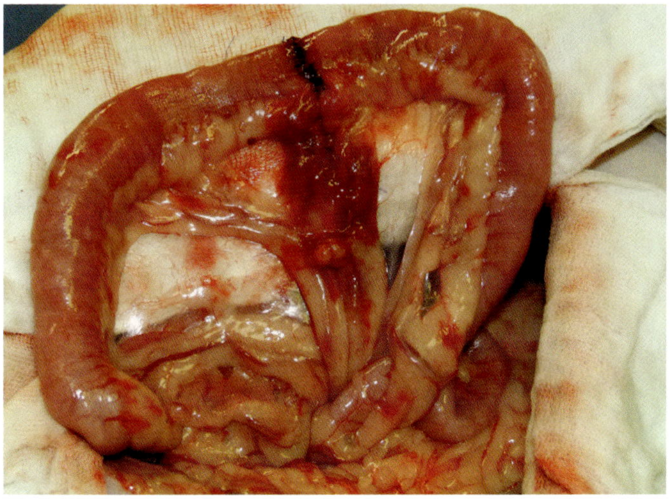

Figure 11.38 Suturing of the mesentery to decrease the risk of intestinal entrapment.

Video 11.19. Suturing of the mesentery using a simple continuous pattern.

Video 11.20. Placement of omentum over the anastomosis site.

Stapled functional end-to-end anastomosis (Fig. 11.42): Several types of anastomoses can be performed with the use of GI stapling systems. When staples, typically made of titanium, are fired, they bend into a B conformation, which improves blood flow to the incision. Two commonly used stapling systems are the GIA (gastrointestinal anastomosis) and the TA (thoracoabdominal) systems (Video 11.21). Five staple heights are available, indicated by the color of the cartridge (grey, white, blue, gold, and green) (see Chapter 6). For GI surgery, the blue and green cartridges are typically used in the intestine and the stomach (usually thicker), respectively. In the blue cartridge, the open staple height is 3.5 mm and 3.8 mm for the TA and GIA systems, respectively, and the closed staple height is 1.5 mm. In the green cartridge, the open staple height is 4.8 mm for both the TA and GIA systems, and the closed staple height is 2.0 mm. Regarding staple length, the GIA system comes in three lengths: 60 mm, 80 mm, and 100 mm, while the TA system sizes are 30 mm, 45 mm, 60 mm, and 90 mm. Another stapling system that could be used for functional end-to-end anastomosis in small dogs (<10 kg) and cats is the Endo GIA stapler with purple cartridges (length 60 mm or 45 mm; medium-thick Tri-Staple 3 mm/3.5 mm/4 mm from inside to outside line).

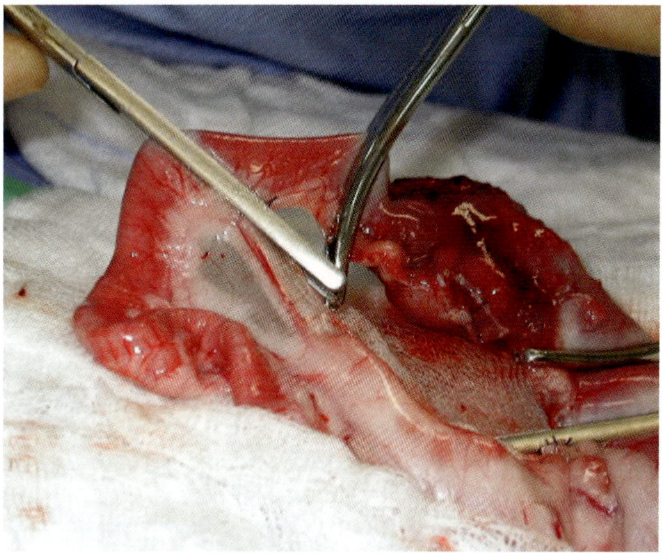

Figure 11.39 Angling the edge of the intestinal segment with the narrower lumen if a disparity exists between the two lumen sizes.

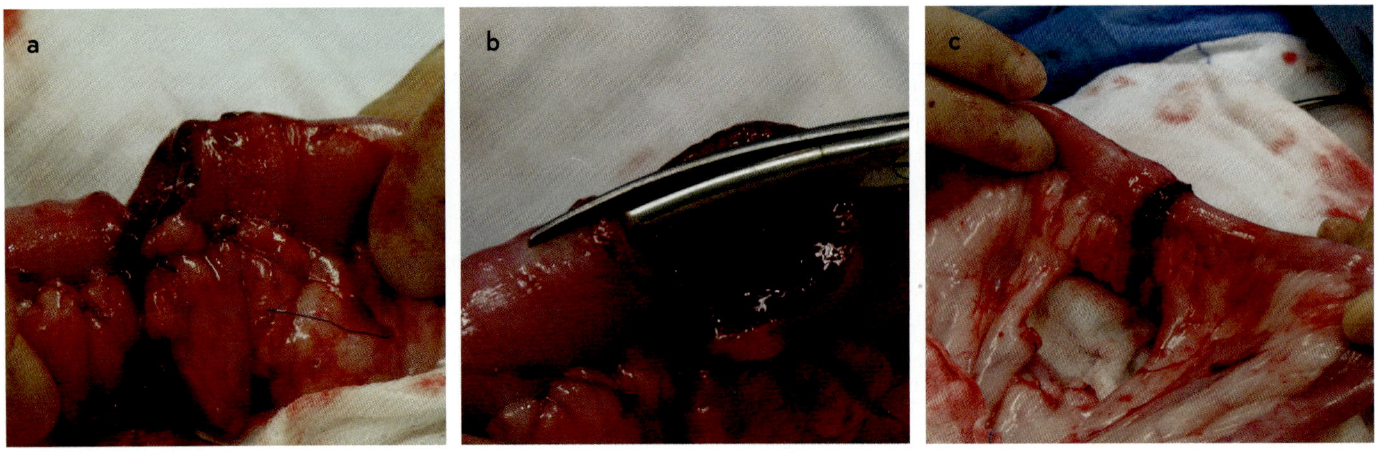

Figure 11.40 Spatulation of the antimesenteric side in case of lumen size disparity.

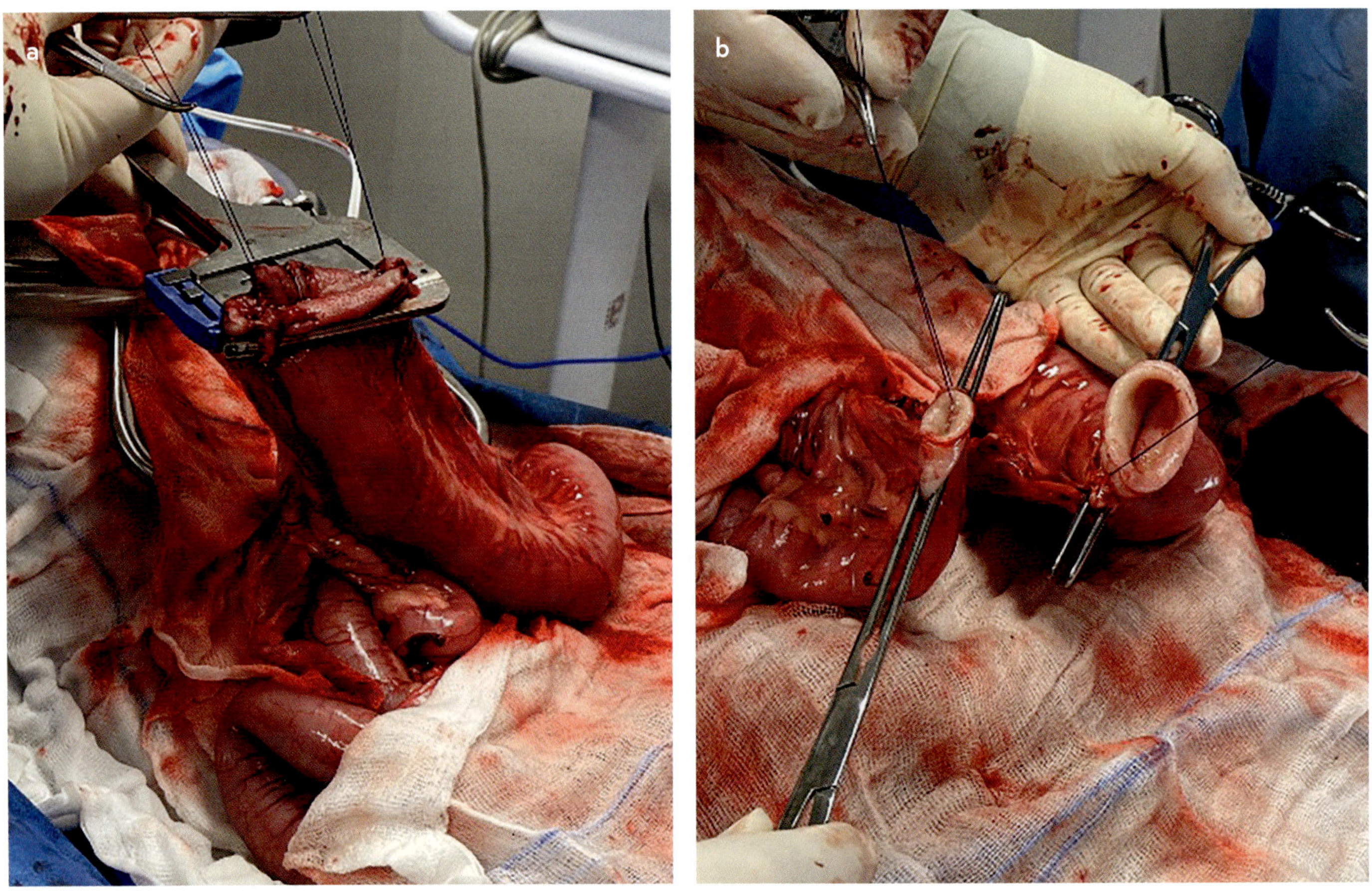

Figure 11.41 Use of stapling devices for cases with a large disparity between bowel lumen sizes.

Video 11.21. Use of two stapling systems, GIA (gastrointestinal anastomosis) and TA (thoracoabdominal), for performing a stapled anastomosis.

1. After performing the intestinal resection, the GIA stapling system is separated into its two arms. The arms are introduced into each bowel loop and closed, with the staple line facing the antimesenteric walls (Fig. 11.43; Video 11.22).

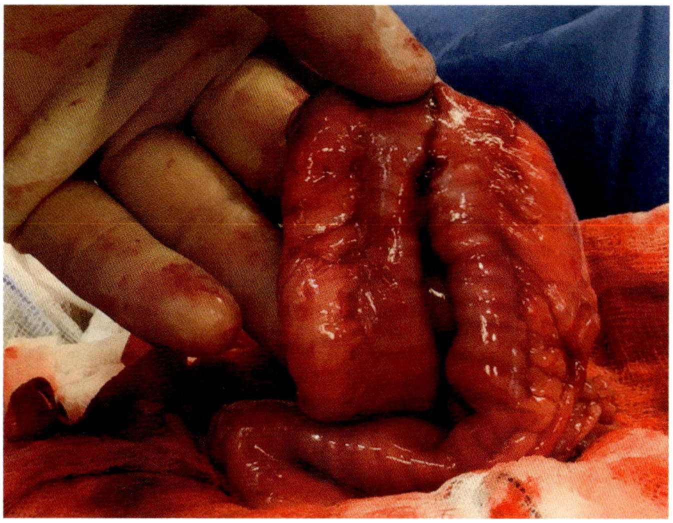

Figure 11.42 Functional end-to-end intestinal anastomosis performed with the use of staples.

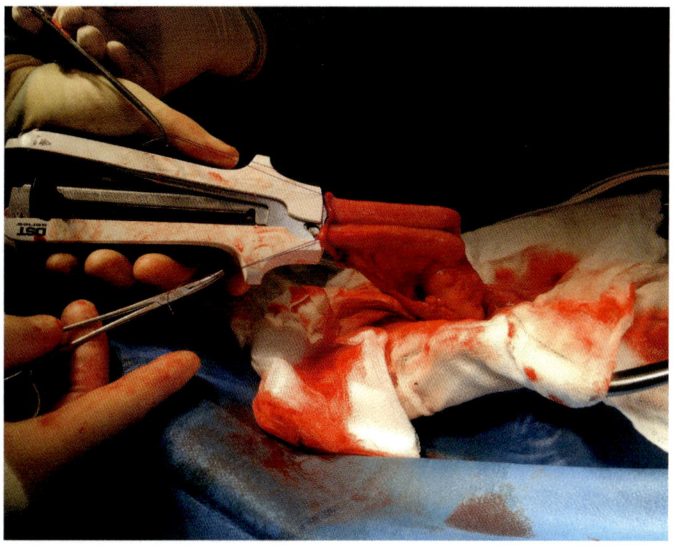

Figure 11.43 Introduction of the arms of the GIA stapling device into each intestinal loop.

Video 11.22. The arms of the GIA stapling device are inserted into each bowel loop and locked, with the staples on the antimesenteric side.

2. Once the GIA system is fired, it releases four staggered staple lines and cuts the intestine longitudinally, creating a lumen between the two intestinal loops. The length of the lumen depends on the length of the GIA arms.
3. The arms of the GIA system are removed, and the cut edges of the intestinal segments are then closed with a TA stapling system (Fig. 11.44; Video 11.23).

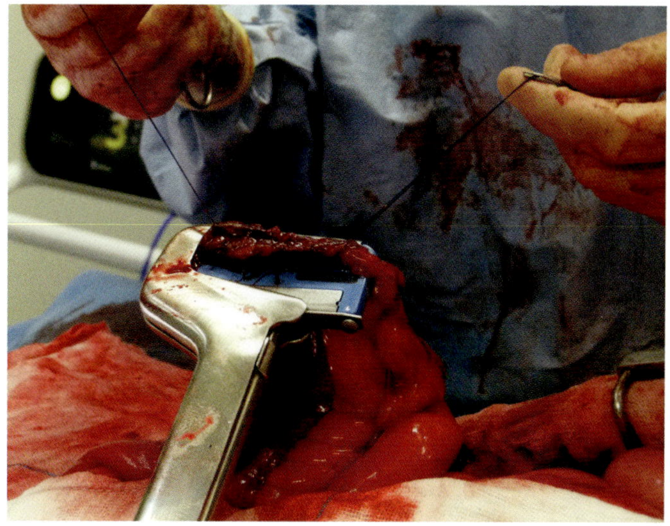

Figure 11.44 Closure of the cut edges of the intestinal segments using a TA stapling system.

Video 11.23. Closure of the cut edges of the intestinal segments using a TA stapling device.

4. The TA system produces an eversion of the intestinal edges. An inverting suture pattern can be performed over the staple line to reduce the risk of adhesion and leakage of intestinal contents (Video 11.24).[28]
5. Two interrupted sutures are placed at the distal junction of the two intestinal loops to decrease tension and reduce the risk of dehiscence along the staple line (Fig. 11.45; Video 11.25).[29]

The advantages of stapling systems compared to sutures are:

- They promote primary healing in the early postoperative period. In the inflammatory phase of healing, the force exerted by sutures decreases until the proliferative phase begins. In contrast, with stapling systems, there is a linear increase in the force exerted by the staples.
- They provide a greater burst strength in the early postoperative period.
- Staple anastomosis is faster to perform, reducing anesthetic time.

Video 11.24. Use of an inverting suture pattern over the staple line.

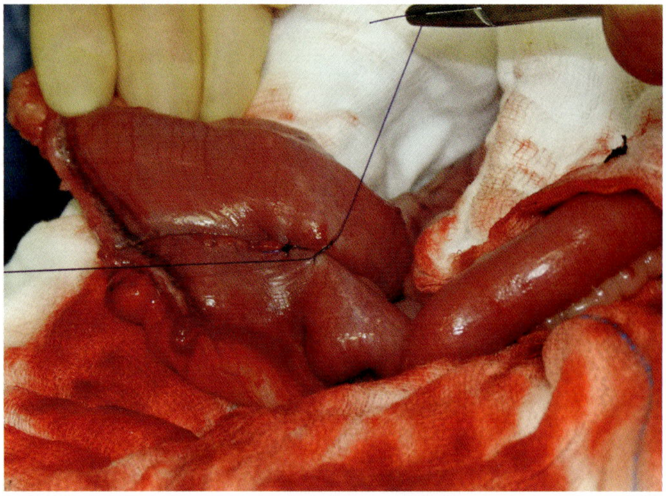

Figure 11.45 Placement of one or two interrupted sutures in the crotch of the anastomosis.

Video 11.25. Placement of two interrupted sutures at the distal junction of the two intestinal loops.

- There is less tissue handling.
- They can be used if there is a disparity in the intestinal lumen sizes.
- Stapled anastomosis is generally more reliable.

In case of septic peritonitis, the risk of anastomosis dehiscence is 35%–38%, while in patients without septic peritonitis the risk is 6%–9%. In patients with peritonitis, the risk of dehiscence of an anastomosis with sutures and with staples is 13%–28.9% and 5%–9.7%, respectively. Therefore, in the presence of septic peritonitis, a stapled anastomosis is likely a better choice.[30,31]

Colonic foreign body

Colonic foreign bodies are usually incidental findings with no clinical signs, and they typically do not require any treatment. However, if a colonic foreign body is causing clinical signs, it can be retrieved using endoscopy or, in case of a sharp object localized in the distal colon, with careful manual manipulation. Surgery should only be attempted if unavoidable.

Linear foreign body

In cats that present immediately after ingesting linear foreign material and show no signs of obstruction or peritonitis, conservative treatment can involve cutting the piece of string attached to the tongue. In 9 out of 19 cats (47%), the string passed through the intestine in 1–3 days; however, the remaining 10 cats required surgery due to deterioration of their condition, and one-third of them had perforation.[32] In dogs, linear foreign material is usually lodged in the pylorus, making surgical treatment necessary. These foreign bodies can affect a large segment of intestine, and if a significant portion needs to be resected, short-bowel syndrome should be considered. Due to the risk of perforation and subsequent septic peritonitis associated with linear foreign bodies, surgical treatment is recommended.

Surgical technique:

1. If the linear foreign body is attached to the tongue, it should be cut before performing abdominal surgery.
2. A midline celiotomy approach is made (see Chapter 3).
3. The plicated intestine is isolated from the abdominal cavity (Fig. 11.46).
4. An enterotomy is performed midway along the site of the plicated intestine on the antimesenteric side.
5. The string is identified, grasped with two hemostats, and then cut in the middle.
6. If the linear foreign body is attached to the pylorus, a gastrotomy at the level of the pylorus is performed. The material is identified and gently pulled from the stomach (Fig. 11.47).
7. Multiple enterotomies may be necessary to safely remove the foreign body. If the piece of string moves and comes out after applying gentle traction, it can be removed; otherwise, another enterotomy must be performed until the string can be safely removed without causing perforation of the intestine (Figs. 11.48 and 11.49).

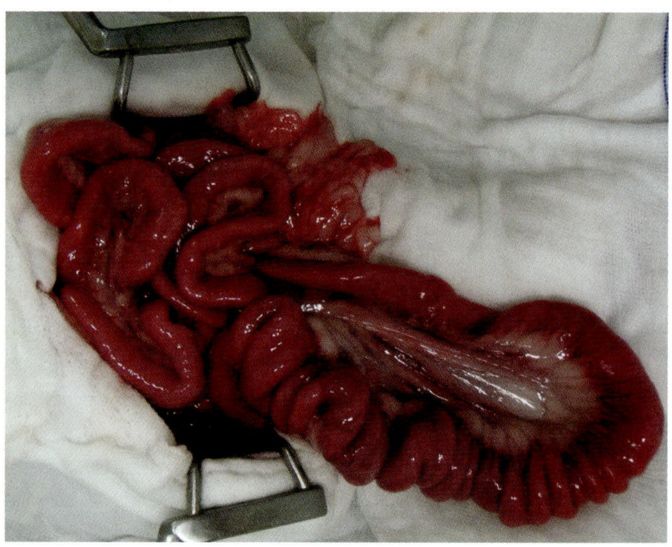

Figure 11.46 Isolation of the plicated section of intestine from the abdominal cavity.

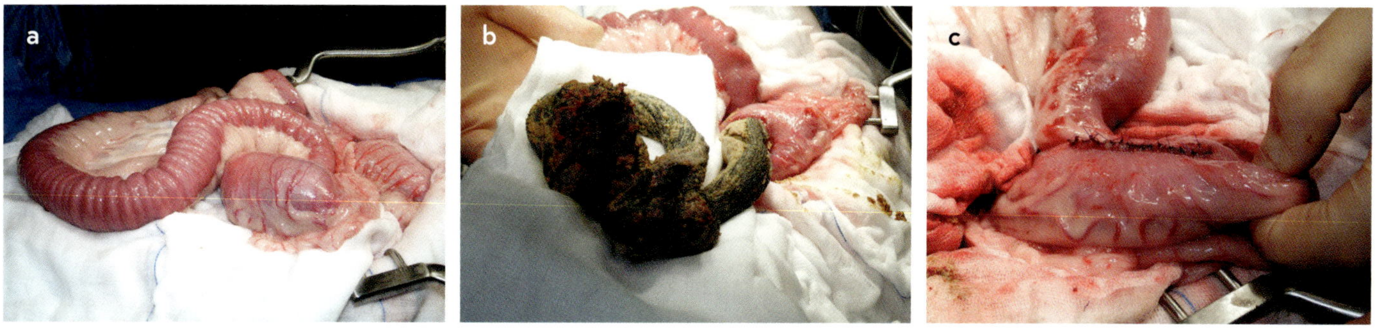

Figure 11.47 (a) Linear foreign body trapped in the pylorus of a dog. (b) A pyloric incision is performed and the linear material removed. (c) Pyloric incision sutured.

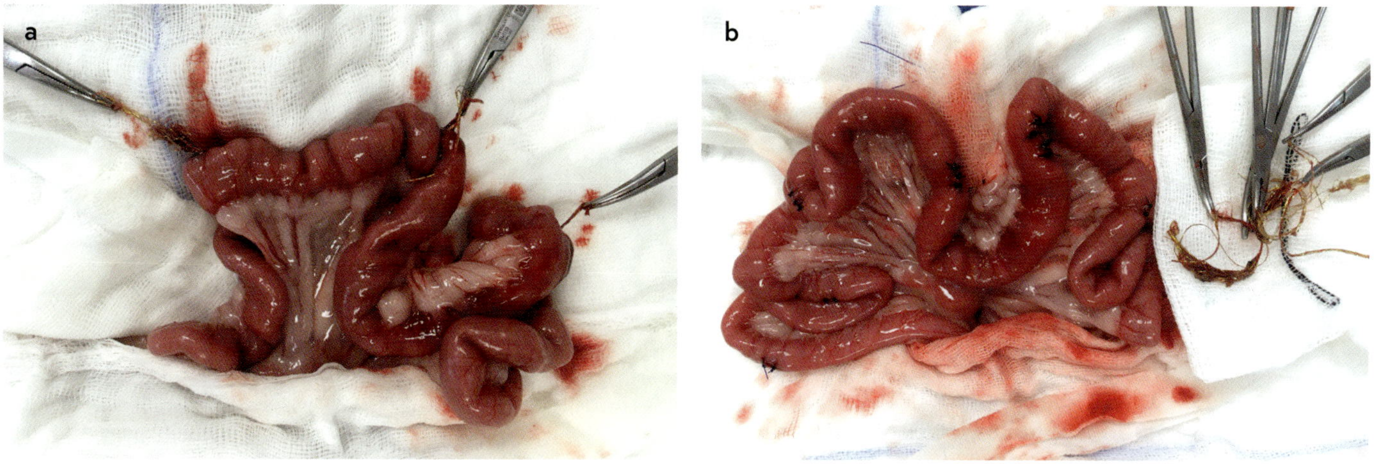

Figure 11.48 Removal of a linear foreign body through multiple enterotomies to avoid damaging the intestine.

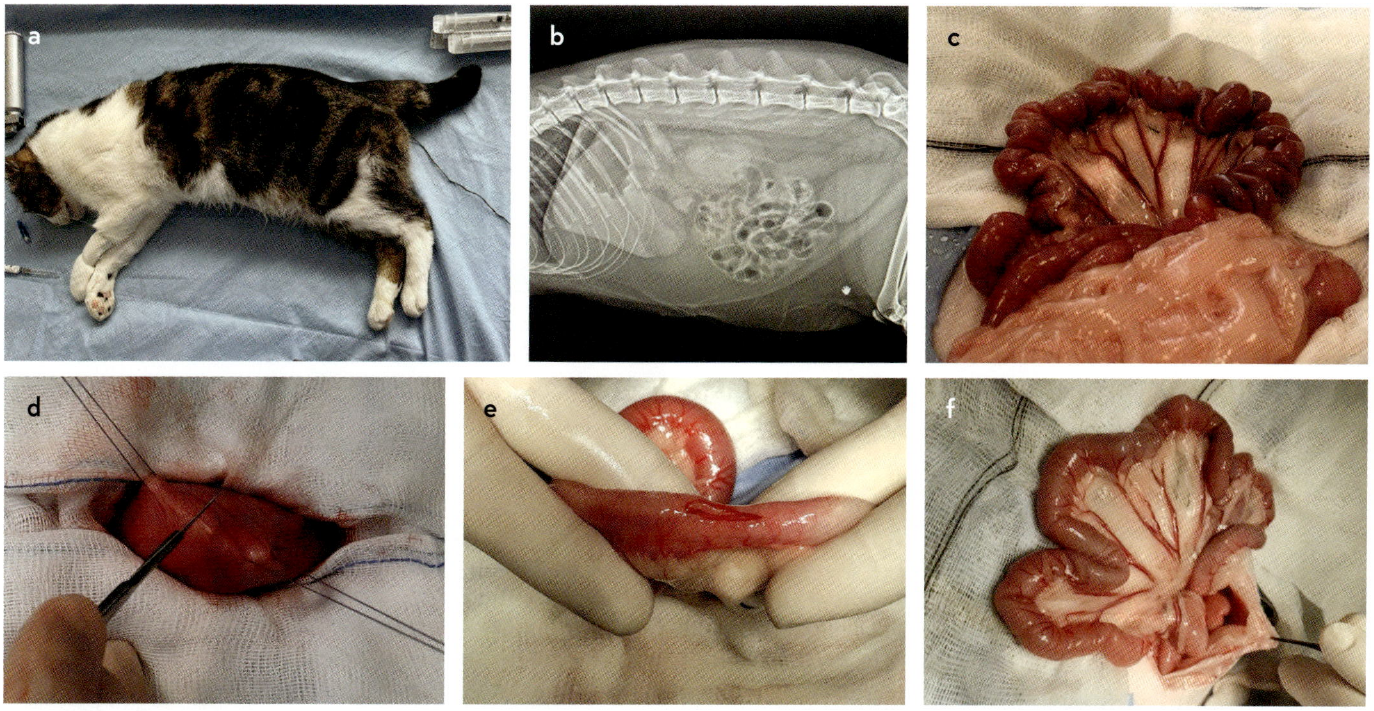

Figure 11.49 Linear foreign body in a cat. (a) The patient presented with kyphosis, and a linear foreign body was visible from the anus. (b) Radiography revealed intestinal plication. (c) Intraoperative image of small intestinal plication secondary to the foreign body. (d,e) Gastrotomy and enterotomy to release the anchor point of the foreign body. (f) Resolution of intestinal plication is observed.

8. After removing the piece of string, the mesenteric side of the intestine is evaluated for perforations.
9. If no perforations are found, the enterotomy incisions can be sutured (see "Enterotomy" section above).
10. If perforations are present, a section of intestine will need to be resected and anastomosed (see "Enterectomy" section above).
11. The abdomen is copiously lavaged and closed routinely.

Postoperative management

After surgery, correction of fluid, electrolytes, and acid–base disturbances should be continued. If peritonitis was present, it should be treated with antibiotics and an abdominal closed-suction drain placed (see Chapter 16). If the patient is not vomiting, water and food can be offered 12 hours after anesthetic recovery. Appropriate analgesia should be provided.

Outcome

The prognosis after surgical retrieval of gastric foreign bodies is excellent. For intestinal foreign bodies, the prognosis is generally good, although it can become more complicated if there is necrotic tissue or septic peritonitis. The prognosis for cats with linear foreign bodies is good, with perforations being rare but increasing the risk of mortality if present. The prognosis for dogs with linear foreign bodies is guarded, as the likelihood of perforation and death is higher than in cats. Intestinal resection and anastomosis are required in more than 40% of dogs. Septic peritonitis following small intestinal surgery has been reported to occur in 7%–16% of cases, and factors such as the presence of peritonitis, intestinal foreign bodies, hypoalbuminemia, use of blood products, and delayed enteral feeding have been identified as possible predictors of GI leakage.[30]

Intussusception

Intestinal intussusception is a relatively common GI disorder in dogs and cats. It is characterized by the telescoping and invagination of one segment of the intestine (intussusceptum) into the lumen of an adjacent segment of intestine (intussuscipiens).[33] Intussusception is believed to be caused by changes in intestinal motility, often triggered by other conditions such as inflammation, infection (bacterial, parasitic, viral), neoplasia, foreign body, and surgery. The most frequently reported types of intussusception are ileocolic in dogs[33–35] and jejunojejunal in cats.[36] Imaging may be required to confirm the diagnosis. Appropriate emergency stabilization and surgical intervention are typically necessary.

Clinical presentation and diagnosis

The most common clinical signs of intussusception include anorexia, lethargy, vomiting, bloody diarrhea, and abdominal pain.[33–35] The severity and type of clinical signs partially depend on patient factors, the duration of the intussusception, and whether the obstruction is complete or incomplete.[33–35] Common physical examination findings associated with intussusception include dehydration, abdominal pain, hypothermia (in cats), presence of an abdominal mass, intestinal thickening, or distension.[34,36] While radiography may be a good initial screening test for GI disease, it is not a reliable method for diagnosing intussusception.[33] Ultrasound is the preferred diagnostic imaging modality due to its high specificity (97.8%), sensitivity (100%), and accuracy (98.4%).[37] Ultrasonographic findings typically include concentric rings in the transverse section (Fig. 11.50), forming a target-like structure consisting of a hyperechoic or anechoic center surrounded by multiple hyper- and hypoechoic concentric rings. Finally, careful attention should be paid to find or rule out the possible cause of intussusception to improve the success of treatment and avoid recurrence.

Treatment

Although some intussusceptions may resolve spontaneously, or after analgesic premedication and general anesthesia, definitive treatment generally involves surgery. Following appropriate patient stabilization, an abdominal exploratory laparotomy is warranted. The surgical technique is dictated by intraoperative findings and includes manual reduction or en bloc resection and anastomosis of the intussusception.

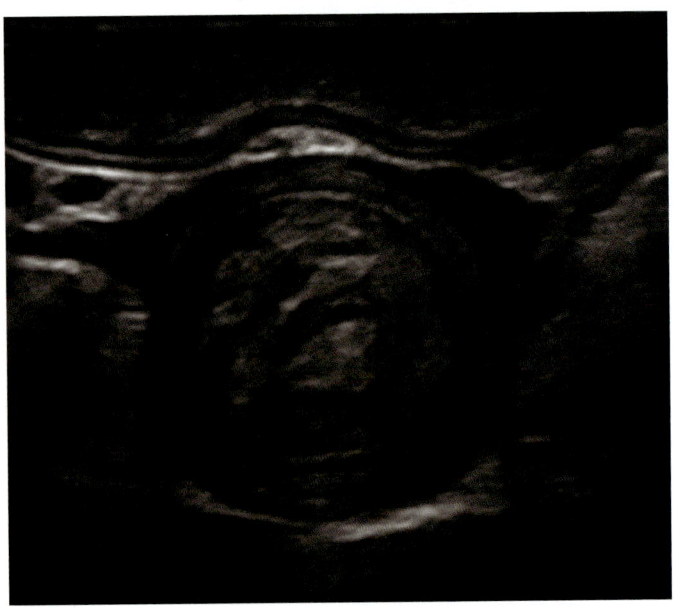

Figure 11.50 Ultrasound image of an intestinal intussusception showing concentric rings in the transverse section.

Surgical treatment

1. A midline celiotomy approach is made (see Chapter 3).
2. Complete assessment of the GI tract should be performed. In some cases, spontaneous resolution of intussusception is possible.
3. After identifying the intussusception, manual reduction with very gentle traction on the intussusceptum is attempted (Fig. 11.51; Video 11.26).
4. Resection and anastomosis are recommended when portions of the intestine are likely to be necrotic, nonviable, or not reducible (see "Enterectomy" section above) (Fig. 11.52; Video 11.27). Subjective criteria for evaluating intestinal viability include intestinal wall thickness, intestinal color (Fig. 11.53), and the presence of peristalsis (pinch test) and vascular pulsation.
5. In selected cases, an enteroplication technique may be performed to reduce the incidence of future recurrences. However, it should be considered that a study investigating the complications and recurrence rates in 35 dogs with intussusception found no significant differences in the rate of recurrence between patients who did or did not undergo en-

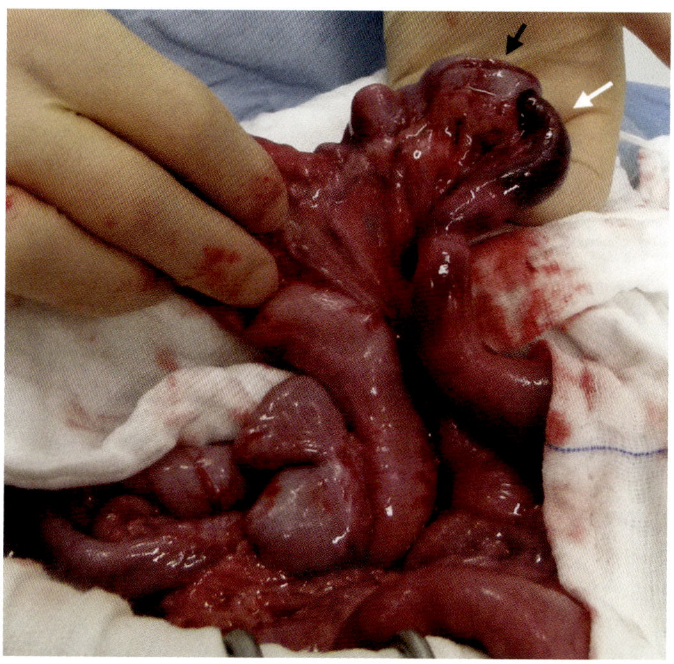

Figure 11.51 Intraoperative image of an intestinal intussusception in a dog, showing the intussusceptum (white arrow) and the intussuscipiens (black arrow).

Video 11.26. Manual reduction of an intestinal intussusception.

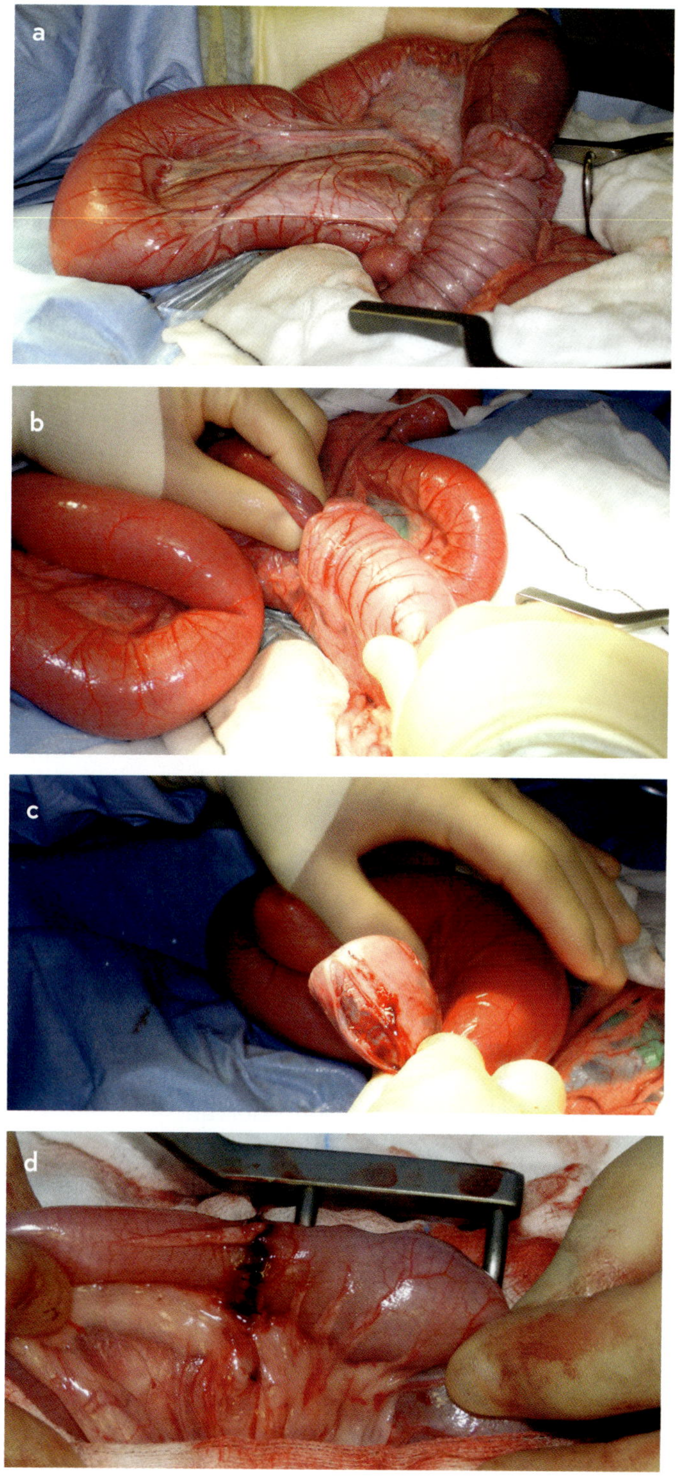

Figure 11.52 (a) Intestinal intussusception in a dog. (b) Manual reduction. (c) Intestinal antimesenteric edge laceration. (d) Enterectomy.

Video 11.27. Resection and functional end-to-end anastomosis with Endo GIA of a nonreducible intestinal intussusception in a cat.

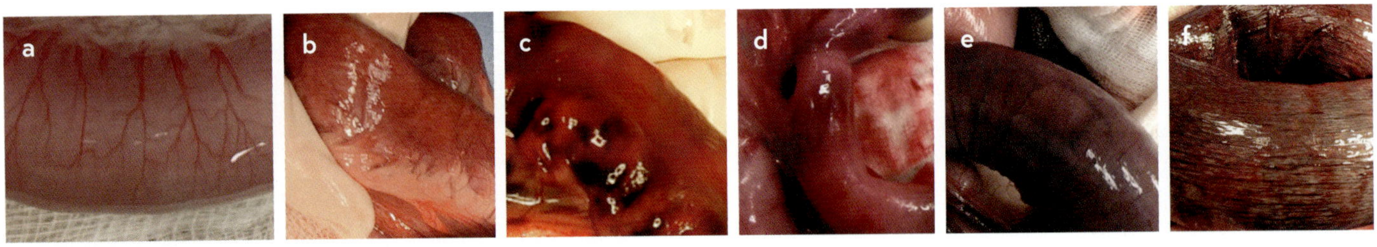

Figure 11.53 Assessment of intestinal viability based on color, ranging from (a) normal viable to (f) nonviable necrotic.

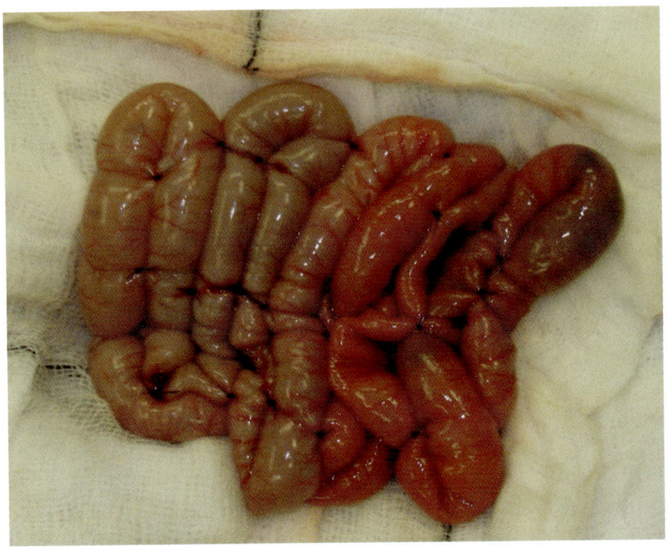

Figure 11.54 Enteroplication of the small intestine.

teroplication. Moreover, life-threatening complications related to enteroplication, such as strangulation and obstruction, were observed.[38,39]

a. The small intestine is arranged in gentle loops side by side from the duodenocolic ligament to the level of the ileum.
b. Adjacent loops of intestine are sutured together midway between the mesenteric and antimesenteric borders with simple interrupted sutures, engaging the submucosa (Fig. 11.54).

6. For ileocolic intussusception associated with cecal inversion, the following treatment techniques are possible:
   - Manual reduction.
   - Resection and anastomosis of necrotic, nonviable, or not reducible sections (see "Enterectomy" section above).
   - Antimesenteric colotomy to facilitate reduction of the intestine and cecum, followed by typhlectomy of the necrotic/nonviable cecum using a stapler or blade incision and suturing of the colon (Fig. 11.55).
7. Histopathologic examination of the resected intestinal section should be performed.

Postoperative management

After surgery, correction of fluid, electrolyte, and acid–base disturbances should be continued. If peritonitis is present, it should be treated with antibiotics and an abdominal closed-suction drain can be placed (see Chapter 16). If the patient is not vomiting, water and food can be offered 12 hours after anesthetic recovery.

Outcome

The prognosis for animals that have undergone uncomplicated reduction or resection of small intestinal intussusception is good.[34] Recurrence rates range from 3% to 27%.[38,39] Recurrence is usually noted within 3 days of surgery but has been reported up to 3 weeks after surgery.[33] It appears that recurrence may be more frequent in patients undergoing manual reduction rather than resection and anastomosis, but no other specific risk factors for recurrence have been identified.[39] Enteroplication may decrease recurrence rates, but it can be associated with serious complications.[38,39]

Gastric dilatation–volvulus

Gastric dilatation–volvulus (GDV) is a life-threatening disease in dogs that occurs most commonly in large-breed, deep-chested animals. It involves the trapping of air within the lumen of the stomach, which rotates on its axis, resulting in a rapid increase of intraluminal pressure, gastric malpositioning, compression of the diaphragm and caudal vena cava, and impaired respiratory and cardiovascular function. The exact sequence of events—whether the stomach rotates first or distension develops first—remains uncertain, and there is supportive evidence for both theories.[40–43] Although various risk factors have been studied, the etiology and pathophysiology of GDV are not completely understood. Specific risk factors identified in dogs include purebred large or giant breed, high thoracic depth:width ratio, history of GDV in a first-degree relative, feeding few meals per day, rapid eating, aggressive or fearful temperament, small food particle size, increased hepatogastric ligament length, and exercise or stress after a meal.[40–44]

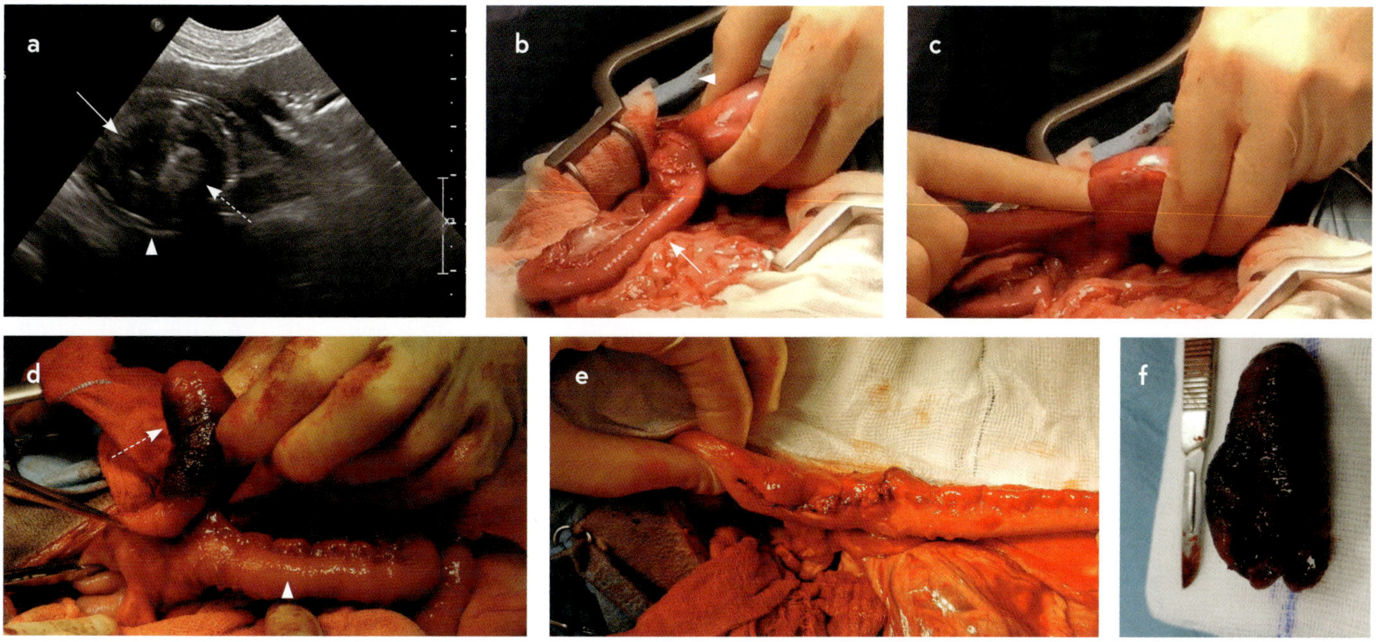

Figure 11.55 (a) Ultrasound image in transverse section showing cecal inversion and ileocolic intussusception (colon, white arrowhead; ileal intussusceptum, white arrow; inverted cecum, dashed white arrow). (b) Inverted cecum in association with ileocolic intussusception (colon, white arrowhead; ileum, white arrow). (c) Manual reduction failed to resolve the intussusception. (d) Antimesenteric proximal colotomy for reduction of the intussusception. Note the inverted necrotic cecum (dashed white arrow). The ileum was healthy, with minimal serosal inflammation (white arrowhead). (e) After typhlectomy, the colon was sutured using a simple interrupted pattern. (f) Necrotic cecum after excision.

The pathophysiology of GDV is complex and involves multiple organ systems. Gastric distension leads to increased abdominal pressure and decreased venous return, resulting in cardiogenic shock. Pressure on the diaphragm hampers inspiration, leading to decreased oxygen delivery. Portal hypertension causes venous stasis, mucosal damage, bacterial translocation through the GI tract, and decreased clearance of bacteria and endotoxins. Increased intragastric pressure reduces blood flow in the gastric wall, leading to gastric wall necrosis. After repositioning the stomach and restoring blood blow, reperfusion injury can occur.[40–44]

Clinical presentation and diagnosis

Dogs with GDV commonly present with clinical signs of gastric distension, nonproductive retching, hypersalivation, restlessness, anxiousness, and stretching. Sign severity depends on the duration of the condition and the stage of shock at the time of presentation. Physical examination findings vary based on disease severity and shock stage. Radiographs with the dog in right lateral recumbency are usually used to confirm the diagnosis. Pylorus malpositioning, with gas entrapped, can be visualized as a typical double bubble or reverse C appearance (Fig. 11.56). Laboratory findings are primarily related to hypotension and its effects. Hemoconcentration, a stress leukogram, and thrombocytopenia may be observed. Hepatocellular damage can lead to increased alanine aminotransferase (ALT) and total bilirubin levels. Azotemia with elevated blood urea nitrogen (BUN) and creatinine levels may be present. Electrolyte disturbances and coagu-

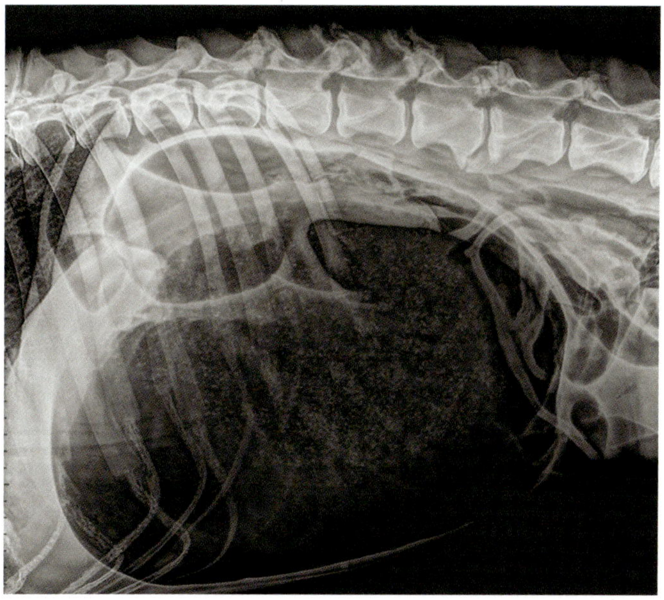

Figure 11.56 Right lateral abdominal radiograph showing gastric dilatation–volvulus. Note the characteristic double bubble or reverse C appearance caused by dorsal displacement of the pylorus.

lation abnormalities can vary among patients. Plasma lactate levels are usually increased in patients with GDV and can potentially serve as a prognostic indicator. Electrocardiographic abnormalities (cardiac ventricular arrhythmias) have been reported in 40%–70% of dogs with GDV.[40–44]

Treatment

Medical management of GDV is aimed at stabilizing the patient before surgery and should be initiated simultaneously with diagnostics. Treatment focuses on restoring perfusion through fluid therapy and on providing analgesia. Venous access is established through at least two large-bore catheters in either the cephalic or jugular veins to facilitate rapid fluid resuscitation. Intravascular volume expansion and maintenance are achieved using a crystalloid solution (e.g., sodium chloride or lactated Ringer's solution at a rate of 45–90 mL/kg/h) combined with a colloid (e.g., hypertonic saline 7% at a dose of 4–5 mL/kg over 5–15 minutes, or hydroxyethyl starch at a dose of 10–20 mL/kg). Systemic parameters such as blood pressure and heart rate should be monitored to assess the response to fluid therapy. Oxygen supplementation is provided using flow-by methods, and the electrocardiogram is monitored for cardiac arrythmias, which can be treated accordingly.[40–44] Broad-spectrum antibiotics and intravenous analgesia, such as methadone, are administered.

Gastric decompression is performed after initiating fluid resuscitation using either orogastric intubation or percutaneous placement of an over-the-needle catheter or trocar into the gas-distended stomach. Most animals tolerate orogastric intubation; however, general anesthesia and endotracheal intubation is strongly recommended to reduce the risk of aspiration pneumonia during gastric decompression. A large-diameter tube with end and side holes is premeasured from the nose to the last rib. The tube is lubricated and passed through the mouth, and the dog is stimulated to swallow the tube into the esophagus. The tube should not be advanced beyond the premeasured and marked point. If passing the tube through the rotated caudal esophageal sphincter is not possible, decompression can be achieved by percutaneous placement of a large-bore needle or catheter (14–16 gauge) caudal to the ribs in the most distended and tympanic area.[41]

The overlying skin should be shaved, cleaned, and disinfected before the procedure.

Once the patient is stabilized, anesthesia is induced for surgical correction of the malpositioned stomach followed by gastropexy. Generally, surgery is initiated as soon as possible; however, a recent study suggested that surgery can be delayed with adequate supportive therapy in selected cases.[45]

Surgical technique

1. A cranial midline celiotomy is performed (see Chapter 3).
2. Identification of the malpositioned and rotated stomach is facilitated by the presence of omentum covering the ventral surface (Fig. 11.57).
3. Prior to derotation, it is essential to achieve full gastric decompression. A nonsterile assistant can pass an orogastric tube through the patient's mouth, and the surgeon can manipulate the tube as it passes from the esophagus into the cardia. This maneuver allows for the emptying of fluid and food from the stomach, facilitating the derotation process.
4. Derotation is performed by locating and retracting the pylorus toward the right side of the abdomen while simultaneously pushing the stomach body dorsally with the other hand. Palpation of the gastroesophageal junction aids in determining whether the stomach is completely derotated. The orogastric tube can also assist in identifying the gastroesophageal junction.
5. Following derotation, a thorough abdominal examination should be performed to identify any additional abnormalities and allow adequate time for reperfusion of the stomach and spleen. Assessment of gastric and splenic viability is crucial and involves visual and tactile inspection. The dorsal side of the stomach wall should also be inspected. Subjective

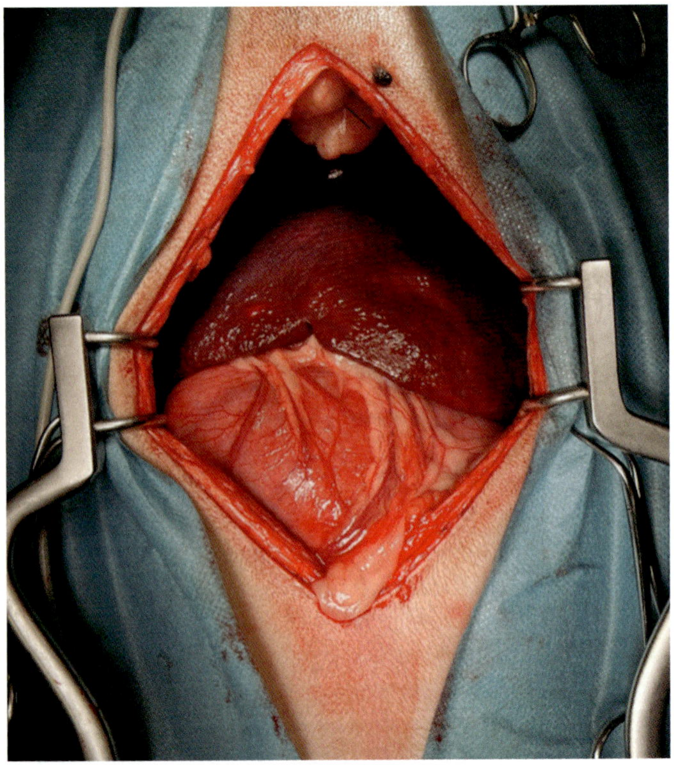

Figure 11.57 Intraoperative image of a rotated stomach covered by omentum. Image courtesy of Krista van Blokland-Post.

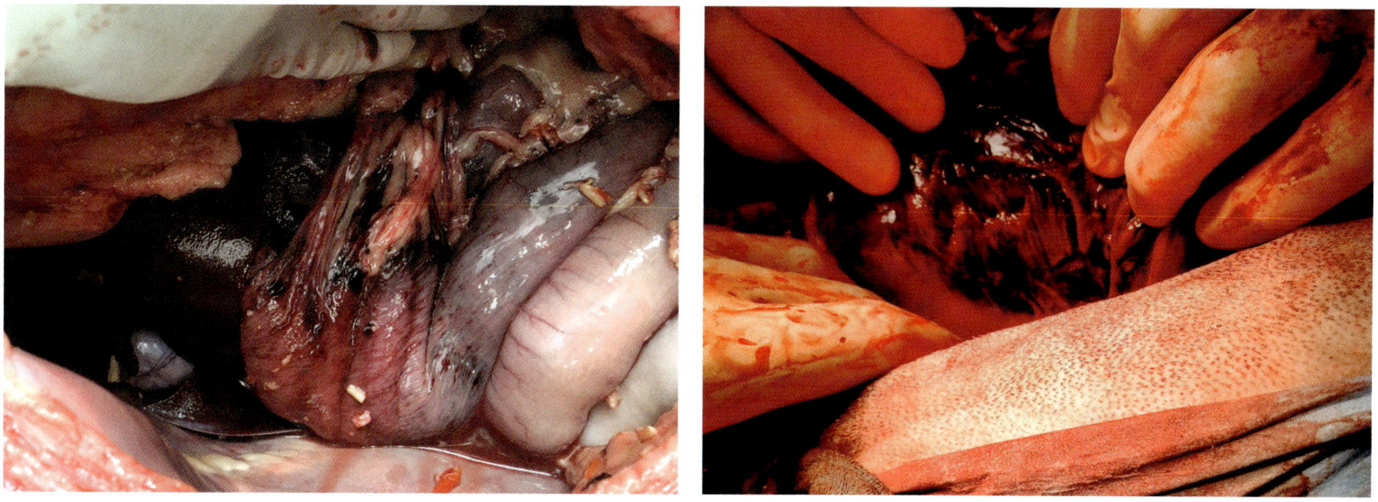

Figure 11.58 Intraoperative images showing gastric necrosis in a patient with gastric dilatation–volvulus. Images courtesy of Lucinda van Stee.

criteria for evaluating stomach viability include gastric wall thickness, serosal surface color, evidence of serosal capillary perfusion, and the presence of peristalsis. Devitalized stomach wall appears thin, gray, or green and should be resected until bleeding occurs (Fig. 11.58).

6. If thrombosis is detected in the splenic vessels, splenectomy may be necessary.
7. Partial gastrectomy may be warranted. The stomach is isolated with moistened swabs to prevent leakage and stay sutures are placed around the proposed resection site. Vessels to the affected area are ligated. The affected tissue is sharply excised with scissors or a scalpel blade, ensuring that the edges bleed actively. The defect is closed using two layers of 2-0 or 3-0 absorbable sutures or a stapling device.
8. Another technique involves invaginating the affected portion of the stomach by folding inward the affected area and suturing healthy tissue over it using two layers of a simple continuous or inverting suture pattern (2-0 or 3-0 absorbable monofilament; e.g., polydioxanone). Although this technique is easier and quicker, it may result in significant melena up to 2 weeks following the procedure.
9. A gastropexy should be performed to create a permanent adhesion between the pyloric antrum and the right abdominal wall. Several gastropexy techniques have been described, including incisional gastropexy, belt-loop gastropexy, modified belt-loop gastropexy, circumcostal gastropexy, modified circumcostal gastropexy, incorporating gastropexy, tube gastropexy, and gastrocolopexy (see below). To ensure a durable adhesion, the muscularis of the stomach must be in contact with the muscles of the abdominal wall. The authors prefer incisional gastropexy due to its simplicity and efficiency.
10. Routine closure of the abdomen is performed.

Surgical technique: Gastropexy

Incisional gastropexy (Video 11.28)[43,44,46]

1. A 4–5 cm seromuscular incision is made in the antrum between the vasculature of the greater and lesser curvatures, without penetrating the gastric lumen (Fig. 11.59).

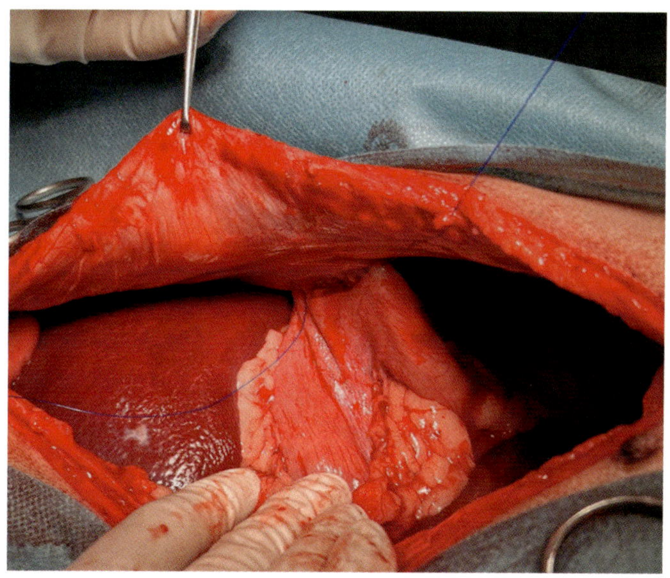

Figure 11.59 Incisional gastropexy between the pyloric antrum and right abdominal wall. Image courtesy of Krista van Blokland-Post.

Video 11.28. Incisional gastropexy.

2. The stomach is manually apposed against the right abdominal wall to estimate the anatomical position of the stomach.
3. A second incision (in a craniocaudal or ventrodorsal direction, as the surgeon prefers) is created on the right abdominal wall at the appropriate site through the peritoneum and transversus abdominis muscle, staying 2–4 cm caudal to the last rib to prevent pneumothorax. The abdominal wall can be lifted with towel clamps or Allis tissue forceps to facilitate appropriate dorsal placement of the incision.
4. The incisions are approximated with two continuous suture lines of 2-0 or 0 absorbable or nonabsorbable monofilament. To aid visualization, the dorsal suture line is closed first (Fig. 11.60).

Belt-loop gastropexy[43,44,46]

1. A seromuscular flap is created in the antrum region by making two parallel 4 cm long incisions 3 cm apart, connecting them in the most cranial aspect.
2. The flap is undermined from the underlying mucosal layer.
3. Two 5 cm long incisions are created in the abdominal wall through the peritoneum and transversus abdominis muscle, 3 cm apart.
4. A tunnel is made between these incisions by undermining the tissue in between.
5. A stay suture is placed in the free end of the flap, and the flap is passed through the tunnel.
6. The flap is sutured back to the site where it was elevated using 2-0 or 3-0 monofilament suture in a simple interrupted or continuous pattern.

Modified belt-loop gastropexy (Fig. 11.61; Video 11.29)[47]

1. Two parallel incisions (4–5 cm long and 2 cm apart) are made through the peritoneum and transversus abdominis muscle on the right abdominal wall, 2 cm caudal to the costal arch and 5 cm from the linea alba. The incisions should be oriented obliquely ventrodorsally and craniocaudally.
2. A tunnel is created between these incisions by undermining the tissue in between.
3. After passing Allis tissue forceps through the tunnel from caudal to cranial, a seromuscular fold of the antral wall is grasped.
4. The forceps with the fold are pulled back through the tunnel, and the fold is sutured to both the greater curvature of the stomach and the cut edge of the abdominal wall with 0 or 2-0 nonabsorbable mono-

Video 11.29. Modified belt-loop gastropexy. Video courtesy of Luca Formaggini.

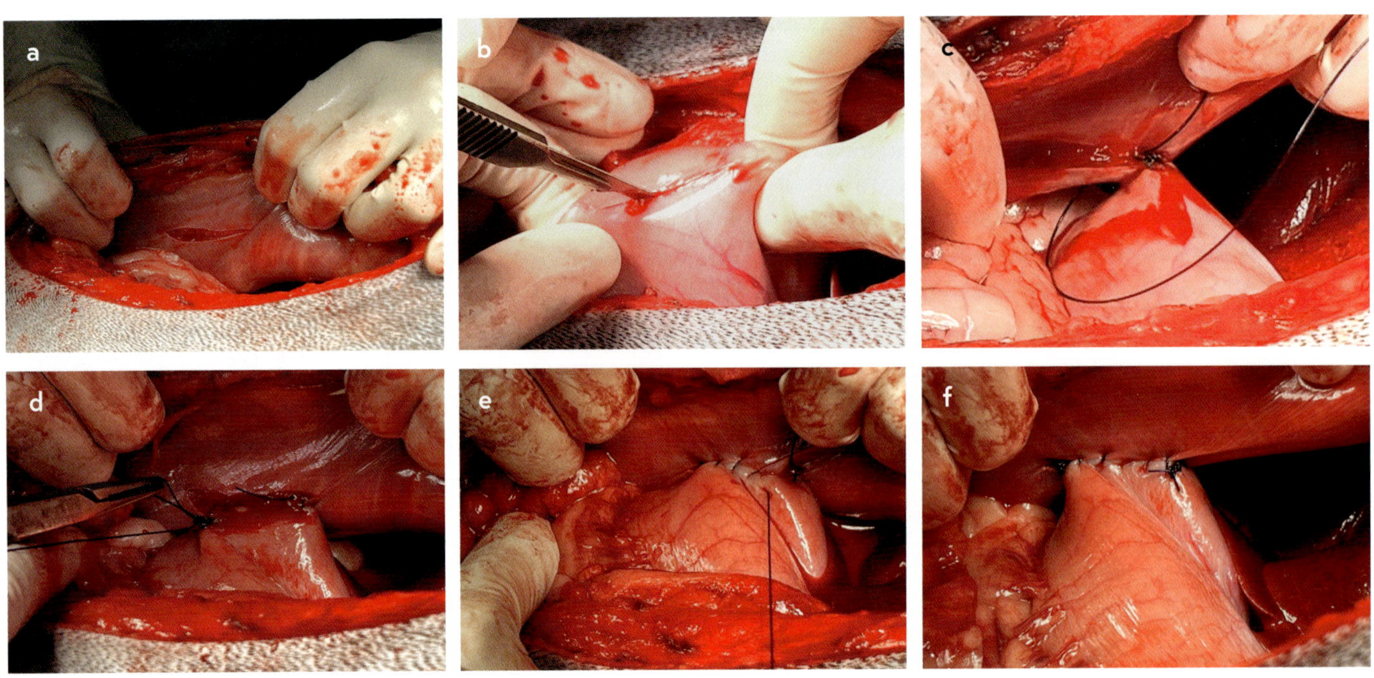

Figure 11.60 Incisional gastropexy. (a) Creation of a 4–5 cm incision in the right abdominal wall, 2–3 cm caudal to the last rib. (b) Creation of a seromuscular incision in the pyloric antrum. (c–f) The incisions are apposed with two continuous suture lines using absorbable or nonabsorbable material.

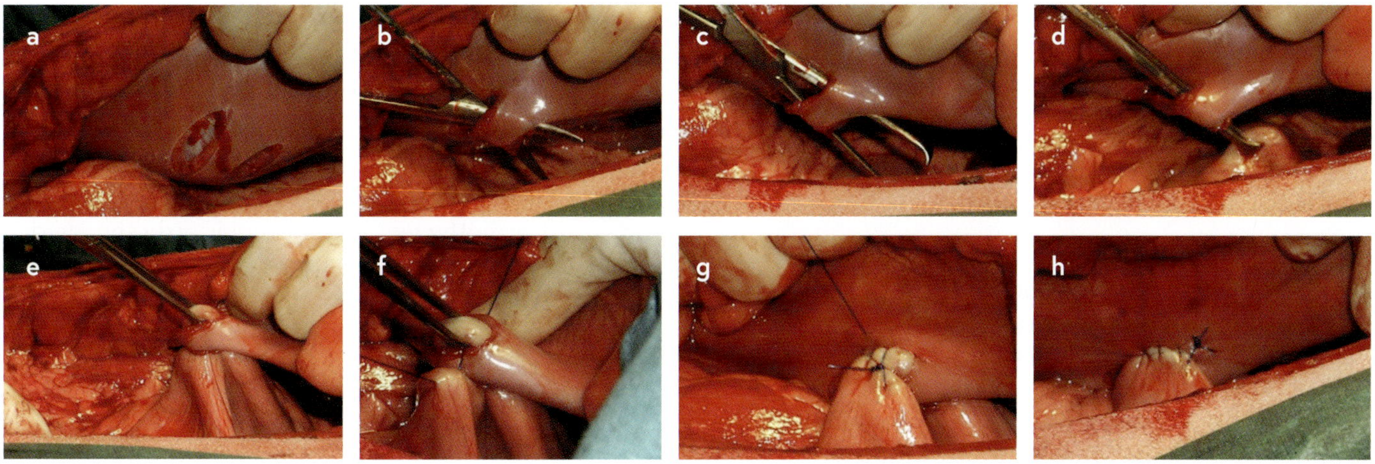

Figure 11.61 Modified belt-loop gastropexy. (a) Creation of two parallel incisions on the right abdominal wall. (b) Creation of a tunnel between the incisions. (c,d) Passage of Allis tissue forceps through the tunnel to grasp a seromuscular fold of the pyloric antrum. (e–h) Pulling back of the forceps and fold through the tunnel and suturing of the fold to the greater curvature of the stomach and the cut edge of abdominal wall in a continuous pattern. Images courtesy of Luca Formaggini and *Journal of the American Animal Hospital Association* 2018; 54(5):239–245.

filament material in a continuous pattern from caudal to cranial. Each bite should include the serosa and muscularis of the stomach, the serosa and muscularis of the fold, the fascia and muscular tissue of the transversus abdominis muscle, and the peritoneum.

Circumcostal gastropexy[43,48] and modified circumcostal gastropexy[49]

1. A seromuscular flap of stomach wall is created as described before. The modified technique involves the use of a seromuscular fold of the antral wall (Fig. 11.62).[49]
2. A 5–6 cm incision is made over the 11th or 12th rib on the right side, at the level of the costochondral junction.
3. The tissue around the rib is bluntly dissected, staying in close contact to the rib. Care should be taken to avoid creation of a pneumothorax or rib fracture.
4. A stay suture is placed in the free end of the flap or fold of the antral wall (modified technique) and the flap is passed from cranial to caudal through the tunnel around the rib.
5. The flap is sutured back to the site where it was elevated in a simple interrupted or continuous pat-

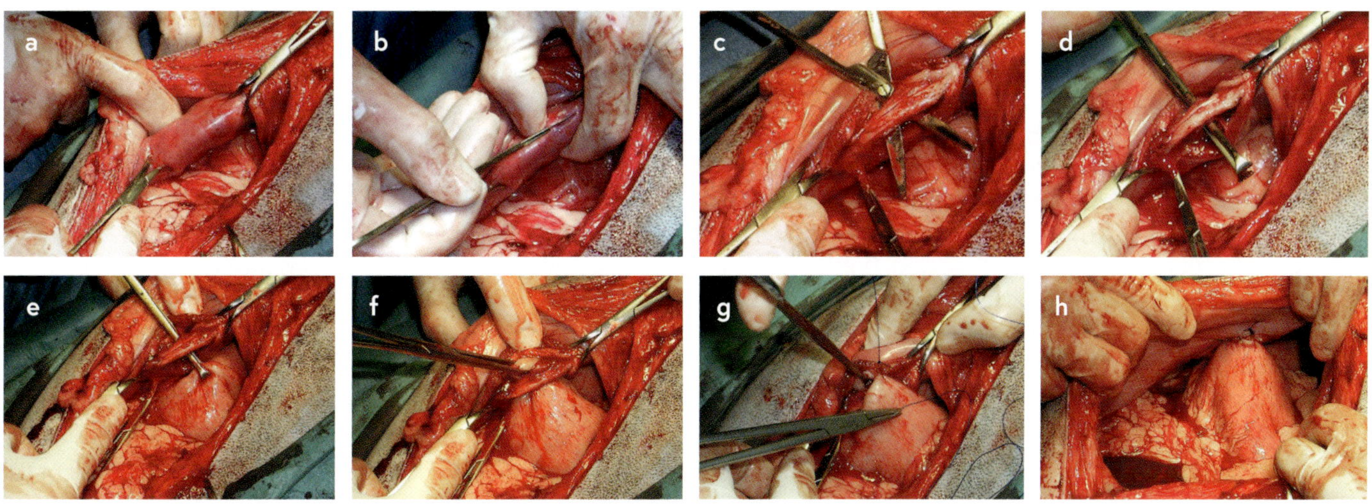

Figure 11.62 Modified circumcostal gastropexy. (a) Isolation and visualization of the last palpable rib. (b) Incision over the isolated rib using a scalpel blade. (c) Creation of a 3 cm wide tunnel under the rib by sharp dissection with a scalpel or scissors. (d) Passage of Allis tissue forceps from lateral to medial through the tunnel under the rib. (e) Grasping of a 3 cm wide fold of stomach in the region of the pyloric antrum using the forceps. (f) Pulling of the fold through the tunnel and wrap around the rib. (g,h) After creating three or four incisions (each 1 cm) through the serosa and muscularis on each side of the fold, the suture is passed through the stomach, the gastric fold, and the abdominal wall. Images courtesy of Luca Formaggini.

tern using 2-0 or 3-0 monofilament. If the modified technique is used, multiple sutures are applied involving the serosa and muscularis of the stomach, the serosa and muscularis of the fold, the fascia and muscular tissue of the transversus abdominis muscle, and the peritoneum.

Incorporating gastropexy[43,50]

Upon abdominal closure, approximately 5 cm of gastric wall of the pyloric antrum should be included in the cranial linea alba closure, with absorbable suture material (2-0 or 3-0 monofilament). This technique is not recommended if other techniques are available due to the high risk of complications (adhesion formation and risk of gastric entry in future surgeries).

Gastrocolopexy[43,48]

The transverse colon is brought in apposition with the greater curvature of the stomach. This technique is less recommended due to the possible risk of recurrence.

1. The greater omentum is tucked dorsolateral to the transverse colon.
2. The surfaces of the stomach and colon are scarified at the proposed pexy site with a number 11 scalpel blade.
3. 10–15 cm of stomach wall is sutured to the colon wall with interrupted polypropylene sutures, spaced approximately 0.5 cm apart, including the serosal and muscular layers only.

Tube gastropexy[51]

1. A skin stab incision is created 3–4 cm caudal to the last rib and lateral to the ventral midline.
2. Using mosquito forceps, the tip of a tube (de Pezzer mushroom-tipped catheter or Foley catheter, 24 or 26 gauge) is passed into the abdominal cavity through the incision.
3. A purse-string suture is preplaced in the pyloric antrum (2-0 absorbable material). A stab incision is made into the stomach through the purse-string suture, and the catheter tip is placed into the lumen. The purse-string suture is tied tightly around the catheter; if using a Foley catheter, the bulb is inflated with saline.
4. Multiple absorbable monofilament pexy sutures (4–5 simple interrupted sutures) are preplaced and tightened around the gastric and abdominal wall incisions.
5. The pexy site is omentalized.
6. The mushroom tip or balloon is drawn up to the stomach wall, and the tube is secured on the outside of the skin with a finger-trap suture (see Chapter 5).
7. The gastropexy tube should remain in place for 10–14 days. The tube is removed by traction and the stoma left to heal by secondary intention.

Postoperative management

After surgery, fluid therapy should be continued to maintain the hydration status and correct any remaining electrolyte imbalances. If the dog recovers well, fluid therapy can be discontinued after 24 hours.[46] Continuous electrocardiography is used to monitor the development of arrhythmias, as ventricular arrhythmias can occur up to 72 hours after surgery. If needed, arrhythmias are treated medically with lidocaine or procainamide. Arterial blood pressure should be monitored, especially in patients with septic shock before surgery or in cases that required gastrectomy, and supported with inotropes to maintain mean arterial pressure above 60 mmHg.[43,44,52]

Parameters such as pulse rate and quality, respiratory rate, temperature, mucous membrane color, capillary refill time, and evidence of abdominal distension should be closely monitored to detect complications at an early stage.[46,52,53]

Postoperative analgesia should be provided with opioids, such as morphine, buprenorphine, methadone, or fentanyl. Additionally, constant-rate infusions of lidocaine or ketamine can be used for adjunctive analgesia. Nonsteroidal anti-inflammatory drugs should be avoided to prevent GI and renal side effects,[50] but they can be prescribed for further postoperative analgesia after discharge once the dog has fully recovered from surgery and remains stable.[46] Feeding can be resumed 12–24 hours postoperatively. Histamine (H_2) receptor blockers and sucralfate can be used in case of gastric mucosal damage or partial gastrectomy.[40,43,46,52]

Outcome

Complications reported after GDV surgery include prolonged hypotension, cardiac arrhythmias, ileus or abnormal gastric motility, vomiting and aspiration pneumonia, peritonitis, sepsis, and disseminated intravascular coagulation, and additional treatment or reoperation may be necessary.[43,44,46,53]

Mortality rates of GDV are around 10%–20%, and approximately 80% of the surgically treated cases survive to discharge.[40,43,54] Negative prognostic factors include hyperlactatemia, the need for splenectomy or partial gastrectomy, gastric perforation and sepsis, increased duration of clinical signs before hospital admission, hypotension, and arrhythmias.[40,43,53] Recurrence rates are similar between surgical techniques, with approximately 8% for incisional gastropexy,[55] 9% for circumcostal gastropexy, and 20% for gastrocolopexy.[48]

Rectal prolapse

Rectal prolapse can be partial or complete. In the former, also known as anal prolapse, only the anal mucosa protrudes through the anal orifice. In the latter, a cylindrical mass comprising all layers of the rectum circumferentially protrudes through the anal orifice.[56] Spontaneous resolution is unlikely due to swelling caused by edema formation. There is a higher incidence of rectal prolapse in younger animals, particularly in those with underlying GI disease such as parasites. Prolapse commonly occurs secondary to tenesmus, which may be due to underlying GI or urogenital disease or as a result of surgery.[56,57]

Clinical presentation and diagnosis

Patients with partial rectal prolapse exhibit red and swollen mucosa protruding from the anus after defecation. Animals with complete rectal prolapse present with an elongated, cylindrical mass protruding from the anus (Fig. 11.63). Initially, the protruding tissue appears swollen and red, but laceration, hemorrhage, necrosis, and ulceration can occur due to trauma and/or self-mutilation. To differentiate rectal prolapse from prolapse of an intussusception of the colon or small intestine, a finger or blunt instrument can be gently passed between the prolapse and the anus. In the case of rectal prolapse, the instrument cannot be passed because the prolapsed tissues converge with the mucocutaneous junction of the anus. Conversely, in cases of intussusception, the instrument can easily be passed 5–7 cm between the rectal wall and the prolapsed tissue (Fig. 11.64).[56,57] The diagnosis of rectal prolapse is relatively straightforward, but identifying the underlying cause can be more challenging. However, it is essential to investigate underlying diseases to achieve a permanent cure and reduce the likelihood of recurrence.

Treatment

In addition to possible diagnostic workup and treatment of the underlying cause, the prolapsed tissue should be treated as an emergency. Manual reduction is often achievable when vital rectal tissue is present. However, if the tissue is necrotic or devitalized, rectal resection and anastomosis are required.

Surgical technique: Manual reduction

1. General or epidural anesthesia is required for this procedure.
2. The mucosal surface is cleaned with a warm isotonic solution.
3. The protruding mass is lubricated, and gentle pressure is applied for reduction.
4. After reduction, an appropriately sized test tube or syringe case is temporarily placed in the anal orifice, and a 3-0 or 2-0 nonabsorbable monofilament pure-string suture is inserted at the mucocutaneous junction to narrow the anal orifice (Fig. 11.65).
5. The purse-string suture is tightened sufficiently to prevent mucosal prolapse while still allowing soft feces to pass through the slightly narrowed orifice.
6. The suture is left in place for 3–5 days. The patient is fed a low-residue diet and given laxatives such as lactulose.
7. In the case of recurrence, colopexy can be performed (Fig. 11.66) (see Chapter 15).[58,59]

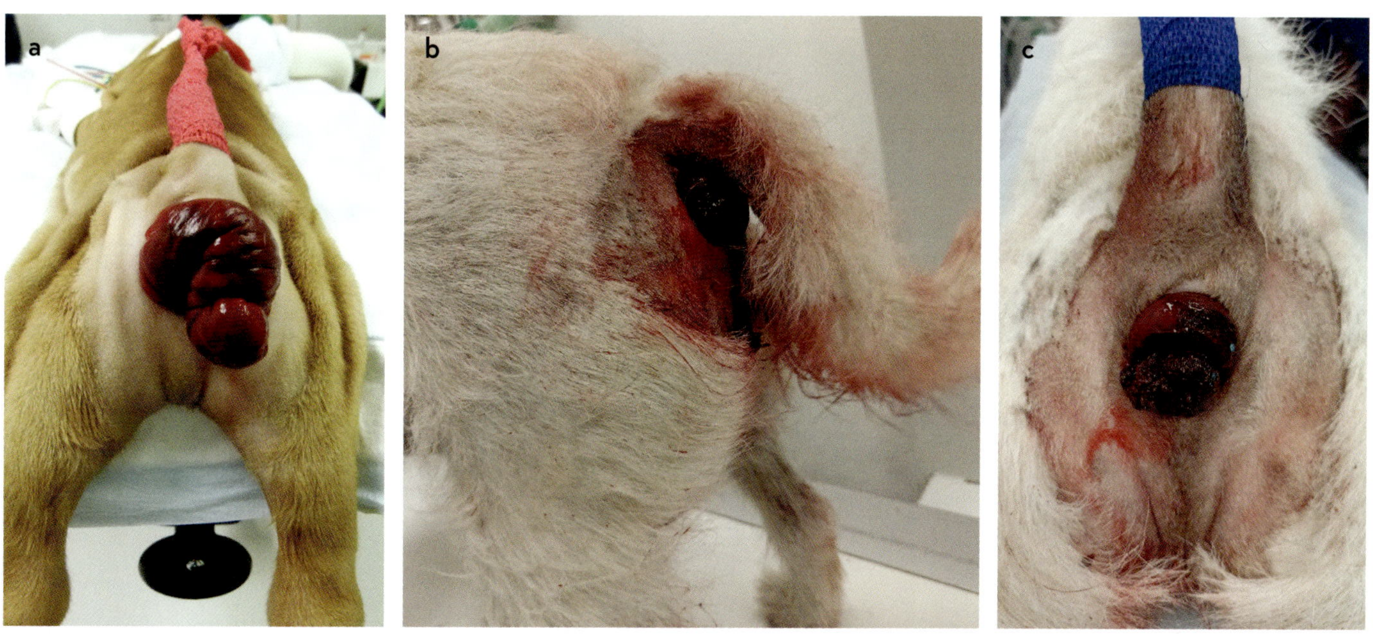

Figure 11.63 (a) Complete rectal prolapse in a dog, presenting as an elongated, cylindrical mass protruding from the anus. (b,c) Rectal prolapse in another case, with hemorrhage, necrosis, and ulceration.

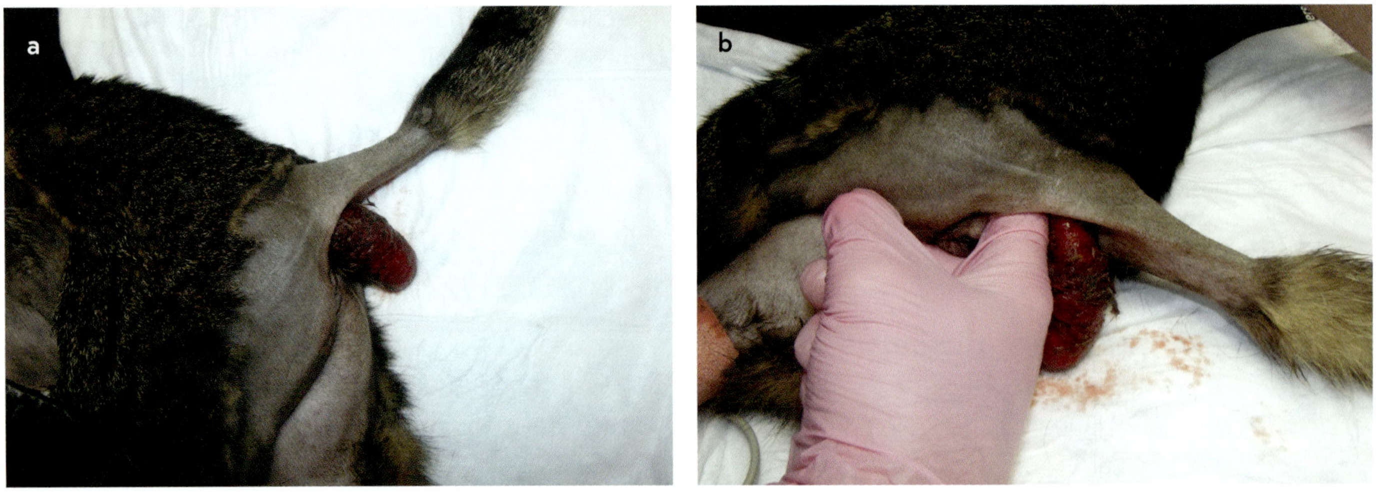

Figure 11.64 Prolapsed intestinal intussusception. Unlike in the case of rectal prolapse, a finger or the blunt end of an instrument can easily be passed between the prolapsed intussusception and the anus.

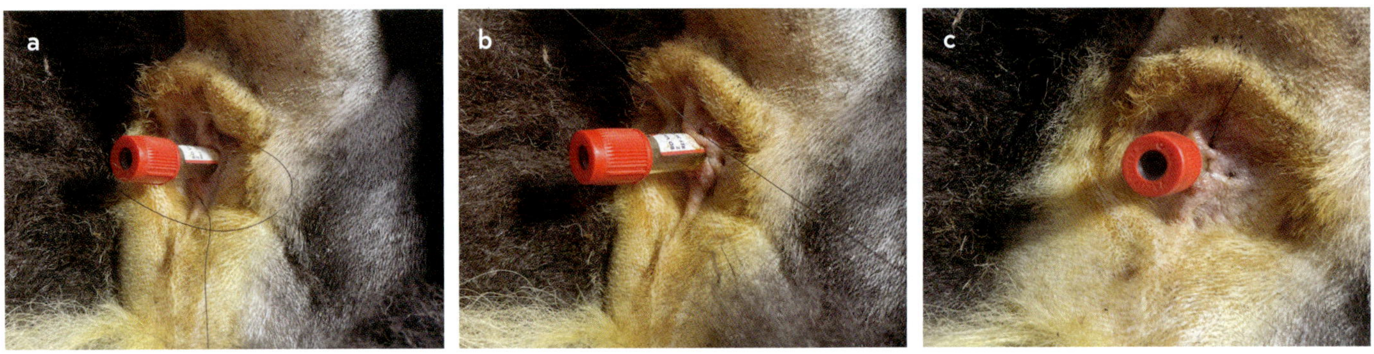

Figure 11.65 Application of a purse-string suture after manual reduction of rectal prolapse. (a) Initial 1 cm bites at the mucocutaneous junction, remaining medial to the anal sac duct opening. (b,c) Subsequent bites around the circumference of the anus, tightening the purse-string suture around an appropriately sized test tube or syringe case to reduce the anal opening to approximately one-third of its original diameter.

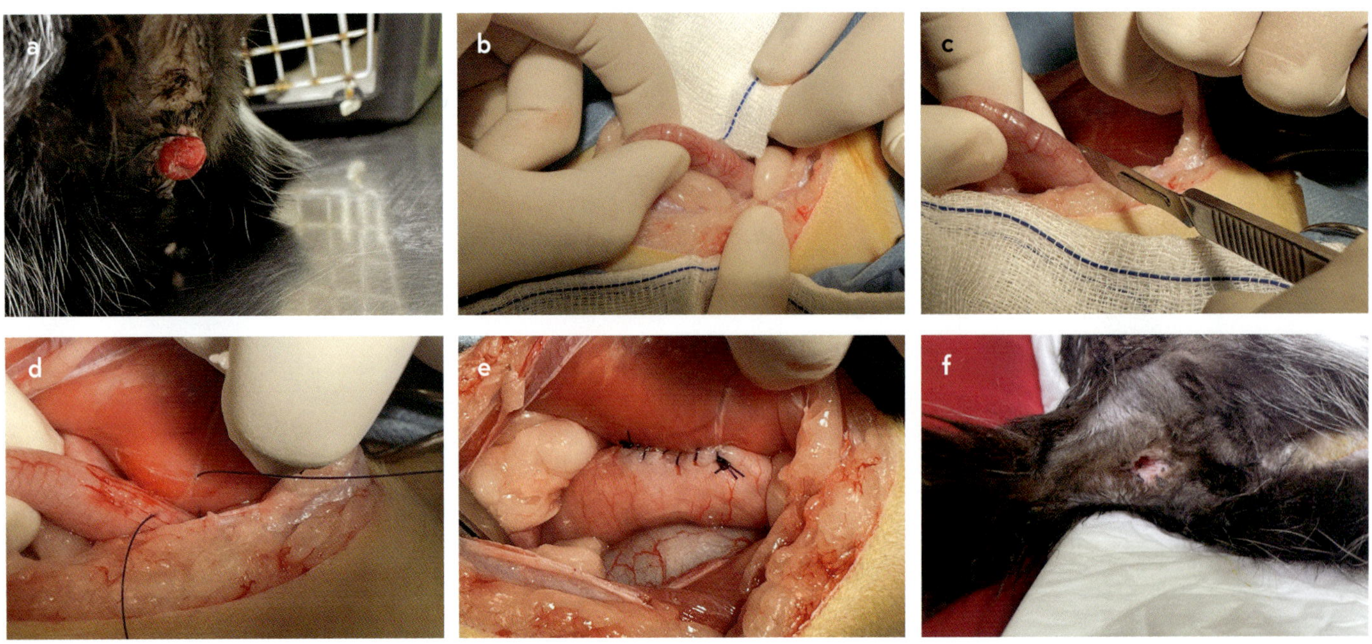

Figure 11.66 Manual reduction and colopexy in a case of recurrent rectal prolapse.

Surgical technique: Rectal resection and anastomosis (Fig. 11.67)

1. General and epidural anesthesia are required for this procedure, as well as perioperative antibiotic therapy.
2. The patient is placed in sternal recumbency, with the pelvic limbs over a padded end of the surgery table and the tail secured in a forward position. The perineal area is surgically prepared and draped.
3. To aid suture placement and prevent contamination, a sponge or test tube can be placed into the rectum.
4. Four full-thickness stay sutures are placed in healthy tissue, spaced 90 degrees apart. These sutures should include both layers of the prolapse.
5. One-third to one-half of the prolapsed tissue is resected 1–2 cm from the anus, caudal to the stay sutures.
6. A single layer of full-thickness simple interrupted sutures, using 4-0 or 3-0 absorbable monofilament material, is used to create an anastomosis. The cut edges are sewn together, taking wide bites to ensure the submucosa is contained within the suture.
7. The remaining tissue is cut and sewn in sections.
8. The stay sutures are removed, and the everted rectum is manually reduced.

Postoperative management

To reduce tenesmus and prevent recurrence after purse-string suture removal, periodic application of a local anesthetic to the rectal tissue has been suggested to prevent further straining. Other treatments to reduce tenesmus and prevent recurrence include anticholinergic-antispasmodic drugs such as dicyclomine and retention enemas with an anti-inflammatory drug such as hydrocortisone or mesalamine (dogs only).[56]

Outcome

The prognosis for rectal prolapse is generally favorable with manual reduction, with or without colopexy. Complications of rectal amputation and anastomosis include incontinence, dehiscence, recurrence of the prolapse, and anorectal stricture (particularly in cats).[56,60]

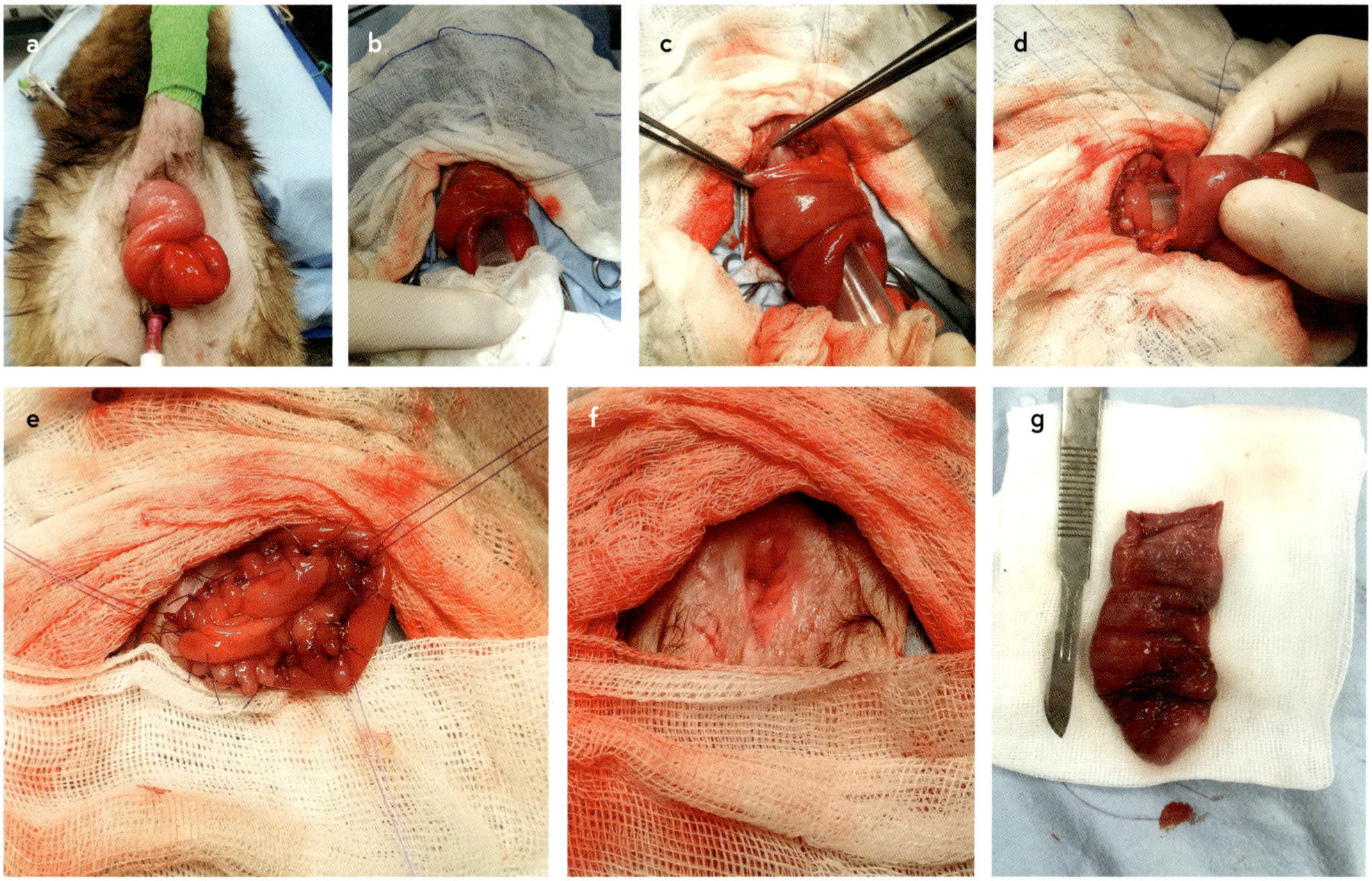

Figure 11.67 Rectal prolapse in an adult cat. (a) Preoperative appearance. (b) Placement of a test tube inside the anus to assist with suturing. Placement of full-thickness stay sutures in healthy tissue, spaced 90 degrees apart, encompassing both layers of the prolapse. (c–e) Resection and anastomosis with a single layer of full-thickness simple interrupted sutures. (f) Final appearance after resection and anastomosis. (g) Prolapsed rectal tissue following excision.

KEEP IN MIND

- Clinical signs vary depending on the location and degree of obstruction caused by a foreign body.
- Ultrasonography is a valuable imaging modality for detecting foreign bodies.
- Exploratory laparotomy is the most common treatment for removing foreign bodies and assessing intestinal viability.
- Proficiency in performing enterotomy and enterectomy is essential when dealing with gastrointestinal foreign bodies.
- After removing a linear foreign body, it is important to assess the affected mesenteric site for signs of perforation.
- Gastric dilatation–volvulus negative prognostic factors include hyperlactatemia, the need for splenectomy or partial gastrectomy, gastric perforation and sepsis, increased duration of clinical signs before hospital admission, hypotension, and arrhythmias.
- In case of rectal prolapse with necrotic or devitalized tissue present, rectal resection and anastomosis is required.
- It is essential to investigate underlying diseases to achieve a permanent cure and reduce the risk of recurrence when treating rectal prolapse.

References

1. Ritter MJ, Stanley BJ. Salivary glands. In: Johnston SA, Tobias KM (eds.). *Veterinary Surgery: Small Animal*, 2nd ed. St. Louis, MO: Elsevier/Saunders; 2018. pp. 1653–1663.
2. Bellenger CR, Simpson DJ. Canine sialocoeles—60 clinical cases. *J Small Anim Pract.* 1992; 33(8):376–380.
3. Cinti F et al. Complications between ventral and lateral approach for mandibular and sublingual sialoadenectomy in dogs with sialocele. *Vet Surg.* 2021; 50(3):579–587.
4. Bobis-Villagrá D et al. Feline sialocoele: Clinical presentation, treatment and outcome in 19 cases. *J Feline Med Surg.* 2022; 24(8):754–758.
5. Benjamino KP, Birchard SJ, Niles JD, Penrod KD. Pharyngeal mucoceles in dogs: 14 cases. *J Am Anim Hosp Assoc.* 2012; 48(1):31–35.
6. Weber WJ, Hobson HP, Wilson SR. Pharyngeal mucoceles in dogs. *Vet Surg.* 1986; 15(1):5–8.
7. White RAS, Lane JG. Pharyngeal stick penetration injuries in the dog. *J Small Anim Pract.* 1988; 29(1):13–35.
8. Griffiths LG, Tiruneh R, Sullivan M, Reid SW. Oropharyngeal penetrating injuries in 50 dogs: A retrospective study. *Vet Surg.* 2000; 29(5):383–388.
9. Doran IP, Wright CA, Moore AH. Acute oropharyngeal and esophageal stick injury in forty-one dogs. *Vet Surg.* 2008; 37(8):781–785.
10. Robinson W, Shales C, White RN. The use of rigid endoscopy in the management of acute oropharyngeal stick injuries. *J Small Anim Pract.* 2014; 55(12):609–614.
11. Leib MS, Sartor LL. Esophageal foreign body obstruction caused by a dental chew treat in 31 dogs (2000–2006). *J Am Vet Med Assoc.* 2008; 232(7):1021–1025.
12. Deroy C, Corcuff JB, Billen F, Hamaide A. Removal of oesophageal foreign bodies: Comparison between oesophagoscopy and oesophagotomy in 39 dogs. *J Small Anim Pract.* 2015; 56(10):613–617.
13. Binvel M et al. Endoscopic and surgical removal of oesophageal and gastric fishhook foreign bodies in 33 animals. *J Small Anim Pract.* 2018; 59(1):45–49.
14. Aertsens A, Hernandez J, Ragetly GR, Poncet CM. Surgical extraction of canine oesophageal foreign bodies through a gastrotomy approach: 12 cases. *J Small Anim Pract.* 2016; 57(7):354–359.
15. Brisson BA et al. Risk factors and prognostic indicators for surgical outcome of dogs with esophageal foreign body obstructions. *J Am Vet Med Assoc.* 2018; 252(3):301–308.
16. Juvet F, Pinilla M, Shiel RE, Mooney CT. Oesophageal foreign bodies in dogs: Factors affecting success of endoscopic retrieval. *Ir Vet J.* 2010; 63(3):163–168.
17. Doran I. Esophageal foreign bodies. In: Aronson LR. *Small Animal Surgical Emergencies*, 1st ed. Willey & Sons; 2016. pp. 22–32.
18. Carey Beer AJ et al. Complications associated with and outcome of surgical intervention for treatment of esophageal foreign bodies in dogs. *J Am Vet Med Assoc.* 2022; 260(6):622–627.
19. Moore AH. Removal of oesophageal foreign bodies in dogs: Use of the fluoroscopic method and outcome. *J Small Anim Pract.* 2001; 42(5):227–230.
20. Sterman AA, Mankin KMT, Ham KM, Cook AK. Likelihood and outcome of esophageal perforation secondary to esophageal foreign body in dogs. *J Am Vet Med Assoc.* 2018; 253(8):1053–1056.
21. Teh H et al. Medical management of esophageal perforation secondary to esophageal foreign bodies in 5 dogs. *J Vet Emerg Crit Care (San Antonio).* 2018; 28(5):464–468.
22. Killen DA, Pridgen WR. Tolerance of the dog to esophageal perforation. *J Surg Res.* 1961; 1:315–317.
23. Burton AG, Talbot CT, Kent MS. Risk factors for death in dogs treated for esophageal foreign body obstruction: A retrospective cohort study of 222 cases (1998–2017). *J Vet Intern Med.* 2017; 31(6):1686–1690.
24. Gianella P, Pfammatter NS, Burgener IA. Oesophageal and gastric endoscopic foreign body removal: Complications and follow-up of 102 dogs. *J Small Anim Pract.* 2009; 50(12):649–654.
25. Graham JP, Lord PF, Harrison JM. Quantitative estimation of intestinal dilation as a predictor of obstruction in the dog. *J Small Anim Pract.* 1998; 39(11):521–524.
26. Tyrrell D, Beck C. Survey of the use of radiography vs. ultrasonography in the investigation of gastrointestinal foreign bodies in small animals. *Vet Radiol Ultrasound.* 2006; 47(4):404–408.

27. Saile K, Boothe HW, Boothe DM. Saline volume necessary to achieve predetermined intraluminal pressures during leak testing of small intestinal biopsy sites in the dog. *Vet Surg.* 2010; 39(7):900–903.
28. Sumner SM, Regier PJ, Case JB, Ellison GW. Evaluation of suture reinforcement for stapled intestinal anastomoses: 77 dogs (2008–2018). *Vet Surg.* 2019; 48(7):1188–1193.
29. Duffy DJ, Chang YJ, Moore GE. Influence of crotch suture augmentation on leakage pressure and leakage location during functional end-to-end stapled anastomoses in dogs. *Vet Surg.* 2022; 51(4):697–705.
30. DePompeo CM et al. Intra-abdominal complications following intestinal anastomoses by suture and staple techniques in dogs. *J Am Vet Med Assoc.* 2018; 253(4):437–443.
31. Snowdon KA, Smeak DD, Chiang S. Risk factors for dehiscence of stapled functional end-to-end intestinal anastomoses in dogs: 53 cases (2001–2012). *Vet Surg.* 2016; 45(1):91–99.
32. Basher AW, Fowler JD. Conservative versus surgical management of gastrointestinal linear foreign bodies in the cat. *Vet Surg.* 1987; 16(2):135–138.
33. Levitt L, Bauer MS. Intussusception in dogs and cats: A review of 36 cases. *Can Vet J.* 1992; 33(10):660–664.
34. Larose PC et al. Clinical findings and outcomes of 153 dogs surgically treated for intestinal intussusceptions. *Vet Surg.* 2020; 49(5):870–878.
35. Rallis TS, Papazoglou LG, Adamama-Moraitou KK, Prassinos NN. Acute enteritis or gastroenteritis in young dogs as a predisposing factor for intestinal intussusception: A retrospective study. *J Vet Med A Physiol Pathol Clin Med.* 2000; 47(8):507–511.
36. Burkitt JM, Drobatz KJ, Saunders HM, Washabau RJ. Signalment, history, and outcome of cats with gastrointestinal tract intussusception: 20 cases (1986–2000). *J Am Vet Med Assoc.* 2009; 234(6):771–776.
37. Patsikas MN et al. Ultrasonographic signs of intestinal intussusception associated with acute enteritis or gastroenteritis in 19 young dogs. *J Am Anim Hosp Assoc.* 2003; 39(1):57–66.
38. Applewhite AA, Hawthorne JC, Cornell KK. Complications of enteroplication for the prevention of intussusception recurrence in dogs: 35 cases (1989–1999). *J Am Vet Med Assoc.* 2001; 219(10):1415–1418.
39. Giuffrida MA, Brown DC. Small intestine. In: Johnston SA, Tobias KM (eds.). *Veterinary Surgery: Small Animal*, 2nd ed. St. Louis, MO: Elsevier Saunders; 2018. pp. 1730–1761.
40. Rosselli D. Updated information on gastric dilatation and volvulus and gastropexy in dogs. *Vet Clin North Am Small Anim Pract.* 2022; 52(2):317–337.
41. Tivers MS, Brockman DJ. Gastric dilation–volvulus syndrome in dogs 1. Pathophysiology, diagnosis and stabilisation. *In practice.* 2009; 31(2):66–69.
42. Monnet E. *Small Animal Soft Tissue Surgery*, 1st ed. Ames, IA: Wiley-Blackwell; 2013.
43. Cornell K. Stomach. In: Johnston SA, Tobias KM (eds.). *Veterinary Surgery: Small Animal*, 2nd ed. St. Louis, MO: Elsevier; 2018. pp. 1700–1730.
44. Monnet E. Gastric dilatation–volvulus syndrome in dogs. *Vet Clin North Am Small Anim Pract.* 2003; 33(5):987–1005.
45. White RS, Sartor AJ, Bergman PJ. Evaluation of a staged technique of immediate decompressive and delayed surgical treatment for gastric dilatation–volvulus in dogs. *J Am Vet Med Assoc.* 2021; 258(1):72–79.
46. Tivers MS, Brockman DJ. Gastric dilation–volvulus syndrome in dogs 2. Surgical and postoperative management. *In practice.* 2009; 31(3):114–119.
47. Formaggini L, Degna MT. A prospective evaluation of a modified belt-loop gastropexy in 100 dogs with gastric dilatation–volvulus. *J Am Anim Hosp Assoc.* 2018; 54(5):239–245.
48. Eggertsdóttir AV et al. Comparison of the recurrence rate of gastric dilatation with or without volvulus in dogs after circumcostal gastropexy versus gastrocolopexy. *Vet Surg.* 2001; 30(6):546–551.
49. Degna MT, Formaggini L, Fondati A, Assin R. Using a modified gastropexy technique to prevent recurrence of gastric dilatation–volvulus in dogs. Presented at the 2nd Annual Surgical Forum of the European College of Veterinary Surgeons, Cambridge, UK, July 1993.
50. Allen P, Paul A. Gastropexy for prevention of gastric dilatation–volvulus in dogs: History and techniques. *Top Companion Anim Med.* 2014; 29(3):77–80.
51. Belch A, Rubinos C, Barnes DC, Nelissen P. Modified tube gastropexy using a mushroom-tipped silicone catheter for management of gastric dilatation–volvulus in dogs. *J Small Anim Pract.* 2017; 58(2):79–88.
52. Bruchim Y, Kelmer E. Postoperative management of dogs with gastric dilatation and volvulus. *Top Companion Anim Med.* 2014; 29(3):81–85.
53. Griffon D, Hamaide A. *Complications in Small Animal Surgery.* Ames, IA: Wiley Blackwell; 2016.
54. O'Neill DG et al. Gastric dilation–volvulus in dogs attending UK emergency-care veterinary practices: Prevalence, risk factors and survival. *J Small Anim Pract.* 2017; 58(11):629–638.
55. Benitez ME, Schmiedt CW, Radlinsky MG, Cornell KK. Efficacy of incisional gastropexy for prevention of GDV in dogs. *J Am Anim Hosp Assoc.* 2013; 49(3):185–189.
56. Baines SJ, Aronson LR. Rectum, anus and perineum. In: Johnston SA, Tobias KM (eds.). *Veterinary Surgery: Small Animal*, 2nd ed. St. Louis, MO: Elsevier; 2018. pp. 1783–1827.
57. Smeak DD. Rectum and anal sac. In: Monnet E, Smeak DD. *Gastrointestinal Surgical Techniques in Small Animals*, 1st ed. Newark, NJ: John Wiley & Sons; 2020. pp. 235–262.
58. Popovitch CA, Holt D, Bright R. Colopexy as a treatment for rectal prolapse in dogs and cats: A retrospective study of 14 cases. *Vet Surg.* 1994; 23(2):115–118.
59. Park J et al. Laparoscopic colopexy for recurrent rectal prolapse in a Maltese dog. *Can Vet J.* 2022; 63(6):593–596.
60. Billet JP. Large intestine surgery. In: Griffon D, Hamaide A. *Complications in Small Animal Surgery*, 1st ed. Ames, IA: Wiley Blackwell; 2016. pp. 435–440.

Chapter 12

Splenic and pancreatic emergencies

Adrien Aertsens, Stephen Martin

Splenic torsion

Splenic torsion is an uncommon, potentially life-threatening condition in dogs but has not been reported in cats.[1] It occurs when the spleen rotates around the gastrosplenic and phrenicosplenic ligaments, leading to occlusion of venous drainage and arterial supply.[1,2] This vascular occlusion causes congestion, thrombosis, and ultimately ischemic necrosis of the spleen.[2–5] Splenic torsion is often seen in conjunction with gastric dilatation and volvulus (referred to as secondary splenic torsion), but it can also be an isolated entity (primary or isolated splenic torsion).[3] Overall, it accounts for 0.5%–3.4% of all splenic conditions.[6,7]

The etiology of splenic torsion is poorly understood but proposed predisposing factors include congenital absence or weakness of the supportive ligaments of the spleen.[8,9] However, the age at presentation of this disease leads to suspect a more acquired progressive laxity of these ligaments as a result of surgery, trauma, or previous episodes of gastric dilatation with or without volvulus.[9,10]

Clinical presentation and diagnosis

Splenic torsion is most commonly reported in large- or giant-breed, deep-chested dogs, with breeds like German Shepherd Dog, Great Dane, and English Bulldog being overrepresented.[1,5] Male dogs are more commonly affected.[1,5] While splenic torsion typically occurs in in middle-aged dogs, it has been reported in dogs as young as 8 months and as old as 16 years.[1,2]

Splenic torsion can be acute or chronic,[1] with clinical signs nonspecific and variable in duration, ranging from hours to several months.[1,5,11] Clinical presentation of patients with acute splenic torsion includes severe abdominal pain, cardiovascular collapse, lethargy, depression, weakness, anorexia, acute gastrointestinal signs, and possible abdominal distention.[1] Chronic splenic torsion can represent a diagnostic challenge. It leads to similar clinical signs, albeit vaguer and more intermittent, including anorexia, vomiting, lethargy, hematuria, diarrhea, polyuria/polydipsia, weight loss, and tenesmus.[1,2]

Physical examination reveals a palpable abdominal mass in approximately 70% of cases, while hemoperitoneum and hypovolemic shock are identified in 31% and 22% of cases, respectively.[1] Tachycardia or premature ventricular contractions are occasionally observed (10%).[1] Anemia, leukocytosis with monocytosis, and leukocytosis and thrombocytopenia can be seen on hematology, while biochemical findings, despite being nonspecific, may include elevated hepatic and pancreatic enzyme concentrations.[5]

Diagnostic imaging plays a crucial role in confirming the clinical suspicion of splenic torsion. Abdominal ultrasonography has traditionally been the preferred imaging modality; characteristic findings include splenomegaly with diffuse hypoechoic parenchyma, atypical splenic position, and splenic intravenous thrombosis and infarctions.[1,2,4] Color Doppler ultrasonography can detect minimal or absent blood flow through splenic hilar vessels.[1,2] Atypical spleen position and free peritoneal fluid are reported in 32% and 46% of cases, respectively.[1] A hilar perivenous hyperechoic triangle, characteristic of a twisted splenic pedicle, can be identified by experienced ultrasonographers (Fig. 12.1).[2] Parenchymal gas shadowing can be seen in chronic torsions.[3]

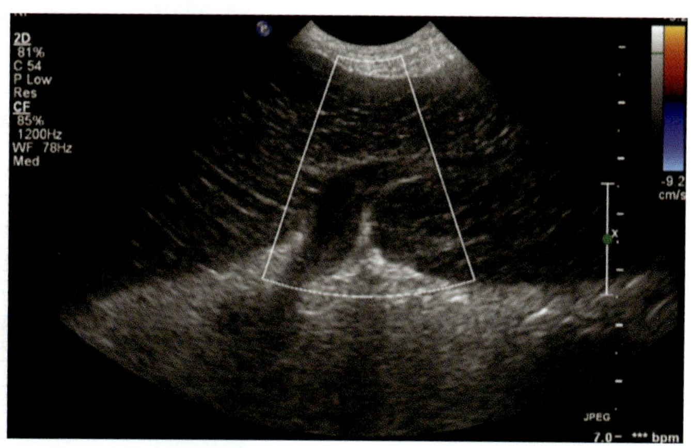

Figure 12.1 Ultrasound image of a large and hypoechoic spleen secondary to venous congestion, with the hilar perivenous hyperechoic triangle typical of a twisted pedicle. Image courtesy of Brad Cotter.

On abdominal radiographs, a midabdominal mass is present, with the lack of a normal splenic silhouette.[9] Splenomegaly and loss of serosal detail due to peritoneal effusion can be seen in 68% and 47% of cases, respectively.[1] A C-shaped spleen can be observed on a lateral abdominal projection. Gas density due to parenchymal necrosis may be present in chronic torsions.[3,5]
On computed tomography (CT) examination, the spleen appears enlarged and has rounded margins, with a characteristic C shape appreciated best on the dorsal plane.[2] The splenic parenchyma is usually homogenous, with a lack of parenchymal and vascular contrast enhancement.[2] If some contrast enhancement is noted, partial splenic torsion should be suspected.[2] A whirl sign, representing the twisted appearance of the soft tissue attenuating vessels of the torsed fibrovascular splenic pedicle, is a very common finding (Fig. 12.2; Video 12.1).[2] Abdominal effusion is commonly identified.[2]

Video 12.1. Multiplanar reformation/reconstruction (MPR) video in the sagittal and dorsal planes showing a splenic torsion in a dog. Note the marked enlargement of the spleen and the whirl sign at the center of the abdomen. Video courtesy of Matteo Rossanese.

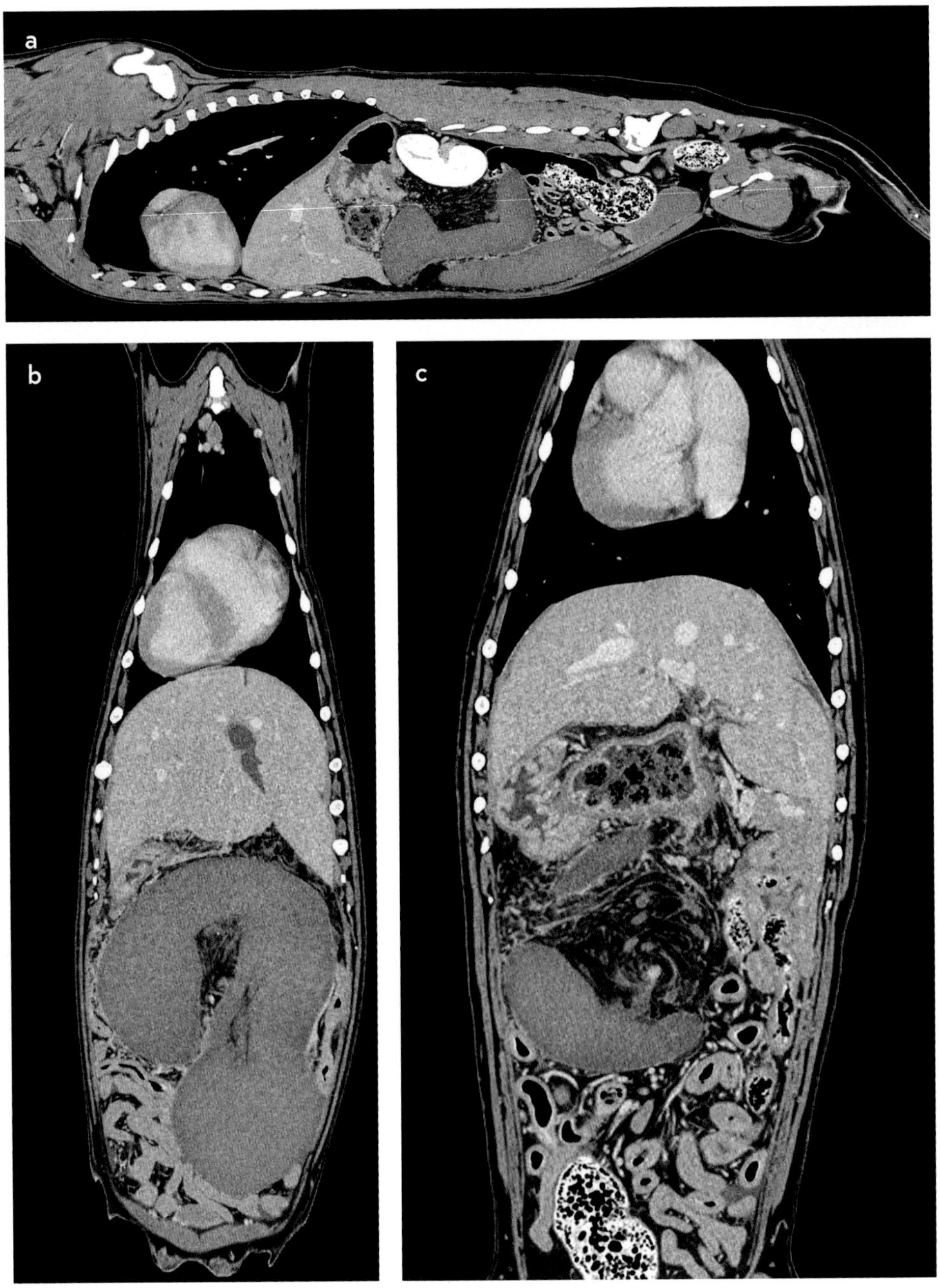

Figure 12.2 Computed tomography images of a dog with splenic torsion. The spleen is enlarged and has rounded margins and a C-shaped appearance. A whirl sign can be seen in image c. Images courtesy of Filippo Cinti.

Treatment

The patient should be stabilized prior to surgery; intravenous fluid therapy, analgesia, and supportive care as needed should be instituted promptly, especially if signs of shock are identified during the initial presentation. Surgery should be performed as soon as the patient is sufficiently stable.

Recommended treatment includes supportive care, exploratory laparotomy, and splenectomy without derotation.[1,10,12,13] Although spontaneous reduction and successful splenic derotation without surgery have been successfully reported, derotation during surgery should not be attempted.[10,13] This could result in intravascular release of thrombi and cellular breakdown products (e.g., free radicals, tumor necrosis factor, and vasoactive compounds) that could induce a distributive shock.[9] Patients with chronic splenic torsion may develop adhesions between the vascular pedicle, omentum, and small intestine.[9] If the patient is stable, prophylactic right-sided incisional gastropexy should be performed due to the potential risk for developing gastric dilatation and volvulus.[1,5]

Surgical technique

1. A midline celiotomy approach is made (see Chapter 3).
2. The spleen is exteriorized to facilitate identification of the twisted pedicle (Figs. 12.3 and 12.4; Video 12.2). No attempt should be made to untwist the spleen.
3. Splenectomy is performed proximal to the torsed tissue using manual suture ligation or a vessel-sealing device (Fig. 12.5).

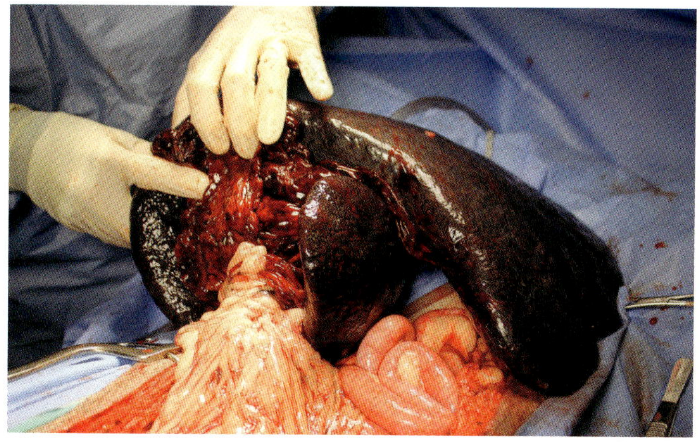

Figure 12.3 Folded C-shaped spleen of a Great Dane. Note the acute change in color of the omentum, which indicates the area to be dissected.

4. If safe, the area of ligation is gradually freed of the omentum and mesentery, allowing identification of the splenic vessels.
5. Each vessel encountered during dissection should be ligated or sealed individually.

Video 12.2. Splenic torsion in a 3-year-old American Bulldog. The spleen is exteriorized and the torsed pedicle identified. Note the marked enlargement and congestion of the spleen. Video courtesy of Matteo Rossanese.

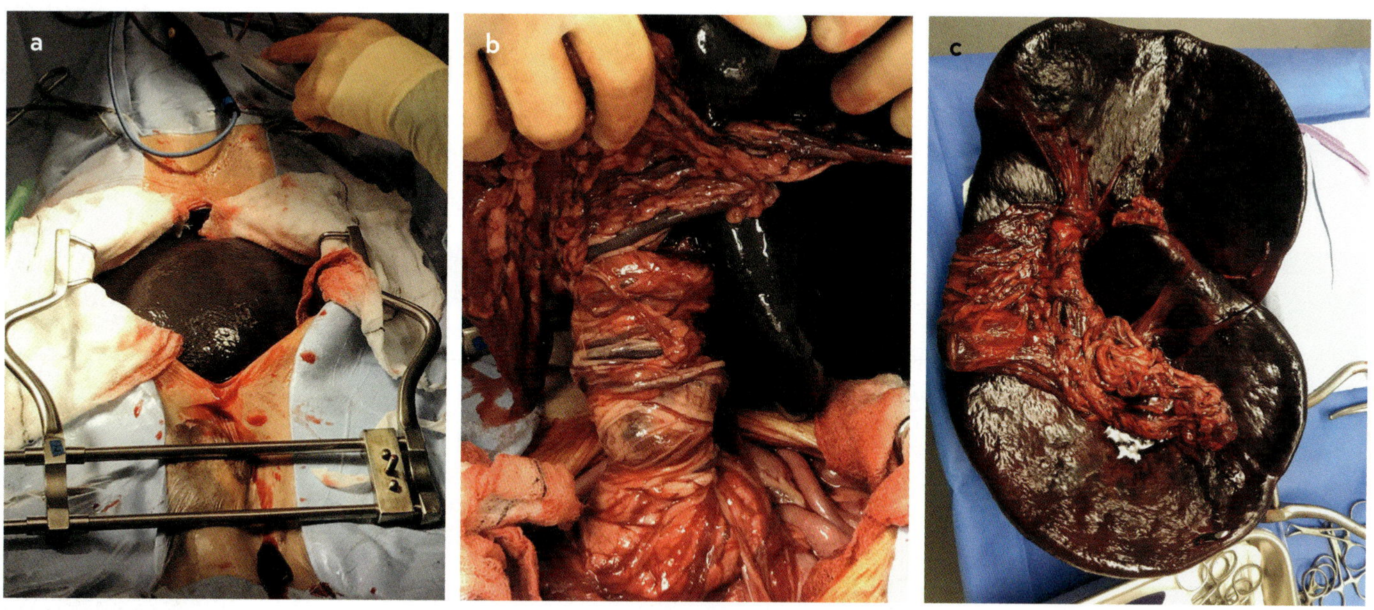

Figure 12.4 Splenic torsion in a 3-year-old American Bulldog. (a) Markedly enlarged spleen visible after midline celiotomy. (b) Torsed fibrovascular pedicle. (c) C-shaped spleen after splenectomy. Images courtesy of Matteo Rossanese.

6. Once identified, the splenic artery and vein are ligated or sealed individually:
   a. The artery is double ligated proximally using 3-0 or 2-0 absorbable mono- or multifilament suture material and transected. Care should be taken to leave a cuff of tissue between the ligatures and the cutting site in order to prevent the sutures from slipping.
   b. The splenic vein is ligated in the same manner.
7. If the splenic artery and vein are not visualized, the pedicle can be ligated en bloc by placing two circumferential ligatures proximal to the torsed pedicle using 0 or 2-0 absorbable mono- or multifilament suture material prior to transection.
8. The pancreas is commonly encountered during dissection (Fig. 12.6). In this case, partial pancreatectomy may need to be performed (see below).
9. The remaining omental fat is transected or ligated if too broad or significant bleeding is expected prior to transection.
10. The spleen is removed and the pedicle is inspected for bleeding.
11. The abdomen is lavaged and suctioned using warmed isotonic saline solution.
12. Complete abdominal exploration is performed.
13. If the patient is sufficiently stable, right-sided gastropexy is performed (see Chapter 11).
14. The abdomen is routinely closed.

Postoperative management

Analgesia and hemodynamic support are provided postoperatively. Intravenous fluid therapy is administered based on the patient's cardiovascular parame-

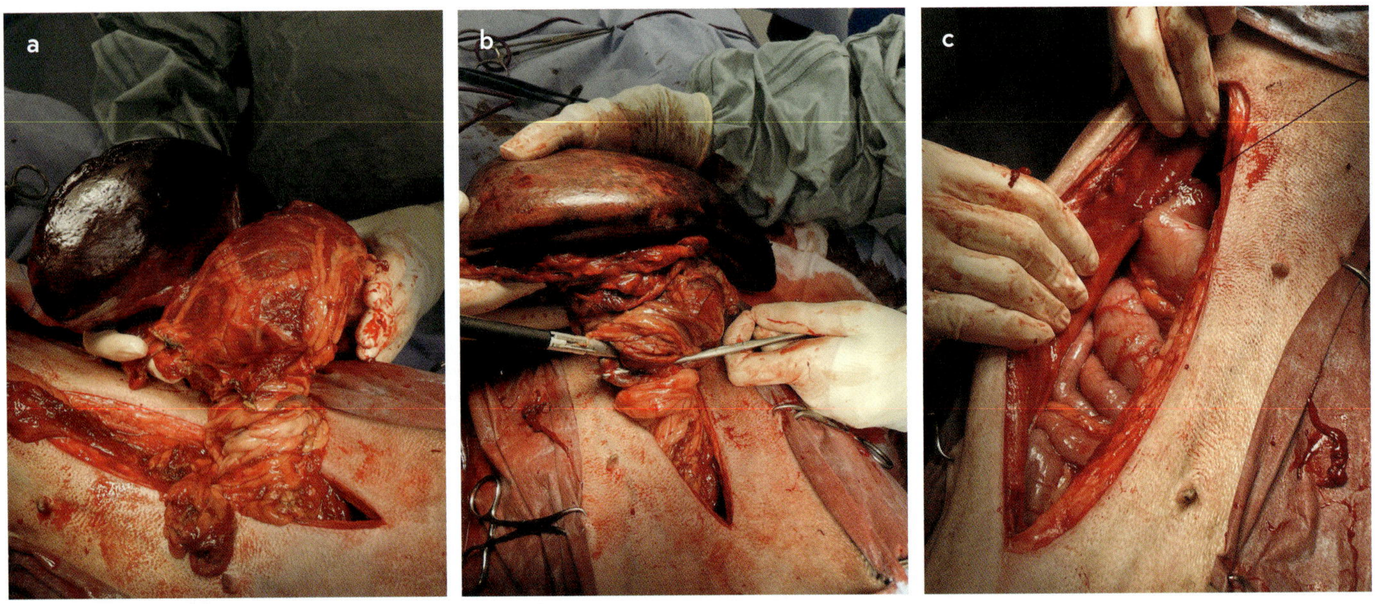

Figure 12.5 Surgical treatment of a splenic torsion in a 6-year-old dog. (a) Exteriorization of the spleen. (b) En bloc ligation of the pedicle with two circumferential ligatures and resection with a vessel-sealing device. (c) Right-sided gastropexy at the end of surgery. Images courtesy of Filippo Cinti.

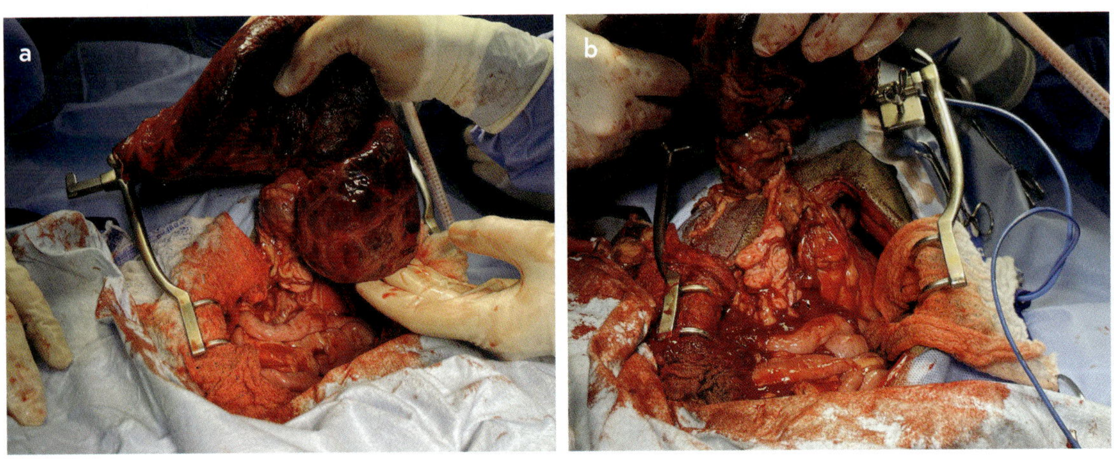

Figure 12.6 (a) Splenic torsion involving the pancreas. (b) Appearance of the pedicle after dissection by gentle tearing of the omentum. The pancreas can be spared, but further dissection has to be performed more distally to allow its retraction away from the pedicle prior to hemostasis.

ters. Opioids (e.g., methadone, fentanyl) can be used to control pain. Nonsteroidal anti-inflammatory drugs, if not contraindicated, can be prescribed for 7–14 days. Paracetamol (acetaminophen) can also be considered.
Continuous electrocardiogram monitoring is used to detect any arrhythmia. Vital parameters including heart rate, blood pressure, respiratory pattern, and temperature as well as packed cell volume, total proteins, and electrolytes must be checked for the first 24–48 hours. Blood products have been used in 26% of dogs undergoing splenectomy for splenic torsion.[1] If gastrointestinal signs were present preoperatively, medical treatment is given accordingly.
Exercise should be restricted for at least 2 weeks after surgery, with 10–15-minute slow on-leash walks allowed 2–3 times daily. Exercise can be gradually increased after the first 2 weeks. The surgical site should be rechecked 10–14 days postoperatively.

Outcome

Intraoperative complications have been reported in up to 28% of cases, including hemorrhage, ventricular arrhythmias, atrioventricular block, and thrombosis, whereas postoperative complications have been described in 35% of dogs, with the most common complications being anemia and ventricular arrhythmias.[1]
Historically, guarded to poor prognosis was given to dogs presented for splenic torsion; however, recent studies have showed a survival rate of over 90% after prompt medical stabilization and surgery.[1,5] Risk factors associated with death within the immediate recovery period are the presence of septic peritonitis at the time of diagnosis, intraoperative hemorrhage, and postoperative respiratory distress.[1] Following hospital discharge, no death attributed to splenic torsion or its management has been reported.[1]
Common histopathologic splenic features reveal only findings consistent with vascular occlusion, including congestion, hemorrhage, and necrosis.[2] No evidence of neoplasia has been reported apart from a case of myelolipoma infiltration.[1]

Pancreatic abscess

Pancreatic abscesses are described as circumscribed collections of necrotic, purulent material, with or without infection in the vicinity of the pancreas. They are infrequently reported in dogs and rare in cats. It has been suggested that pancreatic abscesses develop as a sequela to pancreatitis in dogs; however, they only occur in 1.4%–6.5% of dogs with pancreatitis. The underlying pathophysiology of this process has not been determined in veterinary medicine. Pancreatic abscesses are usually sterile in dogs, and the isolation of microbial agents is much less frequent in canine cases, with only 15%–27% yielding a positive culture compared to 40%–70% in human patients.[14–16] Pancreatic abscesses should be differentiated from other pancreatic mass lesions such as neoplasia or pseudocysts.

Clinical presentation and diagnosis

Most affected animals are middle-aged or older, and dogs are more commonly affected than cats. Patients with a pancreatic abscess may have a history of clinical signs indicating gastroenteritis, which likely was pancreatitis. The clinical signs of pancreatic abscess are generally nonspecific and can resemble those of pancreatitis, including vomiting, weight loss, anorexia, lethargy, and diarrhea. Cranial abdominal pain, abdominal distension, and occasionally pyrexia may be observed on physical examination. Although not usually palpable, a painful mass in the cranial abdomen may be discernible in small or emaciated patients.
Confirmation of diagnosis is based on a combination of a detailed and accurate clinical history, physical examination, laboratory investigation, and diagnostic imaging results.
Initial investigation should include hematology and serum biochemistry, although findings may be inconsistent. However, leukocytosis, neutrophilia with or without left shift, hyperbilirubinemia, elevated canine pancreatic lipase immunoreactivity (cPLI), and/or an elevated C-reactive protein level should prompt further imaging investigation.
On survey abdominal radiographs, the most consistent finding is an ill-defined increase in soft tissue opacity in the right cranial abdominal quadrant, with loss of serosal detail if local peritonitis is present. Gas opacities within the pancreas can also be seen. Abdominal ultrasound is the ideal tool for identifying pancreatic abscesses, and it is more sensitive than abdominal radiographs. However, differentiation between abscesses, pseudocysts, and other fluid-filled lesions is not possible without clinicopathological evaluation of the fluid.[15] The ultrasonographic appearance of pancreatic abscesses varies depending on the type, amount, and consistency of suppurative material and the presence of gas bubbles, but a hypoechoic or fluid-filled mass is typically observed within or adjacent to the pancreas (Fig. 12.7). The abscess wall is usually thick, highly echogenic, and irregular. Local peritonitis, if present, is characterized by a hyperechoic appearance of the pancreas, peripancreatic fat, and omentum.
CT can be extremely useful in differentiating chronic pancreatitis from pancreatic abscessation, with the added advantage of allowing visualization of the extrahepatic biliary tract, local lymph nodes, and both pancreatic limbs. CT features of pancreatic abscessation are similar to those of pancreatitis, with the additional

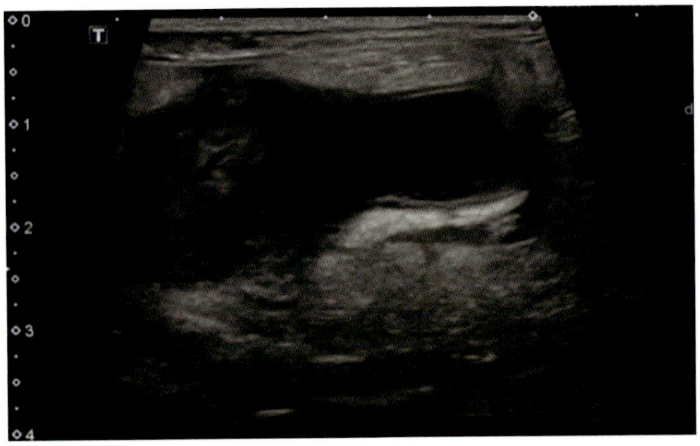

Figure 12.7 Ultrasound image of a pancreatic abscess, seen as a large, fluid-filled structure arising from the left limb of the pancreas and located between the left pancreatic limb and the stomach, with surrounding steatitis. Image courtesy of Brad Cotter.

characteristic of fluid-filled and thick-walled structures in the pancreatic parenchyma that may or may not maintain a rim contrast enhancement (Fig. 12.8). Regardless of the imaging modality used, identifying the abscess location on the pancreas is crucial, as abscesses located on the right pancreatic limb are more challenging to manage surgically (see below).

Diagnostic sampling of pancreatic fluid accumulations is safe and provides cytological and microbiological assessment to differentiate between sterile and septic processes. Cytological evaluation typically reveals a highly cellular population with a predominance of degenerate neutrophils.[16] Fluid samples should be sent for aerobic and anaerobic bacterial culture and antimicrobial susceptibility testing, although positive cultures have only been reported in 15%–27% of cases. Exploratory laparotomy may be required in some patients to make a definitive diagnosis. Ultimate diagnosis of pancreatic abscess relies on histopathological evaluation of samples obtained during surgical management of this pathology.

Treatment

Stabilizing the patient before surgery is crucial. If pancreatitis is present, medical management should be initiated, including intravenous fluid therapy administration, electrolyte abnormalities correction, and treatment with analgesics and antiemetics. If sepsis is suspected, broad-spectrum antibiotics should be administered intravenously. Fresh frozen plasma may be used if coagulopathies are present.

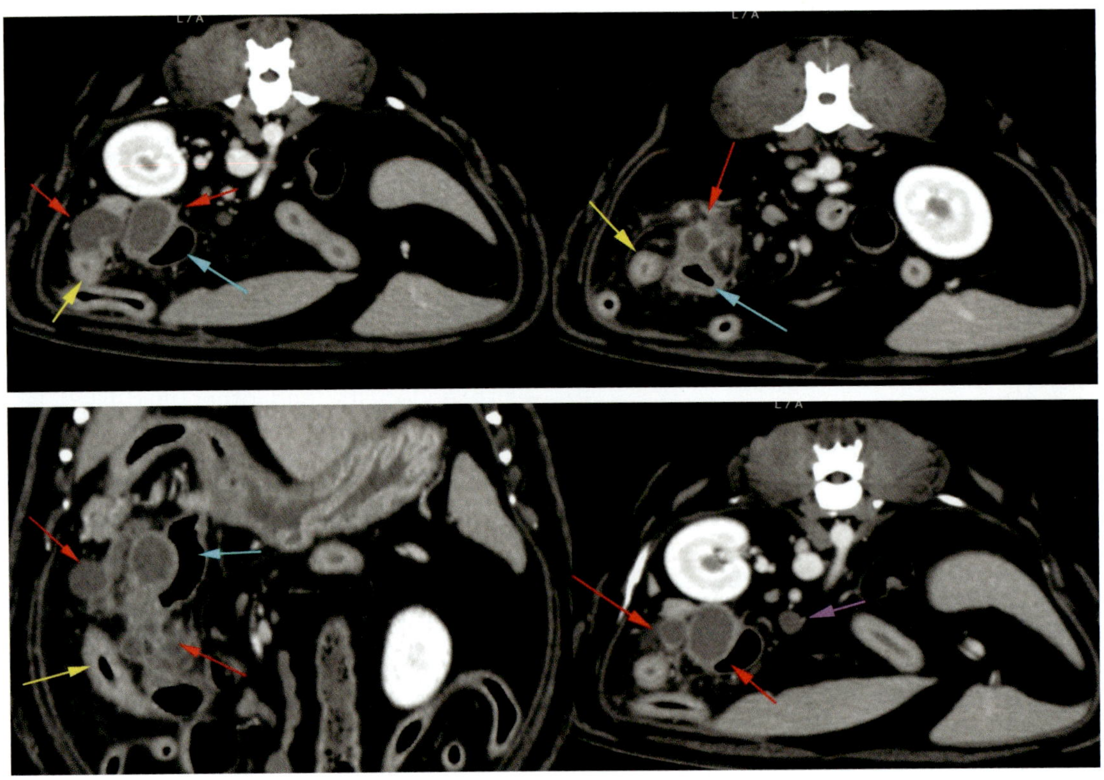

Figure 12.8 Multiplanar reconstruction of the computed tomography image of a confirmed aseptic pancreatic abscess. There is a multicavitated structure with coalescing, thick-walled, fluid-filled cavities in the mid-right abdomen (red arrows). It is located parallel or within the right pancreatic limb, between the duodenum (yellow arrows) and ascending colon (blue arrows). A small lymph node cyst is visible medial to this area (purple arrow). The surrounding mesentery has a streaky appearance, consistent with local peritonitis.

Pancreatic abscesses have historically been considered surgical pathologies; however since the majority of these cases have a sterile abscess ultrasound-guided percutaneous aspiration has been reported. Successful medical management in dogs was reported in a study and included intravenous fluid therapy, gastroprotectants, antiemetics, antinausea medication, opioid analgesia and nutritional support.[16] Antimicrobials were administered in 50% of these dogs.[16]

For cases requiring surgery, the choice of procedure depends on the abscess location and the involvement of surrounding structures. Surgical options include debridement, excision, omentalization, and peritoneal drainage by an open or closed technique. The aim of the surgery is either to remove the abscess en bloc or, if this is not safe, to debride the abscess and establish drainage.

Surgical technique (Fig. 12.9)

1. A midline celiotomy approach is made (see Chapter 3).
2. The abdomen should be gently explored and the pancreas and associated pancreatic mass located (Fig. 12.10). To evaluate the right limb of the pancre-

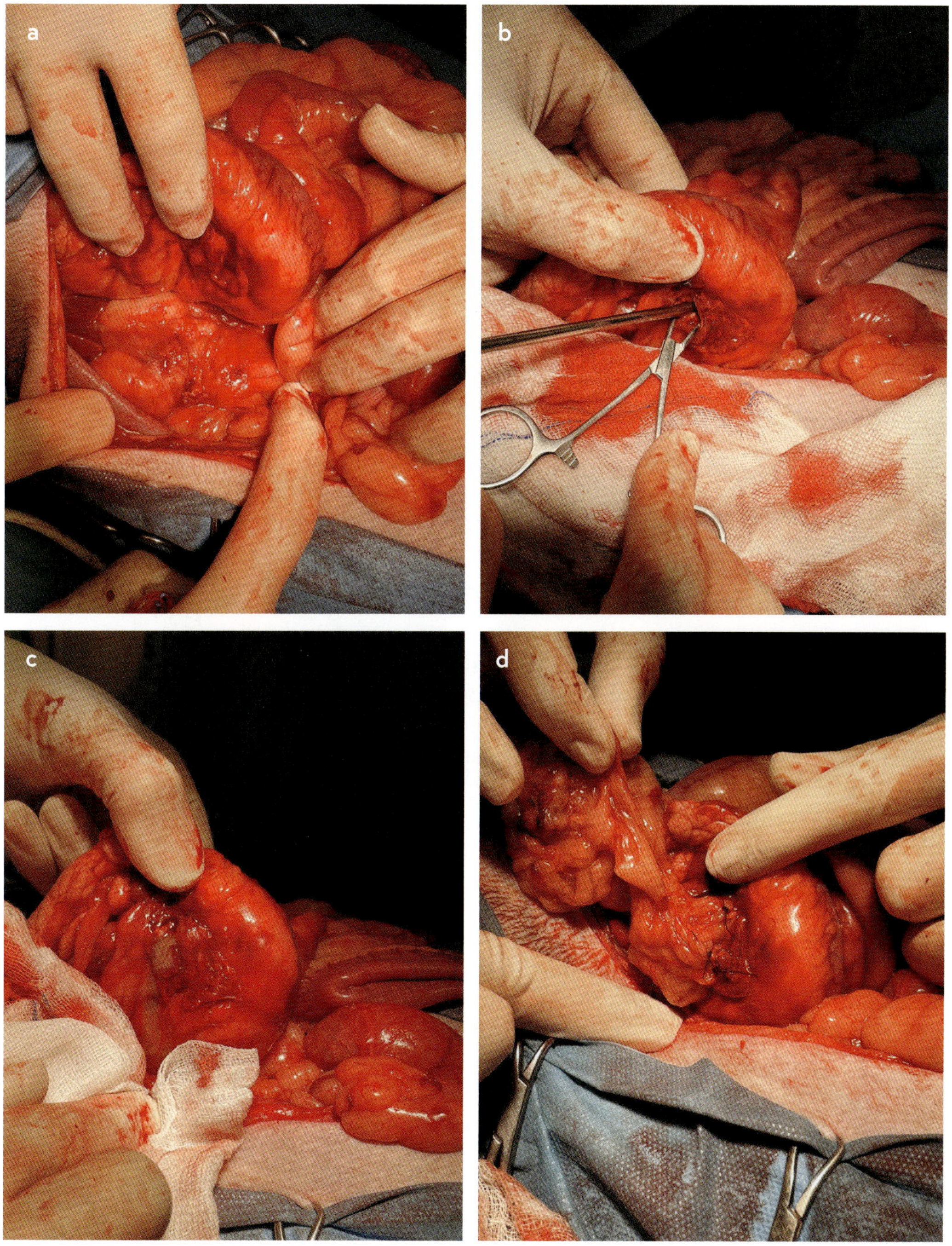

Figure 12.9 Surgical treatment of a pancreatic abscess in a 5-year-old Jack Russel Terrier. (a) Isolation and identification of the abscess. (b,c) Opening of the abscess, aspiration of the content, and debridement and lavage of the necrotic and purulent area. (d) Omentalization of the abscess. Images courtesy of Filippo Cinti.

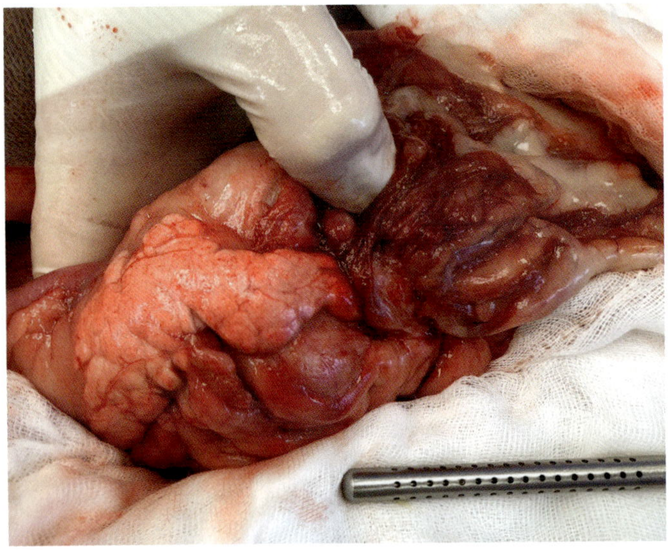

Figure 12.10 Intraoperative image of a pancreatic abscess demonstrating severe local inflammation, with copious local adhesion formation, omental attachment, and pocketing of fluid.

as, the duodenum should be located and retracted ventrally toward the midline. To evaluate the left limb of the pancreas, the omental bursa should be opened.

3. If a discrete pocket of fluid or mass is palpated, the adhesions with the intestine and omentum should be gently disrupted to visualize the lesion.
4. This lesion is isolated with moistened laparotomy swabs to decreased peritoneal contamination.
5. The abscess is opened with a number 11 scalpel blade or entered with the tip of a pair of mosquito forceps, inserted at 90 degrees to the pancreatic surface.
6. The abscess content is suctioned, and the opening is enlarged with a pair of forceps.
7. Samples are taken for histopathological evaluation and bacterial culture and susceptibility testing.
8. The necrotic and purulent areas of the pancreas should be resected and debrided as much as possible with a combination of sharp and blunt dissection, without damaging the pancreatic vascularization and duct.
9. Omentum should be placed on the surface or into the lesion and secured to the abscess wall using 3-0 or 2-0 absorbable monofilament suture material.
10. The abdomen is copiously lavaged with warm sterile saline.
11. Ideally, a closed-suction drain is placed (e.g., Jackson–Pratt abdominal drain).
12. The abdomen is closed routinely.
13. Placement of a feeding tube should be considered (see Chapter 5).

Surgical technique: Partial pancreatectomy

If the lesion originates from the edge of the pancreas and can be safely removed en bloc, partial pancreatectomy may be performed. If the body or the right limb of the pancreas are affected, the bile duct, pancreaticoduodenal artery, and duodenum should be carefully preserved. Conversely, if the left limb of the pancreas is affected, preserving the splenic artery is essential; however, if this artery is compromised, splenectomy may be necessary. Techniques for partial pancreatectomy include blunt dissection and suture fracture. Additionally, stapling techniques and vessel-sealing devices have also been successfully used.

1. The affected area of the pancreas is located and isolated as previously described.
2. The mesoduodenum and omentum on each side of the pancreas are incised.
3. The next step varies depending on the technique used:
   - Suture fracture technique: 2-0 or 3-0 absorbable or nonabsorbable monofilament suture material is passed around the pancreas proximal to the incision, and the suture is tightened crushing the parenchyma and occluding the vessels.
   - Blunt dissection technique: The pancreatic lobules are bluntly dissected using sterile cotton buds or mosquito forceps and the associated ducts and vessels are ligated or sealed.
4. After the pancreatic abscess has been excised, the mesoduodenum is closed using 3-0 or 4-0 absorbable monofilament suture material.

Postoperative management

Pancreatitis is a common and potentially life-threatening complication following pancreatic surgery. During recovery, especially in animals that develop pancreatitis, intravenous fluid therapy, electrolyte abnormality correction, and analgesia are of utmost importance. Opioids such as fentanyl and methadone are safe options, although they may cause side effects including nausea, vomiting, ileus, and constipation. Lidocaine can be combined with opioids to utilize its antiendotoxic and prokinetic effects. Given the risk of local duodenal compromise and anticipated anorexia, nonsteroidal anti-inflammatory drugs should be avoided, while paracetamol (acetaminophen) can be a viable alternative in dogs. Placement of a feeding tube and initiation of enteral nutrition as soon as the patient fully recovers from surgery are recommended to mitigate villus atrophy, bacterial translocation, and pancreatic inflammation.

Antiemetics, proton pump inhibitors, and prokinetics (e.g., metoclopramide, maropitant, ondansetron, omeprazole) are indicated to manage postoperative ileus and pain.

Antibiotic administration should be continued if infection is suspected, and animals should be closely monitored postoperatively for signs of worsening inflammation.

Outcome

The prognosis for animals with pancreatic abscesses is guarded, with reported survival rates between 33% and 86%.[14–18] Severe and often fatal postoperative complications include disseminated intravascular coagulation and septic peritonitis. A recent study reported that seven out of eight dogs undergoing medical treatment for pancreatic abscess survived to discharge, although three subsequently required successful surgical intervention after recurrence of clinical signs.[16] Due to the limited number of studies and the rarity of this pathology, no definitive predictors of mortality have been identified.

KEEP IN MIND

- Splenic torsion is an uncommon but potentially life-threatening condition in dogs.
- A characteristic C-shaped appearance and a whirl sign on diagnostic imaging are indicative of splenic torsion.
- Splenic torsion has a >90% survival rate following appropriate patient stabilization and splenectomy.
- Due to the potential risk of developing gastric dilatation and volvulus in dogs with splenic torsion, prophylactic right-sided incisional gastropexy should be performed.
- Pancreatitis often precedes pancreatic abscessation.
- Pancreatic abscesses are commonly aseptic.
- Timely and efficient surgical management of pancreatic abscesses is essential to optimize clinical outcomes.
- The mortality rate in patients with a pancreatic abscess is >50%.

References

1. DeGroot W et al. Primary splenic torsion in dogs: 102 cases (1992–2014). *J Am Vet Med Assoc.* 2016; 248(6):661–668.
2. Hughes JR, Johnson VS, Genain MA. CT characteristics of primary splenic torsion in eight dogs. *Vet Radiol Ultrasound.* 2020; 61(3):261–268.
3. Richter MC. Liver and biliary Spleen. In: Tobias KM, Johnston SA. *Veterinary Surgery: Small Animal,* 2nd ed. St. Louis, MO: Elsevier; 2018. pp. 1551–1564.
4. Saunders HM, Neath PJ, Brockman DJ. B-mode and Doppler ultrasound imaging of the spleen with canine splenic torsion: A retrospective evaluation. *Vet Radiol Ultrasound.* 1998; 39(4):349–353.
5. Neath PJ, Brockman DJ, Saunders HM. Retrospective analysis of 19 cases of isolated torsion of the splenic pedicle in dogs. *J Small Anim Pract.* 1997; 38(9):387–392.
6. Spangler WL, Culbertson MR. Prevalence, type, and importance of splenic diseases in dogs: 1,480 cases (1985–1989). *J Am Vet Med Assoc.* 1992; 200(6):829–834.
7. Day MJ, Lucke VM, Pearson H. A review of pathological diagnoses made from 87 canine splenic biopsies. *J Small Anim Pract.* 1995; 36(10):426–433.
8. Patsikas MN, Rallis T, Kladakis SE, Dessiris AK. Computed tomography diagnosis of isolated splenic torsion in a dog. *Vet Radiol Ultrasound.* 2001; 42(3):235–237.
9. Weber NA. Chronic primary splenic torsion with peritoneal adhesions in a dog: Case report and literature review. *J Am Anim Hosp Assoc.* 2000; 36(5):390–394.
10. Goldsmid SE, Davis P, Pechman R. Successful derotation of a splenic torsion in a racing greyhound. *J Small Anim Pract.* 1994; 35(2):112–115.
11. Reinhart JM et al. Chronic splenic torsion in two dogs. *J Am Anim Hosp Assoc.* 2015; 51(3):185–190.
12. Sumer F et al. Laparoscopic splenopexy due to wandering spleen: Feasible technique. *Cureus.* 2022; 14(2):e22597.
13. Szatmári V, Péntek G, Vörös K. Spontaneous resolution of splenic torsion in a dog. *Vet Rec.* 2000; 147(9):247–248.
14. Anderson JR, Cornell KK, Parnell NK, Salisbury SK. Pancreatic abscess in 36 dogs: A retrospective analysis of prognostic indicators. *J Am Anim Hosp Assoc.* 2008; 44(4):171–179.
15. Johnson MD, Mann FA. Treatment for pancreatic abscesses via omentalization with abdominal closure versus open peritoneal drainage in dogs: 15 cases (1994–2004). *J Am Vet Med Assoc.* 2006; 228(3):397–402.
16. Talbot CT, Cheung R, Holmes EJ, Cook SD. Medical and surgical management of pancreatic fluid accumulations in dogs: A retrospective study of 15 cases. *J Vet Intern Med.* 2022; 36(3):919–926.
17. Salisbury SK, Lantz GC, Nelson RW, Kazacos EA. Pancreatic abscess in dogs: six cases (1978–1986). *J Am Vet Med Assoc.* 1988; 193(9):1104–1108.
18. Edwards DF et al. Pancreatic masses in seven dogs following acute pancreatitis. *J Am Animal Hosp Assoc.* 1990; 26:189–198.

Chapter 13

Biliary disease

Karla Lee

Surgical emergencies of the biliary system include gallbladder rupture, extrahepatic biliary duct obstruction (EHBDO), and biliary peritonitis. In dogs, gallbladder mucocele, necrotizing cholecystitis, and cholelithiasis are the leading causes of gallbladder rupture and EHBDO requiring surgery, with neoplasia being the major differential diagnosis. Most cats undergoing emergency biliary surgery present with an inflammatory disease, including cholelithiasis, cholangiohepatitis, cholecystitis, and/or pancreatitis, but up to 41% have been reported to have neoplasia. In both dogs and cats, other surgical biliary emergencies include foreign bodies within the common bile duct or duodenum and traumatic or iatrogenic injury to the extrahepatic biliary system. The challenge for the emergency surgeon is to diagnose the primary disease process and to determine whether the patient presents with a surgical or medical emergency.

Bile functions to facilitate the absorption of fats, steroids, and lipid-soluble vitamins from the bowel, to maintain intestinal immune function, and to control the gut microbiota. Bile is also an important excretory pathway for many of its constituents, including drug metabolites, xenobiotics, and environmental toxins. It is synthesized and secreted by hepatocytes into the bile ducts. These bile ducts merge as they pass through the liver before ultimately becoming the hepatic ducts that transport bile from each liver lobe to the common bile duct. The majority of bile then passes via the cystic duct into the gallbladder. The cystic duct joins the common bile duct proximal to the entry of the hepatic ducts. Bile passes from the gallbladder back along the cystic duct into the common bile duct, which enters the wall of the proximal duodenum along its mesenteric surface. The common bile duct runs a short distance intramurally before entering the major duodenal papilla, which opens into the duodenal lumen. This opening into the duodenal lumen is surrounded by the sphincter of Oddi. The major duodenal papilla is located aborad to the gastric pylorus by 3–7 cm in the dog and 2–3 cm in the cat. In the dog, a small branch of the accessory pancreatic duct also terminates within the major duodenal papilla. In the cat, the major branch of the pancreatic duct joins the common bile duct, resulting in a shared opening within the major duodenal papilla.[1–3]

The gallbladder is partially encased by the right medial and quadrate liver lobes. The area of the liver that is adherent to the gallbladder is known as the hepatic fossa. The gallbladder has a single artery (cystic artery), which runs along the cystic duct, and a network of small veins that drain into the portal vein. The gallbladder wall has a mucosa, a smooth muscle layer, and a serosa. The mucosa has a columnar epithelium with short tubular invaginations that extend into the lamina propria and form gland-like structures containing mucin-secreting cells. The mucosa absorbs fluid for bile concentration, secretes fluid to assist gallbladder emptying, and secretes bicarbonate and mucins to protect the gallbladder wall from bile-induced injury. Flow of bile into and out of the gallbladder is dependent on neurohormonal signals. Between meals, gallbladder relaxation and sphincter of Oddi contraction permit gallbladder filling. After a meal, active contraction of the gallbladder and relaxation of the sphincter of Oddi results in outflow of up to 80% of bile into the duodenum over 2 hours.[2,3] Duplex gallbladder has been reported in cats.

Gallbladder mucocele

Gallbladder mucocele is common in dogs, but rare in cats.[2] It is a viscous accumulation of gelatinous material within the gallbladder, with distension of the gallbladder lumen (Fig. 13.1). The principal component of

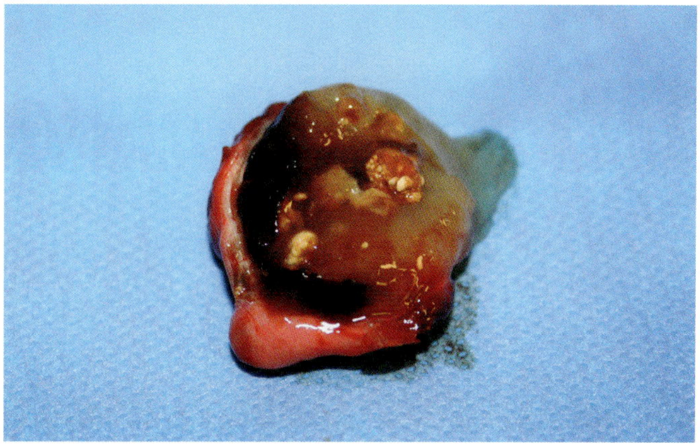

Figure 13.1 Internal contents of a gallbladder with gallbladder mucocele and multiple choleliths.

this material is mucin. Histopathology reveals cystic mucinous hyperplasia, characterized by mucin-filled epithelial cells. Gallbladder volume is increased, and postprandial gallbladder emptying is reduced.

Gallbladder mucocele may require emergency surgery due to progression to obstruction of the cystic and common bile ducts with mucocele contents or necrosis and possible rupture of the gallbladder wall (Fig. 13.2). Common bile duct dilation, suggestive of EHBDO, is reported in 50% of dogs undergoing cholecystectomy for gallbladder mucocele, whereas gallbladder wall necrosis or rupture is reported in 20%–35% of cases.[4–6]

The etiology of gallbladder mucocele is poorly understood. The Border Terrier and Shetland Sheepdog breeds seem to be predisposed, but no genetic link has been found. Other commonly affected breeds include the Cocker Spaniel, Pomeranian, Miniature Schnauzer, Chihuahua, Bichon Frise, Beagle, and Shih Tzu. Dogs with gallbladder mucocele are more likely than those without to have hyperadrenocorticism, hypothyroidism, and hyperlipidemia, but a pathophysiological link has not been identified. Positive bile bacterial cultures have been reported in 2.7%–67% of dogs with gallbladder mucocele. *Enterococcus* and *Escherichia coli* are the most common isolates. Mixed bacterial infections and multidrug-resistant isolates have been reported. Bacterial cholecystitis may contribute to gallbladder wall necrosis and progression of mucocele formation, but no association with etiology or prognosis has been found.[2,4,7]

Clinical presentation and diagnosis

Gallbladder mucocele may be an incidental finding in subclinical dogs. Dogs presenting with clinical gallbladder mucocele are on average 9–11 years old and may have chronic waxing and waning clinical signs or an acute presentation. Clinical signs include vomiting (80%), lethargy (47%), anorexia (46%), diarrhea (18%), abdominal pain (17%), hyporexia (11%), and jaundice (10%). Common biochemical abnormalities include increased alkaline phosphatase, alanine aminotransferase, and gamma-glutamyltransferase activities and increased total bilirubin and cholesterol. Hypoalbuminemia, azotemia, hyperphosphatemia, and hypokalemia have also been reported. Frequent hematological abnormalities include anemia, neutrophilia, and increased number of band neutrophils. Abnormalities in platelet numbers and monocytosis can also be detected.[4,7]

Ultrasound is diagnostic for gallbladder mucocele, characterized by echogenic immobile or nongravity-dependent bile with a stellate and/or finely striated pattern. The stellate pattern describes an echogenic star shape, with a central core and radiating arms, within an anechoic space. The finely striated pattern appears as faint echogenic striations that resemble the cut surface of a kiwi fruit (Fig. 13.3). Biliary sludge, often preceding mucocele, appears as echogenic bile lacking an acoustic shadow and is gravity dependent. CT may show a hyperattenuating gallbladder with centrally distributed

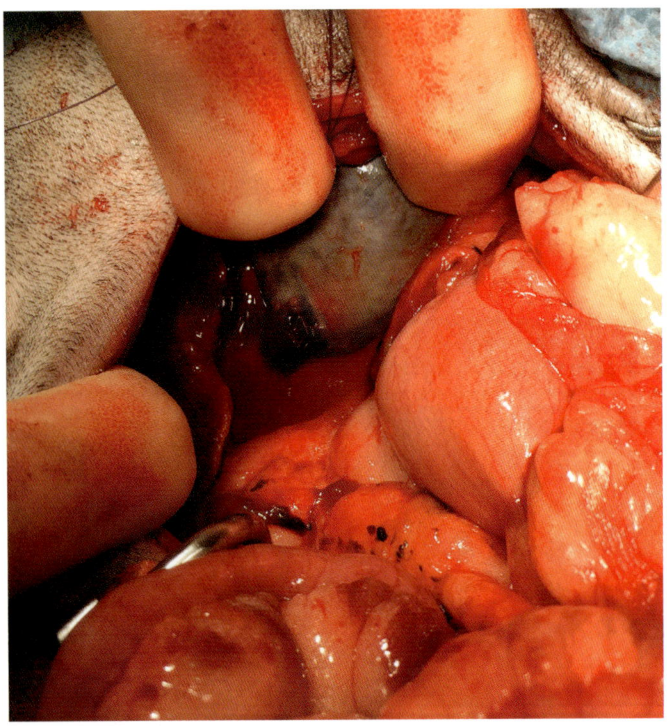

Figure 13.2 Intraoperative image of gallbladder mucocele rupture. Image courtesy of Filippo Cinti.

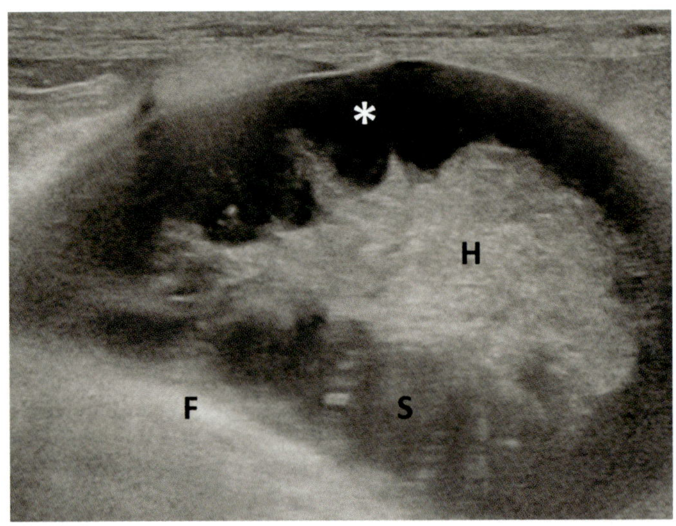

Figure 13.3 Ultrasound image of the gallbladder of an adult Border Terrier with a biliary mucocele, demonstrating both stellate and finely striated patterns. The stellate pattern describes the central immobile hyperechoic material (H) with radiating arms within a largely anechoic space (asterisk). In the bottom half of the image, the anechoic space contains faint echogenic striations (S). Surrounding the gallbladder there is hyperechoic fat (F), which is suspicious for wall necrosis or early perforation. Image courtesy of Helen Dirrig.

mineral, but it has a low specificity for mucocele detection.[8] Ultrasound is also useful for identifying concurrent gallbladder rupture and EHBDO. Indicators of gallbladder rupture include a discontinuous gallbladder wall, pericholecystic peritoneal fluid, and pericholecystic hyperechoic mesentery.[4] EHBDO is characterized by distension of the cystic and common bile ducts, defined as a duct width of 4 mm or more; however, the common bile duct cannot always be fully visualized in dogs.[9]

Treatment

The ultimate treatment of gallbladder mucocele is cholecystectomy, which is recommended as an emergency surgery if EHBDO or gallbladder rupture is suspected. Cholecystectomy is further recommended for animals with clinical signs and/or worsening clinicopathological abnormalities despite medical management (Fig. 13.4). If EHBDO due to mucocele migration is suspected, catheterization and flushing of the common bile duct is typically advised. However, recent studies have demonstrated an increased risk of postoperative pancreatitis and a longer surgical time associated with catheterization. Postoperative medical management, especially in patients with biochemical abnormalities or histopathological evidence of cholangitis and/or hepatitis, is often pursued, but with variable treatment duration.[5,6]

Medical management may be pursued for subclinical gallbladder mucocele. Medical management primarily comprises ursodeoxycholic acid, S-adenosylmethionine (SAMe), and a low-fat diet. Additional treatments may include antibiotics, proton pump inhibitors, antiemetics, and treatments for concurrent endocrinopathies. While medical management alone has been associated with survival times exceeding 12 months, it may carry a less favorable long-term prognosis compared to surgery, due to disease progression and development of life-threatening sequelae. Prophylactic cholecystectomy may therefore be advised in subclinical dogs.[5]

Outcome

In dogs undergoing cholecystectomy for gallbladder mucocele, 14-day mortality rates of up to 38% have been reported, but animals that survive surgery have good longevity.[5] Dogs receiving only medical management have a 4 times greater risk of death compared to those treated with cholecystectomy. Dogs initially managed medically but requiring emergency surgery have a 14 times greater risk of death compared to cholecystectomy dogs.[5] Preoperative gallbladder rupture and bile peritonitis are associated with a 2.7 times greater risk of early mortality,[4] whereas this risk is substantially reduced when cholecystectomy is performed electively or prophylactically in dogs with subclinical mucocele, with reported mortality rates of 2%–5%.[7] Other factors linked to increased mortality include jaundice, elevated bilirubin, hyperadrenocorticism, older age, Pomeranian breed, higher alkaline phosphatase activity, elevated white cell counts, elevated creatinine, and hyperphosphatemia.[4,5,7]

In one study, common bile duct catheterization was associated with intra- and postoperative complication rates of 32.5% and 47%, respectively, resulting in an in-hospital mortality of 14%.[10] In another study, catheterization resulted in intra- and postoperative complication rates of 14% and 23%, respectively, resulting in an in-hospital mortality of 6.7%.[6] Intraoperative com-

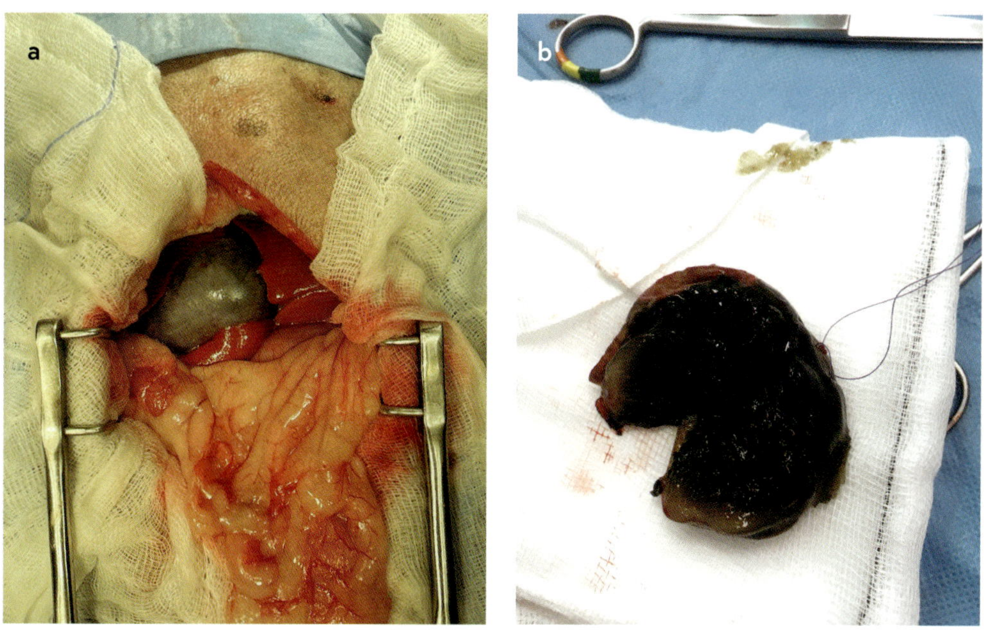

Figure 13.4 (a) Intraoperative image of gallbladder mucocele. (b) Contents of gallbladder mucocele after cholecystectomy. Images courtesy of Filippo Cinti.

plications included difficult bile duct catheterization, gallbladder rupture, tears to hepatic, cystic or common bile ducts, hypotension, hemorrhage, and cardiac arrest. Postoperative complications included pancreatitis, bile peritonitis, persistent biliary stasis, persistent gastrointestinal signs, hypotension, anemia, oxygen requirement, heart failure, pulmonary edema, acute kidney injury, multi-organ dysfunction, acute respiratory distress syndrome, systemic inflammatory response syndrome, disseminated intravascular coagulation, euthanasia, and death. Catheterization was associated with an increased chance of postoperative pancreatitis. Compared to normograde catheterization, retrograde catheterization had a greater incidence of postoperative complications, a slower decline in total bilirubin postoperatively, and an increased chance of postoperative increase in total bilirubin. Complication rates were lower in the presence of a diplomate surgeon.

Cholelithiasis

Cholelithiasis is the presence of solid concretions (choleliths or stones) within the biliary system (Fig. 13.5). Reported cholelith composition in cats and dogs includes 100% calcium bilirubinate, 100% calcium carbonate, 100% calcium oxalate, 100% bilirubin, and mixed composition including, in addition to the aforementioned, bile components, cholesterol, and unspecified bile pigments.[11–14]

Choleliths composed entirely of calcium carbonate are suggested to form in the gallbladder as a result of chronic intermittent cystic duct obstruction, whereas choleliths of a mixed composition are associated with bacterial infection. Concurrent gallbladder disease is reported in up to 100% of dogs and cats, including chronic lymphoplasmacytic and acute suppurative cholecystitis, gallbladder mucocele, acute cholecystitis, and emphysematous cholecystitis. Bacteriology is positive in 75%–100% of dogs and 56%–63% of cats, including *Escherichia coli* and *Enterococcus* spp. Concurrent primary hyperparathyroidism may also be a contributory comorbidity.[11,13]

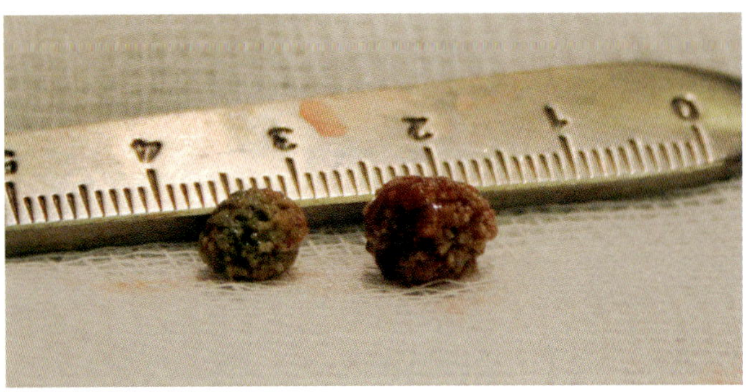

Figure 13.5 Two choleliths removed from the common bile duct of a cat by choledochotomy.

Although cholesterol choleliths have not been specifically identified in dogs and are rarely reported in cats, they are suspected to occur. This is because, unlike other cholelith types, cholesterol choleliths are radiolucent, and 52%–77% of canine choleliths are radiolucent. In addition, 21% of dogs with cholelithiasis had concurrent endocrinopathies, including hypothyroidism and hyperadrenocorticism, which are associated with hypercholesterolemia.[11]

Bilirubin choleliths form in the presence of excess unconjugated bilirubin. They have been reported in Somali cats with hemolytic anemia secondary to pyruvate kinase deficiency. Excess unconjugated bilirubin may also result from ileal dysfunction or resection.[3]

Clinical presentation and diagnosis

Cholelithiasis is likely subclinical in most dogs and cats.[14] Clinical cholelithiasis is due to EHBDO, biliary tree rupture, or acute cholecystitis. It is typically seen in middle-aged to older dogs and cats, but cats can also present at a young age. Small-breed dogs, especially the Cavalier King Charles Spaniel, are reported more frequently. Common presenting clinical signs include vomiting, hyporexia, lethargy, diarrhea, jaundice, abdominal pain, and weight loss. Vomiting and jaundice appear to be consistent findings in case of biliary tree rupture. Pyrexia or hypothermia are commonly seen in cats presenting with EHBDO.[11–13]

Common biochemical abnormalities include increased alkaline phosphatase, alanine transferase, and gamma-glutamyltransferase activities and increased total bilirubin and cholesterol, with derangements being greater in patients with EHBDO or biliary tract rupture. Hypoalbuminemia is also reported in surgical emergencies. Frequent hematological abnormalities include anemia, neutrophilia, increased number of band neutrophils, and monocytosis.[11–13]

Radiopaque choleliths can be seen on abdominal radiographs, but ultrasound is the preferred imaging modality for diagnosis.[15] Choleliths appear as hyperechoic structures within anechoic bile. Acoustic shadowing and a mobile nature help distinguish choleliths from other intraluminal structures, but these findings are not always evident. In dogs, subclinical cholelithiasis is mainly localized to the gallbladder (95%), with 5% localized to the intrahepatic ducts.[11] In both dogs and cats, clinical cholelithiasis is typically localized to the gallbladder and common bile duct.[11,13]

Obstructive choleliths are frequently visualized close to the major duodenal papilla.[13,15] Complete obstruction of the common bile duct results in progressive dilation of the common bile duct within 2 days, intrahepatic ducts within 5–6 days, and interlobar ducts by 7 days. Dilation of the cystic duct is not a consistent finding. Diagnosis of EHBDO secondary to cholelithiasis requires visualization of the cholelith, as duct dilation can persist following relief of obstruction. Concurrent gallbladder abnormalities are almost always seen, including distension, mural thickening, and intraluminal biliary sludge or mucocele.[11,13,15]

Treatment

Subclinical cholelithiasis and clinical cholelithiasis without biliary tract rupture or EHBDO can be treated medically, but there are no guidelines to determine when medical management can be successful.[11] Ursodeoxycholic acid is the cornerstone of medical management. It decreases biliary cholesterol saturation and bile acid toxicity and promotes choleresis. Antibiotics are indicated for bacterial cholecystitis. Additional treatments include SAMe, a low-fat diet, proton pump inhibitors, antiemetics, and management of concurrent endocrinopathies. Medical management with ursodeoxycholic acid has been shown to result in resolution of cholelithiasis and reduction in cholelith number in 50% and 12.5% of dogs, respectively. However, medical management does not prevent progression to gallbladder rupture and EHBDO, emphasizing the need for close monitoring.[11,13]

Surgical treatment for cholelithiasis is dependent on cholelith location and on the presence of concurrent biliary disease. Cholecystectomy is indicated for choleliths confined to the gallbladder, gallbladder rupture, chronically diseased gallbladder, and gallbladder necrosis. In addition, cholecystectomy has been associated with better prognosis in dogs undergoing surgical management for cholelithiasis and may be indicated as a prophylactic measure to reduce recurrence of choleliths in both dogs and cats. However, in the critically ill patient, prophylactic cholecystectomy may detrimentally prolong anesthesia.[11,13]

Choledocholiths (i.e., choleliths within the common bile duct) may be retrieved through the duodenal papilla following sphincterotomy, by cholecystectomy and retrograde saline flushing, or by choledochotomy.[11–13] Sphincterotomy may be the least invasive option, requiring minimal manipulation of the biliary system and thus with fewer biliary-related complications. If cholecystectomy is indicated in presence of choledocholiths, then retrograde flushing may be the simplest approach, if cystic duct anatomy permits. Choledochotomy is the least favorable option due to the risk of early dehiscence and late stricture.[12] However, if the choledocholith is large and the common bile duct is markedly distended, choledochotomy may be the simplest and only feasible option, with the possibility for accurate suture placement and minimal risk of obstructive stricture. Concurrent placement of a biliary stent between the common bile duct and duodenum could aid in biliary system decompression, decreasing the risk of bile leak and stricture.[11–13] A postoperative period of medical management for cholelithiasis, as described above, is often pursued, especially if cholecystectomy is not performed or if there are ongoing biochemical abnormalities or histopathological evidence of cholangitis and/or hepatitis. The recommended duration of treatment is variable.[11,13]

Outcome

Prognosis following surgical management of cholelithiasis is good for survival and resolution of clinical disease, although choleliths may recur. In dogs, a surgical survival rate of 90% has been reported.[11] Major surgical complications include immediate postoperative death and stricture at the major duodenal papilla requiring stenting.[11] Long-term resolution of choleliths has been reported in 71% of cases, with a median survival time of 577 days (range, 0–2266 days).[11] In cats, surgical survival rates of 78% and 82% have been reported, with a median survival time of 24 months (range, 13–27 months).[13,16] However, a reported 36% of cats may experience short- and/or long-term intermittent vomiting.[13]

Neoplasia

Neoplasia of the extrahepatic biliary system is rare in dogs and cats, but it is an important differential diagnosis for EHBDO (Fig. 13.6). The most commonly reported tumor is biliary neuroendocrine carcinoma, but gallbladder lymphoma, pancreatic carcinoma, and neoplasia within the major duodenal papilla are also diagnosed.[17,18] In addition to clinical and biochemical signs of EHBDO, hematemesis may occur due to paraneoplastic gastrin secretion leading to gastric ulceration. Ultrasound reveals a stricture or mass lesion affecting the common bile duct, cystic duct, gallbladder, or adjacent organs. Exploratory laparotomy confirms EHBDO due to a mass lesion. Cholecystectomy, biopsy, biliary stenting, and biliary diversion by cholecystoenterostomy may be indicated. Prognosis is guarded due to a high rate of metastasis. Cats frequently do not survive the immediate postoperative period, with a reported 1-year survival rate of 22%.[18] Dogs, despite a reported metastatic rate of 46%, have a reported median survival time of 3.7 years amongst those that survive surgery. However, 63% have ongoing clinical signs.[17]

Pancreatitis

Acute pancreatitis is a rare cause of severe EHBDO requiring surgical intervention. Clinical and ultrasound findings consistent with EHBDO, combined with a mass-like lesion or thickening at the major duodenal papilla, may be a specific indicator of EHBDO secondary

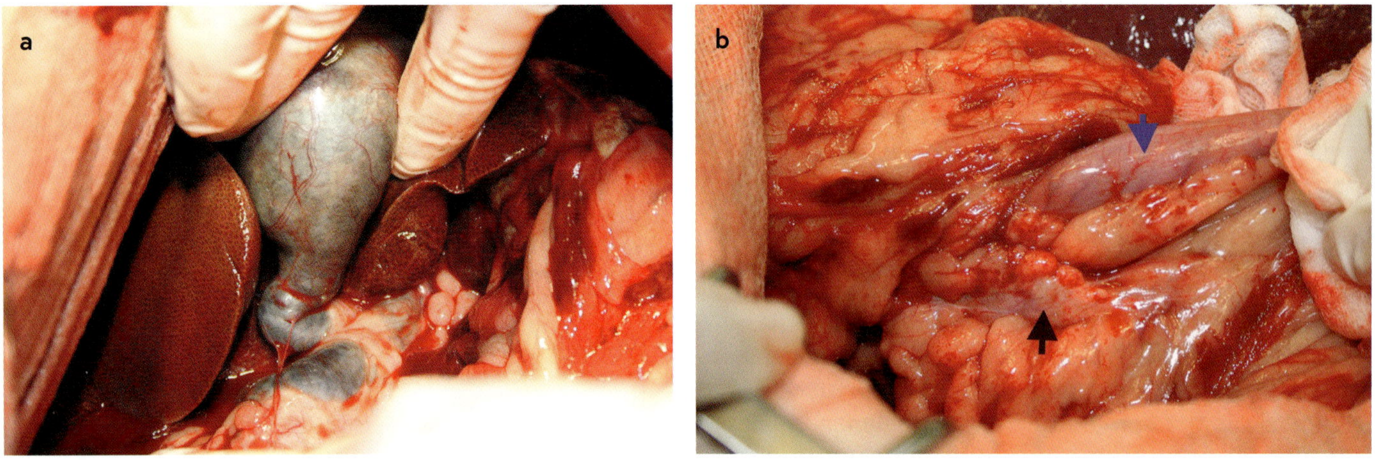

Figure 13.6 Intraoperative photos of a dog with a metastatic soft tissue mass obstructing the entrance of the common bile duct into the duodenum. (a) The gallbladder, cystic duct, and common bile duct are distended. The gallbladder cannot be decompressed by applying gentle pressure with the fingers. (b) A soft tissue mass (black arrow) overlies the entrance of the common bile duct into the duodenum (purple arrow), which is being retracted caudally.

to pancreatitis. Worsening serial ultrasound findings, pancreas cytology consistent with necrosuppurative septic inflammation or necrosis, lack of clinical improvement, or worsening clinical signs are indications for surgery. Cholecystoenterostomy or biliary stenting may be required. Prognosis in cats may be good, with one study reporting a survival rate of 71%.[19]

Trauma

Traumatic injuries to the extrahepatic biliary tract have been reported as a result of gunshots, penetrating trauma, road traffic accidents, dog bites, and iatrogenic injury during thoracostomy tube placement and abdominal surgery. Reported injuries include perforation of the gallbladder and cystic duct, avulsion of the common bile duct from the duodenum, stricture of the common bile duct, and biliary entrapment secondary to diaphragmatic rupture. Injury that results in bile leak tends to present 2–6 days after trauma, while those that result in common bile duct stricture present 7 days post-traumatically. Clinical signs of biliary peritonitis include vomiting, anorexia, and abdominal effusion. Diagnosis is based on bilirubin concentrations of body cavity effusions being more than twice that of serum concentrations. Dogs and cats with traumatic stricture of the common bile duct may present with jaundice as well as other signs of trauma and sepsis including abdominal discomfort, abdominal wall bruising, abdominal effusion, and external wounds. Treatment is aimed at repairing biliary tract rupture or stricture, flushing bilirubin and any associated bacteria out of the abdominal cavity, and providing appropriate antibiotic therapy for bacterial infection if present. Abdominal drain and feeding tubes are frequently indicated. Prognosis can be good if surgical repair is successful (see "Perioperative management" below).[3,20]

Surgical techniques for treatment of biliary disease

Cholecystectomy

Cholecystectomy is the removal of the gallbladder.[13]

1. A midline celiotomy is performed as described in Chapter 3.
2. Exposure and isolation of the gallbladder can be improved by placing:
   - alaparotomic swab cranial to the liver;
   - a stay suture on the apex of the gallbladder; and/or
   - stay sutures on the body of the stomach with caudal traction.
3. The gallbladder is dissected out of the hepatic fossa.
   a. The peritoneal attachments at the margins of the hepatic fossa are sharply released.
   b. Blunt dissection with moist cotton tip applicators, swabs, or a fine Poole suction tip is performed to release the remainder of the gallbladder wall from the hepatic fossa, resulting in circumferential access to the cystic duct. If a Poole suction tip is used, monitoring for blood loss is essential, as this can be underestimated if blood is continuously suctioned from the surgical site. Dissection should not extend into the common bile duct to avoid damage to the hepatic ducts.
   c. Hemostasis of the hepatic fossa can be achieved using electrocautery and topical hemostatic materials.

d. The cystic artery, which runs alongside the cystic duct, may be transected before it is noticed, requiring suture ligation or electrocautery to minimize blood loss. If using electrocautery, care should be taken to avoid collateral injury to the cystic duct, hepatic ducts, and common bile duct.

4. The cystic duct and artery are clamped together with hemostatic forceps and circumferentially ligated using 2-0 or 3-0 absorbable or nonabsorbable suture material (e.g., polypropylene, polyglactin 910, or polydioxanone) (Figs. 13.7 and 13.8). Alternatively, they can be ligated with three or four surgical hemostatic clips placed in alternating directions (Fig. 13.9; Video 13.1).

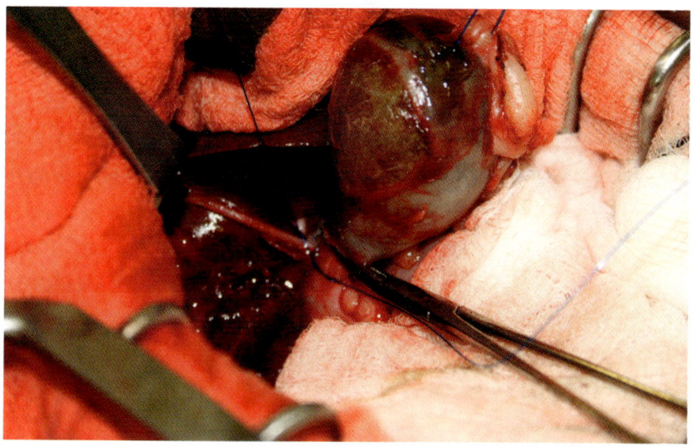

Figure 13.7 Intraoperative photo of cholecystectomy for management of gallbladder mucocele in a dog. After placing a blue stay suture in the gallbladder and releasing the gallbladder from the hepatic fossa, hemostatic forceps are placed around the cystic duct and a circumferential ligature is tied.

Figure 13.8. Cholecystectomy for management of gallbladder mucocele. Images courtesy of Filippo Cinti

Figure 13.9. Cholecystectomy using hemostatic clips. Images courtesy of Benito de la Puerta.

Video 13.1. Cholecystectomy. Video courtesy of Benito de la Puerta.

5. The transected cystic duct should be examined for leak and double ligated if necessary. A transfixing suture may be appropriate if the cystic duct is thickened or dilated and ligature slip is a concern.

Catheterization and flushing of the common bile duct

Gentle pressure on the gallbladder should result in visible expulsion of bile along the common bile duct and into the duodenum. When this is not possible (Fig. 13.6a) or when EHBDO is suspected, catheterization of the common bile duct is indicated. This can be performed normogradely via the cystic duct or retrogradely via the major duodenal papilla. For both, contamination of the abdominal cavity with bile can be limited by isolating the surgical field from the rest of the abdomen with moistened swabs.

For catheterization, a small fine catheter is used, such as a 2.5Fr–5Fr silicone urethral cat catheter or a 5Fr–8Fr latex red rubber catheter.[12,13] Lubrication with an aqueous gel is recommended. If the catheter does not pass easily, it may be possible to assist passage by placement of a hydrophilic guidewire or stiff monofilament suture. The common bile duct should be flushed through with 0.9% sterile saline. Gentle pressure should be applied while simultaneously visualizing the extrahepatic biliary tree to avoid retrograde flushing of material into the hepatic or intrahepatic ducts. For retrograde flushing, outflow of bile duct contents may require removal of the catheter or use of a small catheter to allow passage of fluid around the catheter at the major duodenal papilla.

For normograde catheterization (Fig. 13.10):[10]

1. Catheterization can be performed by cholecystotomy (a 5–10 mm incision is performed at the apex of the gallbladder) or after cholecystectomy.

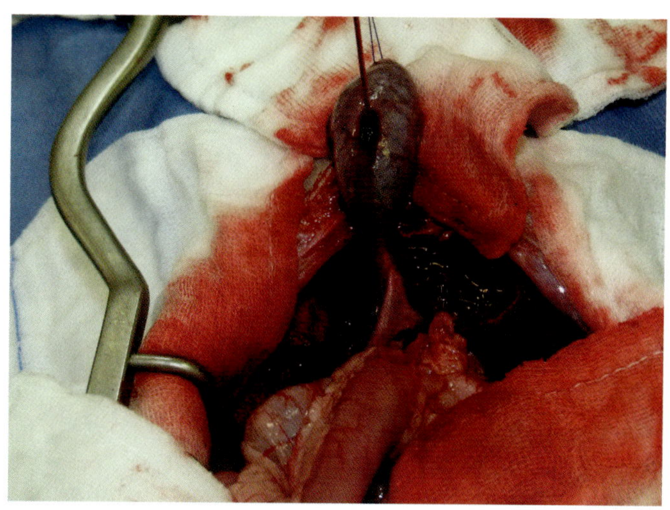

Figure 13.10 Normograde catheterization of the common bile duct after cholecystotomy. Image courtesy of Benito de la Puerta.

2. Bile spill into the abdomen can be reduced by elevating the gallbladder or cystic duct with stay sutures placed adjacent to the site of cholecystotomy or at the opening to the cystic duct.
3. The gallbladder contents are suctioned.
4. Normograde catheterization may be challenging if the angle between the gallbladder infundibulum and cystic duct is very acute.

For retrograde catheterization (Figs. 13.11 and 13.12):[10]

1. A longitudinal incision is made along the antimesenteric surface of the duodenum opposite the major duodenal papilla.
2. The edges of the duodenotomy are elevated and handled with stay sutures.

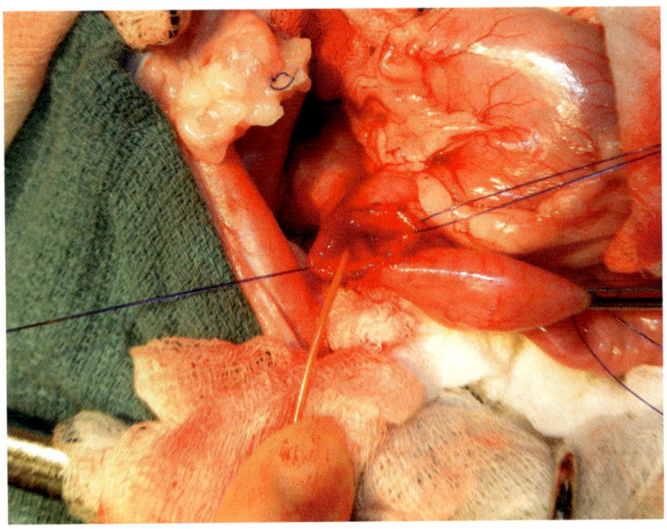

Figure 13.11 Intraoperative photo of catheterization of the common bile duct in a cat with a red rubber catheter. The duodenotomy incision made to access the major duodenal papilla is held open with two stay sutures, and bowel clamps are closing the duodenum aborad.

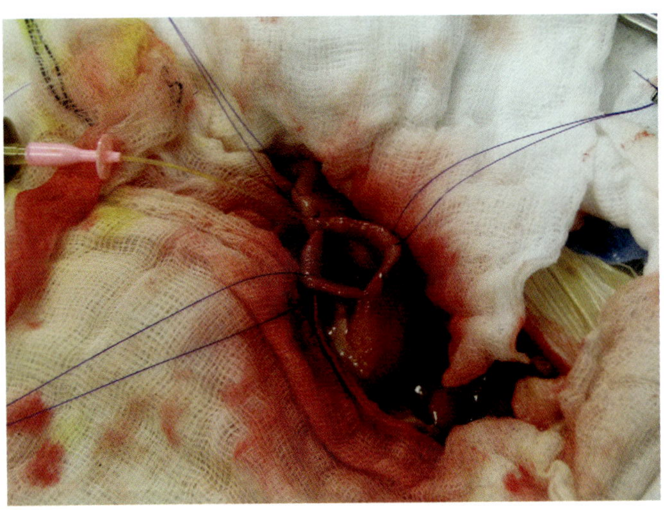

Figure 13.12 Retrograde catheterization of the common bile duct after duodenotomy. Image courtesy of Benito de la Puerta.

3. Leak of intestinal contents is limited by use of atraumatic bowel clamps or an assistant's fingers.
4. The common bile duct is catheterized and flushed with 0.9% sterile saline.
5. Standard repair of duodenotomy is performed with a simple continuous or simple interrupted pattern of 3-0 or 4-0 absorbable suture material (see Chapter 11).

Sphincterotomy of the sphincter of Oddi

Sphincterotomy is the creation of a 2–3 mm longitudinal incision across the sphincter of Oddi at the level of the major duodenal papilla (Fig. 13.13).[13]

1. A 1–2 cm longitudinal incision is made along the antimesenteric surface of the duodenum opposite the major duodenal papilla.
2. The major duodenal papilla is catheterized to provide a guide for sphincterotomy.
3. The incision is made using a scalpel blade or electrocautery, beginning at the natural opening of the major duodenal papilla and extending orally. Electrocautery may be preferred if bleeding is a major concern; use of coagulation/blended (rather than cutting) settings is recommended. Avoid perforation of the duodenum or common bile duct.
4. Standard repair of duodenotomy is performed with a simple continuous or simple interrupted pattern of 3-0 or 4-0 absorbable suture material (see Chapter 11).

Choledochal stenting

Choledochal stenting (Fig. 13.14) is indicated for temporary management of EHBDO if it is hoped that the primary cause for EHBDO will respond to medical management or when biopsy results and a definitive long-term plan are pending.[12,13] Custom-made stents can be prepared using 2.5Fr–8Fr latex red rubber or silicone urethral catheters, cut to an appropriate length.[12,13] Commercial temporary biliary stents with deployment systems are also available. These are commonly made of polyurethane and have flanges on each end or a double pigtail to prevent migration. They are available in a range of sizes (4–12 cm in length, with an expanded diameter of 6–10 mm and 6.5Fr–8.5Fr deployment systems). Stent length within the common bile duct and duodenum should be the shortest possible.

1. An antimesenteric 1–2 cm longitudinal duodenotomy is made to expose the major duodenal papilla.
2. The common bile duct is catheterized and flushed with 0.9% sterile saline.
3. The stent is passed through the major duodenal papilla into the common bile duct just beyond the site of obstruction.
4. If a custom-made stent is used, the stent can be secured to the internal duodenal wall with two circum-

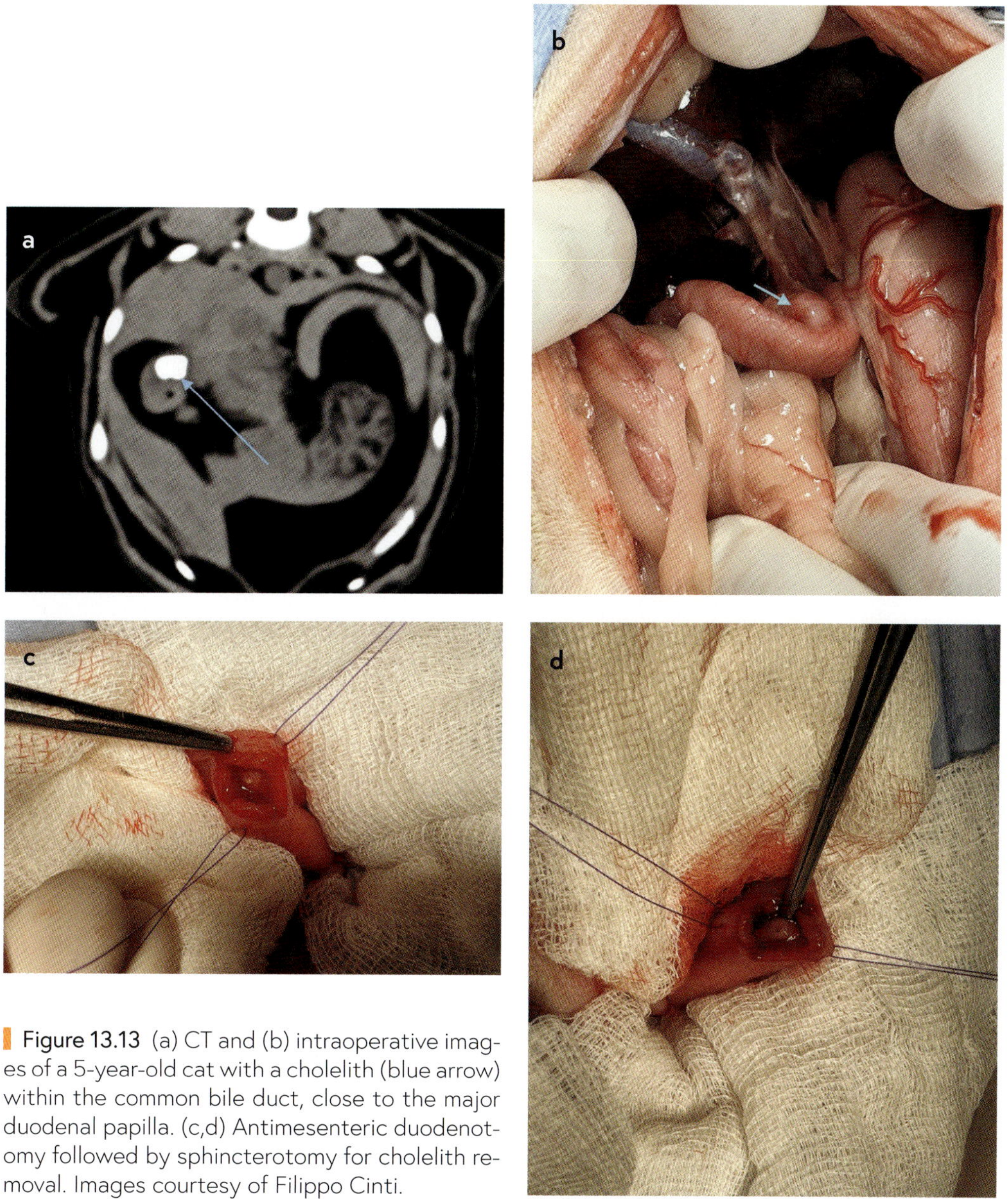

Figure 13.13 (a) CT and (b) intraoperative images of a 5-year-old cat with a cholelith (blue arrow) within the common bile duct, close to the major duodenal papilla. (c,d) Antimesenteric duodenotomy followed by sphincterotomy for cholelith removal. Images courtesy of Filippo Cinti.

ferential sutures placed partial thickness through the duodenal wall to include the submucosa. Absorbable monofilament (3-0, 4-0) suture materials are advised (e.g., polydioxanone or poliglecaprone).

5. Standard repair of duodenotomy is performed with a simple continuous or simple interrupted pattern of 3-0 or 4-0 absorbable suture material (see Chapter 11).

Endoscopic retrieval of the stent should be planned 6–8 weeks after placement due to the risk of occlusion, dislodgement, and reflux of intestinal contents into the biliary system. Since the stent may pass naturally in the stool, the ongoing presence of the stent can be checked by ultrasound. There is also risk of ascending bacterial cholangitis and cholecystitis; therefore, there may be a rationale for prophylactic, as well as ongoing, antibiotics.[13]

Choledochotomy and common bile duct repair

Choledochotomy is the incision of the common bile duct, often necessary in case of cholelithiasis causing obstruction.[12,13] This procedure should be performed only if the calculi cannot be pushed into the gallbladder (for cholecystectomy) nor directed toward the major duodenal papilla (for sphincterotomy).

1. A longitudinal incision is made over the cholelith.
2. The cholelith is removed.
3. Closure is achieved using 4-0 or 5-0 absorbable or nonabsorbable suture material (e.g., polydioxanone, polypropylene, or nylon) in a simple interrupted pattern. The choice of suture material and size should be based on bile duct size and tissue friability. A transverse closure should be considered if excessive luminal narrowing is a concern.

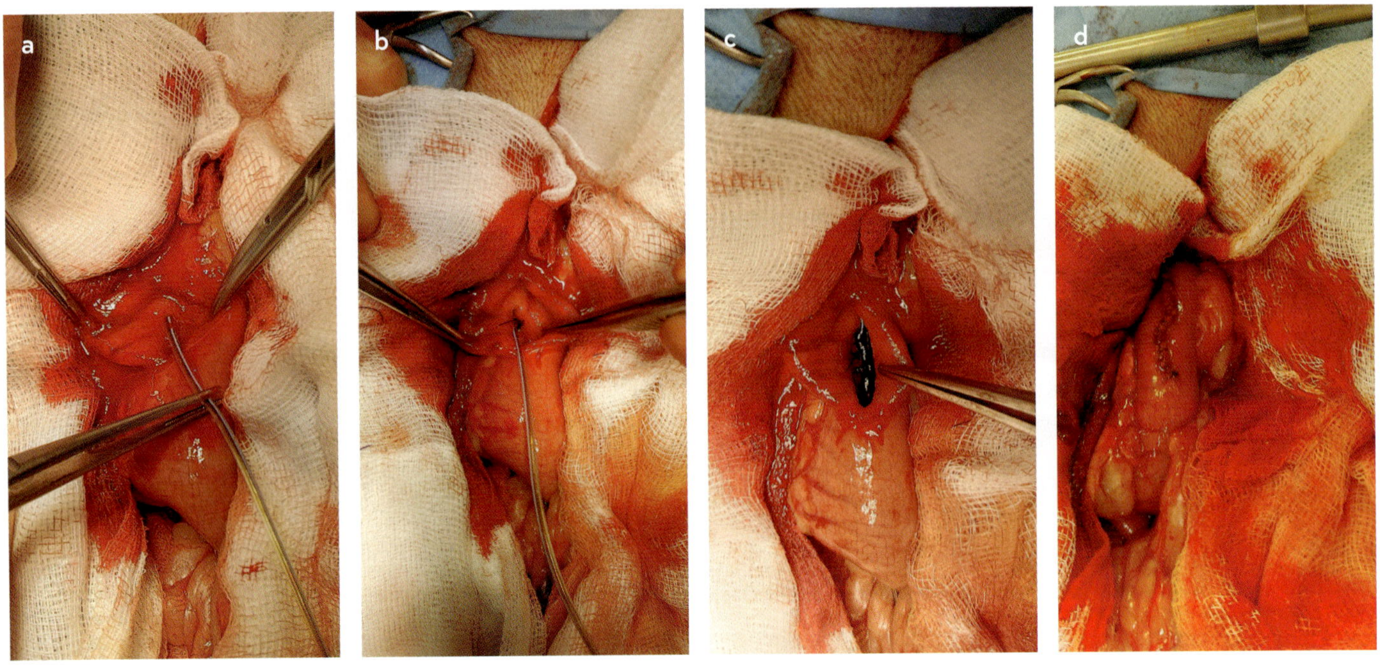

Figure 13.14 Application of a temporary choledocal stent in a 10-year-old dog with distal obstruction of common bile duct. Images courtesy of Filippo Cinti.

Cholecystoenterostomy

Cholecystoenterostomy is indicated for the management of permanent obstruction of the common bile duct (Fig. 13.15; Video 13.2).[13,20] The procedure involves anastomosing the gallbladder lumen to the duodenum (cholecystoduodenostomy) or to a section of jejunum (cholecystojejunostomy). A simple continuous or interrupted pattern of 3-0 or 4-0 delayed absorbable monofilament suture material is appropriate. The use of a 30 mm endoscopic gastrointestinal anastomosis stapler for cholecystoduodenostomy has been described in dogs; however, long-term follow-up was not reported.

Video 13.2. Cholecystoduodenostomy. Video courtesy of Benito de la Puerta.

1. The gallbladder is released from the hepatic fossa, as described above for cholecystectomy.
2. The surgical field is carefully isolated with moistened laparotomy swabs.
3. An incision is made along the longitudinal axis of the gallbladder, and the bile is suctioned.
4. A corresponding incision is then created on the antimesenteric surface of the duodenum for cholecystoduodenostomy or on a section of jejunum for cholecystojejunostomy.
5. The gallbladder wall is sutured to the seromuscular layer of the corresponding intestinal incision to create a new stoma using a simple continuous pattern of 3-0 or 4-0 absorbable monofilament material on both sides. The stoma is expected to contract down to 50% of its original size; therefore, stoma size should be maximized.
6. An additional simple interrupted suture can be added at each end of the stoma to pexy the gallbladder to the intestine.

Specific immediate complications after this surgery include dehiscence and obstruction of the stoma leading to life-threatening bile leak and EHBDO. Other postop-

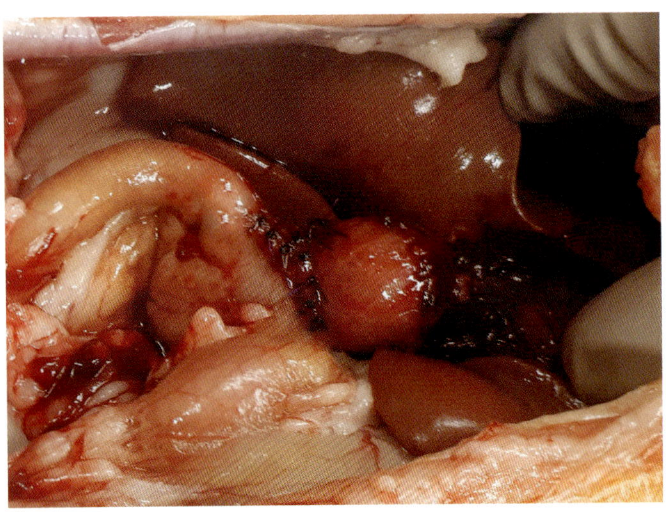

Figure 13.15 Intraoperative image of a completed cholecystoduodenostomy in a cat. The pink spherical gallbladder at the center of the image is sutured to the pale pink duodenum to the left.

erative complications include recurrent cholangiohepatitis characterized by pyrexia, anorexia, and lethargy, chronic diarrhea secondary to exocrine pancreatic insufficiency, chronic vomiting, chronic weight loss, and stricture requiring revision surgery. Long-term medical treatment is frequently indicated, including antibiotics, pancreatic enzyme supplements, and low-fat prescription diets. These chronic, recurrent problems frequently lead to euthanasia or death.[12,20,21]

Perioperative management

Postoperative medical management of each underlying disease is covered under the "Treatment" sections above. Additionally, perioperative care needs to incorporate management of the consequences of biliary obstruction and inevitable bile spill at surgery, as well as monitoring, treatment, and mitigation of reported perioperative complications, including persistent hypotension, acute kidney injury, anemia, dysregulated coagulation, and pancreatitis.[3]

Biliary obstruction is associated with loss of the normal functions of bile, among which are the control of intestinal immunity, the absorption of fat-soluble nutrients, and the excretion of toxins. Biliary obstruction is therefore associated with endotoxemia, dysregulated coagulation, decreased immunity (which may lead to systemic inflammatory response syndrome), septic shock, and multiple organ failure.[3] Biliary leak results in biliary peritonitis and is frequently associated with bacterial infection. Bile is cytotoxic and results in a severe inflammatory process exacerbated by infection, which may also lead to systemic inflammatory response syndrome, septic shock, and multiple organ failure.[3] Intensive care monitoring and treatment is therefore required. Antibiotics targeting *Escherichia coli* and *Enterococcus* are indicated, pending results of bile or tissue culture.

Postoperative bile leak requires exploratory surgery. If the risk of postoperative bile leak is considered high or if there is a preoperative diagnosis of septic peritonitis, placement of an abdominal drain at surgery is indicated for monitoring and ongoing abdominal drainage. Diagnosis of postoperative bile peritonitis is based on rising serum bilirubin concentration and a bilirubin concentration in peritoneal fluid more than 2.5 times that of serum.[3]

Persistent and frequently unresponsive hypotension is a commonly reported anesthetic complication of biliary surgery.[22] Unresponsiveness to treatment results in persistent hypotension into the postoperative period and can progress to fatal cardiorespiratory arrest. Treatment of intraoperative hypotension should be achieved with intravenous fluid boluses, constant-rate infusions of positive inotropes and/or vasopressors dosed to effect, and reduction in inhalant anesthetic agents. Reduction in inhalant anesthetics may be achieved by careful consideration of analgesia, with the incorporation of epidural opioids, local anesthetics, and constant-rate intravenous infusions of analgesics into the anesthetic plan.

Acute kidney injury is characterized by elevation in serum creatinine concentrations. This may result from preoperative dehydration and intraoperative kidney hypoperfusion secondary to unresponsive hypotension. Careful preoperative rehydration and management of intraoperative hypotension are indicated. Anemia is frequently seen in dogs and cats presenting for emergency biliary surgery, and clinically significant hemorrhage is a commonly reported intraoperative complication. This may be compounded by dysregulated coagulation. Pretreatment with vitamin K and perioperative treatment with fresh frozen plasma or packed red blood cells may be indicated.

Prompt diagnosis of pancreatitis using laboratory testing and institution of supportive care including antiemetics, proton pump inhibitors, analgesics, and intravenous fluid therapy is indicated. Feeding is also critical in patients with pancreatitis and in dogs undergoing biliary surgery due to frequently reported hypoproteinemia, emphasizing the need for intraoperative placement of a feeding tube.[20–22]

KEEP IN MIND

- Emergency biliary surgery is indicated for gallbladder rupture, extrahepatic biliary duct obstruction unresponsive to medical management, and biliary peritonitis.
- Irrespective of the cause, biliary surgical emergencies present similarly. Common clinical signs include vomiting, hyporexia, lethargy, jaundice, and abdominal pain. Frequent clinicopathological abnormalities include elevations in liver enzyme activities, increased total bilirubin, anemia, and high band neutrophil numbers. However, not all biliary emergencies will demonstrate the typical signs of jaundice and elevated total bilirubin.
- Ultrasound is key to diagnosis of biliary emergencies.
- Serial ultrasound examinations and serum biochemistries may be required to detect progression of disease or failure of medical management, indicating the need for surgical intervention.
- Success of emergency biliary surgery is dependent on surgeon experience, careful choice of the surgical technique based on the individual patient, and detailed attention to anesthetic protocols and perioperative care.

References

1. Furneaux RW. A series of six cases of sphincter of Oddi pathology in the cat (2008–2009). *J Feline Med Surg.* 2010; 12(10):794–801.
2. Kesimer M et al. Excess secretion of gel-forming mucins and associated innate defense proteins with defective mucin unpackaging underpin gallbladder mucocele formation in dogs. *PLoS One.* 2015; 10(9):e0138988.
3. Thompson BJ, Sherman RA. Comprehensive review of biliary peritonitis. *Top Companion Anim Med.* 2021; 44:100532.
4. Jaffey JA et al. Gallbladder mucocele: Variables associated with outcome and the utility of ultrasonography to identify gallbladder rupture in 219 dogs (2007–2016). *J Vet Intern Med.* 2018; 32(1):195–200.
5. Parkanzky M et al. Long-term survival of dogs treated for gallbladder mucocele by cholecystectomy, medical management, or both. *J Vet Intern Med.* 2019; 33(5):2057–2066.
6. Piegols HJ et al. Association between biliary tree manipulation and outcome in dogs undergoing cholecystectomy for gallbladder mucocele: A multi-institutional retrospective study. *Vet Surg.* 2021; 50(4):767–774.
7. Jaffey JA et al. Effect of clinical signs, endocrinopathies, timing of surgery, hyperlipidemia, and hyperbilirubinemia on outcome in dogs with gallbladder mucocele. *Vet J.* 2019; 251:105350.
8. Besso JG, Wrigley RH, Gliatto JM, Webster CR. Ultrasonographic appearance and clinical findings in 14 dogs with gallbladder mucocele. *Vet Radiol Ultrasound.* 2000; 41(3):261–271.
9. Wilson K et al. Dogs with biliary rupture based on ultrasound findings may have normal total serum bilirubin values. *Vet Radiol Ultrasound.* 2021; 62(2):236–245.
10. Putterman AB et al. Influence of normograde versus retrograde catheterization of bile ducts in dogs treated for gallbladder mucocele. *Vet Surg.* 2021; 50(4):784–793.
11. Allan F, Watson PJ, McCallum KE. Clinical features and outcomes in 38 dogs with cholelithiasis receiving conservative or surgical management. *J Vet Intern Med.* 2021; 35(6):2730–2742.
12. Baker SG, Mayhew PD, Mehler SJ. Choledochotomy and primary repair of extrahepatic biliary duct rupture in seven dogs and two cats. *J Small Anim Pract.* 2011; 52(1):32–37.
13. Simpson M, Neville-Towle J, Lee K, Rossanese M. Cholecystectomy in 23 cats (2005–2021). *Vet Surg.* 2022; 51(1):109–116.
14. Ward PM et al. Cholelithiasis in the dog: Prevalence, clinical presentation, and outcome. *J Am Anim Hosp Assoc.* 2020; 56(3):152.
15. Larson MM. Ultrasound imaging of the hepatobiliary system and pancreas. *Vet Clin North Am Small Anim Pract.* 2016; 46(3):453–480.
16. Eich CS, Ludwig LL. The surgical treatment of cholelithiasis in cats: A study of nine cases. *J Am Anim Hosp Assoc.* 2002; 38(3):290–296.
17. O'Brien KM et al. Clinical, histopathologic, and immunohistochemical features of 13 cases of canine gallbladder neuroendocrine carcinoma. *J Vet Diagn Invest.* 2021; 33(2):294–299.
18. Patnaik AK, Lieberman PH, Erlandson RA, Antonescu C. Hepatobiliary neuroendocrine carcinoma in cats: A clinicopathologic, immunohistochemical, and ultrastructural study of 17 cases. *Vet Pathol.* 2005; 42(3):331–337.
19. Mayhew PD, Weisse CW. Treatment of pancreatitis-associated extrahepatic biliary tract obstruction by choledochal stenting in seven cats. *J Small Anim Pract.* 2008; 49(3):133–138.
20. Ludwig LL, McLoughlin MA, Graves TK, Crisp MS. Surgical treatment of bile peritonitis in 24 dogs and 2 cats: A retrospective study (1987–1994). *Vet Surg.* 1997; 26(2):90–98.
21. Mehler SJ, Mayhew PD, Drobatz KJ, Holt DE. Variables associated with outcome in dogs undergoing extrahepatic biliary surgery: 60 cases (1988–2002). *Vet Surg.* 2004; 33(6):644–649.
22. Monticelli P, Stathopoulou TR, Lee K, Adami C. Life-threatening perianaesthetic complications in five cats undergoing biliary tract surgery: Case series and literature review. *J Feline Med Surg.* 2017; 19(6):717–722.

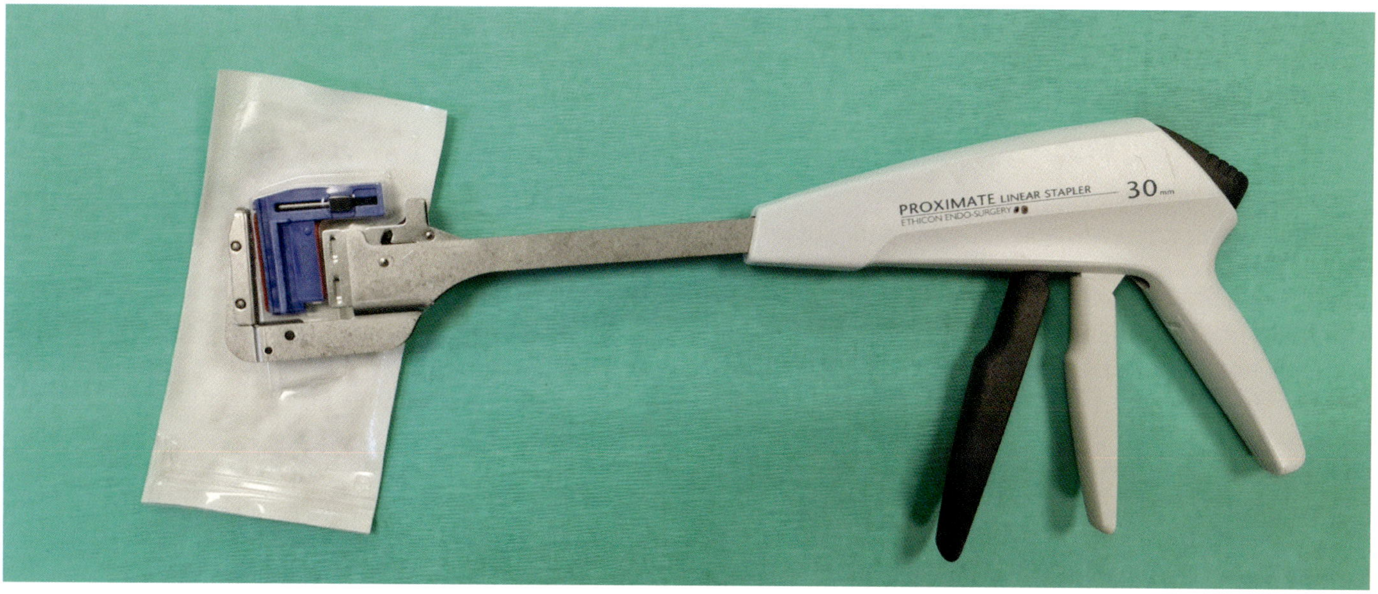

Figure 14.4 TA 30 stapler (blue cartridge, open leg length 3.5 mm) (Ethicon).

first 2 days following surgery. Daily blood tests should be conducted with a focus on coagulation, platelet count, electrolytes, glucose, blood gases, hematocrit, total protein, and albumin. Intravenous fluid therapy is administered in the postoperative period until vital signs stabilize and eating resumes. The administration of fresh frozen plasma or intravenous colloids may be considered if the serum albumin concentration drops below 2.0 g/dL.[17] Opioids (e.g., methadone, fentanyl) can be used to control pain. If not contraindicated, patients are prescribed nonsteroidal anti-inflammatory drugs for 7–14 days. Paracetamol can also be considered in dogs. Antibiotics (empirical intravenous, then switched to oral antibiotics based on culture and sensitivity results) are administered for a minimum of 7 days postoperatively. Exercise should be restricted for at least 2 weeks after surgery, with 10–15-minute slow on lead walks allowed 2–3 times daily. Exercise can be gradually increased after the first 2 weeks. The surgical site should be rechecked 10–14 days postoperatively.

Outcome

In the absence of disseminated intravascular coagulation, hemoabdomen, pneumonia, or other life-threatening postoperative complications, the overall postoperative survival rate for dogs with liver lobe torsion undergoing liver lobectomy is reported to be 84%.[2,5–7,9–12]

Liver abscess

Liver abscesses occur infrequently in dogs and cats, mainly affecting middle-aged to older dogs, with no clear breed or sex predisposition. A definitive cause is not always identified, but reported etiologies include extrahepatic infections (e.g., chronic bacterial infections with septicemia, pancreatitis, pneumonia) and damage to the hepatic parenchyma (e.g., trauma, torsion, neoplasia, previous biopsy). Underlying preexisting endocrine disorders (e.g., diabetes mellitus, hyperadrenocorticism), prolonged use of phenobarbital or corticosteroids, and gallbladder rupture have also been associated with the development of liver abscesses.[18–23]

Clinical presentation and diagnosis

Patients often present with nonspecific clinical signs such as lethargy, anorexia, vomiting, diarrhea, abdominal pain, dehydration, and fever. Cats typically exhibit a lower prevalence of pyrexia (23% vs. 86%) and abdominal pain (31% vs. 57%) when compared to dogs.[21,24] In 75%–85% of cases, blood tests reveal neutrophilia, sometimes accompanied by a left shift.[21,22] The biochemistry panel often shows elevated levels of serum alkaline phosphatase, alanine aminotransferase, and aspartate aminotransferase. Hypoalbuminemia is observed in 64% of dogs and 79% of cats.[22,24] Bacterial infection is present in 69%–90% of cats and dogs with liver abscesses.[21,22,24]

Abdominal ultrasound is a sensitive technique to diagnose liver abscess, revealing poorly echogenic and centrally cavitated lesions; however, hypoechoic, hyperechoic, or heterogeneous masses have also been described.[22] Solitary abscesses are observed in 77% of cases.[21] However, in cats, hepatic abscessation often presents as multiple macroscopic or microscopic nodules.[24] The majority of liver abscesses in dogs are located in the left lobes, while in cats they are more commonly found in the right lobes.[21,24] Cytology plays a crucial role in confirming the diagnosis. Examination of the cellular population reveals suppurative inflammation with degenerated neutrophils, and phagocytosed bacteria may be observed within the neutrophils.[17]

Treatment

Systemic antibiotics are frequently used in the treatment of liver abscesses. The choice of antibiotics is based on culture and sensitivity testing results, but empirical treatment can be initiated with penicillins, clindamycin, or a combination of metronidazole and an aminoglycoside or fluoroquinolone.[22] These antimicrobials target the most common causative agents of liver abscesses, which include *Escherichia coli*, *Staphylococcus* spp., *Enterococcus* spp., *Micrococcus*, *Proteus mirabilis*, *Klebsiella pneumoniae*, *Staphylococcus epidermidis*, *Staphylococcus intermedius*, *Clostridium* spp., *Lactobacillus*, *Serratia* sp., and *Citrobacter freundii*.[21,25] Approximately 55% of cases involve more than one organism.[21] The presence of *E. coli* as the most commonly isolated microbe suggests an ascending biliary infection.[23]

Ultrasound-guided percutaneous drainage and alcoholization of liver abscesses, a technique described in human medicine, has shown positive outcomes, including shorter hospital stays.[26] In some cases, (partial) liver lobectomy (see "Liver tumors" section below) or debridement and omentopexy may be considered, especially when abscesses are associated with neoplasia,[17] or as part of the treatment approach.

Surgical technique: Ultrasound-guided percutaneous drainage and alcoholization[23]

1. Under general anesthesia and ultrasonographic guidance, a 20-gauge needle is placed inside the abscess.
2. The abscess content is aspirated completely.
3. A 95% ethanol solution (ethanol volume should be 50% of aspirated exudate volume) is injected within the abscess and left in situ for 3 minutes before aspiration.

Surgical technique: Liver abscess omentalization

1. A standard midline celiotomy and abdominal exploration are performed (see Chapter 3).
2. The affected lobe is isolated with moistened laparotomy swabs to avoid contamination.
3. After locating the abscess, a stab incision is performed in the center of the abscess with a number 11 scalpel blade.
4. The abscess is drained using a Poole suction tip.
5. The abscess is then debrided and lavaged with sterile saline solution.
6. For omentalization of the abscess, the bursal portion of the greater omentum is surgically opened, and the omentum is anchored into the remnant of the abscess capsule with two or three simple interrupted sutures (3-0 or 4-0 absorbable monofilament material).

Caution is necessary, as some liver abscesses are associated with neoplasia. In this case, liver lobectomy should be performed.[17]

Postoperative management

The postoperative treatment following surgical resection or drainage and omentalization is comparable to the one described in the "Liver lobe torsion" section above. The ultrasound-guided percutaneous drainage and alcoholization is a safe, cost effective, and rapid technique that does not require postoperative admission. Administration of enrofloxacin for 1 month is suggested after the alcoholization procedure.[23]

Outcome

The outcome of liver abscess treatments in canine and feline patients varies, with different approaches yielding distinct results. Surgical intervention in dogs has been associated with a reported survival rate of 71%. However, it is crucial to note that almost 50% of the dogs in one study did not undergo surgical intervention, experiencing either spontaneous mortality or euthanasia.[22] Prognosis in cases involving percutaneous drainage and omentalization is favorable, with a 100% abscess resolution rate and an absence of complications observed in all patients (5 dogs and 1 cat).[23]

In a retrospective study encompassing 49 dogs diagnosed with liver abscess, treatment outcomes varied. Among them, 8 dogs received medical treatment, while 41 underwent surgical intervention. Notably, in the medically treated group, 3 dogs were still alive 1 year after treatment. In the surgically treated group, 35 dogs survived until discharge. However, the information on the 1-year survival of 13 dogs is somewhat unreliable due to a substantial loss of subjects during the follow-up period.[25]

In another study involving surgical treatment for liver abscesses in 38 dogs, a noteworthy finding emerged. One-third of the patients underwent multiple lobectomies, with some undergoing this procedure earlier due to anatomical considerations rather than multifocal disease. Despite a perioperative mortality rate of 21%, it is crucial to highlight that if patients survived until discharge, the long-term prognosis was favorable.[26] In contrast to dogs, feline mortality following surgical treatment is higher, approximately 79%. This difference is likely attributed to the higher occurrence of multiple macroabscesses in cats, in combination with a higher likelihood of sepsis at the time of diagnosis.[27]

Liver trauma

Hepatic trauma typically arises as a consequence of blunt trauma due to collision, gunshot, or bite wounds, or other penetrating injuries. In cases involving trauma to the liver parenchyma and major blood vessels, the patient will present with a hemoabdomen.

Clinical presentation and diagnosis

Liver trauma can lead to significant hemorrhage from the parenchyma or through rupture of the blood supply. As the volume of effusion increases, abdominal enlargement may become evident and free intra-abdominal fluid may be detected through ballottement. Abdominal distension may interfere with normal ventilation and may result in tachypnea or respiratory distress. Animals with peritonitis often display signs of abdominal pain, although abdominal tenderness may not always be detected.[28] Ultrasonographic examination of abdominal parenchymatous organs can aid in identifying the underlying cause of peritoneal effusion. Point-of-care ultrasound (POCUS) to detect free abdominal fluid complemented with abdominocentesis and peritoneal fluid analysis can confirm a hemoabdomen.[29] These examinations establish the diagnosis and determine the necessity for surgical intervention (see Chapter 16).

Treatment

Patients suspected of having liver trauma should first be stabilized through the administration of intravenous crystalloids and colloids, as necessary to address hypotension, along with intravenous analgesics. It is crucial to note that trauma causing bleeding from the liver likely requires comprehensive investigation for concomitant injuries, including those affecting the diaphragm, orthopedic structures, and neurological components. In cases of diffuse mild hemorrhage from the liver parenchyma, supportive care and conservative management is often successful. It is essential to stabilize the patient, continually assess vital parameters, measure serial packed cell volume and total solids, and monitor the abdominal circumference. If there are indicators of ongoing hemorrhage and the patient fails to stabilize despite appropriate therapy, surgical intervention is warranted. General anesthesia and monitoring (blood pressure, ECG, $ETCO_2$), intravenous fluid support, and perioperative antibiotics are required for this procedure.

Surgical technique

1. A standard midline celiotomy and abdominal exploration are performed (see Chapter 3).
2. The liver lobes, vascular structures, and bile tract are carefully evaluated for lacerations and any source of bleeding.
3. To treat a liver lobe laceration, the following can be performed:
   - Application of pressure to tamponade the bleeding vessel.
   - Use of a mechanical hemostatic agent (e.g., gelatin, cellulose) or an active hemostatic agent (thrombin–gelatin matrix).
   - Partial liver lobectomy.
   - Complete liver lobectomy.

More specific information can be found in the "Liver tumors" section below.

Postoperative management

Postoperative continuous ECG monitoring and blood pressure monitoring are recommended during the first 2 days following surgery. Intravenous fluid therapy is administered in the postoperative period until vital signs stabilize and eating resumes. Daily blood tests should be conducted with a focus on coagulation, platelet count, electrolytes, glucose, blood gases, hematocrit, total protein, and albumin. Additionally, the administration of fresh frozen plasma or intravenous colloids may be considered if the serum albumin concentration is below 2.0 g/dL.[17] In cases of acute blood loss, full blood transfusion or autotransfusion should be considered.

Outcome

In the authors' experience, the majority of liver trauma cases are effectively treated in a conservative fashion, especially in the absence of other concomitant injuries. Factors linked to mortality in cases with severe hemoabdomen include tachycardia, the need for substantial transfusion of blood products, and the onset of respiratory complications attributed to suspected pulmonary thromboembolism or acute respiratory distress syndrome.[30]

Liver tumors

Primary liver tumors originate from hepatocytes, bile duct epithelial cells, neuroendocrine cells, and connective tissue cells. Liver tumors arising from hepatocytes include hepatocellular carcinomas, adenomas, or hyperplastic nodules. Neuroendocrine cells or the epithelium lining the bile ducts may give rise to carcinomas or adenomas, whereas sarcomas develop from connective tissue cells.[31] In the context of hepatocellular tumors, hepatocellular adenomas are more prevalent in cats, while hepatocellular carcinomas are more frequently diagnosed in dogs. A classification is made between massive, nodular, and diffuse forms, and only the latter and some nodular forms are considered inoperable;[15] intraoperative mortality can occur due to tumor exsanguination but is reported to be low, approximately 5%. In most dogs, these tumors are localized in the left and central liver lobes, with reported incidences of 68% in the left liver division, 20% in the central division, and 12% in the right division.[37] A multicenter retrospective study on feline primary nonhematopoietic malignant liver tumors demonstrated that in cats most intrahepatic tumors were left-sided (54.2%), with the left medial lobe being primarily affected (25%).[38]

Regarding biliary tumors, bile duct adenocarcinomas are more common than adenomas, and they metastasize to local lymph nodes, lungs, abdominal organs, and bones in 66%–88% of cases.[32,39] In general, bile duct tumors are more common in cats, with biliary cystadenomas being the most prevalent.[40,41]

Carcinoids, classified as neuroendocrine tumors, are mostly diffuse, with involvement of the gallbladder and metastases to lymph nodes,[33,34,42,43] lungs, intestines, and peritoneal cavity. Finally, hepatic sarcomas are usually metastases originating from a primary tumor elsewhere, including hemangiosarcoma, leiomyosarcoma, fibrosarcoma, osteosarcoma, malignant mesenchymoma, and chondrosarcoma.[44–48]

Clinical presentation and diagnosis

Nonspecific clinical signs such as weight loss, reduced appetite, vomiting, and polyuria/polydipsia are identified in 28%–71% of patients.[32,35–37,39,49] A mass may be detected by abdominal palpation in approximately half of the dogs with a hepatic carcinoma.[37] In a retrospective study in dogs, anemia was present in 54% of patients, whereas microcytosis and leukocytosis accounted for 31% and 27%, respectively. Thrombocytosis was present in 46% of cases. Serum biochemical findings included elevated concentrations of alkaline phosphatase (95%), alanine aminotransferase (88%), aspartate aminotransferase (66%), gamma-glutamyltransferase (54%), and cholesterol (31%). More incidental findings were decreased levels of total protein (5%), albumin (7%), and glucose. Coagulation profiles showed abnormalities in approximately 20% of cases.[37]

Most animals with a hepatic tumor will not be presented as emergency cases unless the tumor starts bleeding due to necrosis or external trauma. The diagnosis is best established through abdominal ultrasonography, which allows differentiation between diffuse, nodular, or single massive neoplasms.[31] Contrast-enhanced ultrasound is not reliable in distinguishing between malignant and benign masses.[50] Preoperatively, the histological diagnosis may be confirmed by ultrasound-guided fine needle aspiration or multiple core biopsies.[51–53] However, a solitary massive neoplasm may be excised entirely and histopathologically typified after surgery, as it usually involves hepatocellular carcinoma (Fig. 14.5). Based on the current literature, a multiphase multiplanar CT scan is recommended for preoperative planning and assessing the thorax and abdomen for metastases and lymphadenopathy.[31]

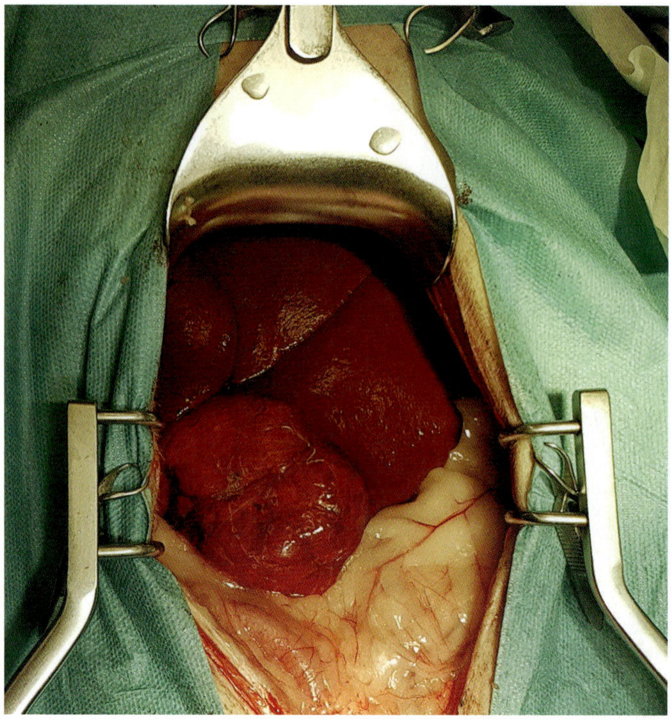

Figure 14.5 Hepatocellular carcinoma in the left lateral liver lobe of a 12-year-old crossbred female before liver lobectomy.

Treatment

Based on the type of tumor, surgical resection of the affected liver lobe(s) is the treatment of choice, and meticulous dissection techniques can render apparent inoperable masses amenable to successful excision.[37] It is important to consider that tumor compression of the vena cava may precipitate hypotension. In addition to anesthetic preparations for hypotension, preoperative administration of fresh frozen plasma is crucial in the presence of abnormal coagulation, and having blood products readily available is paramount in the event of severe intraoperative hemorrhage.[31]

Surgical technique: Liver lobectomy

As a reminder of surgical anatomy, the liver is organized in three divisions:

- Right division: Right lateral lobe and caudate process of caudate lobe, supplied and drained by the right portal branch and right hepatic vein.
- Central division: Right medial and quadrate lobes and papillary process of caudate lobe. In dogs with a galbladder tumor a combination of a central division lobectomy and cholecystectomy may be necessary (Fig 14.8).
- Left division: Left medial and left lateral lobes.

The surgical approach is as follows:

1. A midline celiotomy is performed as described in Chapter 3.

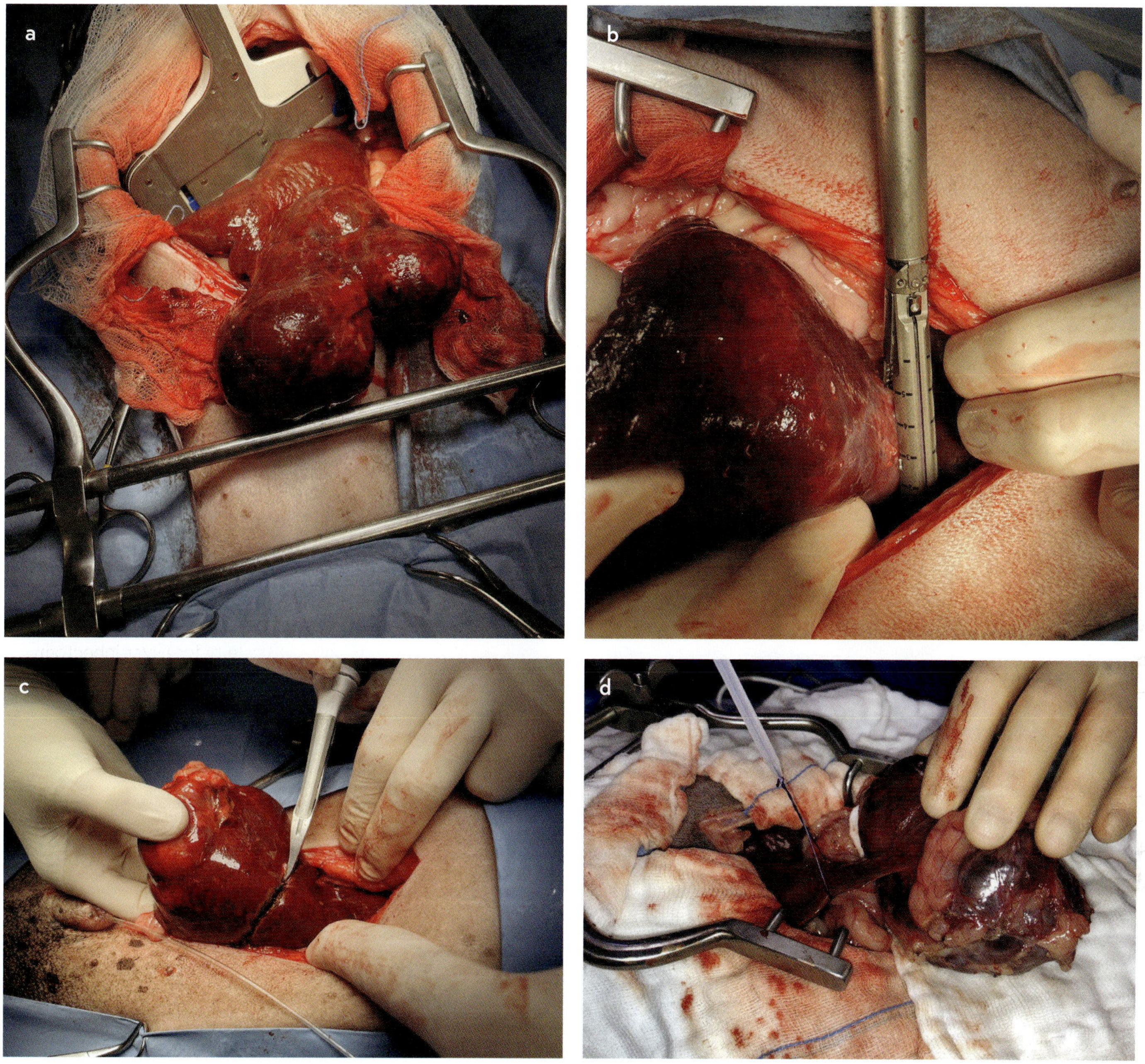

Figure 14.6 Liver lobectomy with (a) TA stapler, (b) Endo GIA, (c) harmonic sealing device, and (d) Endoloop. Images a–c courtesy of Filippo Cinti. Image d courtesy of Rosario Vallefuoco.

2. The liver lobe is exposed and isolated. This can be improved by:
   - Placing laparotomy swabs cranial to the liver.
   - Placing stay sutures on the body of the stomach, with caudal traction.
   - Transecting the triangular ligaments to facilitate lobe manipulation.
   - Performing a paracostal approach, usually necessary for masses involving the right division.
   - Performing a caudal median sternotomy and a partial ventrodorsal midline incision of the diaphragm. Eliminating the negative intrathoracic pressure results in a caudal shift of the cranial abdominal organs. This is rarely needed.
3. The liver lobe is resected. Numerous surgical techniques have been elucidated;[31] the most commonly used methods are described below (Fig. 14.6). For extensive hilar resections, the reader is referred to the references.[31,62]
   - One or two guillotine ligatures (circumferential ligature or Miller's knot, with 3-0 or 2-0 absorbable monofilament suture) or 2-0 Polysorb pretied ligation loop (or Endoloop) at the hilus of the liver lobe can be used in cats and small dogs (Fig. 14.7).[8]

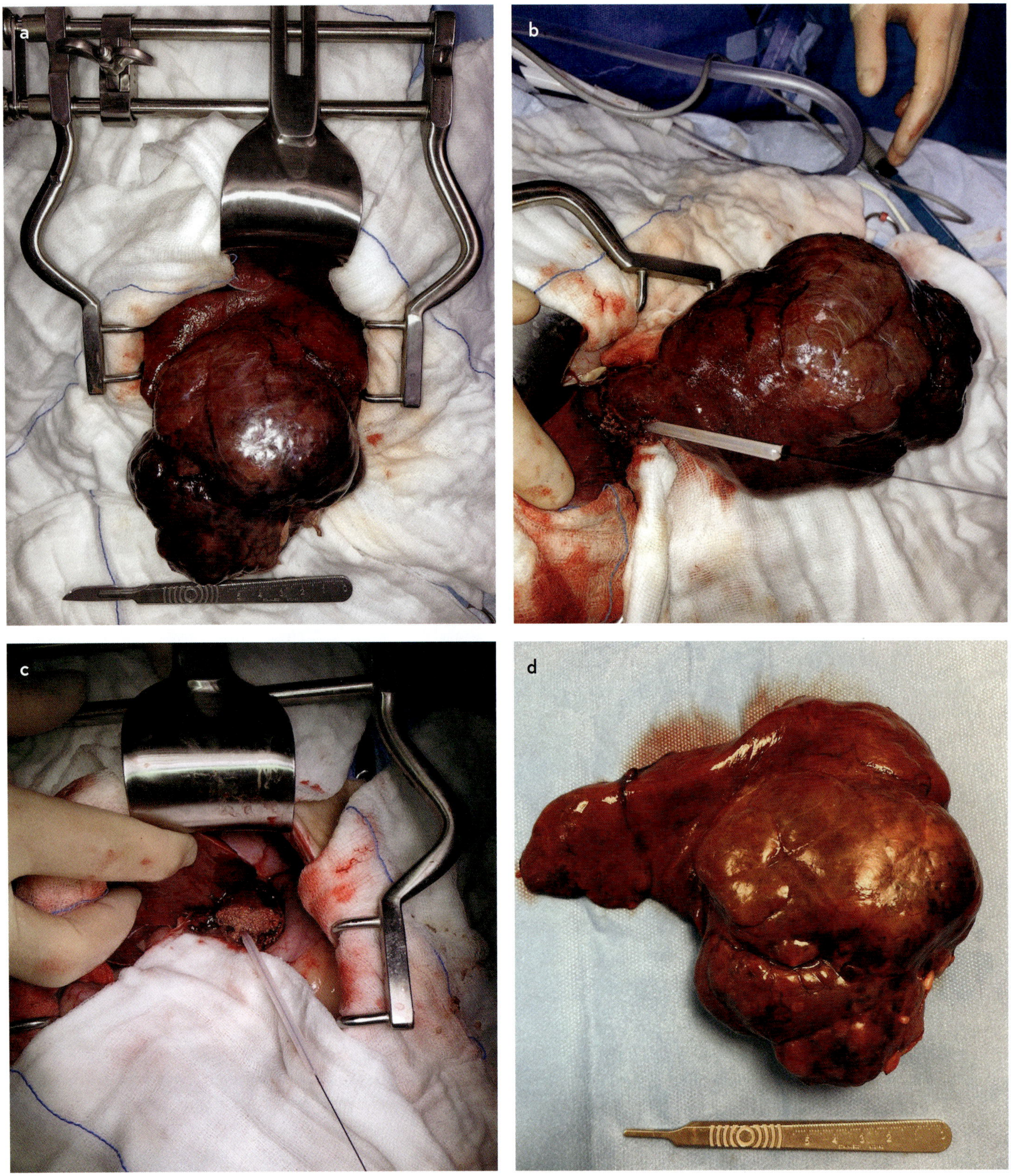

Figure 14.7 (a) Hepatic mass in the left lateral liver lobe. (b) Liver lobectomy with Endoloop. (c) Image after liver lobe excision. (d) Liver lobe excised. Images courtesy of Rosario Vallefuoco.

- Digital fracturing and ligation of separated vasculobiliary structures, which implies skeletonization of vasculobiliary structures to simplify their ligation (with vascular clips or simple interrupted absorbable monofilament sutures) (Fig. 14.8).[31]
- Use of stapling devices. Although this is common practice, it should be taken into consideration that the diameter of most lobar arteries is 1.5 mm or smaller, and the use of the TA 30 and 60 stapler (blue cartridge, two staggered rows of staples with 1.5 mm closed height) can cause significant arterial hemorrhage.[31,54,58] Therefore, it is advised to use the TA 30 V3 stapler with three staggered rows of staples, with a closed height of 1.0 mm; however, the disadvantage of this device is its narrow opening, which makes placement around the hilus challenging. This practical problem can be solved by using the Endo GIA stapler, with a staple leg length of 2.5 mm for medium to large dogs and 2.0 mm for small dogs and cats. Different lengths of staple lines are available (30, 45 and 60 mm) and make this device a good option for liver lobectomy involving the left hepatic division (see Chapter 6).[55]
- Use of vessel-sealing devices (Harmonic, Enseal, LigaSure), alone or in combination with other techniques (circumferential suture, Endoloop, stapler).

4. The liver lobe is excised with a number 11 scalpel blade or Metzenbaum scissors at least 5 mm from the sutures or staple line.
5. The surgical site is checked for bleeding. Some generalized oozing or bleeding is common. This can be readily resolved by applying pressure (laparotomy swabs) for at least 5 minutes or using additional methods of hemostasis (e.g., absorbable gelatin compressed sponge, absorbable oxidized regenerated cellulose).
6. The abdomen is lavaged with warm sterile saline if considered necessary.
7. Abdominal closure is routine.

A study comparing five surgical techniques (suction combined with TA stapler, ultrasonic surgical aspirator, SurgiTie, LigaSure, and skeletonization of the lobar vessels before individually clipping them) concluded that all were safe to use in small animals up to 26 kg. Skeletonization and individually clipping the vessels resulted in the highest blood loss of all techniques but was still below 7.5% of total blood volume.[16] The 2-0 Polysorb

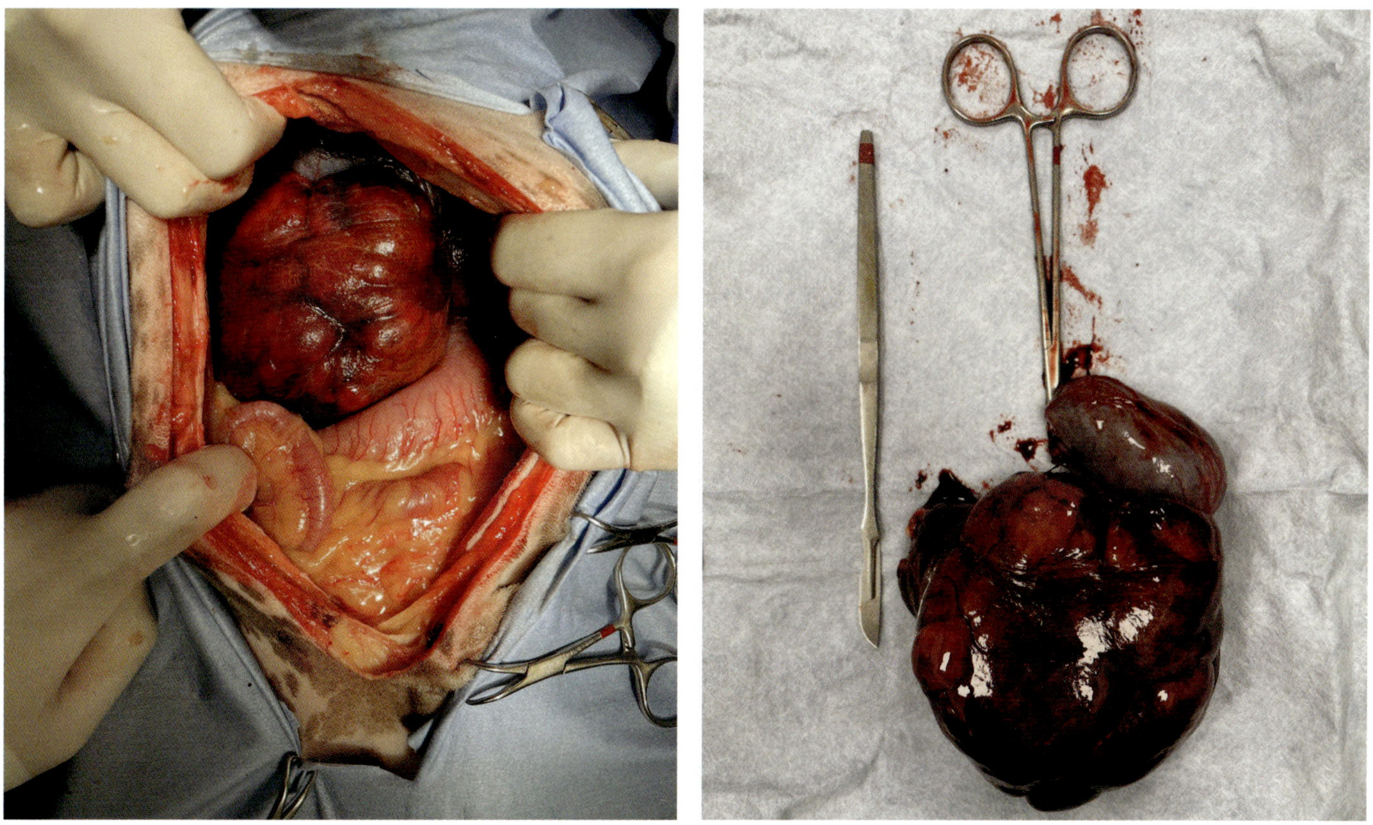

Figure 14.8 Central division liver lobectomy and cholecystectomy in a dog with liver and gallbladder tumors. Images courtesy of Filippo Cinti.

pretied ligation loop (SurgiTie) is a cost-effective and rapid method that can be used for liver biopsy and resection of twisted liver lobes and neoplastic tissue. When considering liver tissue resection, it is recommended to utilize the pretied ligating loop when the circumference of the lobe measures less than 80 mm.[15] The Cavitron ultrasonic surgical aspirator is a safe and feasible technique for nodulectomy and complex lobectomy while preserving the major blood vessels with minimal complications.[56] In case of severe hemorrhage, digital occlusion of the portal vein and hepatic artery (Pringle maneuver) can be used to temporarily reduce blood flow to the liver lobes (<20 minutes), allowing provisional hemorrhage control.

Postoperative management

Cardiovascular support and effective pain management are of paramount importance. During the initial 24–48 hours following surgical intervention, intravenous fluid therapy is recommended. If the serum albumin concentration drops below 2.0 g/dL, supplementation with colloids or plasma is advised. Consequently, daily hematological assessment, including hematocrit and total protein, is advised. Ideally, this evaluation should also encompass electrolytes, blood urea nitrogen, glucose, blood gases, and platelet counts. Minimal antimicrobial prophylaxis is utilized; antibiotics may be prescribed for 5 days postoperatively to prevent growth of clostridia, which typically reside in the liver.[31]

Outcome

Regarding hepatocellular tumors in dogs, median survival exceeds 1460 days following surgery, whereas it is approximately 270 days without surgery. A low local recurrence rate is reported, and high levels of alanine aminotransferase and aspartate aminotransferase are associated with a poorer prognosis.[37] In 6.5% (8/124) of dogs, no correlation was found between mass location and mortality. However, right divisional masses were more prone to intraoperative complications, while postoperative complications were not observed more often compared with other localizations.[37,57] Surgical intervention is not considered optimal for addressing diffuse and nodular forms of hepatocellular carcinoma. This is primarily due to the frequent occurrence of incomplete surgical resection and a high metastatic rate.[14]

Cats who undergo liver lobectomy demonstrate a significantly longer median survival time (375 days vs. 16 days without surgery). Additionally, in cases of hepatocellular carcinoma, the median survival time was 868 days. Liver lobectomy is linked to extended survival times and a positive prognosis in cats with hepatocellular carcinoma.[38]

The prognosis associated with benign cystadenoma is highly favorable when managed through surgical excision,[41,58,59] whereas the prognosis for malignant biliary tumors is poor, with a high mortality rate.[41] Cats with bile duct carcinomas have an acceptable prognosis, with a median survival time of 270 days after surgical treatment.[38]

In both cats and dogs, neuroendocrine carcinomas represent aggressive tumors characterized by an exceedingly unfavorable prognosis. Due to their diffuse nature, surgical excision is typically not a viable option.[14] When the condition is limited to the gallbladder, cholecystectomy might be feasible, with extended survival demonstrated in a limited number of instances.[60,61]

The preferred treatment approach for sarcomas entails surgical resection of the affected liver lobe. However, the prognosis remains highly uncertain in the majority of cases due to the prevalent incidence of metastatic disease.[14]

KEEP IN MIND

- Liver lobe torsion typically involves one hepatic lobe, with the left lateral being the most commonly affected.
- Liver abscesses are frequently associated with comorbidities. Bacterial infection is documented in 69%–90% of cases involving liver abscesses in cats and dogs.
- Liver trauma can result in hemoabdomen. If conservative treatment is not sufficient, surgical intervention is necessary and yields a good prognosis.
- Surgery is the preferred treatment for liver tumors. In the case of hepatocellular tumors, only the diffuse form is considered inoperable.

References

1. Tomlinson J, Black A. Liver lobe torsion in a dog. *J Am Vet Med Assoc.* 1983; 183(2):225–226.
2. Tate PS. Hepatic torsion and dislocation with hypotension and colonic obstruction. *Am Surg.* 1993; 59(7):455–458.
3. McConkey S, Briggs C, Solano M, Illanes O. Liver torsion and associated bacterial peritonitis in a dog. *Can Vet J.* 1997; 38(7):438–439.
4. Downs MO et al. Liver lobe torsion and liver abscess in a dog. *J Am Vet Med Assoc.* 1998; 212(5):678–680.
5. Sato AF, Solano M. Radiographic diagnosis: Liver lobe entrapment and associated emphysematous hepatitis. *Vet Radiol Ultrasound.* 1998; 39(2):123–124.
6. Sonnenfield JM et al. Radiographic and ultrasonographic findings of liver lobe torsion in a dog. *Vet Radiol Ultrasound.* 2001; 42(4):344–346.
7. Swann HM, Brown DC. Hepatic lobe torsion in 3 dogs and a cat. *Vet Surg.* 2001; 30(5):482–486.
8. Martin RA, Lanz OI, Tobias KM. Liver and biliary system. In: Slatter D (ed.). *Textbook of Small Animal Surgery*, 3rd ed. Philadelphia, PA: WB Saunders; 2003.
9. Schwartz SG, Mitchell SL, Keating JH, Chan DL. Liver lobe torsion in dogs: 13 cases (1995–2004). *J Am Vet Med Assoc.* 2006; 228(2):242–247.
10. von Pfeil DJ, Jutkowitz LA, Hauptman J. Left lateral and left middle liver lobe torsion in a Saint Bernard puppy. *J Am Anim Hosp Assoc.* 2006; 42(5):381–385.
11. Bhandal J, Kuzma A, Starrak G. Spontaneous left medial liver lobe torsion and left lateral lobe infarction in a Rottweiler. *Can Vet J.* 2008; 49(10):1002–1004.
12. Lee KJ et al. Liver lobe torsion in a Shih-tzu dog. *J Small Anim Pract.* 2009; 50(3):157.
13. Singh M et al. Hepatic lobe torsion and gastric–dilation volvulus in a dog. *Aust Vet Pract.* 2002; 32(4):174–178.
14. Mayhew PD, Weisse C. Liver and biliary system. In: Johnston SA, Tobias KM (eds.). *Veterinary Surgery: Small Animal*, 2nd ed. Missouri, MO: Elsevier; 2018.
15. Cuddy LC, Risselada M, Ellison GW. Clinical evaluation of a pre-tied ligating loop for liver biopsy and liver lobectomy. *J Small Anim Pract.* 2013; 54(2):61–66.
16. Risselada M et al. Comparison of 5 surgical techniques for partial liver lobectomy in the dog for intraoperative blood loss and surgical time. *Vet Surg.* 2010; 39(7):856–862.
17. Degner DA, Bhandal J. Liver lobe torsion and abscess. In: Monnet E (ed.). *Small Animal Soft Tissue Surgery*, 2nd ed. Hoboken, NJ: Wiley Blackwell; 2023.
18. Lord PF, Carb A, Halliwell WH, Prueter JC. Emphysematous hepatic abscess associated with trauma, necrotic hepatic nodular hyperplasia and adenoma in a dog: A case history report. *Vet Radiol.* 1982; 23(2):46–49.
19. Grooters AM, Sherding RG, Biller DS, Johnson SE. Hepatic abscesses associated with diabetes mellitus in two dogs. *J Vet Intern Med.* 1994; 8(3):203–206.
20. Grooters AM, Sherding RG, Johnson SE. Hepatic abscesses in dogs. *Compend Contin Educ Vet.* 1995; 6:833–839.
21. Schwarz LA, Penninck DG, Leveille-Webster C. Hepatic abscesses in 13 dogs: A review of the ultrasonographic findings, clinical data and therapeutic options. *Vet Radiol Ultrasound.* 1998; 39(4):357–365.
22. Farrar ET, Washabau RJ, Saunders HM. Hepatic abscesses in dogs: 14 cases (1982–1994). *J Am Vet Med Assoc.* 1996; 208(2):243–247.
23. Zatelli A et al. Percutaneous drainage and alcoholization of hepatic abscesses in five dogs and a cat. *J Am Anim Hosp Assoc.* 2005; 41(1):34–38.
24. Sergeeff JS, Armstrong PJ, Bunch SE. Hepatic abscesses in cats: 14 cases (1985–2002). *J Vet Intern Med.* 2004; 18(3):295–300.
25. Burke JE et al. Hepatic abscessation in dogs: A multicenter study of 56 cases (2010–2019). *J Vet Emerg Crit Care (San Antonio).* 2023; 33(6):665–675.
26. Dickerson V et al. Outcome in 38 dogs surgically treated for hepatic abscessation. *Vet Surg.* 2023; 52(1):127–133.
27. Center SA. Hepatobiliary infections. In: Greene CE (ed.). *Infectious Diseases of the Dog and Cat.* Philadelphia, PA: WB Saunders; 1990.
28. Richter MC. Spleen. In: Johnston SA, Tobias KM (eds.). *Veterinary Surgery: Small Animal*, 2nd ed. Missouri, MO: Elsevier; 2018.
29. Boysen SR et al. Evaluation of a focused assessment with sonography for trauma protocol to detect free abdominal fluid in dogs involved in motor vehicle accidents. *J Am Vet Med Assoc.* 2004; 225(8):1198–1204.
30. Lux CN et al. Perioperative outcome in dogs with hemoperitoneum: 83 cases (2005–2010). *J Am Vet Med Assoc.* 2013; 242(10):1385–1391.
31. Degner DA, Walshaw R. Liver tumors and partial hepatectomy. In: Monnet E (ed.). *Small Animal Soft Tissue Surgery*, 2nd ed. Hoboken, NJ: Wiley Blackwell; 2023.
32. Patnaik AK, Hurvitz AI, Lieberman PH. Canine hepatic neoplasms: A clinicopathologic study. *Vet Pathol.* 1980; 17(5):553–564.
33. Patnaik AK, Hurvitz AI, Lieberman PH, Johnson GF. Canine hepatocellular carcinoma. *Vet Pathol.* 1981; 18(4):427–438.
34. Patnaik AK, Lieberman PH, Hurvitz AI, Johnson GF. Canine hepatic carcinoids. *Vet Pathol.* 1981; 18(4):445–453.
35. Magne ML, Withrow SJ. Hepatic neoplasia. *Vet Clin North Am Small Anim Pract.* 1985; 15(1):243–256.
36. Kosovsky JE, Manfra-Marretta S, Mathiesen DT, Patnaik AK. Results of partial hepatectomy in 18 dogs with hepatocellular carcinoma. *J Am Anim Hosp Assoc.* 1989; 25(2):203–206.
37. Liptak JM et al. Massive hepatocellular carcinoma in dogs: 48 cases (1992–2002). *J Am Vet Med Assoc.* 2004; 225(8):1225–1230.
38. Brandstetter V et al. Feline primary nonhematopoietic malignant liver tumours: A multicenter retrospective study (2000–2021). *Vet Comp Oncol.* 2023; 21(2):191–199.
39. Trigo FJ, Thompson H, Breeze RG, Nash AS. The pathology of liver tumours in the dog. *J Comp Pathol.* 1982; 92(1):21–39.
40. Post G, Patnaik AK. Nonhematopoietic hepatic neoplasms in cats: 21 cases (1983–1988). *J Am Vet Med Assoc.* 1992; 201(7):1080–1082.
41. Lawrence HJ, Erb HN, Harvey HJ. Nonlymphomatous hepatobiliary masses in cats: 41 cases (1972 to 1991). *Vet Surg.* 1994; 23(5):365–368.
42. Patnaik AK, Lieberman PH, Erlandson RA, Antonescu C. Hepatobiliary neuroendocrine carcinoma in cats: A clinicopathologic, immunohistochemical, and ultrastructural study of 17 cases. *Vet Pathol.* 2005; 42(3):331–337.
43. Patnaik AK et al. Canine hepatic neuroendocrine carcinoma: An immunohistochemical and electron microscopic study. *Vet Pathol.* 2005; 42(2):140–146.
44. Patnaik AK, Liu S, Johnson GF. Extraskeletal osteosarcoma of the liver in a dog. *J Small Anim Pract.* 1976; 17(6):365–370.
45. Jeraj K et al. Primary hepatic osteosarcoma in a dog. *J Am Vet Med Assoc.* 1981; 179(10):1000–1003.

46. McDonald RK, Helman RG. Hepatic malignant mesenchymoma in a dog. *J Am Vet Med Assoc.* 1986; 188(9):1052–1053.
47. Kapatkin AS, Mullen HS, Matthiesen DT, Patnaik AK. Leiomyosarcoma in dogs: 44 cases (1983–1988). *J Am Vet Med Assoc.* 1992; 201(7):1077–1079.
48. Chikata S et al. Primary chondrosarcoma in the liver of a dog. *Vet Pathol.* 2006; 43(6):1033–1036.
49. Strombeck DR. Clinicopathologic features of primary and metastatic neoplastic disease of the liver in dogs. *J Am Vet Med Assoc.* 1978; 173(3):267–269.
50. Burti S et al. Contrast-enhanced ultrasound features of malignant focal liver masses in dogs. *Sci Rep.* 2020; 10(1):6076.
51. Roth L. Comparison of liver cytology and biopsy diagnoses in dogs and cats: 56 cases. *Vet Clin Pathol.* 2001; 30(1):35–38.
52. Cole TL et al. Diagnostic comparison of needle and wedge biopsy specimens of the liver in dogs and cats. *J Am Vet Med Assoc.* 2002; 220(10):1483–1490.
53. Wang KY, Panciera DL, Al-Rukibat RK, Radi ZA. Accuracy of ultrasound-guided fine-needle aspiration of the liver and cytologic findings in dogs and cats: 97 cases (1990–2000). *J Am Vet Med Assoc.* 2004; 224(1):75–78.
54. Schmiedt CW. Suture material, tissue staplers, ligation devices, and closure methods. In: Johnston SA, Tobias KM (eds.). *Veterinary Surgery: Small Animal*, 2nd ed. Missouri, MO: Elsevier; 2018.
55. Szwec D, Singh A, Gatineau M. Hepatic lobectomy in dogs using a stapling device with a vascular cartridge: A retrospective study of 13 cases. *N Z Vet J.* 2023; 71(5):259–266.
56. Sellier C et al. Use of a cavitron ultrasonic surgical aspirator for parenchyma-sparing and complex liver resections in dogs. *Vet Surg.* 2020; 49(4):800–810.
57. Moore VW, White J, Marchevsky AM. Association between divisional location and short-term outcome of liver mass resection in 124 dogs. *Vet Surg.* 2023; 52(4):513–520.
58. Nyland TG, Koblik PD, Tellyer SE. Ultrasonographic evaluation of biliary cystadenomas in cats. *Vet Radiol Ultrasound.* 1999; 40(3):300–306.
59. Trout NJ et al. Surgical treatment of hepatobiliary cystadenomas in cats: five cases (1988–1993). *J Am Vet Med Assoc.* 1995; 206(4):505–507.
60. Lippo NJ, Williams JE, Brawer RS, Sobel KE. Acute hemobilia and hemocholecyst in 2 dogs with gallbladder carcinoid. *J Vet Intern Med.* 2008; 22(5):1249–1252.
61. Willard MD, Dunstan RW, Faulkner J. Neuroendocrine carcinoma of the gallbladder in a dog. *J Am Vet Med Assoc.* 1988; 192(7):926–928.
62. Covey JL et al. Hilar liver resection in dogs. *Vet Surg.* 2009; 38(1):104–111.

Chapter 15

Abdominal hernias

Filippo Cinti, Paolo Buracco

True abdominal hernias

An abdominal hernia is considered "true" when the anatomical limit of the wall defect (hernial ring) is confined within a normal opening in the abdominal wall.[1,2] Most true abdominal hernias are congenital and include defects in the region of the umbilicus and inguinal and femoral canals.[1,2] The true abdominal hernia consist of a hernial ring (a full-thickness defect of the abdominal wall), hernial sac (peritoneum), and hernial content (tissue herniated). Large hernial rings or small defects rarely cause clinical problems requiring emergency treatment. However, if the content of a true hernia is irreducible or painful, or if there is concern for organ incarceration (entrapment of organs or tissue) or strangulation (organ or tissue ischemia due to compromised blood supply), an emergency surgical treatment is warranted.[1,2]

Umbilical hernias

Clinical presentation and diagnosis

The umbilical opening closes rapidly after birth. Its congenital persistence may allow the herniation of abdominal organs. Animals with umbilical hernias in which only fat or omentum is herniated are frequently asymptomatic, except for a soft, small, nonpainful swelling.[1,2] Rarely, intestines or other structures may become displaced into the hernia. Physical examination with the animal in dorsal recumbency often facilitates the identification and reduction of the herniated contents and the identification of the hernial ring. Additionally, careful evaluation for other congenital anomalies, such as cryptorchidism, ventricular septal defects, inguinal hernia, or peritoneopericardial diaphragmatic hernia, should be performed. Further investigations including radiology and/or ultrasonography are normally not necessary unless multiple congenital defects are suspected, or in cases of incarcerated hernias, or when clinical signs suggest possible strangulation or obstruction (Fig. 15.1).[1,2]

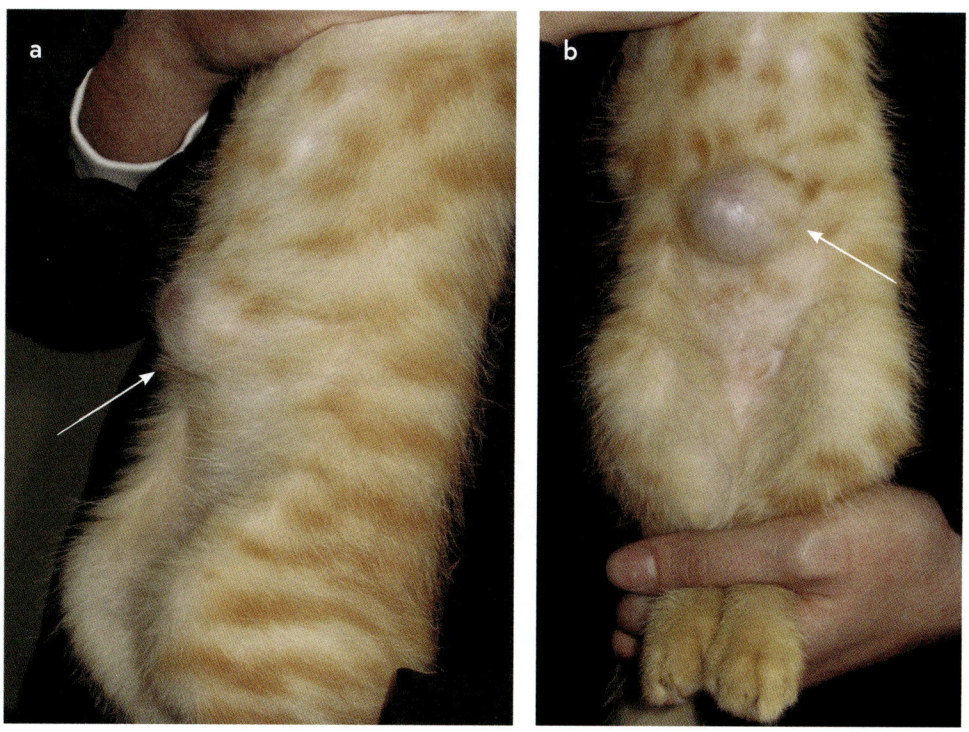

Figure 15.1 Appearance of an umbilical hernia (arrow) containing falciform fat in a young cat.

Treatment

In puppies, small (<2–3 mm), reducible hernias that contain only falciform fat are treated conservatively because the defect may close spontaneously as late as 6 months of age. Early emergency surgical exploration should be considered in patients with large, dilated organs, clinical signs of strangulation/incarceration, or free abdominal fluid.[1,2]

Surgical technique (Fig. 15.2)

1. The ventral abdomen is clipped and prepped routinely, as for spaying.
2. A ventral midline skin incision is made.
   - For small hernias containing only fat, the incision is made directly over the hernial sac.
   - For large, complicated hernias, an elliptical incision is made around the base of the sac to remove redundant tissue.
   - For strangulated/incarcerated hernias, the incision should start caudally, with careful elevation of the skin from the hernial content, and extend cranially to avoid any iatrogenic damage to viscera.
3. The subcutaneous tissue is dissected from the hernial sac.
4. The herniated content is reduced/treated:
   - If only fat is present in the hernial sac, with or without adhesions, the neck of the hernia is ligated, and the sac and remaining content are excised.
   - If the hernial contents are healthy, the sac is opened and the content is inspected and then reduced.
   - If the hernia contains incarcerated or devitalized organs, the hernial ring is enlarged along the linea alba to cautiously inspect and resect any devitalized parts.
5. The sac is excised, and the hernial ring is debrided if adhesions or scar tissue obscure the edges of the linea alba during closure.
   - The hernial ring is closed with a simple interrupted or simple continuous suture of 3-0 to 0 long-lasting absorbable monofilament material.
   - In rare cases of excessive tension, different techniques can be adopted:
     - Tension-relieving suture
     - Releasing incision in the external rectus fascia
     - Rectus advancement (separation of anatomic component)
     - Prosthetic material (mesh)
6. The subcutis and skin are closed routinely.

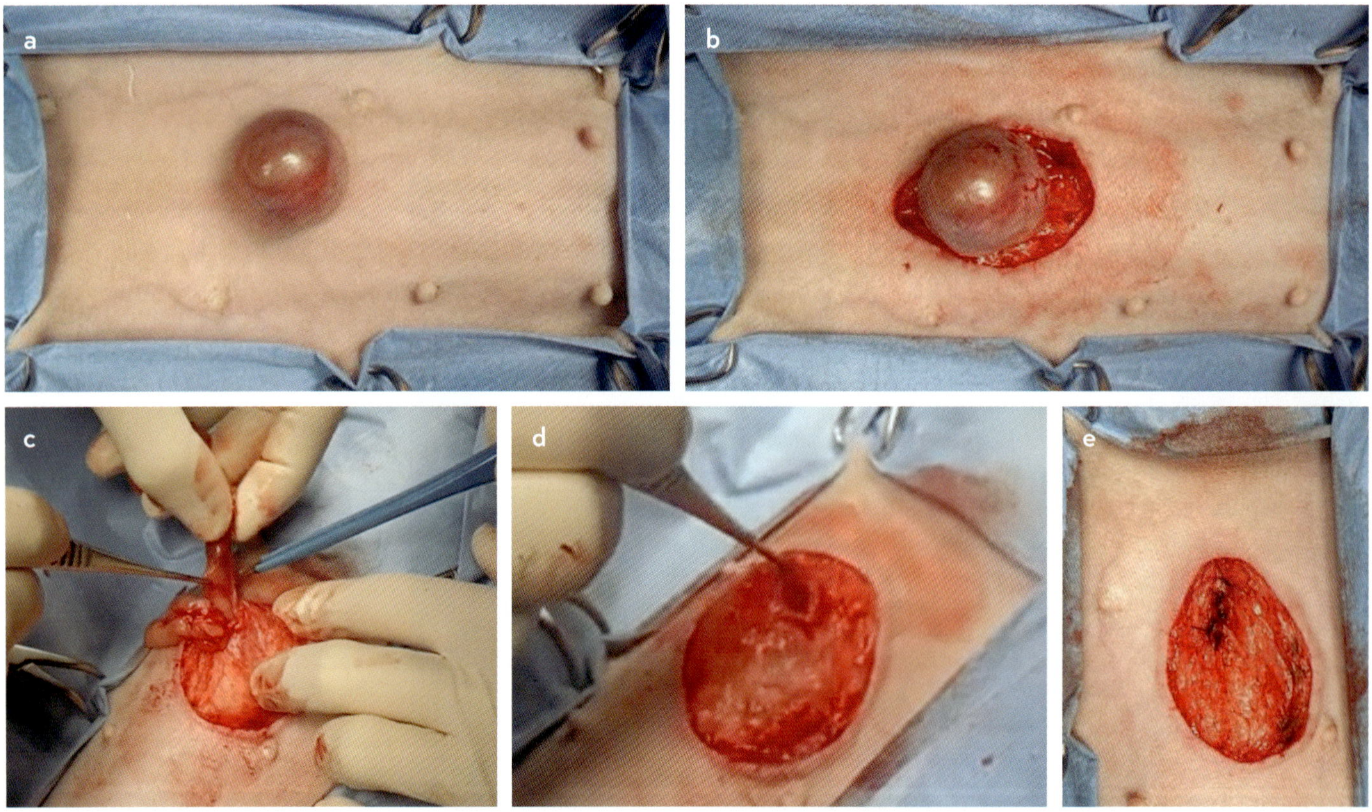

Figure 15.2 Surgical treatment of an umbilical hernia. (a,b) Skin incision around the mass. (c) Opening of the hernial sac and removal of strangled omentum. (d) Debridement of the hernial ring. (e) Closure of the umbilical defect.

Postoperative management

Minimal postoperative care is required after uncomplicated surgery. Standard wound care and removal of sutures after 10–12 days; exercise should be restricted for 1–2 weeks.[1]

Outcome

Patients with uncomplicated umbilical hernias have an excellent prognosis, and postoperative complications are uncommon. Hernias may recur if the suture material is inadequate (too fine) or if the sutures are poorly placed (too close to the edges of the incision, too far from each other, or if the rectus fascia is not properly engaged). These animals may require revision surgery for incisional hernia repair.[1]

Inguinal and scrotal hernias

Clinical presentation and diagnosis

Inguinal (Fig. 15.3) and scrotal hernias (Fig. 15.4) occur through the inguinal ring. Scrotal hernias involve the displacement of tissue into the vaginal process alongside the contents of the spermatic cord. The enlargement of the inguinal canal, either congenital or traumatic, allows the herniation of abdominal contents. While inguinal hernias commonly contain fat and omentum, other structures such as the uterus, intestine or urinary bladder may herniate in dogs. Inguinal hernias are more frequently observed in female dogs.[1–5]

Organs can herniate alongside (direct hernia) or within (indirect hernia) the vaginal process. Clinical signs vary depending on the size and contents of the hernia, ranging from painless swelling to visceral obstruction, or entrapment shock, and even death. Inguinal hernias predominantly occur on the left side (93%),[3] and, in one study, bilateral hernias have been reported in 17% of dogs.[1,2]

Diagnosis is achieved by clinical examination (palpation of the hernia) and imaging investigations (radiography, ultrasonography, or computed tomography). In male dogs, scrotal hernias should be differentiated from testicular torsion, infection, hydrocele, or neoplasia. Strangulation/incarceration of the hernia contents is more common in male dogs with scrotal hernias. Scrotal hernias often cannot be reduced and may require emergency treatment, especially in younger dogs (Video 15.1).[1,2,4-6]

Video 15.1. Clinical presentation of a scrotal hernia in a young dog. Video courtesy of Rosario Vallefuoco.

Treatment

Inguinal and scrotal hernias should be repaired promptly, as delayed surgery can lead to a more complex operation and an increased risk of complications. If necessary, patients should be stabilized before surgery,[1,3,5] but the timing of the procedure depends on the severity of the clinical signs. Emergency surgery is reserved for animals showing signs of visceral strangulation/incarceration, peritonitis, or herniated gravid uterus. Animals presenting with gastrointestinal signs such as vomiting or diarrhea should be suspected of having an ischemic intestine, and enterectomy should be planned as soon as possible.[1,2,5,6]

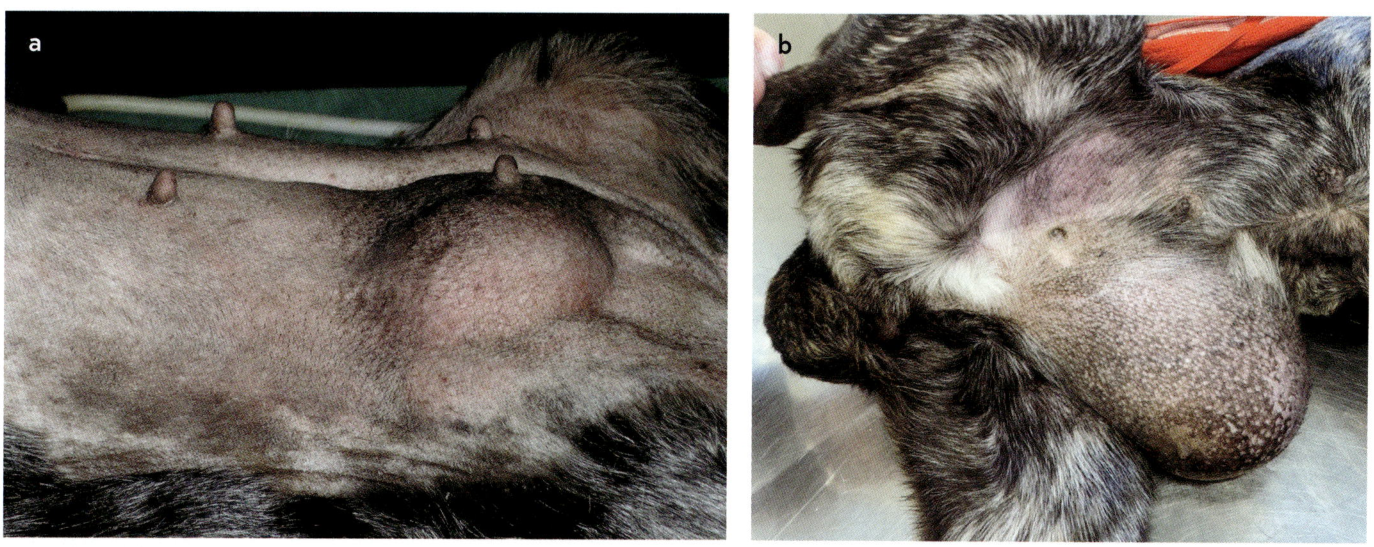

Figure 15.3 (a) Right-sided inguinal hernia. (b) Left-sided inguinal hernia.

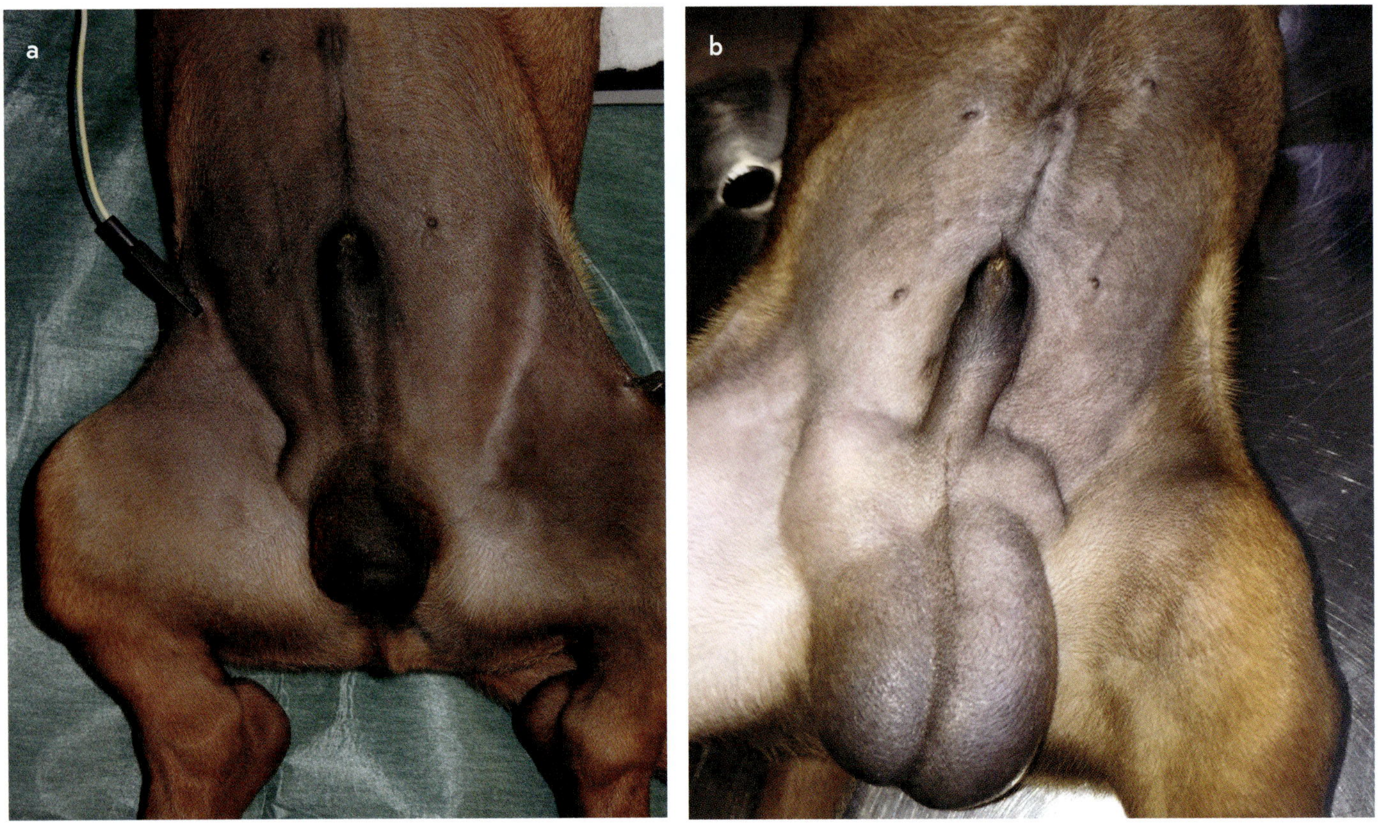

Figure 15.4 (a) Right-sided scrotal hernia. The swelling is present in the right scrotal area and in the region just cranial to the scrotum. (b) Bilateral scrotal hernia. Note the bilateral swelling of the scrotum and just cranial to it.

Surgical technique: Inguinal hernia repair (Figs. 15.5–15.7, Video 15.2)

1. The ventral abdomen is routinely clipped and prepped.
2. Before surgery and under general anesthesia, both inguinal rings should be palpated to determine if the condition is unilateral or bilateral.
3. The skin incision depends on the type of hernia:
   - For unilateral hernias, the skin incision is made directly over the superficial inguinal ring.
   - For bilateral hernias, two separate inguinal incisions or one long ventral midline incision are made, followed by undermining and retraction of the skin toward the hernia to be repaired.
   - A ventral midline celiotomy is required in patients with strangulated/incarcerated viscera or when ovariohysterectomy is necessary.
4. Blunt and sharp dissection with Metzenbaum scissors is necessary to separate the subcutaneous tissue from the hernial sac.
5. The hernial content is reduced:
   - For small, soft, reducible hernias, the hernial content should be gently reduced into the abdominal cavity.

Video 15.2. Surgical technique for inguinal hernia repair.

   - If the hernial content is viable but trapped, the hernial sac should be opened and the cranial part of the inguinal canal (beginning with the external abdominal oblique muscle and, if necessary, the transversus abdominis and internal abdominal oblique muscles) enlarged.
   - If the hernial content is ischemic, nonviable, or swollen, the hernial sac should be opened, the inguinal canal enlarged, and a ventral midline celiotomy performed. A complete abdominal inspection should be performed with the intent to excise all devitalized tissues.
6. The hernial sac is closed and resected.
7. The inguinal canal should be closed with interrupted sutures using 2-0 or 3-0 absorbable or nonabsorbable (the authors routinely use nonabsorbable suture) monofilament material, starting cranially and ensuring correct apposition of the external ab-

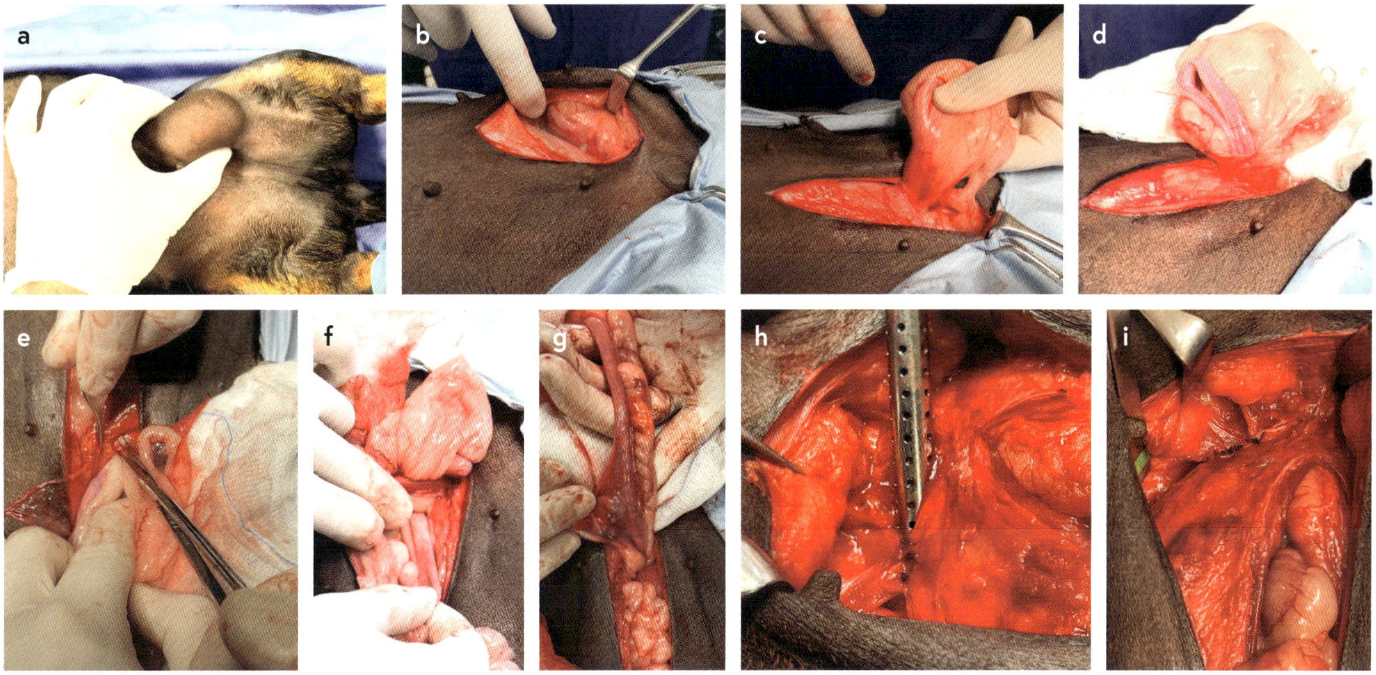

Figure 15.5 Repair of an inguinal hernia. (a) Palpation of the inguinal hernia and inguinal ring. (b,c) Ventral midline skin incision and dissection of the hernial sac from the subcutaneous tissue. (d) The hernial sac is isolated and opened to expose the contents (uterus). (e) To facilitate hernial content reduction, the hernial ring is opened cranially. (f) Combined ventral midline celiotomy for hernial content reduction. (g) Ovariohysterectomy. (h,i) Reduction of the hernial ring size with simple interrupted sutures, leaving a caudal gap for the passage of the pudendal vessels and genitofemoral nerve.

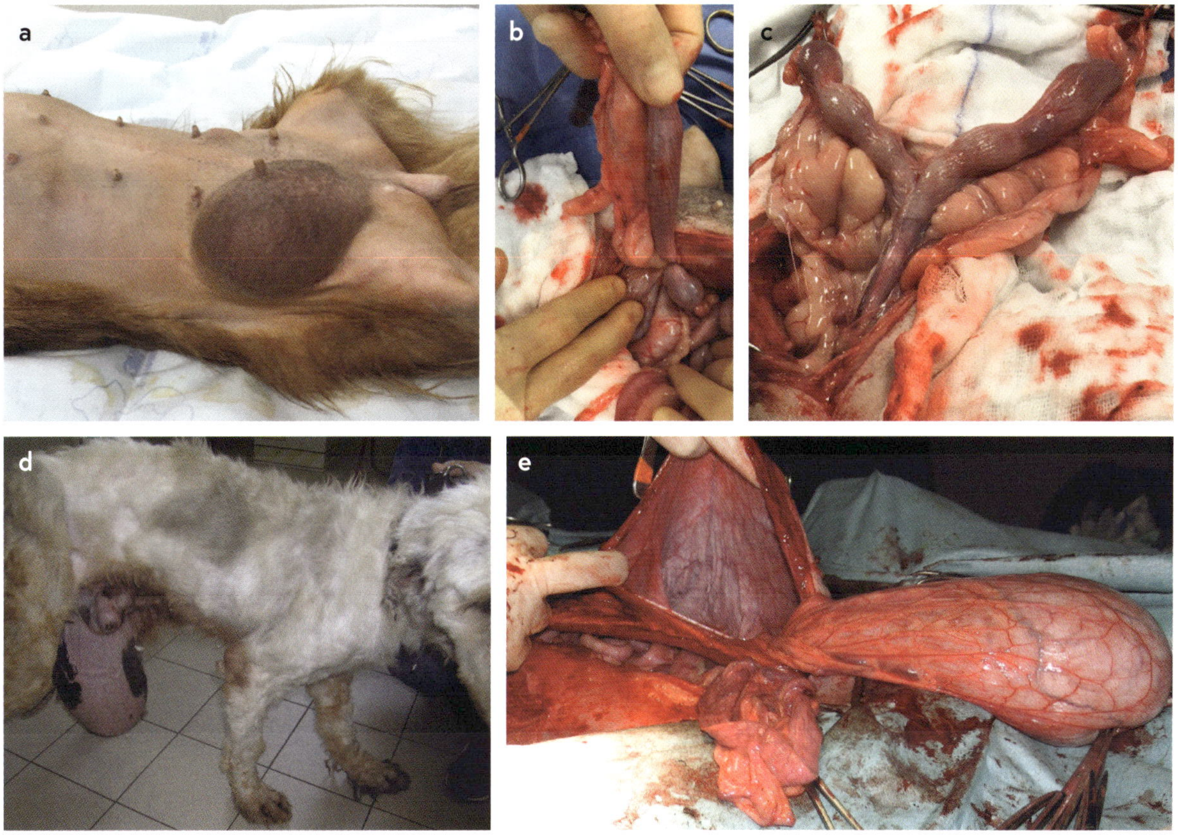

Figure 15.6 Inguinal hernia contents. (a–c) Large uterus (pyometra). (d,e) Bladder. Images a–c courtesy of Benito de la Puerta.

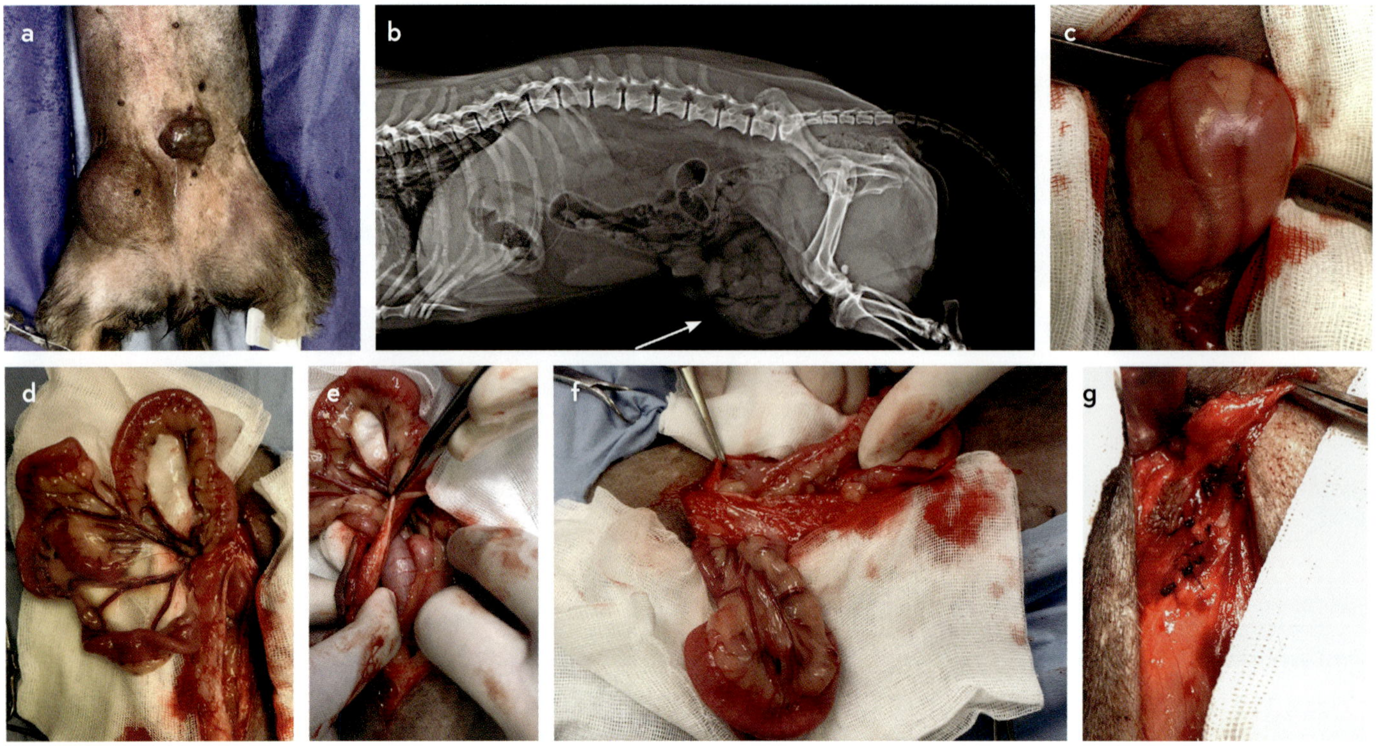

Figure 15.7 (a) Right-sided inguinal hernia containing small intestine. (b) Lateral abdominal radiograph showing gas-filled bowel loops (arrow) within the hernia. (c) Small intestine in hernial sac. (d–f) Opening of the hernial sac with a combined abdominal approach for hernial content reduction and abdominal inspection. (g) Reduction of the hernial ring size.

dominal oblique aponeurosis from side to side. A spacer, such as a Poole suction tube or a pair of closed Metzenbaum scissors, should be positioned in the caudal portion of the inguinal canal, leaving a caudal gap for the passage of the pudendal vessels, the genitofemoral nerve, and, in intact males, the spermatic cord.

8. In rare cases of large, recurrent inguinal hernias with weak regional tissues,[1] two techniques are considered for the reconstruction of the inguinal canal:
   - The use of an ipsilateral cranial sartorius muscle flap.[7]
   - The use of an onlay prosthetic mesh material.
9. The subcutaneous dead space should be carefully obliterated:
   - The subcutaneous tissue is closed in multiple layers using 3-0 or 4-0 absorbable monofilament suture material, tacking the aponeurosis layer of the external abdominal oblique muscle.
   - An active closed-suction drain can be applied for 3–4 days.
   - A soft compression bandage can be applied for 3–4 days.
10. Neutering intact animals is recommended, as the defect may be heritable in some breeds.
11. The skin is apposed routinely.

Surgical technique: Scrotal hernia repair (Figs. 15.8 and 15.9)

1. Approach for the initial incision:
   - For uncomplicated hernias, a lateral approach in the inguinal area is used, and extra-abdominal repair is recommended.
   - For complicated irreducible hernias, a paramedian caudal abdominal approach is performed. Alternatively, a combination of lateral and paramedian caudal abdominal approach can be considered.
2. The hernial sac is exposed and opened.
3. The hernial contents should be examined and the healthy viscera repositioned in the abdominal cavity.
4. In cases requiring intestinal resection and anastomosis, this is performed extra-abdominally after enlarging the hernial ring and recruiting adjacent healthy intestine for repair. A paramedian caudal abdominal approach is recommended for careful examination of the abdominal organs.
5. Castration is strongly recommended.
6. The hernial sac is closed and resected. Closure of the hernial ring is performed as previously described for inguinal hernias.

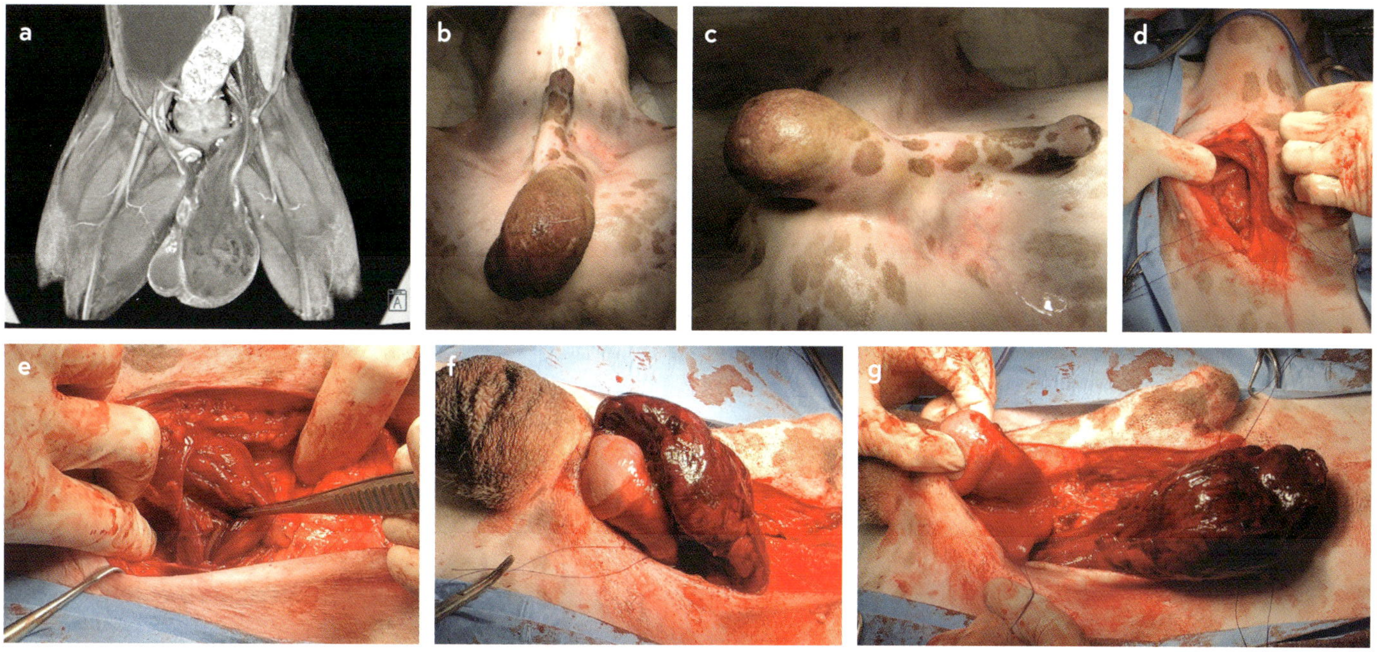

Figure 15.8 Repair of a left-sided scrotal hernia when castration is not intended. (a) Computed tomography and (b,c) clinical appearance of the hernia. (d) Skin incision over the inguinal ring. (e) Approach to the inguinal canal, incision of the hernial sac (parietal vaginal tunic), and inspection and resection of hernial contents (necrotic omentum). (f) The testicle is preserved, and the enlarged vaginal process is closed. (g) Simple interrupted suture of the cranial part of the inguinal ring. Images courtesy of Giovanna Bertolini, Marta Cecchetto, and Lluis Ferré Dolcet.

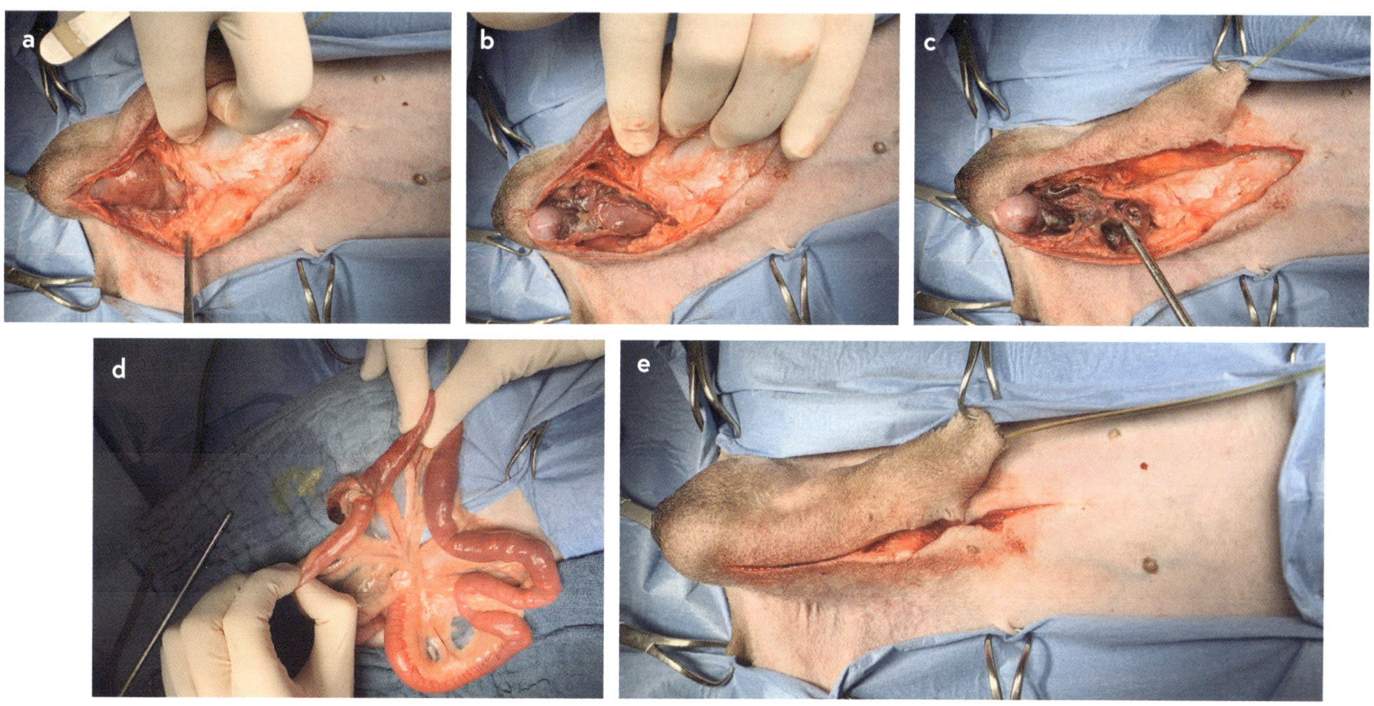

Figure 15.9 Repair of a left-sided scrotal hernia. (a–c) Skin incision over the inguinal ring and hernial contents reduction. (d) Necrotic small intestine. Enterectomy of the necrotic area of the small intestine and removal of the left testicle were performed. (e) Closure of the hernial ring and skin.

7. If the testicle is preserved, the size of the enlarged neck of the hernial sac (parietal vaginal tunic) is reduced using interrupted sutures. The inguinal ring is closed with interrupted sutures, leaving the caudal aspect open to allow unconstricted passage of the spermatic cord, external pudendal vessels, and nerve branches.
8. In cases of severe contamination, the surgical wound is washed and samples for aerobic and anaerobic bacterial culture and antimicrobial susceptibility testing are obtained.
9. Placement of a closed-suction drain system may be necessary in some cases, while in others a tie-over bandage with sterile sponges for 3–4 days may be preferable.
10. The skin is closed routinely.

Postoperative management

Analgesia is usually provided for several days. Exercise should be limited for the first 15–25 days after surgery. Animals that underwent intestinal resection and anastomosis should be monitored for signs of enteric wound dehiscence.[2]

Outcome

Patients with reducible inguinal or scrotal hernias have a good to excellent prognosis.[5] Strangulated/incarcerated hernias requiring emergency surgery carry a more guarded prognosis. One study reported a postoperative complication rate of 17% and a mortality rate of 3% in animals with inguinal hernias.[4] The most common complications include swelling, incisional infection, seroma, dehiscence, peritonitis, sepsis, and vomiting. Scrotal dermatitis and hematoma are the most common local complications after scrotal hernia repair. Recurrence is uncommon. Early diagnosis and surgical repair reduce the risk of complications and improve outcome.[1,2]

Femoral hernias

Clinical presentation and diagnosis

Femoral hernia is a rare condition in small animals. The femoral canal is located in the caudal abdominal wall, just lateral to the inguinal ligament. It consists of two separate spaces, the muscular and femoral lacunae, within the boundaries of the inguinal ligament and pelvis. Blunt or iatrogenic trauma is the most frequent cause of femoral hernia.[1] The clinical presentation is similar to that of inguinal hernias, and misdiagnosis is common. The hernia swelling typically develops on the medial aspect of the thigh but may also extend to the inguinal area (Fig. 15.10).

Diagnosis is based on palpation of the femoral ring after reduction of the herniated contents into the abdomen. Femoral hernias are located caudal to the inguinal ligament and ventrolateral to the pelvic brim. Diagnostic aids are similar to those used for other abdominal hernias.[1]

Treatment

A femoral hernia should be suspected in all traumatized animals presenting with swelling in the inguinal area. Good knowledge of the regional anatomy is essential to avoid damaging vital structures and ensure successful surgical repair. Due to the high risk of strangulation/incarceration of the hernial contents, early surgical treatment is warranted.[1]

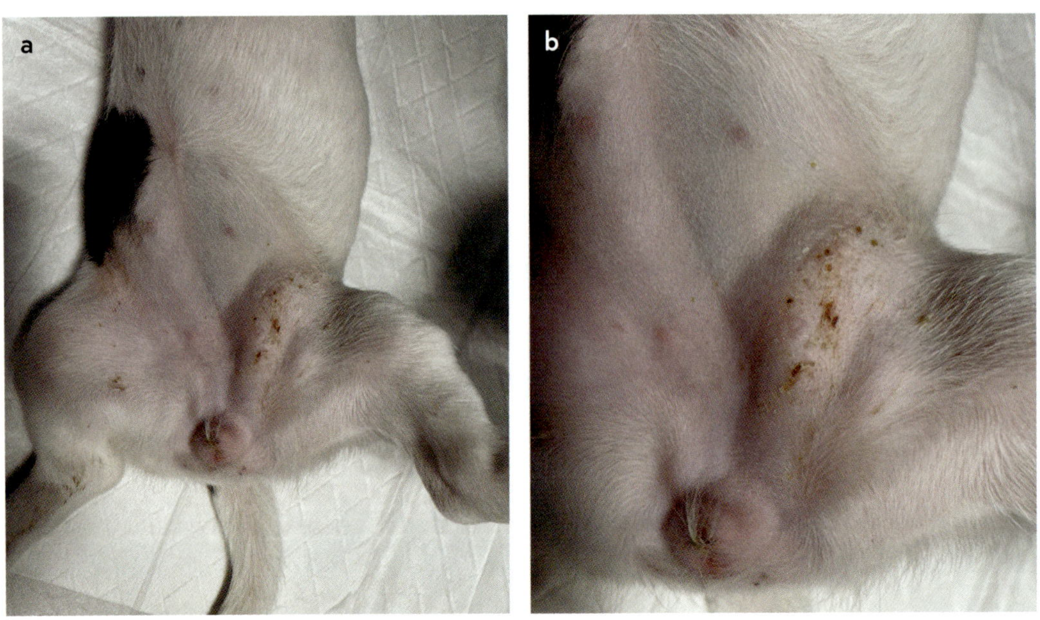

Figure 15.10 Traumatic left-sided femoral–inguinal hernia in a puppy.

Surgical technique (Figs. 15.11 and 15.12)

1. Surgical preparation is similar to that described for abdominal hernias.
2. Before surgery and under general anesthesia, both inguinal and femoral rings should be palpated to determine the location of the hernia.
3. The skin incision depends on the hernia:
   - For uncomplicated hernias, the incision is made parallel to the inguinal ligament.
   - For irreducible or complicated hernias, a combined external and caudal abdominal approach should be used.

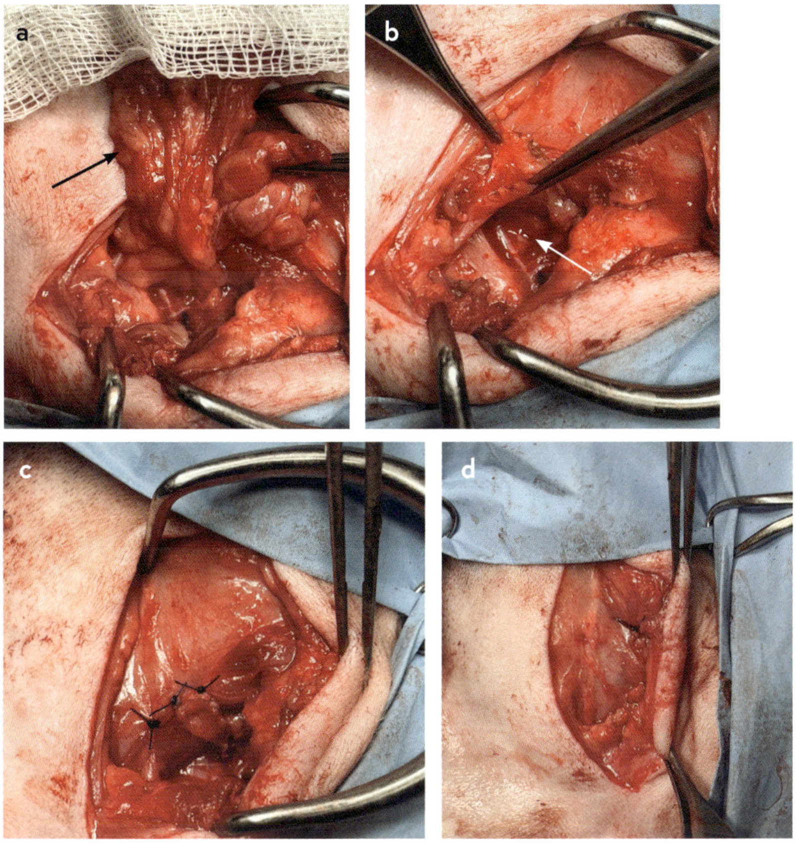

Figure 15.11 Hernia repair in the patient from the previous figure. (a) Opening of the hernial sac and reduction of the hernial content (omentum [black arrow]). (b) Identification of the lacerated inguinal and femoral canals (white arrow). (c,d) Closure of the femoral and inguinal rings.

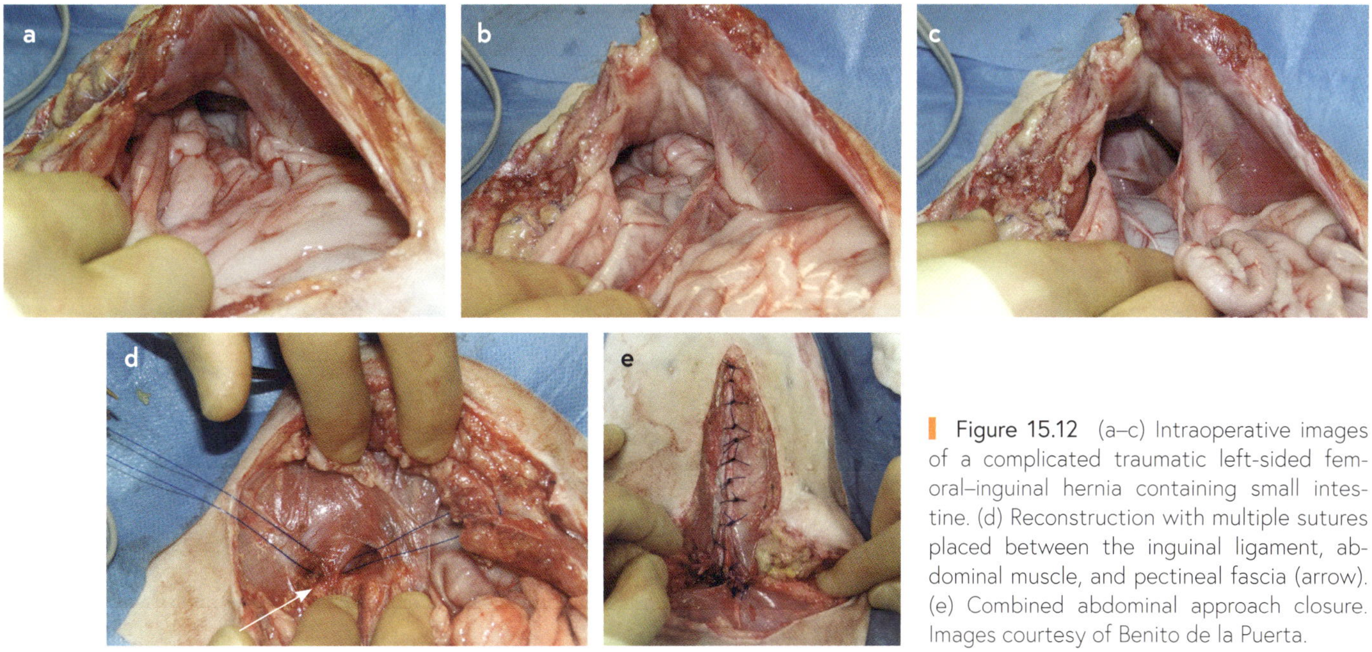

Figure 15.12 (a–c) Intraoperative images of a complicated traumatic left-sided femoral–inguinal hernia containing small intestine. (d) Reconstruction with multiple sutures placed between the inguinal ligament, abdominal muscle, and pectineal fascia (arrow). (e) Combined abdominal approach closure. Images courtesy of Benito de la Puerta.

4. Blunt and sharp dissection using Metzenbaum scissors is necessary to separate the subcutaneous tissue from the hernial sac.
5. The hernial sac is opened and the hernia contents are reduced into the abdomen.
6. The hernial sac is then ligated and transected.
7. If the inguinal ligaments are intact, for closure of the femoral canal, multiple simple interrupted sutures using 2-0 or 3-0 absorbable monofilament material are preplaced between the inguinal ligament and the pectineal fascia.
8. In case of a complicated hernia, a caudal abdominal approach is initially used to carefully explore the abdominal organs. A second approach to the femoral canal is then needed for closure, as described above.
9. The subcutaneous dead space is obliterated as described for inguinal hernias.

Postoperative management

Exercise restriction and wound care are required after surgery. In cases of complicated hernia repair, hobbles are placed between the hind limbs at the level of the hocks for 14 days to protect wound healing. Common complications include pelvic limb swelling, edema, wound dehiscence, and inflammation. Distal limb swelling usually resolves within a few days; massages, hot compressions, and leash walking may aid in recovery. Surgical exploration of the femoral canal is recommended if limb swelling persists or if there is severe pain and femoral neurologic deficit.[1]

Outcome

The prognosis is generally excellent, and recurrence is uncommon.[1]

Traumatic and incisional abdominal hernias

Traumatic and incisional abdominal hernias are characterized by the protrusion of abdominal contents through a defect in the abdominal or thoracic body wall, typically caused by trauma.[1,2] These hernias are classified based on their anatomical location (e.g., paracostal, dorsal, prepubic). Unlike true hernias, traumatic and incisional hernias lack a hernial sac and are often associated with the formation of adhesions. Blunt trauma with increased intra-abdominal pressure is considered the most common cause of abdominal hernias, although penetrating wounds, poor tissue healing, and inadequate surgical closure can also lead to herniation.[1,2] Paracostal hernias typically occur at the boundaries of the external abdominal oblique and transversus abdominis muscles, extending along the caudal margin of the ribs (Fig. 15.13).[1,2] Diaphragmatic hernias fre-

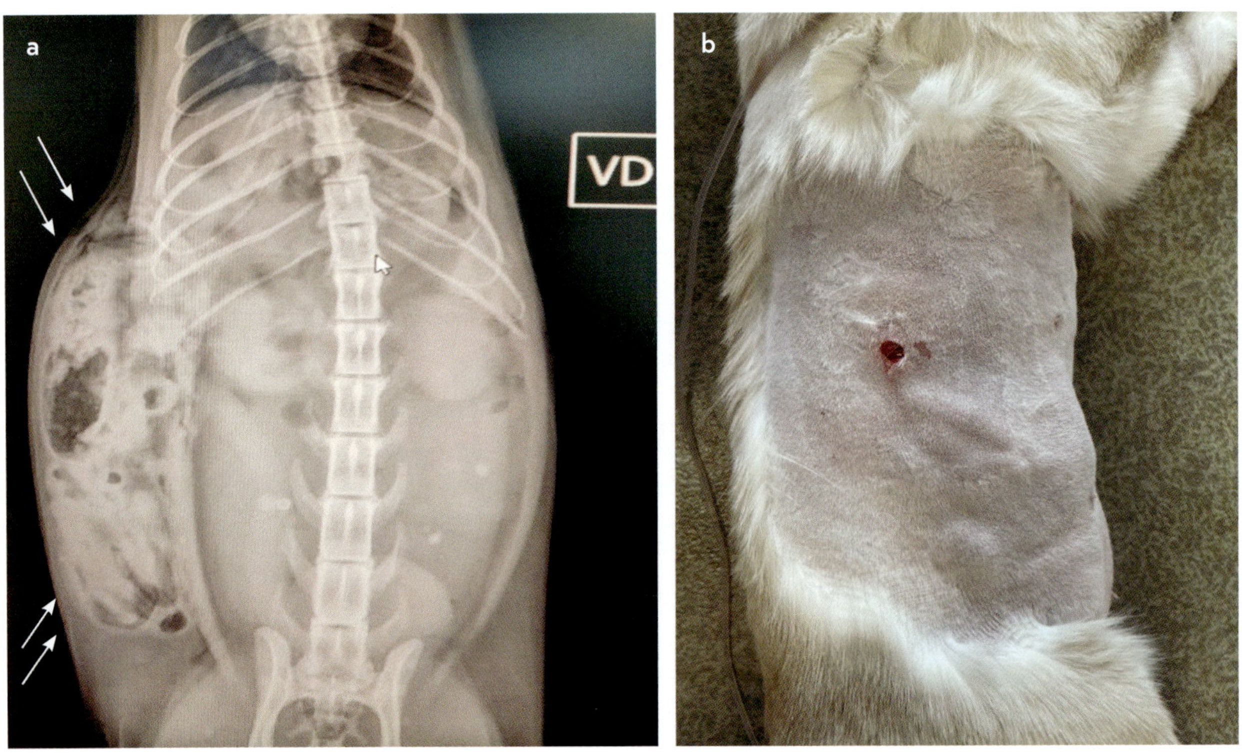

Figure 15.13 (a) Ventrodorsal radiograph of a cat with a paracostal hernia caused by bite wound trauma. The arrows indicate the limits of the hernia. (b) External appearance of the bite wound. Images courtesy of Diego Rossetti.

quently coexist with hernias in this location and should be treated accordingly.

Dorsal abdominal hernias commonly occur at the origin of the transversus abdominis muscle with avulsion from the transverse processes of lumbar vertebrae (Fig. 15.14). Prepubic hernias occur due to the rupture of the prepubic tendon, which is the tendinous insertion of the external and internal abdominal oblique muscles, rectus abdominis, and transversus abdominis muscles on the pubic rim (Fig. 15.15).[1] These hernias may be associated with inguinal or femoral hernias.[1,8]

Other hernia locations can occur due to muscle and tendons tearing at the site of trauma.[9] Abdominal cavity penetration has been reported in up to 79% of dogs presented with multiple superficial wounds.[10] Prompt exploration of penetrating abdominal wounds (e.g., caused by bites, sticks, gunshots, knives) is recommended in animals presenting with multiple superficial wounds that may penetrate the abdominal cavity. This allows for the identification and treatment of concurrent injuries to intra-abdominal organs.[1,2]

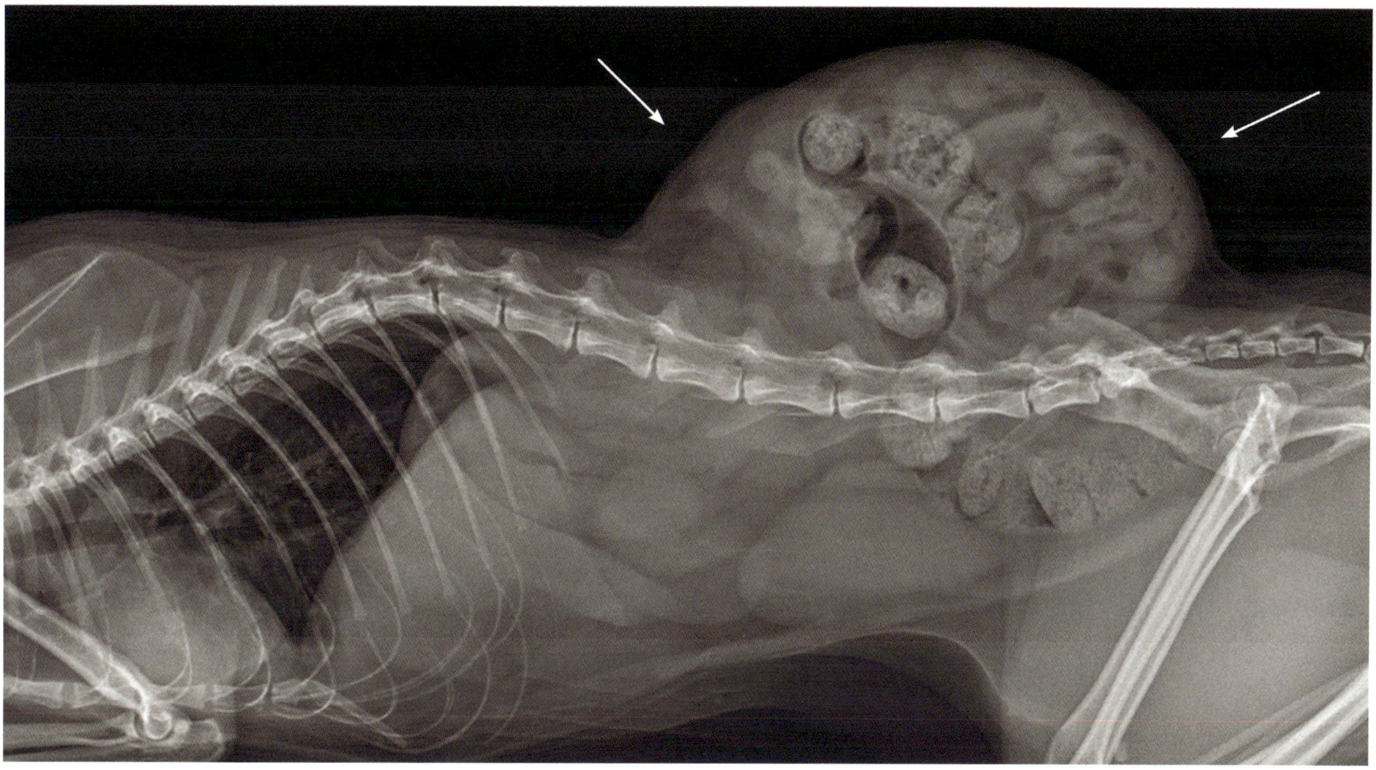

Figure 15.14 Lateral radiograph of a cat with a dorsal abdominal hernia caused by bite trauma.

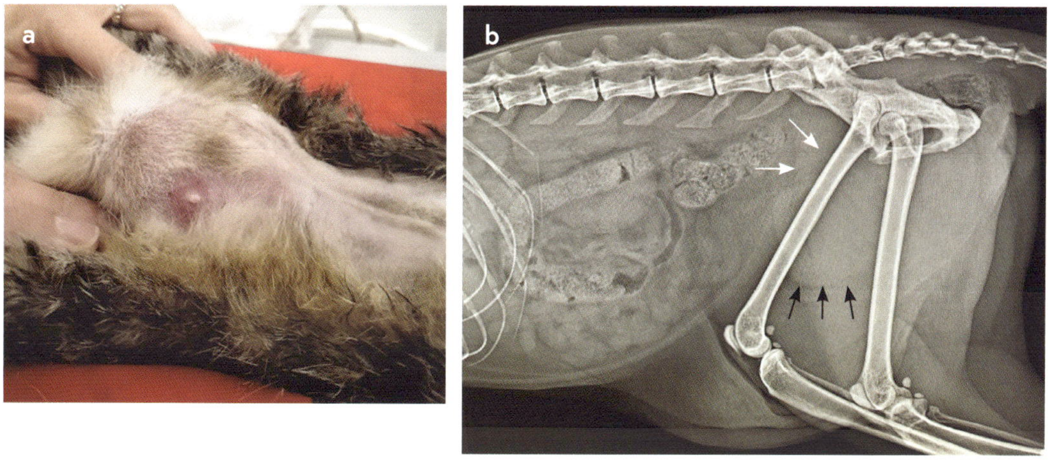

Figure 15.15 Abdominal hernia in a cat after vehicular trauma. (a) Presence of a bulging mass beneath the skin in the caudal abdomen. (b) Lateral radiograph showing the loss of the abdominal strip (white arrows) and the bladder herniated in the subcutaneous space (black arrows).

Traumatic hernias

Clinical presentation and diagnosis

The most common clinical sign of a traumatic abdominal hernia is the presence of a swelling beneath the skin or an asymmetry in the abdominal contour. The size, consistency, or appearance/disappearance of the bulge depend on the content of the hernia.[2] Animals with an abdominal wall hernia often display concurrent injuries that present with specific clinical signs related to the affected organs or systems, such as dysuria/anuria (bladder herniation), lameness or neurologic signs (fractures, vertebral luxation/fracture, intervertebral disc disease).[1,2,11]

Diagnosis of abdominal wall hernias can be challenging, especially when the hernial ring cannot be easily palpated. After stabilizing the patient, radiography and ultrasonography may help demonstrate a defect in the abdominal musculature, intraperitoneal free air, or organ herniation into the subcutaneous space (Fig. 15.16).[2] However, recent studies suggest that whole-body computed tomography is the preferred method in severely traumatized patients, as it provides comprehensive information and reduces the risk of missing injuries compared to traditional diagnostic tests.[12]

Treatment

In animals presenting immediately after acute trauma, evaluation and treatment of life-threatening problems take priority. Open wounds should be protected with bandages until emergency life support and a complete physical examination can be performed.[2] The optimal time for surgical repair of acute closed hernias in stable patients is controversial. Some authors prefer to delay the surgical correction for several days to allow for revascularization of acutely traumatized tissues, reduc-

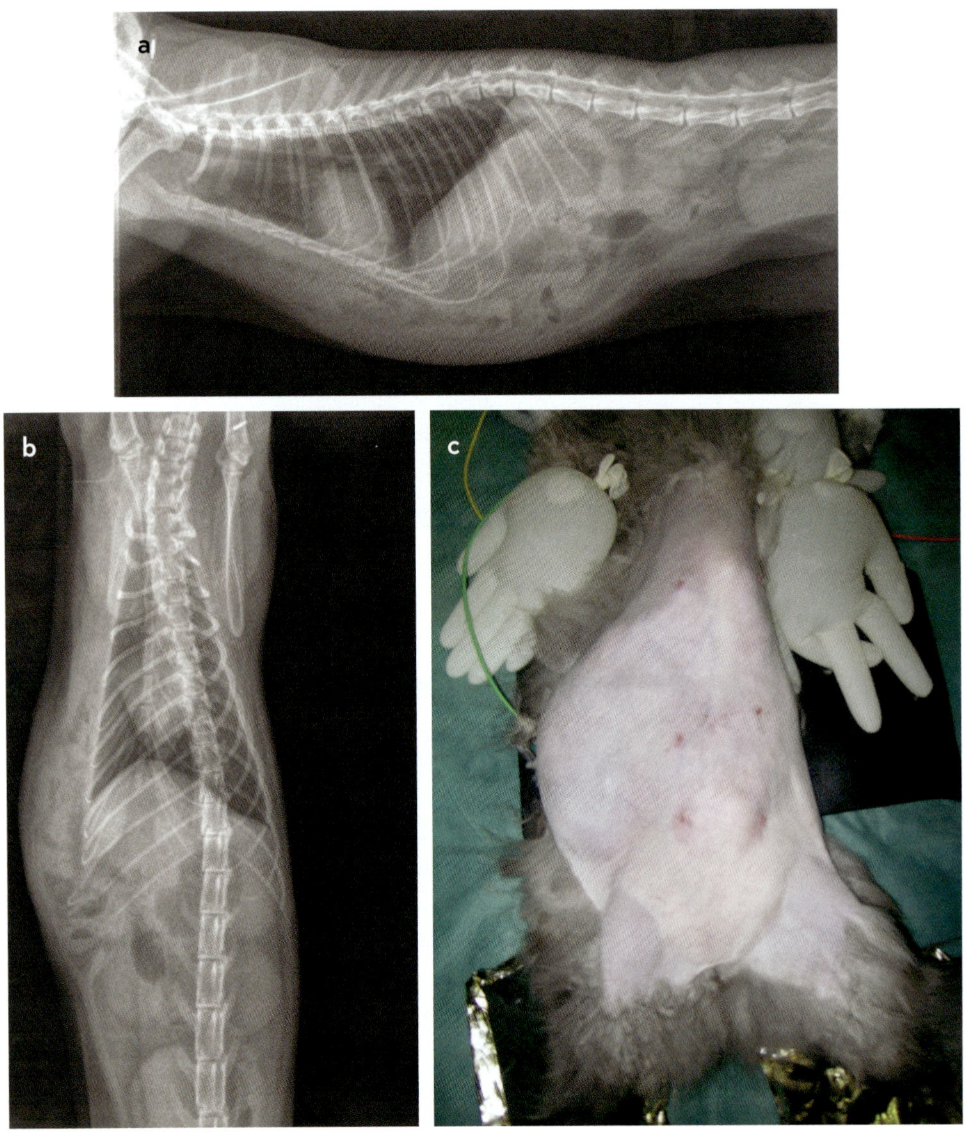

Figure 15.16 (a) Lateral and (b) ventrodorsal radiographs of a cat with a right-sided traumatic abdominal hernia. (c) Clinical presentation. Note the asymmetry of the abdominal contour.

ing the risk of infection and closure failure.[1,13] However, an excessive delay should be avoided, as contraction of the abdominal musculature and adhesion formation may complicate herniorrhaphy.

Emergency surgery is indicated for strangulated/incarcerated hernias, unsatisfactorily stabilized patients, or those showing rapid clinical deterioration.[10] Penetrating abdominal wounds should be explored soon after resuscitative measures. Concurrent injuries to intra-abdominal organs have been reported in 65% of animals with penetrating abdominal wounds.[10] Surgery should initially address the traumatized organ before repairing the hernia.

Surgical technique

1. An extensive area of the skin should be prepared for surgery, as the exact location and extension of acute traumatic hernias are often unknown.
2. The approach varies depending on the type of hernia:
   - A ventral midline approach should be considered for acute hernias with ill-defined borders or potential multiple hernias.
   - A direct approach over the hernial ring, with or without a ventral midline approach, is used for chronic hernias.
3. The hernial content is reduced and the herniated organs are carefully explored. Necrotic/devitalized organs are treated accordingly.
4. In case of an open and contaminated hernia, all foreign material must be meticulously removed.
5. The hernial ring should be examined and any devitalized and infected tissue carefully debrided/excised.
6. Herniorrhaphy: the focus of the surgery is to restore the continuity of the abdominal wall musculature, with attention given to restoring the fascial layers as much as possible.
   - Paracostal hernias: Simple interrupted or continuous sutures using 2-0 or 3-0 absorbable monofilament material, including the last rib and the external abdominal oblique and transversus abdominis muscles (Fig. 15.17).
   - Dorsal hernias: The retroperitoneal space should be explored. Sutures are applied with 2-0 or 3-0 absorbable monofilament material, including the transversus abdominis and epaxial muscles.
   - Prepubic hernias: Repair of the cranial prepubic tendon avulsion.
     - If a small caudal portion of the tendon is present (attached to the cranial pubis), simple interrupted sutures (2-0 or 0 absorbable or nonabsorbable monofilament material) are placed between the caudal and cranial prepubic tendon portions (Fig. 15.18).
     - Most commonly, two or three holes are predrilled in the cranial pubis using a 1.5–2.0 drill bit. Sutures are preplaced through the pubic holes and the remnants of the prepubic tendon using a tension-relieving suture pattern (vertical mattress, horizontal mattress, and cruciate pattern) with 2-0 or 0 absorbable or nonabsorbable monofilament material. Furthermore, if the caudal prepubic tendon is still anchored to the pubis, additional sutures are placed between the cranial and caudal prepubic tendon portions (Figs. 15.19 and 15.20).
     - In prepubic hernia repair, absorbable or nonabsorbable sutures can be used; some authors suggest the latter because the prepubic tendon regains only 20% of its original strength by 21 days following surgery and 80% by 1 year.[8]
     - Modified dorsal recumbency position; the hind limbs are flexed and pulled medially and cranially. This creates truncal ventroflexion and reduces the size of the defect, ultimately resulting in reduction of tension during repair (Fig. 15.21).
     - Reconstruction of larger defects requires the augmentation of the avulsed cranial prepubic tendon using a mesh cuff or double-layer mesh (polypropylene); augmenta-

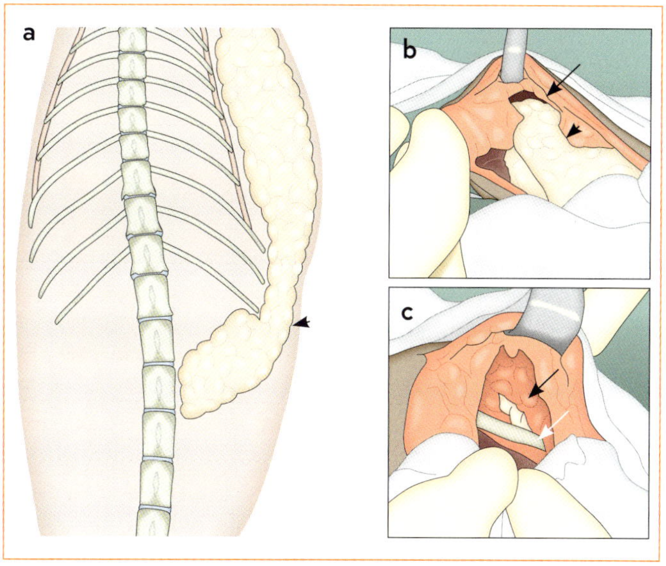

Figure 15.17 Illustrations showing (a) a dorsoventral and (b,c) intraoperative views of a right paracostal hernia, with the omentum (black arrowhead) herniated laterally into the subcutaneous tissue. Paracostal hernias develop when the external abdominal oblique and transversus abdominis muscles (black arrow) separate from their rib or costal cartilage origin (white arrow). In image c, the omentum has been reduced and the paracostal defect will be closed with single interrupted or continuous sutures involving the last rib (white arrow) and the external abdominal oblique and transversus abdominis muscles (black arrow).

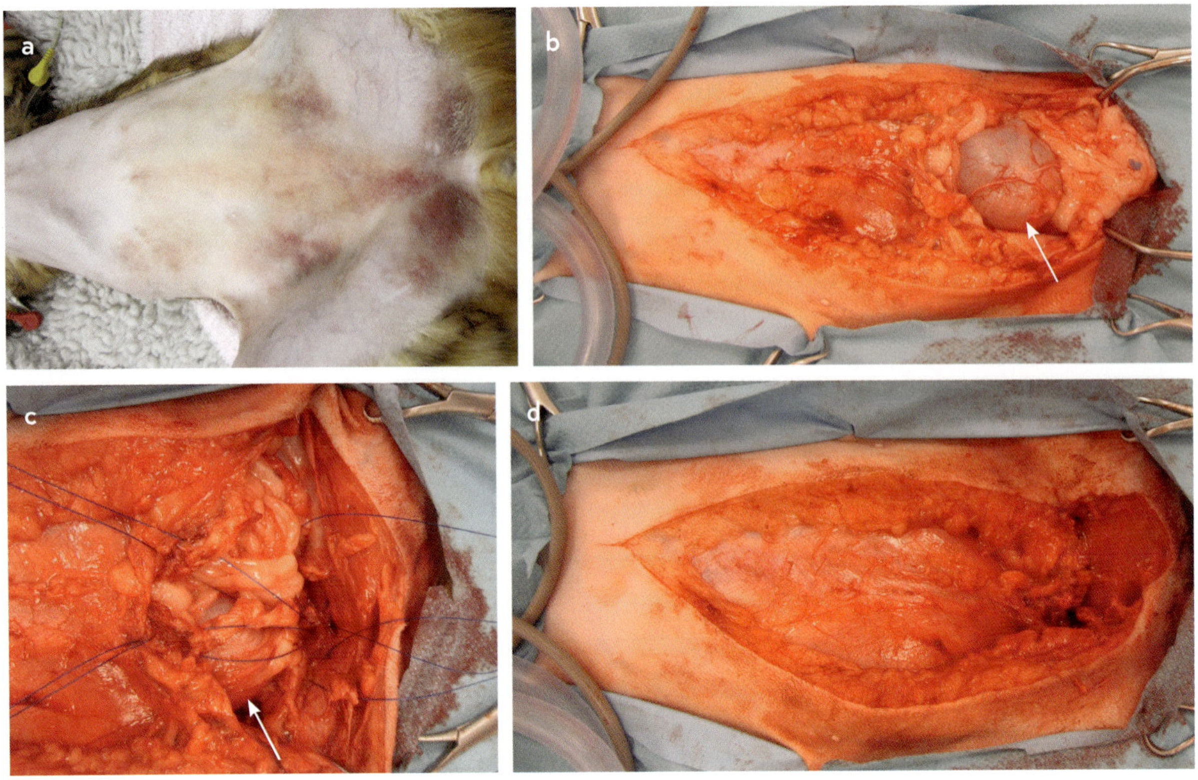

Figure 15.18 (a) Cat with a bulging mass and bruising in the caudal abdomen secondary to vehicular trauma. (b) Bladder herniation in the caudal abdomen (white arrow). (c,d) A small caudal stump of the prepubic tendon was still present, and multiple simple interrupted sutures were applied between the caudal and cranial stumps of the prepubic tendon. Images courtesy of Tim Charlesworth.

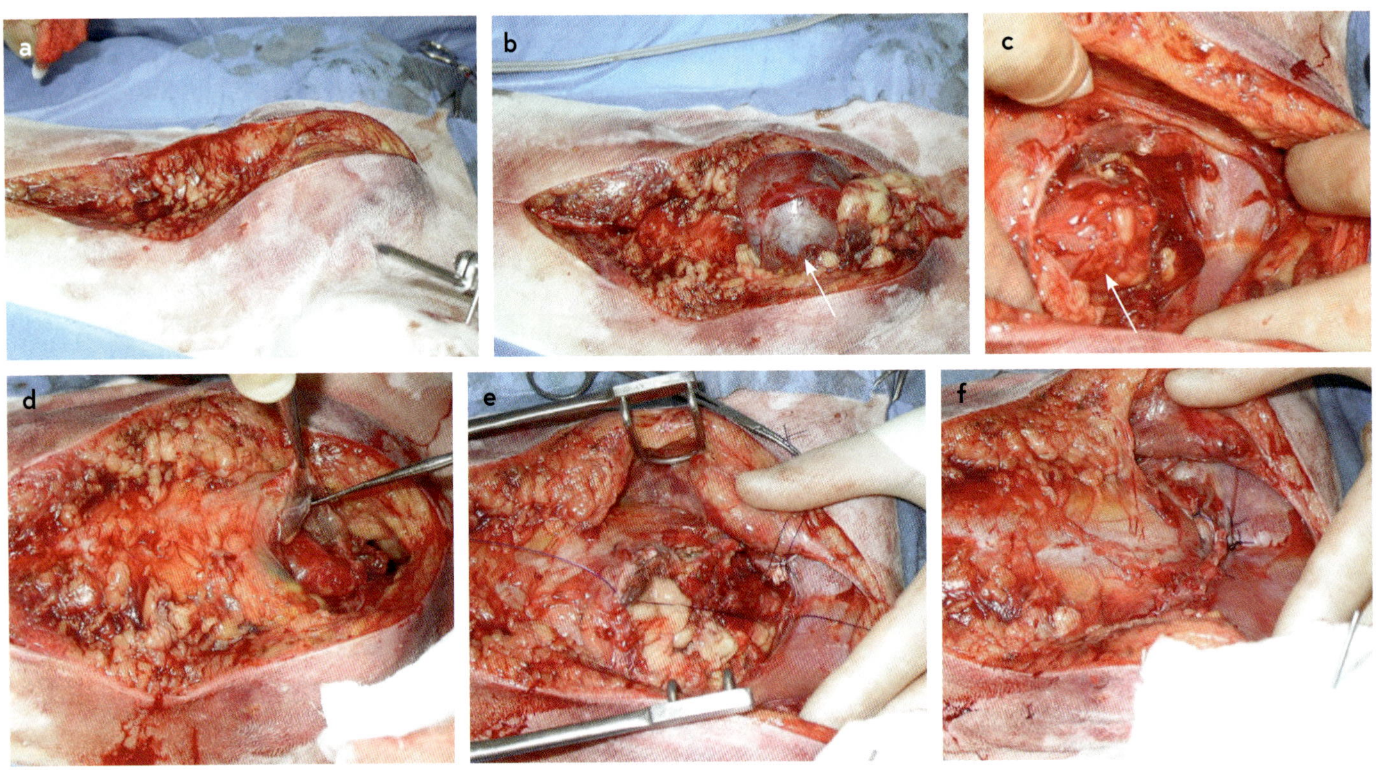

Figure 15.19 (a–c) Traumatic rupture of the prepubic tendon with bladder herniation (white arrow). (d,e) Multiple sutures were preplaced through the pubic holes and the remnants of the cranial prepubic tendon in a tension-relieving pattern. (f) Final appearance of the reconstruction of the caudal abdominal hernia. Images courtesy of Benito de la Puerta.

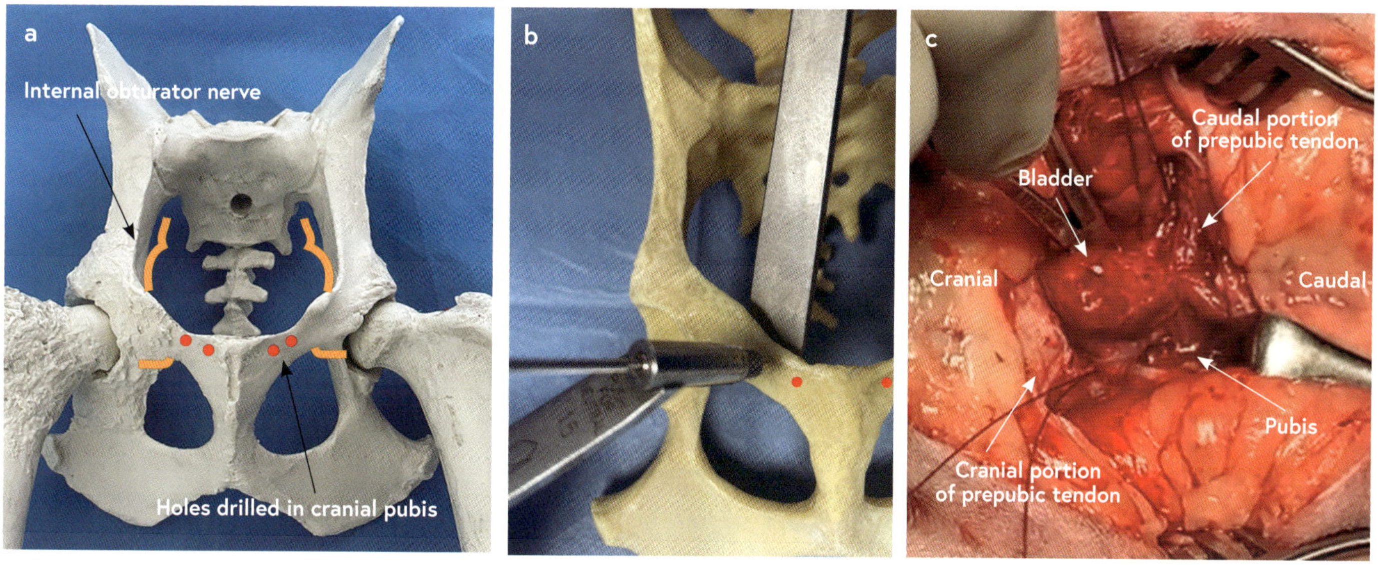

Figure 15.20 Prepubic tendon repair. Holes are drilled into the cranial pubis, through which sutures will be passed to anchor the avulsed tendon to the bone. (a,b) Model. (c) Intraoperative image.

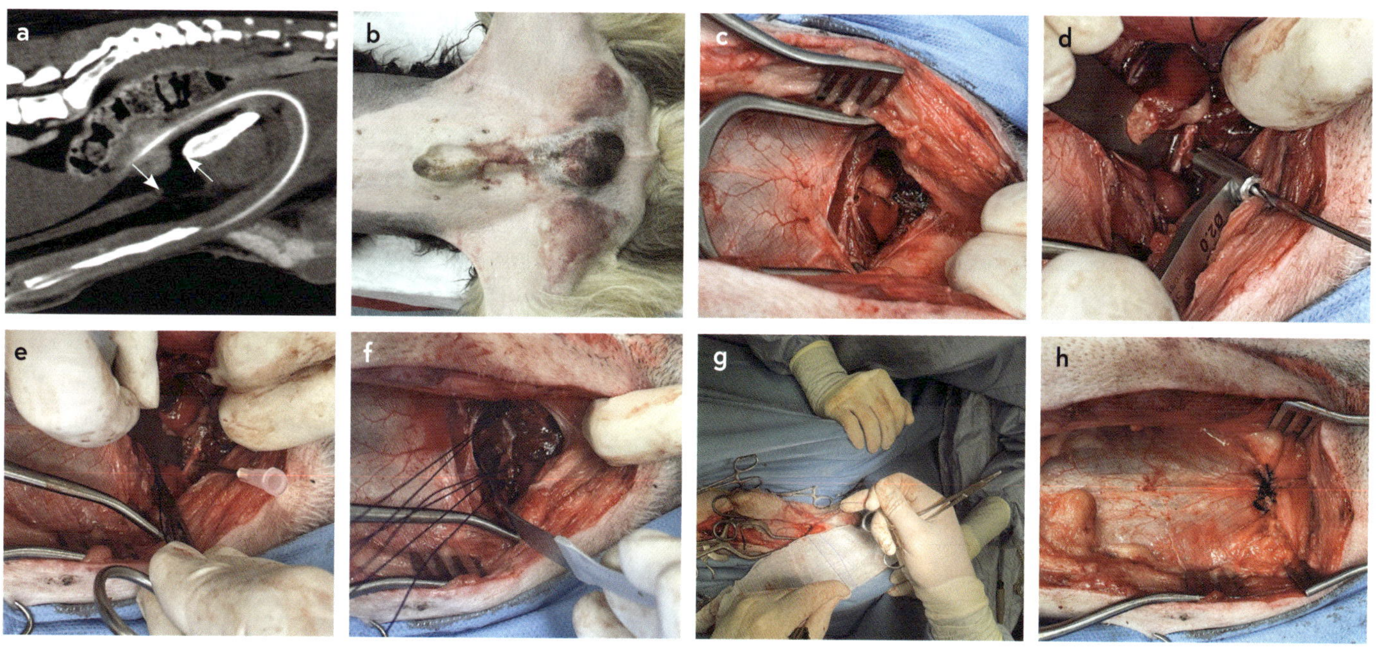

Figure 15.21 (a) Computed tomography image of an 8-year-old dog with traumatic rupture of the prepubic tendon (arrows) after vehicular trauma. (b) Caudal abdomen hematoma. (c) Paraprostatic fat herniation. (d–f) Prepubic tendon repair with holes drilled into the cranial pubis, through which sutures are passed to anchor the avulsed tendon to the bone. (g) Modified dorsal recumbency, with the hind limbs flexed and pulled mediocranially. This creates truncal ventroflexion and reduces the size of the defect, ultimately resulting in reduction of tension during repair. (h) Multiple sutures are added to complete prepubic tendon repair. Image a courtesy of Michelangelo Benvenuti.

tion may also be achieved by a cranial (or entire, if necessary) sartorius muscle flap.[50]

- Lateral abdominal hernias: The abdominal wall is explored and the hernial ring debrided. Closure is achieved using simple interrupted sutures with 2-0 or 3-0 absorbable monofilament material (Fig. 15.22). Reconstruction of large abdominal wall defects can be achieved using different techiques:[1,7,14–21]
  - Cranial or entire sartorius muscle flap
  - External oblique myofascial flap
  - Internal oblique muscle flap
  - Rectus abdominis flap
  - Latissimus dorsi flap

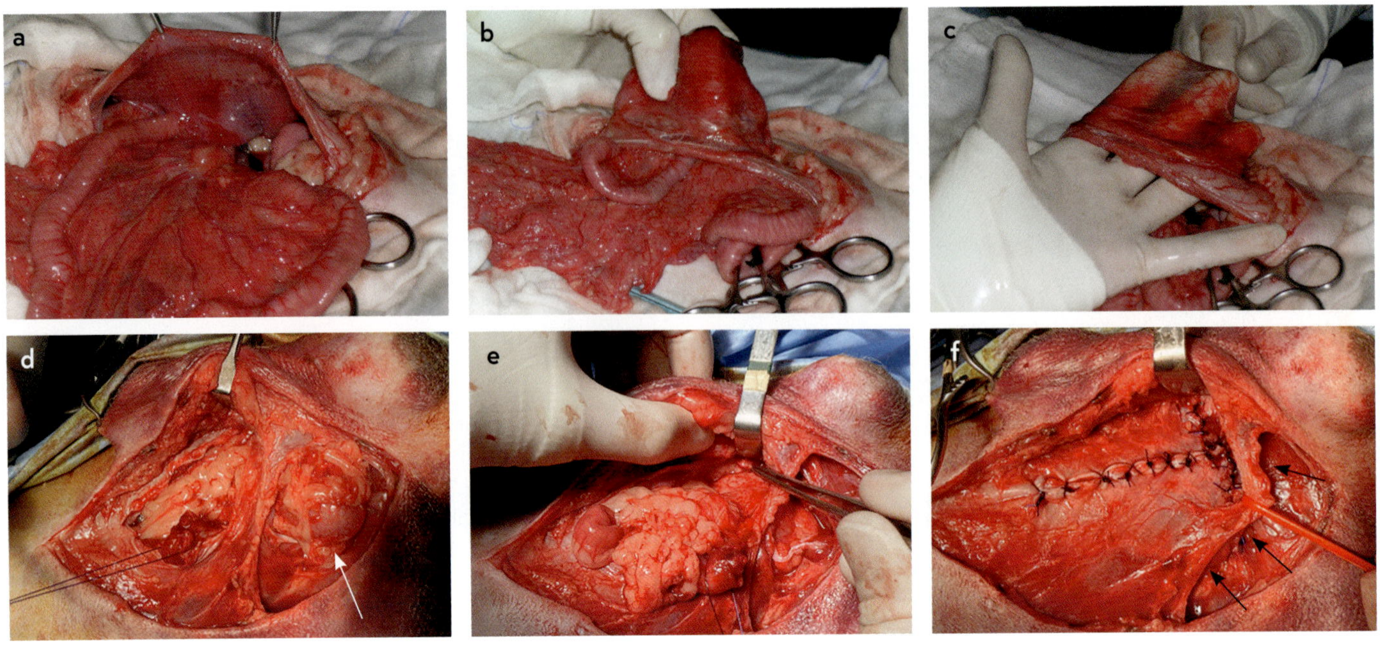

Figure 15.22 (a–c) Traumatic lateral abdominal hernia in a cat. The small intestine was herniated through the abdominal wall defect. The hernial content was reduced and the abdominal wall ring was debrided and closed with multiple simple interrupted sutures. (d–f) Caudal abdominal hernia in a dog after a road traffic accident. Presence of multiple abdominal wall wounds and herniation of abdominal contents (bladder [white arrow]). Reconstruction of the abdominal wall and preservation of the spermatic cord of the right testicle (black arrows).

- Vacuum-assisted closure
- Synthetic mesh

7. A closed-suction drain is applied in case of a large or contaminated wound defect.
8. The subcutis and skin are closed routinely.

Postoperative management

Exercise should be limited during the recovery period, typically for the first 5–6 weeks. Analgesia is administered for 5–14 days postoperatively. Antibiotics are administered if there is evidence of infection and based on aerobic and anaerobic bacterial culture and antimicrobial susceptibility testing.

Outcome

The rate of hospital discharge for patients with traumatic body wall hernia ranged from 73% to 80% in one study,[11] and up to 100% in another study.[22] Postoperative complications may include hematoma or seroma formation, incisional or body wall infection, recurrence, and entrapment of underlying viscera during suture placement.[2] Major complications should be treated promptly to ensure successful outcomes.

Incisional hernias and evisceration

Clinical presentation and diagnosis

Incisional hernia refers to a hernia that occurs at the site of a previous surgical incision in the abdominal wall. It is more commonly observed in midline incision compared to other sites and usually occurs in the early postoperative period (1–7 days).[1] Acute wound failure due to technical errors is the primary cause of incisional hernias. In humans, the reported rate of herniation after laparotomy ranges from 11% to 20%, while in horses it ranges from 1% to 17%.[23–26] Port-site hernias following laparoscopic procedures occur in approximately 1.5% of human patients[27] and 0.6% of small animals.[28] Animals can remain asymptomatic or show signs including discomfort/pain, ventral abdominal swelling, or signs associated with bowel obstruction and/or strangulation.[1] Diagnosis is usually based on the patient's clinical history and physical examination. Abdominal palpation of the incision line can determine a lack of continuity of the abdominal wall. Imaging techniques may be needed in some cases, especially in early stages, obese animals, or complex cases. Ultrasonography, radiography, and computed tomography can help to characterize the abdominal wall defect and plan the surgical approach and the extent of the repair.[1,2]
Most incisional hernias require prompt repair unless they are chronic and easily reducible. Delayed treatment can lead to evisceration, which dramatically alters the prognosis.[1]
Abdominal evisceration is defined as the herniation of abdominal viscera through the body wall, resulting in external exposure. The most common cause of evisceration in both animal and human patients is postoperative dehiscence following laparotomy or trauma (Figs. 15.23 and 15.24). Animals with evisceration have exposed ab-

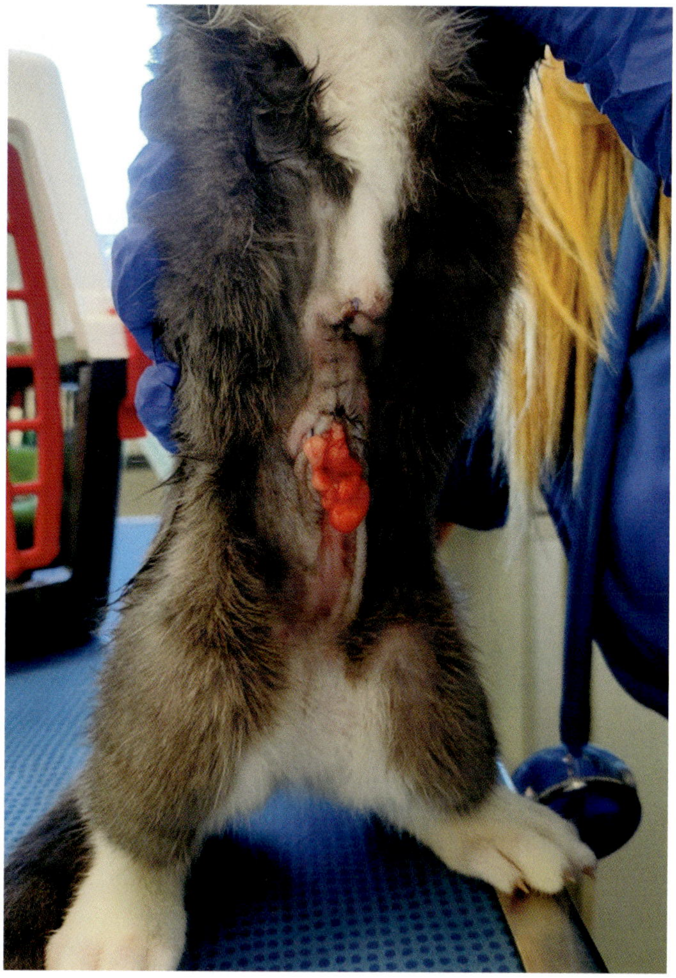

Figure 15.23 Incisional hernia with omental evisceration 3 days after abdominal surgery. Image courtesy of Diego Rossetti.

dominal viscera, increasing the risk of contamination. Early emergency surgical intervention is crucial for a relatively favorable prognosis.[1,22]

Treatment

Surgical technique: Incisional hernia repair

Acute incisional hernias:

1. The patient should be stabilized and the hernia content supported/protected with a bandage if necessary.
2. The skin incision should be reopened and the area thoroughly explored to determine the cause of the herniation.
3. Any previous suture material should be removed.
4. Nonabsorbable suture material should be preferred in patients with impaired wound healing (e.g., diabetes mellitus, hyperadrenocorticism, cachexia, hypoalbuminemia), while absorbable monofilament suture material may be used in healthy or contaminated wounds.
5. The hernial contents are inspected and reduced into the abdominal cavity.
6. If necessary, devitalized tissue and fat around the hernial ring edges are excised before closure.
7. It is extremely important to correctly identify the strongest holding layer of the abdominal wall (abdominal fascia) and place sutures more than 5 mm from the edge and 3–5 mm apart.
8. If necessary, an active closed-suction drain is placed into the subcutaneous tissue, and the subcutis and skin are closed routinely.

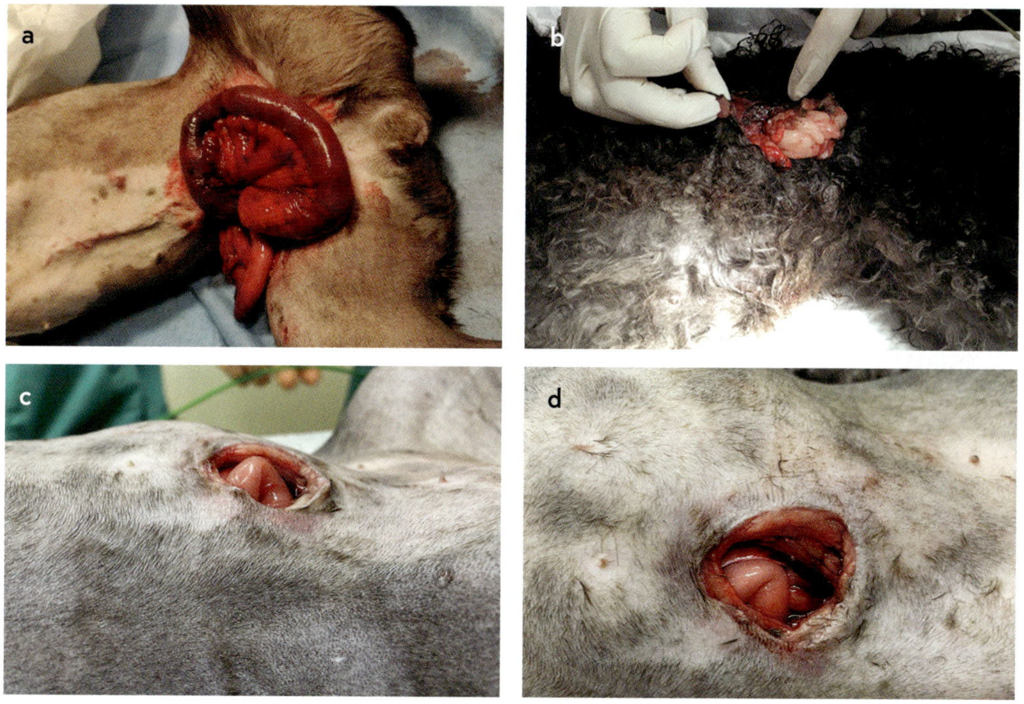

Figure 15.24 (a) Dog with caudal abdominal evisceration after bite wound trauma. (b) Toy-breed dog with abdominal flank evisceration after bite wound trauma. (c,d) Cat with abdominal trauma and evisceration after knife injury. Image a courtesy of Valeria Toneatti. Images c and d courtesy of Matteo Rossanese.

Chronic incisional hernias:

1. The hernia is approached over the original incision area.
2. Adhesions between the subcutaneous tissue and the abdominal organs, if present, are freed. The hernial contents should be evaluated and reduced into the abdominal cavity.
3. The edges of the hernial ring are debrided using a number 11 scalpel blade or a pair of Metzenbaum scissors.
4. A simple interrupted suture with long-lasting absorbable or nonabsorbable monofilament material is used.
5. For the reconstruction of large abdominal wall defects, refer to the section on traumatic hernias above.
6. If necessary, an active closed-suction drain is placed into the subcutaneous tissue, and the subcutis and skin are closed routinely.

Surgical technique: Evisceration repair (Fig. 15.25)

1. Prompt initial emergency treatment must be provided first (by owner or referral veterinarian). The exposed organs are copiously lavaged with saline (or tap water if saline is not available) and replaced in the abdominal cavity if possible. The incision is then protected with a bandage. Alternatively, in case it is not possible to replace the viscera into the abdominal cavity, they should be lavaged and protected with a clean bandage. An Elizabethan collar should be used to prevent self-mutilation of exposed organs.
2. The patient should be stabilized before surgery and carefully monitored to prevent self-trauma. Appropriate fluid therapy and administration of blood products and antibiotics can be included in the initial stabilization of the patient.
3. The abdominal cavity is explored and copiously lavaged with a warm sterile isotonic crystalloid solution (saline or lactated Ringer's solution).
4. All nonviable/severely traumatized tissue should be excised if possible.
5. The decision to close the abdominal wall defect and overlying tissues varies based on the extent and location of tissue damage and wound contamination observed during surgery:
   - In cases of acute herniation and minimal tissue damage or contamination, primary closure of the abdomen is appropriate.
   - In cases of moderate contamination, placement of a Jackson–Pratt drain should be considered (see Chapter 5).
   - In cases of septic peritonitis or severe contamination, vacuum-assisted closure or open peritoneal drainage can be used (see Chapter 16).
6. Sutures are applied using long-lasting absorbable or nonabsorbable monofilament material.

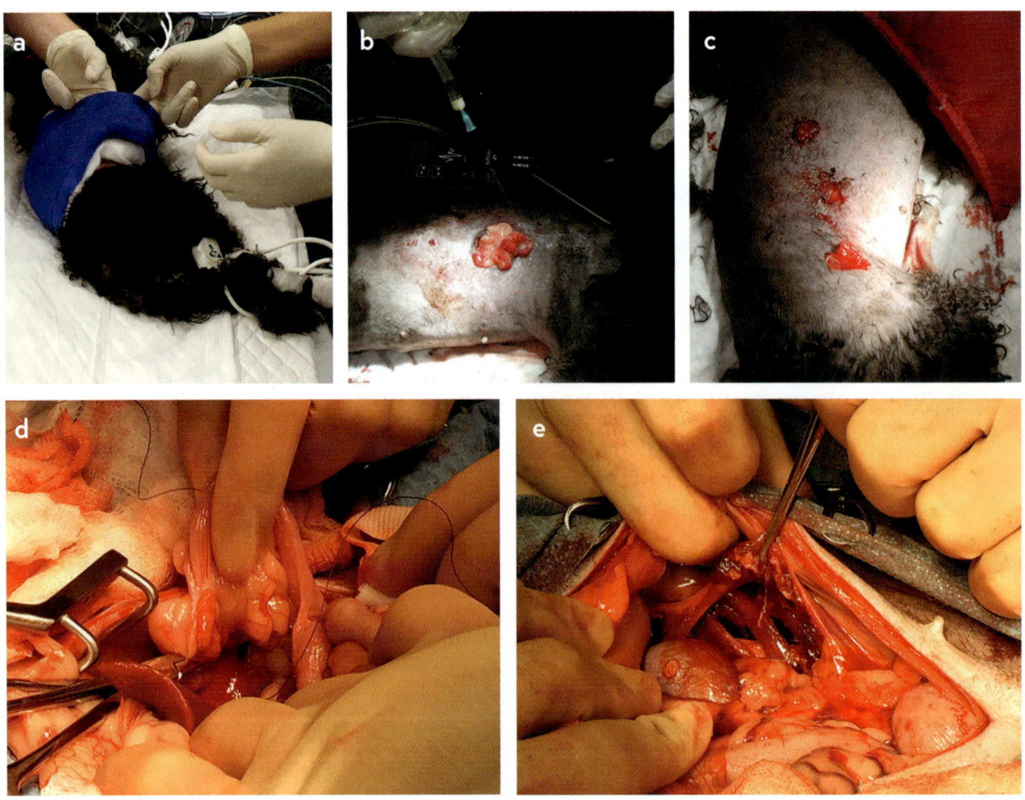

Figure 15.25 Bite wound trauma in a dog. (a) Removal of bandage (early emergency treatment). (b,c) Copious lavage of exposed organs and medication of abdominal wounds after careful examination of the chest and abdomen. (d,e) Ovariohysterectomy and closure of abdominal wound defects after exploration of the abdominal cavity and reduction of eviscerated organs (omentum and uterus).

Postoperative management

Exercise should be restricted for at least 2 weeks following surgery. Careful wound management is crucial to detect early signs of infection. Seroma and hematoma formation should be monitored to prevent infection, especially if a mesh or myofascial flap have been used. Active monitoring and prompt treatment are required if the patient develops signs of shock and septic peritonitis.[1]

Outcome

Most patients with incisional hernias have a good to excellent prognosis after repair, provided the underlying causes are addressed and damage to the abdominal viscera is minimal.

The prognosis after evisceration depends on the extent of injury and the procedures required for the exposed organs.[1] Overall, patients with sepsis and severe peritoneal contamination have guarded to poor prognosis, with a mortality rate exceeding 40%.[29] However, in a case series, all 12 cats and dogs with evisceration and gross abdominal contamination survived to discharge.[22] Factors associated with a prolonged hospitalization included evisceration secondary to trauma, high lactate concentration on admission, and small body size. While major abdominal evisceration injuries can be devastating, prompt medical management and surgical intervention can lead, in these cases, to a relatively good prognosis.[22]

Perineal hernias

Perineal hernia (PH) is a common pathological condition affecting mainly intact male dogs. It is caused by weakness or failure of the pelvic diaphragm muscles, resulting in the loss of lateral (and more rarely ventral) support to the rectum. This condition leads to the herniation of the rectum and pelvic and/or abdominal organs into the perineal subcutaneous space. While PH can occur in female dogs, it is rare in female cats.[30] Predisposing conditions causing tenesmus (rectal/perianal, prostatic, and bladder/urethral diseases) may play a role in its development.[31–34]

Regional deformation or swelling is often clinically evident on one or both sides of the perineum due to fecal accumulation or, less commonly, prostate gland or bladder entrapment. The contents of the hernia may include serous or serosanguinous fluid, perineal fat, deviated or sacculated rectal wall, and other structures such as the prostate gland, extraparenchymal prostatic cysts, urinary bladder, and intestines.[31–34]

Medical management, including digital fecal evacuation and stool softeners, may provide temporary resolution of the clinical signs, but most animals require herniorrhaphy for a complete functional recovery. In patients with impacted or strangulated small intestine or with an obstructed or retroverted bladder, PH is considered a surgical emergency.[31–34]

Clinical presentation and diagnosis

Most animals with PH present with a painless perineal swelling lateral to the anus. The consistency of the swelling upon palpation depends on the contents, ranging from deformable (fecal material) to elastic (inflammation or solid organ herniation) or fluctuant (bladder, fluid collection, prostatic cysts). In addition to tenesmus and irregular fecal evacuation, affected animals may display signs such as dyschezia, rectal prolapse, stranguria or anuria, and vomiting.[31–33]

The definitive diagnosis of PH is based on findings on clinical examination and rectal examination. Digital rectal examination reveals a unilateral or bilateral weakened pelvic diaphragm in most affected animals, except when bladder and/or prostate gland herniation is present.[32] In these cases, rectal deviation or sacculation may be masked. In cases of PH, the examiner's finger, directed laterally, can usually be visible under the perineal skin lateral to the anus (Fig. 15.26). Digital rectal palpation may be challenging if there is fecal impaction, and fecal evacuation is recommended before a second examination is performed, often with the use of sedation.[31–33] Other diagnostic tools, such as abdominal or perineal radiography and ultrasonography, may help evaluate the size and location of the prostate gland and determine whether the bladder or intestine are displaced into the PH.[31,32] Advanced imaging techniques, such as contrast studies, computed tomography, or magnetic resonance imaging, may provide additional information but are only used in selected cases.[31,32] Positive-contrast urethrocystography may be useful to assess the integrity of the lower urinary tract, particularly the bladder (Fig. 15.27).

PH can be anatomically classified as caudal (the most common type, between the levator ani and external anal sphincter muscles), dorsal (between the levator ani and coccygeal muscles), sciatic or lateral (between the coccygeal muscle and the sacrotuberous ligament), and ventral (rare, among the ischiourethral, ischiocavernosus, and bulbospongiosus muscles) (Fig. 15.28).

Treatment

Various surgical techniques have been reported for the treatment of PH. Appositional herniorrhaphy is often not possible due to the atrophy of the levator ani and/or coccygeal muscles and should be discouraged.[31] The most common technique is internal obturator muscle transposition. Additional techniques, including gluteal muscle transposition, semitendinosus muscle transpo-

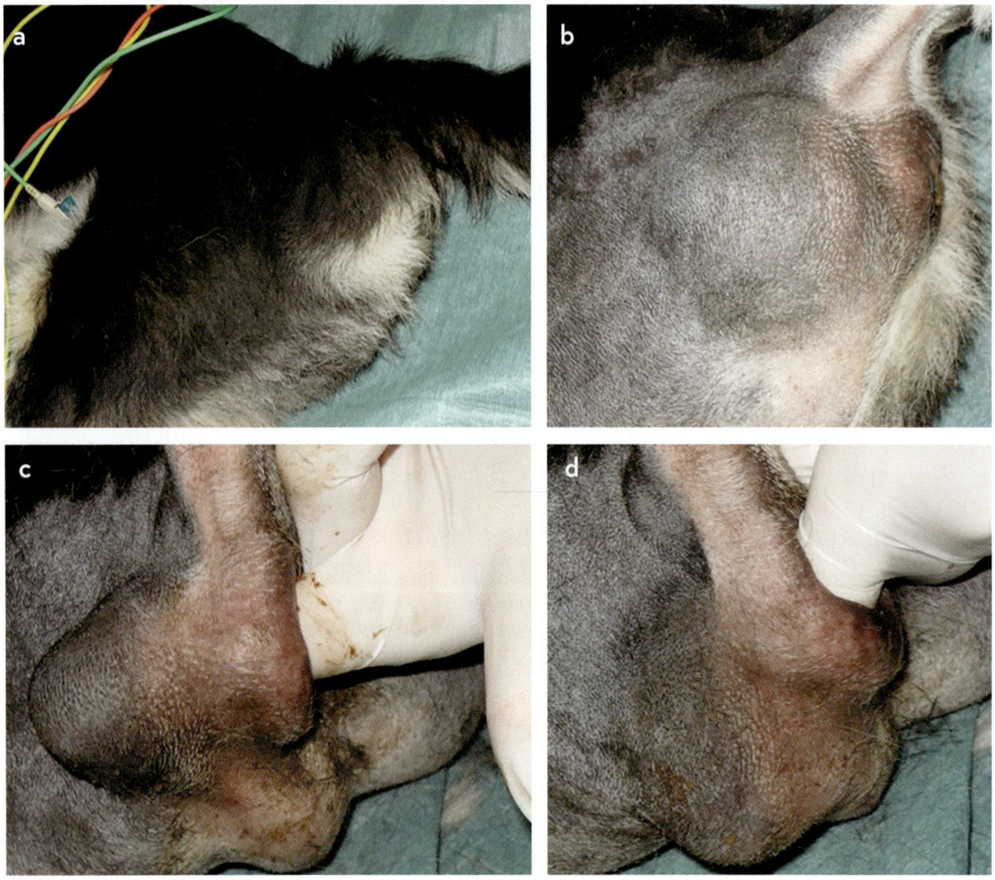

Figure 15.26 (a,b) Left lateral perineal swelling in a dog with perineal hernia. (c) Lateral and (d) ventral digital rectal examination. The tip of the examiner's finger is in the rectal sacculation and can be seen elevating the skin over the pararectal fossa.

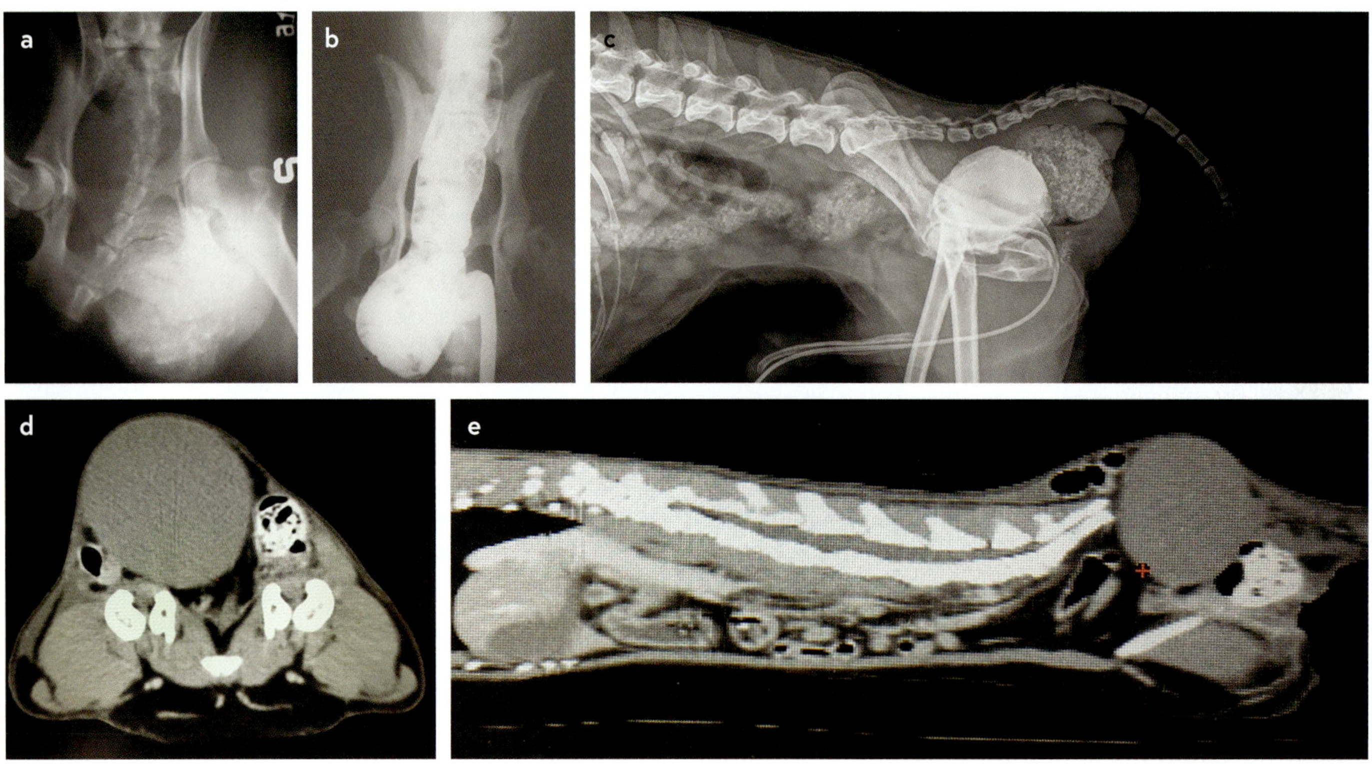

Figure 15.27 (a,b) Radiographic contrast study of a perineal hernia. (c) Retrograde urethrocystogram demonstrating bladder retroflexion into the perineal area; fecal accumulation is also visible caudal to the bladder. (d,e) Computed tomography images of a cat that sustained caudal abdominal/pelvic trauma showing herniation of the bladder into the perineal area.

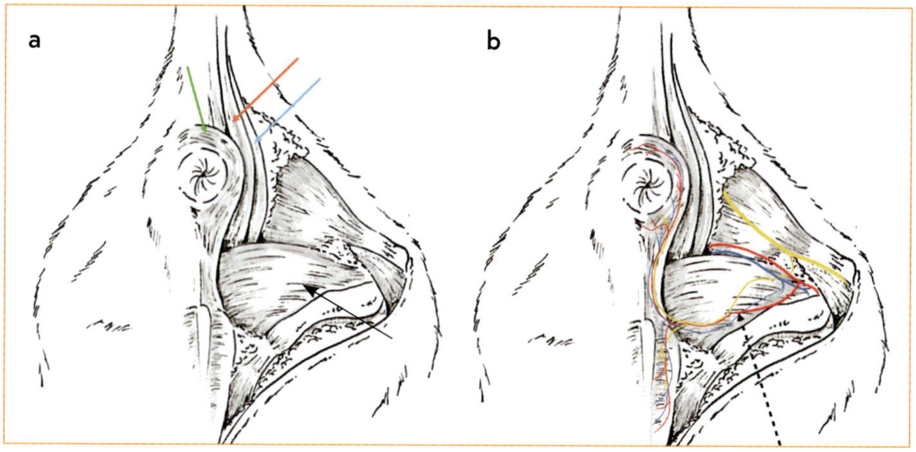

Figure 15.28 Anatomy of the pelvic diaphragm. (a) Coccygeal muscle (blue arrow), levator ani muscle (red arrow), external anal sphincter muscle (green arrow), internal obturator muscle (black arrow). (b) Pudendal vessel and nerve bundle (dotted arrow). Drawings by Fabio Esposito.

sition, incorporation of sacrotuberous ligament, or a combination of these techniques, may be utilized to augment internal obturator muscle transposition. Synthetic implants and different biomaterials have also been used. Bilateral herniorrhaphy can be performed during the same anesthetic episode. In cases with a seemingly unilateral hernia, digital exploration often reveals weakness of the contralateral pelvic diaphragm (incipient PH), suggesting the need for bilateral herniorrhaphy. Complicated PHs with rectal prolapse and bladder and/or prostate displacement may require additional procedures such as colopexy, vasopexy, and, less frequently, cystopexy.[31–33,35–39]

If the patient is unable to urinate, incarceration or strangulation of the urinary bladder may have occurred due to its retroflexion into the hernial sac. Bladder retroflexion, which has been reported in 20%–29% of patients, is diagnosed by unsuccessful bladder catheterization, ultrasonography (abdominal and perineal), contrast radiography, or perineal puncture.[30–32] If an obstruction is present, immediate treatment is indicated. If the bladder is too full and gentle catheterization is unsuccessful, manual repositioning of the bladder into the abdomen may not be possible, requiring decompression by ultrasound-guided perineal puncture (Fig. 15.29). Additionally, in case of bladder entrapment in the PH, a concomitant ipsilateral rectal prolapse may be present. After bladder repositioning, a Foley urinary catheter should be left in place to maintain bladder decompression and avoid re-obstruction before surgery.[32] Preoperative blood testing and urinalysis are recommended, especially if the urinary obstruction persists for more than 36–48 hours.

If the urinary bladder cannot be repositioned due to adhesion to the perineal fascia despite decompression, immediate surgical correction is indicated. The prognosis depends on the condition of the bladder wall and/or renal damage secondary to obstruction. Cystopexy has been recommended in one study to avoid recurrence,[40] while another study does not support this approach.[41] Castration is always recommended in addition to herniorrhaphy due to the high recurrence rate (2.7 times higher) of PH in dogs that are not castrated at the time of herniorrhaphy.[42]

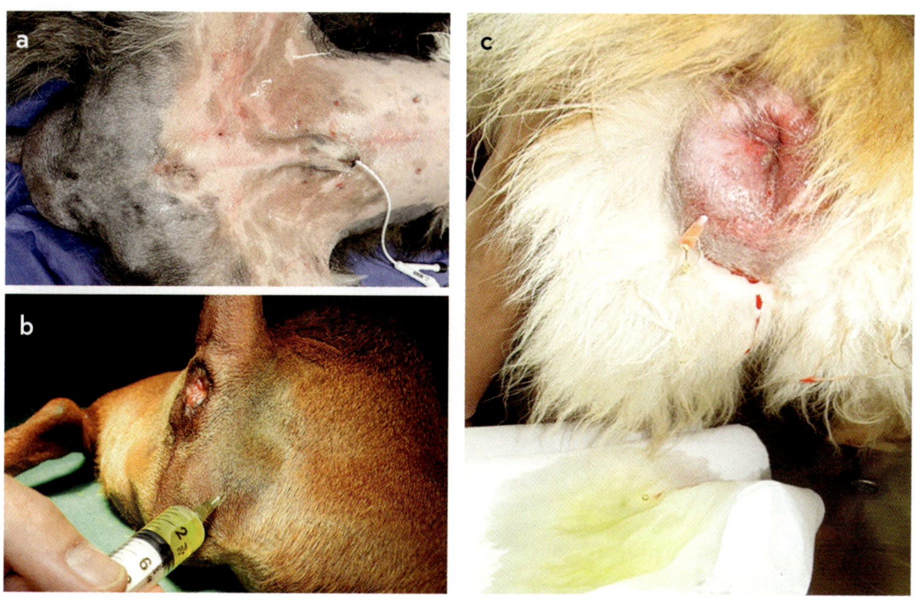

Figure 15.29 Patients with bladder retroflexion into the hernial sac. Immediate therapy to relieve the obstruction must be initiated in these cases. (a) The first option is transurethral catheterization of the bladder. (b,c) If this is not successful, paracentesis through the perineal skin should be performed.

Surgical technique: Internal obturator muscle transposition (Video 15.3)

This procedure is considered the gold standard for PH correction and includes the placement of appositional sutures dorsally combined with ventral transposition of an internal obturator muscle flap.

1. The patient is prepared for surgery as follows (Fig. 15.30):
   - Both the perineum and the base of the tail are clipped and prepped for surgery.
   - Manual evacuation of the rectum and anal sacs is recommended. A roll of gauze is placed in the terminal rectum and a purse-string suture is placed around the anus.
   - The urethra is catheterized using a rigid 6Fr–10Fr urinary catheter in dogs; 3Fr–5Fr in cats.
   - The patient is placed in sternal recumbency, with the pelvic limbs over the padded end of the operating table and the tail secured in a cranial position.

Video 15.3. Left-sided perineal hernia in an 8-year-old crossbreed dog treated with the internal obturator muscle transposition technique.

2. A curvilinear skin incision is made lateral and parallel to the anus (2–4 cm), starting dorsally at the base of the tail and extending at least 2 cm ventrally to the ischiatic tuberosity.
3. After subcutaneous undermining and opening of the hernial sac (perineal fascia), free serous fluid is often released. If necessary, the inflamed perineal and/or paraprostatic fat can be excised.
4. After gentle manipulation of the herniated content, a gauze pad may be positioned within the hernia to keep the herniated organs in the pelvic canal and improve the visibility of the surgical site (Fig. 15.31).

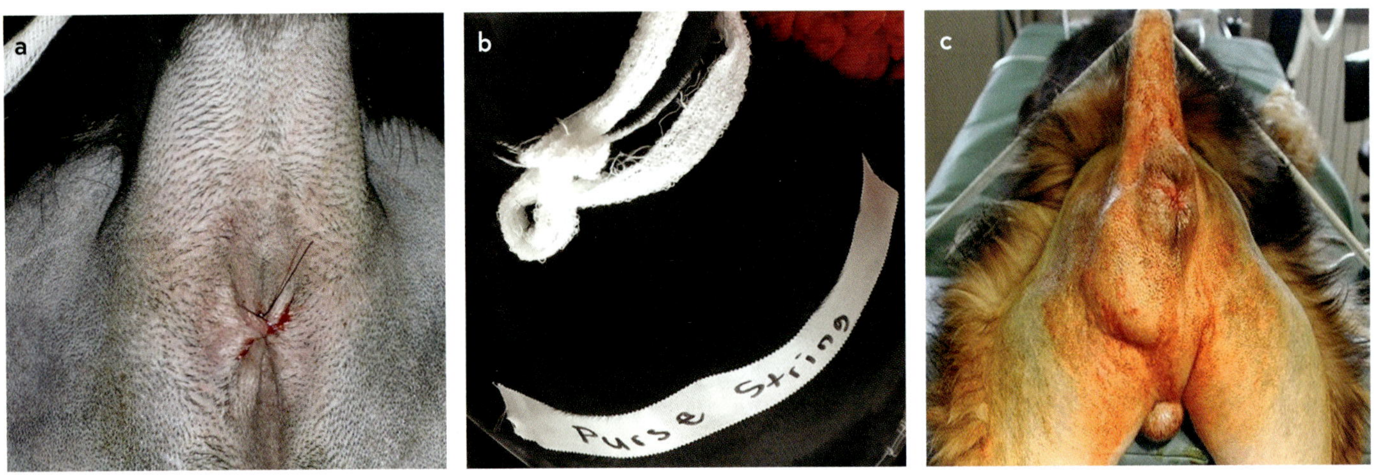

Figure 15.30 Preparation of patients for internal obturator muscle transposition. (a) The perineum and the base of the tail are clipped, and a purse-string suture is placed around the anus. (b) A piece of tape is used to indicate that the patient had an anal purse-string suture applied; it is removed at the end of surgery, after purse-string suture removal. (c) Patient positioning in sternal recumbency, with the hind legs over the padded end of the operating table and the tail secured in a cranial position.

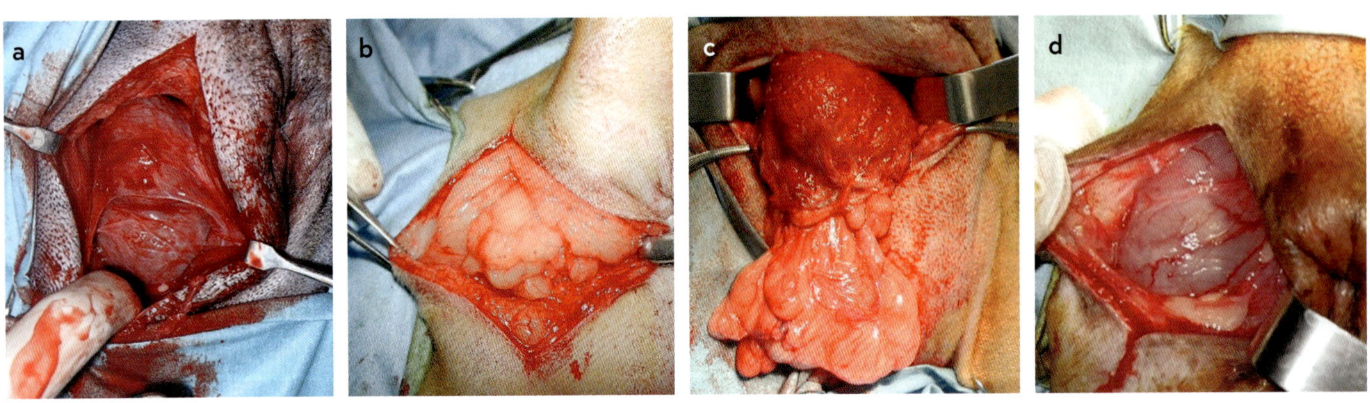

Figure 15.31 Different perineal hernia contents. (a) Deviated rectum or rectal dilatation. (b) Retroperitoneal fat. (c) Prostate gland. (d) Urinary bladder.

5. The muscles of the pelvic diaphragm and the neurovascular bundle dorsal to the internal obturator muscle should be identified (Fig. 15.32).
6. The caudal border of the internal obturator muscle is identified and incised along the caudal aspect of the ischium. A periosteal elevator is then inserted between the muscle and the bone. The internal obturator muscle is elevated off the ischium up to the caudal edge of the obturator foramen (Fig. 15.33).
7. To improve muscle flap mobilization and reduce tension at the suture site, the tendon of the internal obturator muscle is transected with a number 11 scalpel blade. To avoid damaging the sciatic nerve, the tendon should be transected medial to the lateral edge of the bone. Care should also be paid to the caudal gluteal artery.
8. After muscle flap preparation, the muscle is transposed dorsomedially into the perineal defect.
9. To avoid any damage to the urethra, further elevation of the caudomedial edge of the muscle is discouraged. Palpation of the urinary catheter is helpful in detecting the urethra.
10. Palpation under the muscle flap with the index finger is useful to ensure that the flap has been freed from its lateral and caudomedial attachments.

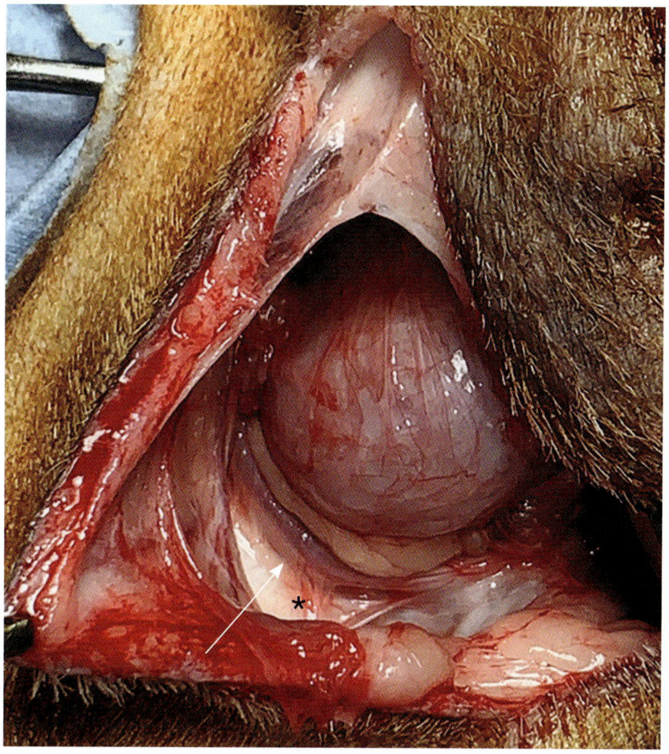

Figure 15.32 Neurovascular bundle (internal pudendal vessels and nerve) (arrow) dorsal to the internal obturator muscle (asterisk).

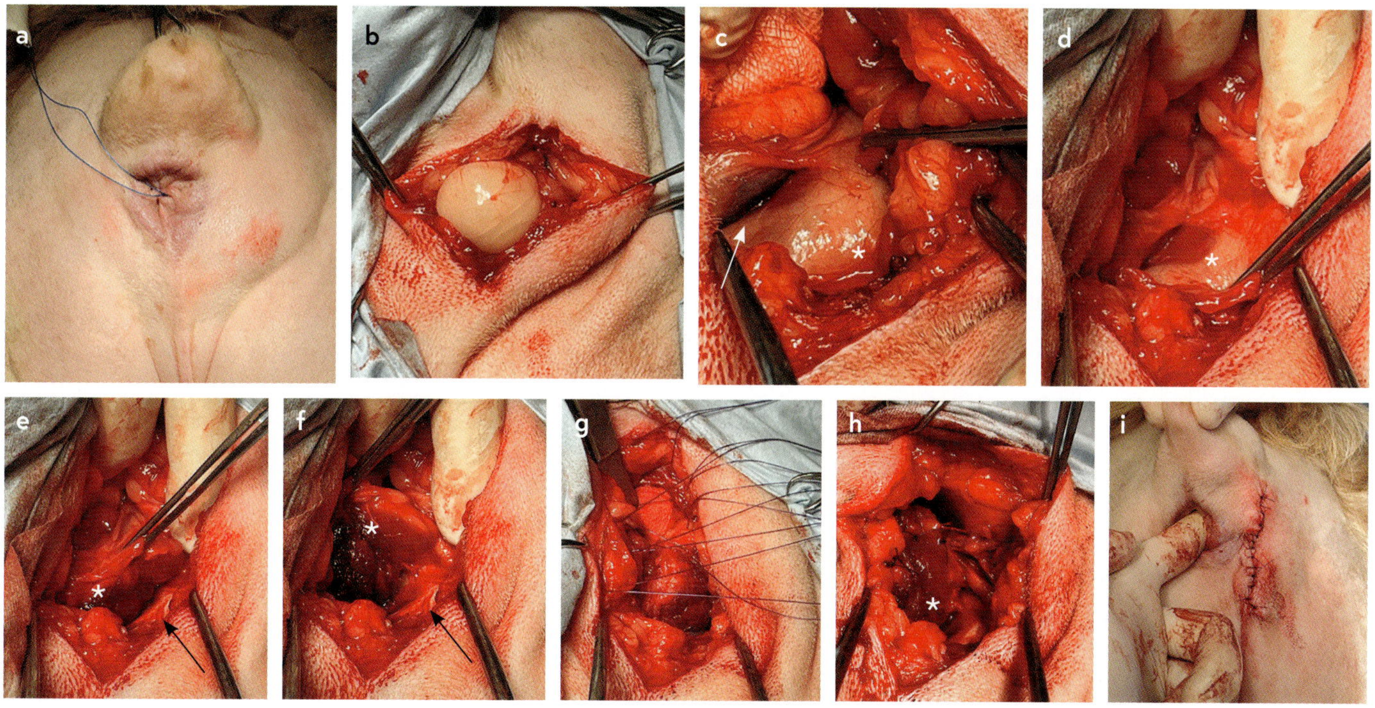

Figure 15.33 Internal obturator muscle transposition technique in a patient with a right-sided perineal hernia. (a) Patient preparation. (b) Skin incision over the hernia. (c) Reduction of hernial contents and identification of the internal obturator muscle (asterisk) and neurovascular bundle (white arrow). (d–f) Incision of the internal obturator muscle along the caudal aspect of the ischium and elevation from the ischiatic table (black arrow). (g) Preplacement of interrupted sutures from dorsal to ventral. (h) Completed herniorrhaphy. (i) Rectal examination after anal purse-string suture removal to confirm the rectal wall is appropriately supported.

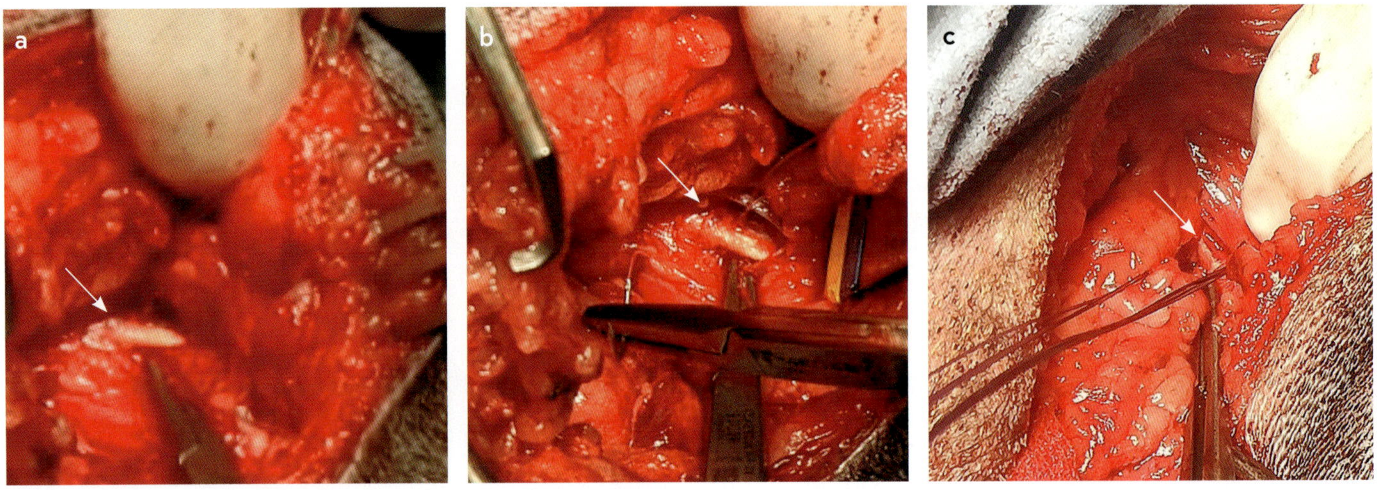

Figure 15.34 Perineal hernia repair with sacrotuberous ligament incorporation. (a) Isolation of the sacrotuberous ligament (arrow) with right-angle forceps. Placement of the sutures (b) through or (c) around the proximal half of the ligament. Care should be taken to avoid injury to or suture entrapment of the sciatic nerve or vessels lying near the sacrotuberous ligament.

11. Multiple interrupted sutures of 3-0 to 0 (depending on the patient's size) absorbable or nonabsorbable monofilament material are preplaced from dorsal to ventral.
    - Four to five sutures are placed between the coccygeal and external anal sphincter muscles. If the sacrotuberous ligament is incorporated, the sutures are placed through or around the proximal half of this ligament to avoid damage to the sciatic nerve (Fig. 15.34).[32,36]
    - The caudal edge of the transected internal obturator muscle is sutured to the coccygeal (laterally) and external anal sphincter (more medially) muscles. In this step, attention should be paid not to incorporate any of the structures of the neurovascular bundle into the sutures.
12. Once all the sutures have been preplaced, they are tied from dorsal to ventral; sutures involving the internal obturator muscle elevate the muscular flap when tied and close the larger ventral hernial opening. If a gauze pad has been used, it must be removed after the first one or two sutures have been tied.
13. The subcutis and skin are closed routinely.

Surgical technique: Semitendinosus muscle transposition (Figs. 15.35–15.37, Video 15.4)

The semitendinosus muscle flap technique is used as a salvage procedure when other procedures have failed or for repair of ventral PHs (if colopexy did not result in functional improvement and there is persistent fecal impaction). This flap is usually combined with other surgical techniques and can be employed ipsilaterally or contralaterally or, if needed, bilaterally.[32,39] Castration is recommended and can be performed before or after the herniorrhaphy.

Video 15.4. Semitendinosus muscle transposition technique for perineal hernia repair.

1. The same preoperative patient preparation is required as described previously, including both perineal areas and caudal aspect of the thighs.
2. The skin incision depends on the hernia:
    - For ipsilateral PHs, the standard incision performed for internal obturator muscle transposition is made and prolonged distally along the caudal thigh.
    - For contralateral PHs, the standard longitudinal incision is continued first transversally below the perianal region and then along the caudal aspect of the contralateral thigh, creating an S-shaped incision.
3. The hernial contents are reduced as previously described. The internal obturator muscle transposition procedure is performed (see above) before semitendinosus muscle transposition.
4. The semitendinosus muscle (type III muscle, with two main vascular pedicles, one proximal and one distal) is identified and isolated. During isolation, care should be paid to avoid any trauma to the proximal part of the muscle and to the caudal gluteal artery and vein. The muscle may be transected at any level from midbelly to distal just proximal to the stifle, as needed. The flap to be transposed may consist of the entire muscle or, based on a modified technique,[39] be limited to the medial half of the

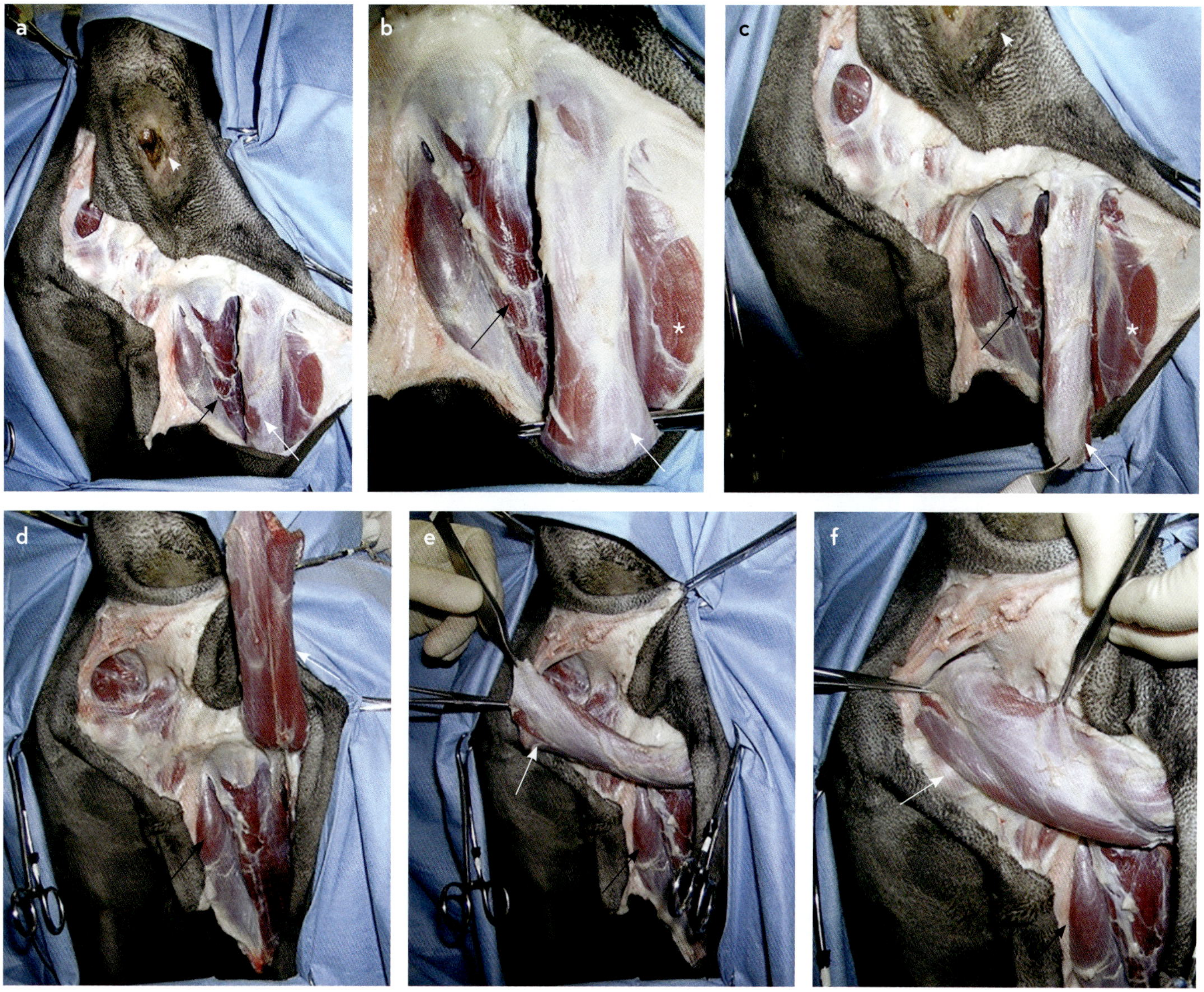

Figure 15.35 Cadaveric model for contralateral semitendinosus muscle transposition. (a) Continuation of the standard longitudinal incision first transversally below the anus (white arrowhead) and then along the caudal aspect of the contralateral thigh (S-shaped incision). (b–d) Identification and isolation of the entire semitendinosus muscle (white arrow), maintaining its proximal attachment. (e,f) Medial transposition of the entire muscle, passing ventral to the anus up to the opposite lateral perineum. Biceps femoris (asterisk), semimembranosus muscle (black arrow).

longitudinally split muscle. Using the modified technique, the semitendinosus muscle is isolated and then bluntly split longitudinally in two parts, sparing both the proximal and distal vascular pedicles. Only the medial part of the muscle is transected, at its distal end (proximal to the popliteal lymph node). The distal medial stump is sutured to the intact lateral muscular part, while the transected medial half of the muscle is transposed.

5. The muscle flap is then transposed:
   - If used ipsilaterally, the semitendinosus flap is reflected dorsally 180 degrees.
   - For contralateral or ventral PHs, the entire or the split muscle is transposed medially, passing ventral to the anus up to the opposite lateral perineum.
6. Multiple interrupted sutures of 3-0 to 0 (depending on the patient's size) absorbable monofilament material are preplaced. Sutures should include the semitendinosus flap, the coccygeal muscle and/or the sacrotuberous ligament, the ventrolateral aspect of the external anal sphincter muscle, and, more cranially, the internal obturator, ischiourethral and bulbospongiosus muscles. Attention should be paid not to incorporate the urethra into any of the sutures.
7. The subcutis and skin are closed routinely.

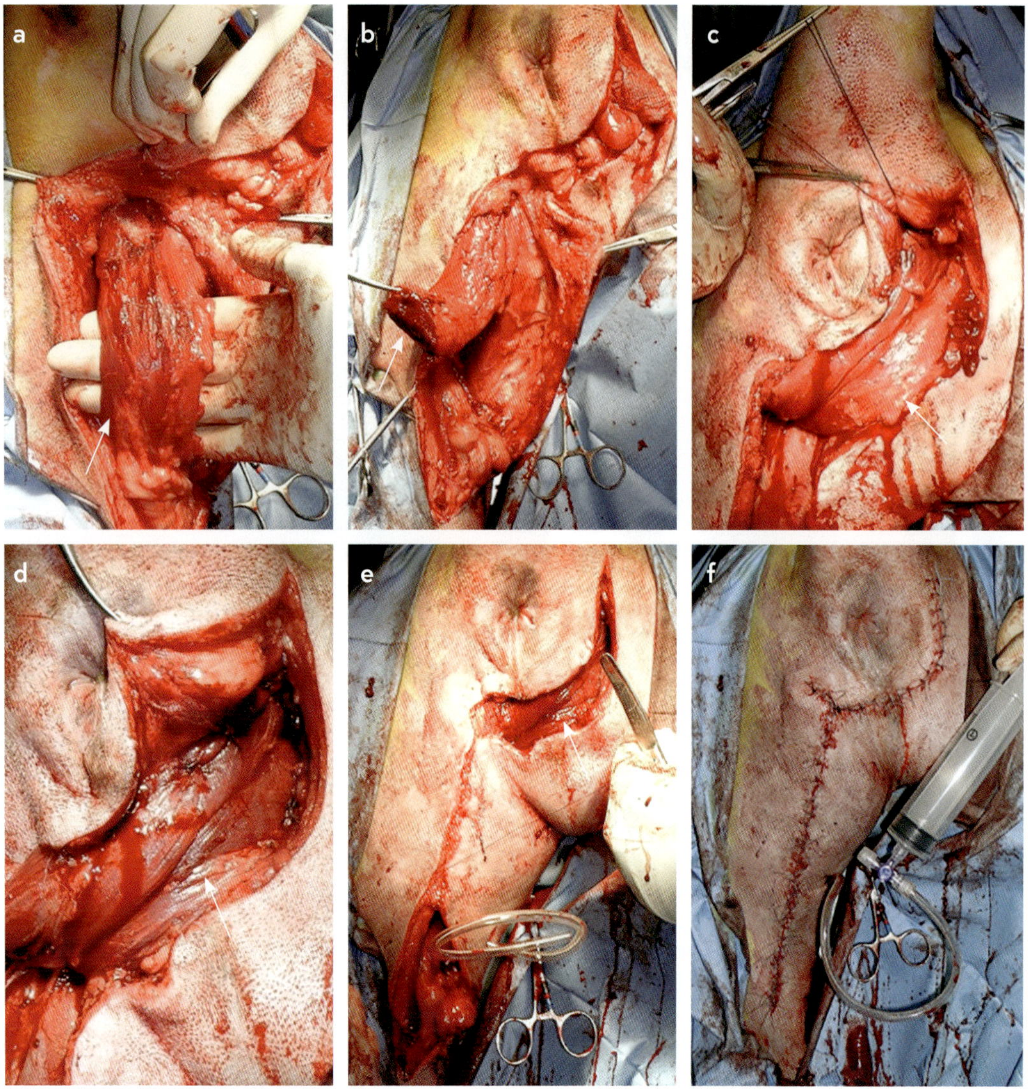

Figure 15.36 Perineal hernia treated with entire semitendinosus muscle transposition. (a) Isolation of the contralateral semitendinosus muscle (arrow) after reduction of the hernia and internal obturator muscle transposition. (b) Distal transection of the muscle. (c) Muscle transposition ventral to the anus and on the right perineal area. (d) Suture of the transected portion of the muscle to the perineal and internal obturator muscles and, in some cases, to the sacrotuberous ligament. (e,f) Application of an active drain and skin closure.

Surgical technique: Superficial gluteal muscle transposition (Fig. 15.38)

Unilateral superficial gluteal muscle transposition has been described in the treatment of dorsal PHs, while bilateral flaps have been recently suggested for ventral PH repair.[32,33,37] Castration of intact male dogs is recommended.

1. The same preoperative patient preparation is required as previously described, including the perineum, the region over the hip, the lateral pelvis, and the proximal thigh.
2. The incision extends from the cranial edge of the ilium across the upper thigh, over the perineal swelling, and down to a point at the level of or below the ischium. A second perpendicular incision is made from the midpoint of the first incision down over the greater trochanter.
3. The herniated contents are repositioned. Concomitant transposition of the internal obturator muscle can be performed if necessary.
4. The fascia lata is incised along the cranial edge of the biceps femoris muscle.
5. The insertion of the superficial gluteal muscle on the third trochanter is exposed.
6. The superficial gluteal muscle tendon is transected and the muscle isolated.
7. The dorsal and ventral aspects of the muscle are undermined to expose the cranial aspect of its origin on the gluteal and caudal fascia.
8. The superficial gluteal muscle flap is then elevated over the internal obturator muscle flap and its tendon sutured to the ischial periosteum, close to the base of the penis, and to the other perineal muscles using 2-0 or 3-0 absorbable monofilament in a simple interrupted pattern.
9. For ventral PH repair, bilateral superficial gluteal muscle transposition can be performed:

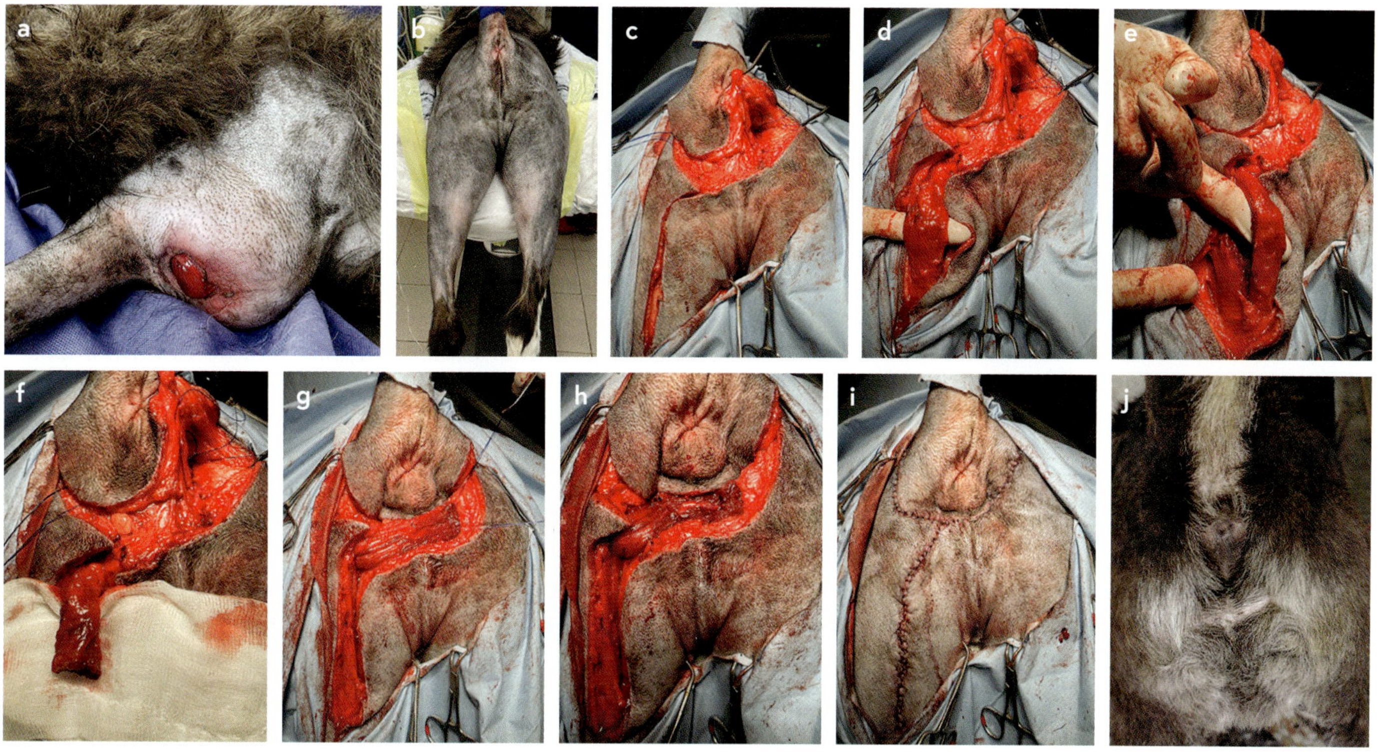

Figure 15.37 Bilateral ventral perineal hernia treated with split semitendinosus muscle transposition. (a,b) Patient preparation. (c) Skin incision for bilateral herniorrhaphy with internal obturator muscle transposition. (d) Preparation of the semitendinosus muscle for hernia repair. Isolation of the muscle. (e) Blunt longitudinal splitting of the muscle in two parts using scissors. (f) Distal transection of the medial part of the muscle, proximal to the popliteal lymph node. (g,h) Transposition of the transected medial half of the muscle and suture to the perineal area. (i) Skin closure. (j) Appearance at recheck 1 month after surgery.

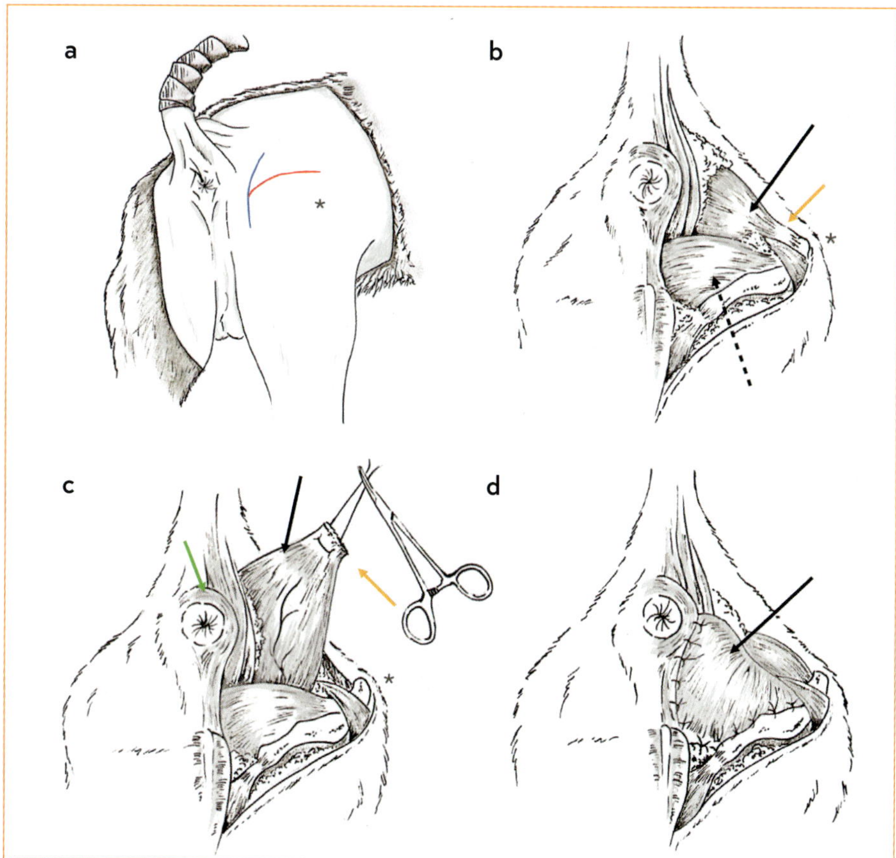

Figure 15.38 (a) Skin incision for traditional herniorrhaphy (blue line). Additional incision for superficial gluteal muscle transposition (red line). (b) The tendon (yellow arrow) of the superficial gluteal muscle (black arrow) is isolated below the biceps femoris muscle and cut at its insertion on the greater trochanter (asterisk). (c,d) The muscle is rotated into the perineal defect and sutured to the internal obturator muscle (dotted arrow), external anal sphincter muscle (green arrow), and sacrotuberous ligament. Drawings by Fabio Esposito.

- Both superficial gluteal muscles are mobilized.
- The origins of both superficial gluteal muscles are transected, except for the muscle fibers inserted on the first caudal vertebra and sacrotuberous ligament.
- The muscles are rotated over the surgical site.
- The insertion of the muscle of one side is pulled ventral to the anus and sutured to the insertion of the contralateral muscle flap and surrounding muscles and soft tissues.
- If no soft tissue is available for suturing, the suture material can be passed through bone tunnels drilled in the ischium (1.5–2.0 drill bits).

10. The subcutis and skin are closed routinely.

Surgical technique: Pexy

Colopexy, cystopexy, and vasopexy in conjunction with castration have also been used as adjunctive procedures for PH repair to reduce the risk of recurrence or in case of bladder retroflexion and rectal prolapse.[32,33,43] In patients with complicated PHs, herniorrhaphy can be performed at the same time of the pexy or delayed for 2–3 weeks in an attempt to decrease hernia-associated inflammation and complications.[32,33,43]

Video 15.5. Colopexy technique in a 5-year-old crossbreed dog.

Colopexy (Fig. 15.39, Video 15.5)

1. A caudal midline abdominal approach is made.
2. The left border of the abdominal wall incision is grasped with towel clamps and everted to expose the peritoneal surface.
3. The descending colon is pulled cranially to resolve any rectal sacculation, deviation, or prolapse. A nonsterile assistant can verify the correct position

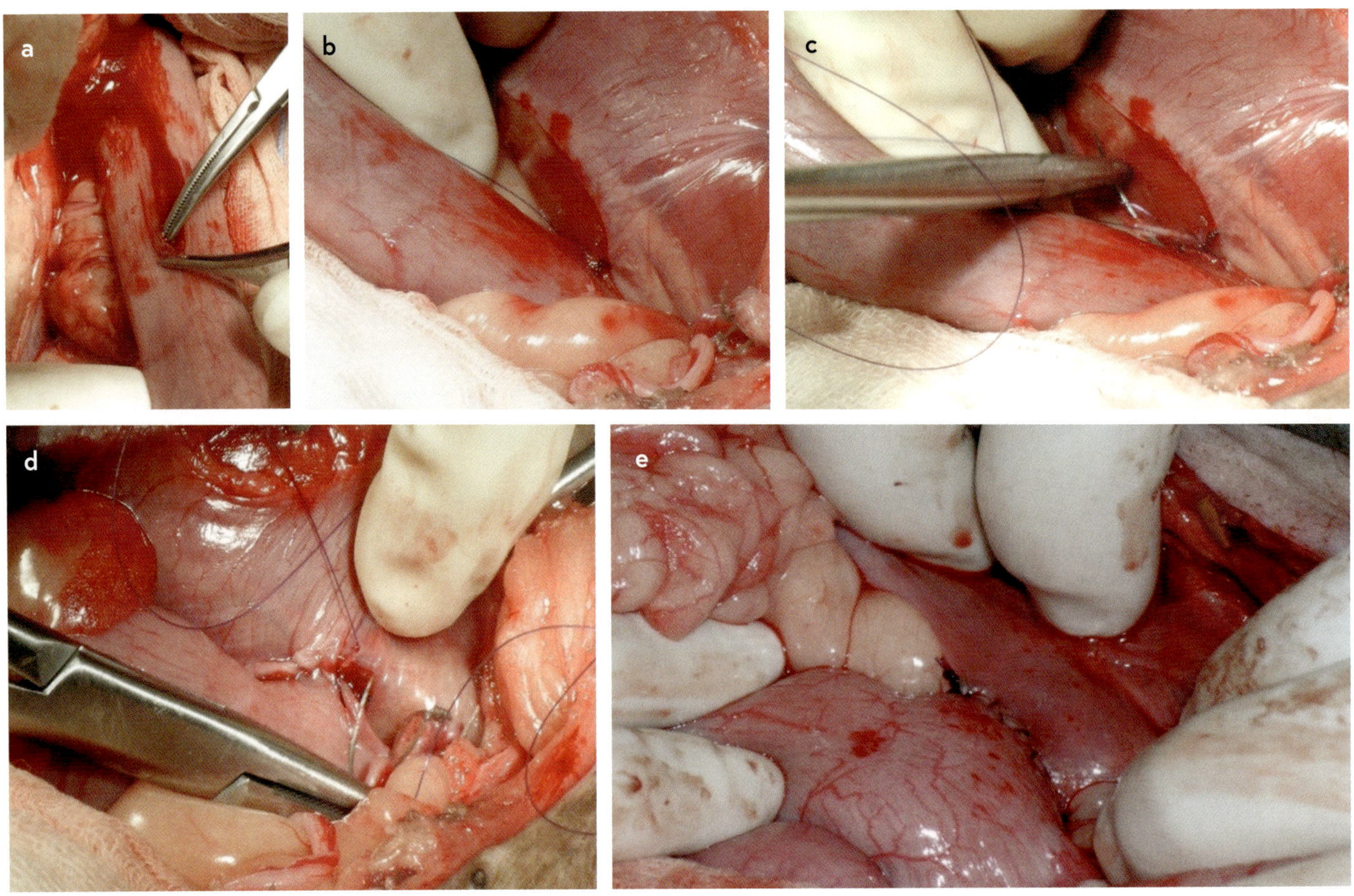

Figure 15.39 Colopexy. (a) Incision (4–6 cm) of the antimesenteric colonic serosa. (b–d) Suture of the colon to the abdominal wall in a simple continuous pattern, starting at the dorsal part of the incision. The ventral part of the incision is sutured similarly to ensure direct apposition of the incised surfaces of the colon and abdominal wall. (e) Final appearance of colopexy.

of the rectum by digital rectal examination beneath the sterile drapes.

4. Colopexy is performed via incision (4–6 cm long) or scarification of the antimesenteric colonic serosa. Fixation is done at the level of the left ventrolateral abdominal wall by placing interrupted sutures of 2-0 or 3-0 long-lasting absorbable monofilament material from the incised body wall to the scarified or incised surface of the descending colon.
   - The abdominal wall bite must include the transversus abdominis muscle.
   - The colon bite must include the submucosa, avoiding penetration of the mucosa.
   - A total of five to eight sutures should be placed about 0.5–1 cm apart, taking 0.5–1 cm bites on each side. Alternatively, two simple continuous sutures lines may be used.
5. The abdomen is closed routinely.

Vasopexy (Fig. 15.40, Video 15.6)

Vasopexy should be performed after colopexy.

1. The urinary bladder should be decompressed by urethral catheterization or cystocentesis before surgery.
2. Open prescrotal castration is performed, with separate ligation of the testicular vessels and vas deferens. Preservation of as much length as possible of the vasa deferentia should be attempted.
3. A caudal celiotomy is performed.

Video 15.6. Vasopexy technique.

4. Cranial traction is applied to the urinary bladder and prostate gland, putting them back in their normal anatomical position. A stay suture can be placed on the cranial aspect of the bladder to help in manipulation.
5. Both vasa deferentia should be identified at the level of the ipsilateral inguinal rings (or where they exit from the prostate gland).
6. Gentle traction is applied to each vas deferens until they exit from the inguinal canal into the abdominal cavity.
7. Both vasa deferentia are isolated from the ligated vessels and peritoneal attachment.
8. A stay suture (3-0 Prolene) or a hemostat clamp is placed at the end of each vas deferens. Mild to moderate traction is applied to both vasa deferentia to pull the bladder and prostate gland cranially.
9. A 1.5–2.5 cm tunnel is created from cranial to caudal under the transversus abdominis muscle along the ventrolateral abdominal wall, at the level of both sides of the empty bladder, near its apex.
10. The vas deferens on each side is pulled in a caudal

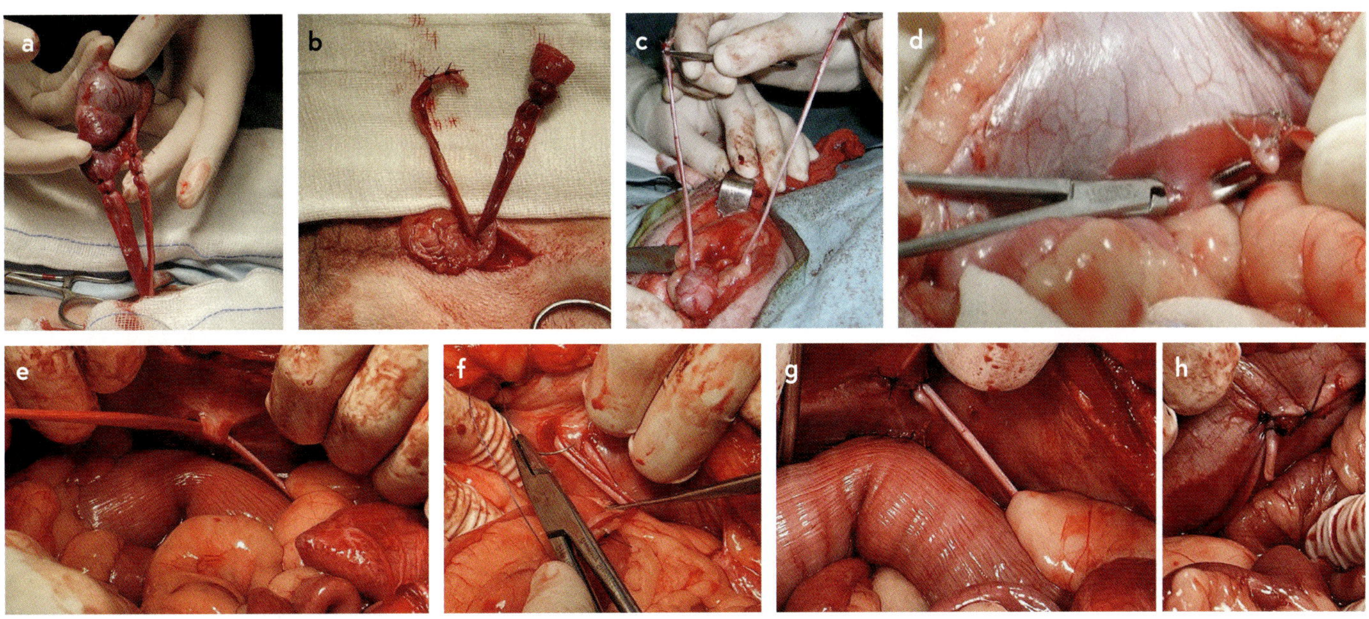

Figure 15.40 Vasopexy. (a,b) Open prescrotal castration. (c) Identification and isolation of the vasa deferentia after caudal celiotomy. (d,e) Intramuscular tunneling of the vas deferens in a caudal to cranial direction. (f–h) Backward turning of the vas deferens and suturing to itself and to the abdominal wall. The same procedure is repeated on the other vas deferens.

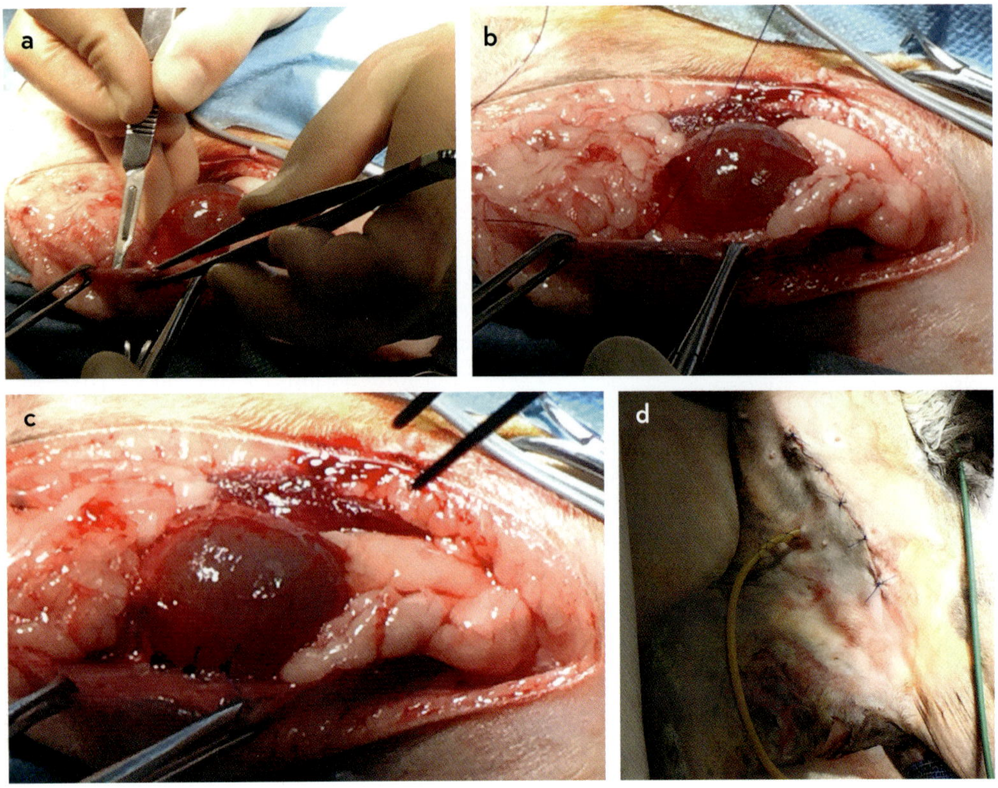

Figure 15.41 Cystopexy. (a) Incision of the bladder apex and right-side abdominal wall. (b,c) Multiple simple interrupted sutures between the bladder and right abdominal wall. (d) Concomitant cystostomy tube placement.

to cranial direction through the intramuscular tunnel and then turned backward. Each vas deferens is sutured to itself and to the abdominal wall using three or four interrupted sutures of 3-0 long-lasting absorbable monofilament material.

Cystopexy (Fig. 15.41)[43,44]

1. The urinary bladder should be decompressed by urethral catheterization or cystocentesis before surgery.
2. A caudal celiotomy is performed.
3. Cystopexy is performed between the bladder neck on the right side (or the bladder apex) and the right lateral abdominal body wall.
   - A 1–2 cm area of bladder neck serosa and a corresponding area of the right lateral abdominal wall are scarified using a number 11 scalpel blade. A pexy is performed with three or four simple interrupted or cruciate mattress sutures using 3-0 long-lasting absorbable monofilament material. Each suture should include the transversus abdominis muscle and the seromuscular layer of the bladder.
   - If the pexy involves the apex of the bladder, multiple rows of interrupted nonabsorbable sutures (3-0 Prolene) are placed between the seromuscular layer of the bladder apex and the right lateral abdominal body wall without scarification. In some cases, a cystostomy tube can be placed to keep the bladder empty and improve the healing of the pexy.

Postoperative management

Before recovery, the purse-string suture must be removed and a digital rectal examination should be performed to confirm adequate repair of the PH. Additionally, urethral and rectal integrity should be checked; no sutures should penetrate the rectum. A low-residue diet and a stool softener, such as lactulose, help reduce straining, which can result in rectal prolapse and suture weakening. An Elizabethan collar is recommended for at least 1 week to prevent self-trauma, and walking is encouraged.

Outcome

The complication rate after PH repair ranges from 15% to 61%.[32,33] Complications include swelling, wound infection, tenesmus, rectal prolapse, anorexia, fecal or urinary incontinence, and hernia recurrence. The risk of wound infection can be reduced by using perioperative antibiotics and maintaining strict asepsis during the procedure. Revision surgery is likely required in case of surgical site infection associated with the inadvertent incorporation of an anal sac during suture placement.

Tenesmus and subsequent rectal prolapse (2%–13%) are also possible postoperative complications.[32,33] Treatment options include stool softeners, analgesia, and even acepromazine to reduce straining. In some cases, colopexy and/or surgical resolution of rectal prolapse may also be necessary.

The recurrence rate of PH ranges from 0% to 70% but decreases to 0%–36% if internal obturator muscle transposition is used.[32,40] Several factors appear to contribute to the risk of recurrence, including the surgeon's experience, previous surgical PH repairs, type of suture material used, poor local tissue strength, amount of tension applied to the sutures, ongoing predisposing factors, and neuter status.[32,33] Possible treatment options in case of PH recurrence include pexies, prosthetic mesh, internal obturator muscle flap, semitendinosus muscle flap, or superficial gluteal muscle flap.[32,33]

Fecal incontinence is uncommon, and if it occurs, it may already have been present preoperatively, especially in long-standing PH cases, or it may be the result of iatrogenic damage to the caudal rectal nerve during surgery. Fecal incontinence caused by unilateral neurologic trauma is usually transient and may resolve within a few weeks through reinnervation from the other side of the external anal sphincter muscle. Transient incontinence may also result from surgical trauma to the external anal sphincter. Permanent fecal incontinence can be the consequence of bilateral damage to the pudendal or caudal rectal nerves, or to the entire external anal sphincter muscle.[32,33,45,46] Other reported major complications after PH repair that need prompt diagnosis and surgical treatment include urethral damage (especially if a urethral catheter was not placed), prostate injury (inadvertent prostatectomy), and sciatic nerve laceration or incorporation into the sutures (resulting in transient or permanent sciatic nerve paresis/paralysis).[51,52]

A potential complication of pexies is the recurrence of clinical signs due to poor surgical technique, breakdown of the pexy, or persistence of the underlying condition. Penetration into the colonic lumen during colopexy may lead to contamination of the abdominal cavity and peritonitis.[33,43,44] To avoid this, it is preferable to scarify the colonic serosa instead of incising it. Excessive cranial tension at the pexy site may also result in colonic wall necrosis or breakdown of the pexy. Possible postoperative complications of cystopexy include bladder atony due to neurovascular damage, recurrence of bladder herniation, stranguria, dysuria, hematuria, and temporary or permanent urinary incontinence.[33,43,44] For these reasons, the need for cystopexy is still debated.[40,41]

Perineal hernia in the cat

Perineal hernia is uncommon in cats, with only isolated reports in the literature. As in dogs, the cause of this type of hernia in cats remains unclear. The herniated contents are the same as described for dogs. Surgical repair is the preferred treatment; however, medical management may be effective in patients with minimal clinical signs. Treatment options are similar to those available for dogs, such as internal obturator muscle transposition or even the semitendinosus muscle flap.[47,48] It is important to remember that the sacrotuberous ligament is absent in cats. The most common postoperative complication is tenesmus.[49] In one study, 12/32 cats experienced short-term tenesmus after surgery, which resolved spontaneously in 9/12 cats (75%). The long-term outcome is good in most (74%) cats treated surgically (Fig. 15.42).[49]

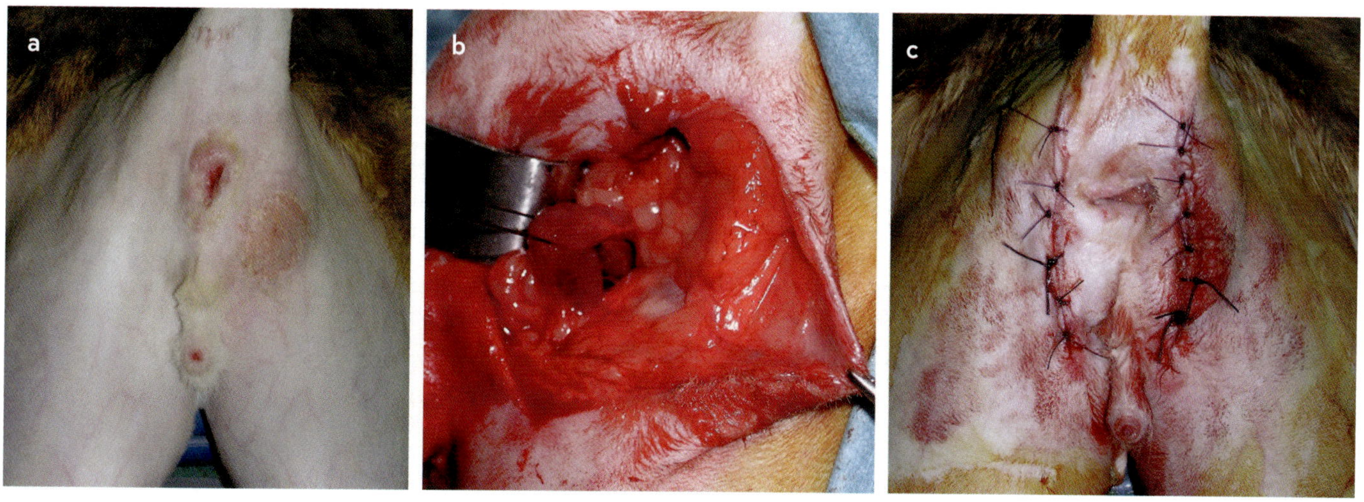

Figure 15.42 Bilateral perineal hernia in a cat. (a) Preoperative, (b) intraoperative, and (c) postoperative images.

KEEP IN MIND

- If the contents of a true hernia are irreducible or painful, emergency surgical treatment is warranted due to the possibility of organ incarceration or strangulation.
- Diaphragmatic hernias are often found concurrently with traumatic/incisional paracostal hernias and should be investigated and treated adequately.
- Patients with a hernia presenting immediately after acute trauma must be evaluated for life-threatening problems first. The time for surgical repair of traumatic hernias depends on their severity. While the repair of acute closed hernias in stable patients may be delayed, emergency surgery is needed in case of strangulated/incarcerated hernias, patient instability, or rapid clinical deterioration.
- Prompt repair of incisional hernias is usually required; otherwise, evisceration may occur, with potentially fatal consequences.
- Patients with a perineal hernia and clinical signs of impacted/strangulated intestines or an obstructed/retroverted urinary bladder require immediate emergency surgery.

References

1. Smeak DD. Abdominal wall reconstruction and hernias. In: Johnston SA, Tobias KM (eds.). *Veterinary Surgery: Small Animal*, 2nd ed. St. Louis: Elsevier; 2018. pp. 1564–1591.
2. Smeak DD. True abdominal hernias. In: Aronson LR (ed.). *Small Animal Surgical Emergencies*, 2nd ed. Wiley; 2022. pp. 178–189.
3. Itoh T, Kojimoto A, Kojima K, Shii H. Retrospective study on clinical features and treatment outcomes of nontraumatic inguinal hernias in 41 dogs. *J Am Anim Hosp Assoc.* 2020; 56(6):301.
4. Waters DJ, Roy RG, Stone EA. A retrospective study of inguinal hernia in 35 dogs. *Vet Surg.* 1993; 22(1):44–49.
5. Bellenger CR. Inguinal and scrotal herniation in 61 dogs. *Aust Vet Pract.* 1996; 26:58–59.
6. Manderino D, Bucklan L. Complete small-bowel obstruction caused by scrotal hernia in a dog. *Mod Vet Pract.* 1987; 68:365–366.
7. Weinstein MJ, Pavletic MM, Boudrieau RJ, Engler SJ. Cranial sartorius muscle flap in the dog. *Vet Surg.* 1989; 18(4): 286–291.
8. Beittenmiller MR, Mann FA, Constantinescu GM, Luther JK. Clinical anatomy and surgical repair of prepubic hernia in dogs and cats. *J Am Anim Hosp Assoc.* 2009; 45(6):284–290.
9. Risselada M, de Rooster H, Taeymans O, van Bree H. Penetrating injuries in dogs and cats. A study of 16 cases. *Vet Comp Orthop Traumatol.* 2008; 21(5):434–439.
10. Shamir MH et al. Dog bite wounds in dogs and cats: A retrospective study of 196 cases. *J Vet Med A Physiol Pathol Clin Med.* 2002; 49(2):107–112.
11. Shaw SR, Rozanski EA, Rush JE. Traumatic body wall herniation in 36 dogs and cats. *J Am Anim Hosp Assoc.* 2003; 39(1):35–46.
12. Sepuya RG et al. Comparing diagnostic findings and cost of whole body computed tomography to traditional diagnostic imaging in polytrauma patients. *J Vet Emerg Crit Care (San Antonio).* 2022; 32(3):334–340.
13. Mudge M, Hughes LE. Incisional hernia: A 10 year prospective study of incidence and attitudes. *Br J Surg.* 1985; 72(1):70–71.
14. Mejia S, Boston SE, Skinner OT. Sartorius muscle flap for body wall reconstruction: Surgical technique description and retrospective case series. *Can Vet J.* 2018; 59(11):1187–1194.
15. Feng YC, Chen KS, Chang SC. Reconstruction with latissimus dorsi, external abdominal oblique and cranial sartorius muscle flaps for a large defect of abdominal wall in a dog after surgical removal of infiltrative lipoma. *J Vet Med Sci.* 2016; 78(11):1717–1721.
16. Alexander LG, Pavletic MM, Engler SJ. Abdominal wall reconstruction with a vascular external abdominal oblique myofascial flap. *Vet Surg.* 1991; 20(6):379–384.
17. Cronin A, Hall JL. A novel internal abdominal oblique muscle flap to close a major abdominal wall defect. *J Small Anim Pract.* 2021; 62(1):55–58.
18. Archipow W, Lanz OI. Rectus abdominis muscle flap for repair of prepubic tendon rupture in 8 dogs. *Can Vet J.* 2011; 52(11):1215–1218.
19. Pavletic MM. Introduction to myocutaneous and muscle flaps. *Vet Clin North Am Small Anim Pract.* 1990; 20(1):127–146.
20. Argenta LC, Morykwas MJ. Vacuum-assisted closure: A new method for wound control and treatment: Clinical experience. *Ann Plast Surg.* 1997; 38(6):563–576.
21. Ferreira F et al. Sequential closure of the abdominal wall with continuous fascia traction (using mesh or suture) and negative pressure therapy. *Rev Col Bras Cir.* 2013; 40(1):85–89.
22. Gower SB, Weisse CW, Brown DC. Major abdominal evisceration injuries in dogs and cats: 12 cases (1998–2008). *J Am Vet Med Assoc.* 2009; 234(12):1566–1572.
23. Luijendijk RW et al. A comparison of suture repair with mesh repair for incisional hernia. *N Engl J Med.* 2000; 343 (6):392–398.
24. Bellón JM et al. Midline abdominal wall closure: A new prophylactic mesh concept. *J Am Coll Surg.* 2006; 203(4):490–497.
25. Whitfield-Cargile CM et al. Comparison of primary closure of incisional hernias in horses with and without the use of prosthetic mesh support. *Equine Vet J Suppl.* 2011; 43(Suppl 39):69–75.
26. Magee AA, Galuppo LD. Comparison of incisional bursting strength of simple continuous and inverted cruciate suture patterns in the equine linea alba. *Vet Surg.* 1999; 28(6):442–447.
27. Owens M, Barry M, Janjua AZ, Winter DC. A systematic review of laparoscopic port site hernias in gastrointestinal surgery. *Surgeon.* 2011; 9(4):218–224.
28. Pope JF, Knowles TG. Retrospective analysis of the learning curve associated with laparoscopic ovariectomy in dogs and associated perioperative complication rates. *Vet Surg.* 2014; 43(6):668–677.

29. Bentley AM, Otto CM, Shofer FS. Comparison of dogs with septic peritonitis: 1988–1993 versus 1999–2003. *J Vet Emerg Crit Care*. 2007; 17(4):391–398.
30. Hayashi AM et al. Retrospective study (2009–2014): Perineal hernias and related comorbidities in bitches. *Top Companion Anim Med*. 2016; 31(4):130–133.
31. Gill SS, Barstad RD. A review of the surgical management of perineal hernias in dogs. *J Am Anim Hosp Assoc*. 2018; 54(4):179–187.
32. Baines SJ, Aronson LR. Rectum, anus, and perineum. In: Johnston SA, Tobias KM (eds.). *Veterinary Surgery Small Animal*, 2nd ed. St. Louis, MO: Elsevier; 2018. pp. 1783–1827.
33. Bellenger CR, Canfield RB. Perineal hernia. In: Slatter DH (ed.). *Textbook of Small Animal Surgery*, 3rd ed. Philadelphia, PA: Saunders; 2003. pp. 487–497.
34. Hosgood G, Hedlund CS, Pechman RD, Dean PW. Perineal herniorrhaphy: Perioperative data from 100 dogs. *J Am Anim Hosp Assoc*. 1995; 31(4):331–342.
35. Bernardé A, Rochereau P, Matres-Lorenzo L, Brissot H. Surgical findings and clinical outcome after bilateral repair of apparently unilateral perineal hernias in dogs. *J Small Anim Pract*. 2018; 59(12):734–741.
36. Cinti F, Rossanese M, Pisani G. A novel technique to incorporate the sacrotuberous ligament in perineal herniorrhaphy in 47 dogs. *Vet Surg*. 2021; 50(5):1023–1031.
37. Bitton E et al. Use of bilateral superficial gluteal muscle flaps for the repair of ventral perineal hernia in dogs: A cadaveric study and short case series. *Vet Surg*. 2020; 49(8):1536–1544.
38. Carbonell Rosselló G, Turner A, Macias C, Ramírez JM. Combined transposition of internal obturator and superficial gluteal muscles for perineal hernia treatment in dogs: 17 cases (2017–2020). *J Small Anim Pract*. 2023; 64(2): 96–102.
39. Morello E et al. Modified semitendinosus muscle transposition to repair ventral perineal hernia in 14 dogs. *J Small Anim Pract*. 2015; 56(6):370–376.
40. van Sluijs FJ, Sjollema BE. Perineal hernia repair in the dog by transposition of the internal obturator muscle. I. Surgical technique. *Vet Q*. 1989; 11(1):12–17.
41. Grand JG, Bureau S, Monnet E. Effects of urinary bladder retroflexion and surgical technique on postoperative complication rates and long-term outcome in dogs with perineal hernia: 41 cases (2002–2009). *J Am Vet Med Assoc*. 2013; 243(10):1442–1447.
42. Hayes HM, Wilson GP, Tarone R. The epidemiologic features of perineal hernia in 771 dogs. *J Am Anim Hosp Assoc*. 1978; 14:703–707.
43. Maute AM, Koch DA, Montavon PM. Perineal hernia in dogs: Colopexy, vasopexy, cystopexy and castration as an alternative therapy in 32 dogs. *Eur J Compan Anim Pract*. 2003; 13:104–109.
44. Risselada M et al. Retroflexion of the urinary bladder associated with a perineal hernia in a female cat. *J Small Anim Pract*. 2003; 44(11):508–510.
45. Sjollema BE, van Sluijs FJ. Perineal hernia in the dog: Developments in its treatment and retrospective study in 197 patients [in Dutch]. *Tijdschr Diergeneeskd*. 1991; 116 (3):142–147.
46. Matthiesen DT. Diagnosis and management of complications occurring after perineal herniorrhaphy in dogs. *Compend Contin Educ Pract Vet*. 1989; 11:797–822.
47. Welches CD, Scavelli TD, Aronson MG, Matthiesen DT. Perineal hernia in the cat: A retrospective study of 40 cases. *J Am Anim Hosp Assoc*. 1992; 28:431–438.
48. Vnuk D et al. Application of a semitendinosus muscle flap in the treatment of perineal hernia in a cat. *Vet Rec*. 2005; 156(6):182–184.
49. Hubers MWL et al. Outcome of surgical treatment of perineal hernia in cats: 36 cases (2013–2019). *J Small Anim Pract*. 2022; 63(10):776–783.
50. Mejia S, Boston SE, Skinner OT. Sartorius muscle flap for body wall reconstruction: Surgical technique description and retrospective case series. *Can Vet J*. 2018; 59(11):1187–1194.
51. Häußler TC, Thiel C, Fischer A, Kramer M. Inadvertent iatrogenic prostatectomy and urethrectomy in 2 dogs. *Tierarztl Prax Ausg K Kleintiere Heimtiere*. 2019; 47(4):282–289.
52. Sereda C, Fowler D, Shmon C. Iatrogenic proximal urethral obstruction after inadvertent prostatectomy during bilateral perineal herniorrhaphy in a dog. *Can Vet J*. 2002; 43(4): 288–290.

Chapter 16

Peritonitis

Rosario Vallefuoco, Mark Longley

Septic peritonitis

Peritonitis is defined as inflammation of the peritoneal cavity. In veterinary medicine, the reported classification of peritonitis includes primary, secondary, or recurrent secondary (based on the underlying cause), acute or chronic (based on the chronology), localized or generalized (based on the extent), and septic or aseptic (based on the presence of infectious agents).[1,2]

Primary peritonitis, or spontaneous bacterial peritonitis, is an infection of the peritoneum without an identifiable inciting intra-abdominal infectious process or known history of penetrating trauma. It has been postulated that this peritoneal infection occurs via hematogenous dissemination, via bacterial translocation[3] or due to bacteremia associated with portosystemic shunt.[4] Primary peritonitis can have a viral origin, as for feline infectious peritonitis (FIP), associated with coronavirus infection. However, primary bacterial and fungal peritonitis has also been reported in dogs[3] and cats.[5]

Secondary peritonitis results from introduction of external bacteria into the peritoneal cavity. Full-thickness perforation and leakage of bacteria from the gastrointestinal (GI) tract is the most common cause of secondary peritonitis in dogs (60%–63%) and cats (47%) (Fig. 16.1).[6–8] However, bacterial contamination from intra-abdominal infectious processes of other organs (e.g., liver, gallbladder, pancreas, spleen, lymph nodes, genitourinary tract) can also occur. Secondary peritonitis caused by fungal organisms is relatively rare.[9]

Recurrent secondary peritonitis relates to an infection of the peritoneal cavity following a perceived successful surgical control of secondary peritonitis.[2]

Aseptic peritonitis is associated with the exposure of the peritoneum to sterile fluids (e.g., gastric, biliary, urine, chyle, pancreatic enzymes) or foreign material including surgical materials (e.g., surgical glove powder, suture, cotton swabs, surgical sponges). This group also includes sclerosing encapsulating, parasitic, and protozoal peritonitis as well as primary or metastatic neoplasms of the peritoneum. In small animal practice, acute generalized secondary septic peritonitis is the most common form of peritonitis. It is a life-threatening condition that requires an early diagnosis, appropriate medical stabilization, and emergency surgical treatment.

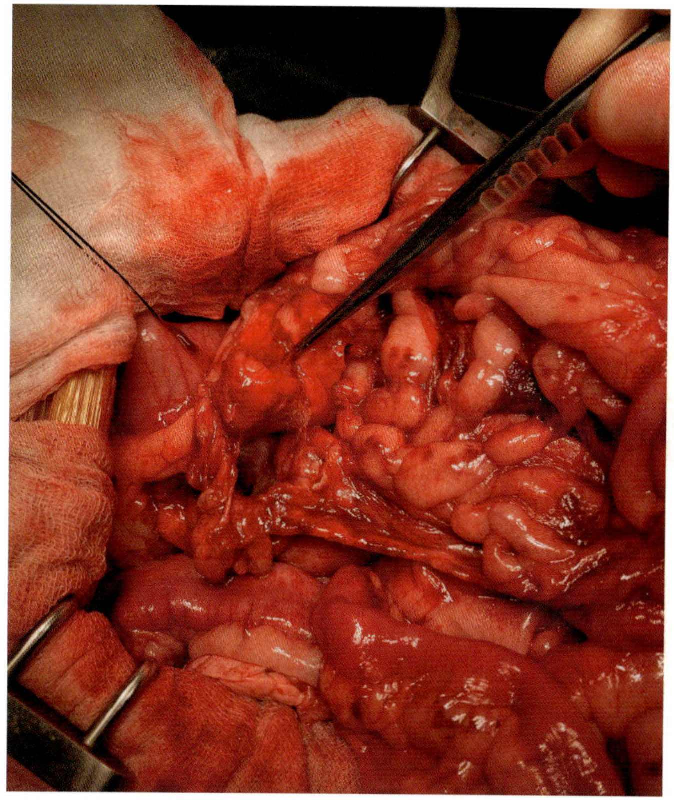

Figure 16.1 Septic peritonitis secondary to a gastric perforation. The stomach is elevated by a stay suture, and the gastric perforation is showed with the help of a DeBakey forceps. The omentum and the serosal aspect of the organs are inflamed and hyperemic.

Clinical presentation and diagnosis

Clinical presentation of dogs and cats with septic peritonitis is variable, often not specific and is dependent on the underlying infectious process. Anorexia, vomiting, depression, and lethargy are common clinical signs. The "pray position" may be adopted by some animals to relieve abdominal pain or distension. Pyrexia is not consistent, and cats are often hypothermic.[10] Abdominal pain can be appreciated on palpation, but it is less consistent in feline patients.[10] Dehydration is common and is caused by reduced fluid intake and by fluid loss due to vomiting and peritoneal effusion. Peritoneal effusion is a consistent finding, but it can be challenging

to appreciate on physical examination (ballottement) in case of small volumes of free abdominal fluid (<10 mL/kg). Patients with septic peritonitis often present in a progressive status of hypovolemic and cardiovascular shock and may already show signs of systemic inflammatory response syndrome. In the early stages, injected mucous membranes, strong pulses, reduced capillary refill time, moderate tachycardia, and fever may be noted. In the later stages, progressive hypovolemia, severe tachycardia, weak pulses, prolonged capillary refill time, pale mucous membranes, and hypothermia are present.
The diagnosis of septic peritonitis is based on the detection and examination of free peritoneal fluid. However, definitive diagnosis can sometimes be challenging to obtain, and other diagnostic tests may be necessary to support the suspicion of septic peritonitis.
Hematology, serum biochemistry, blood gas analysis, and urinalysis are recommended in cases of septic peritonitis. The findings are generally not specific. However, it is crucial to have a baseline to assess the treatment and progression of the patient. Neutrophilia with a left shift is a common hematologic abnormality, but neutropenia can be also present. Increased values of urea, creatinine, and liver enzymes are possible as a consequence of the primary problem or secondary to hypovolemia and decreased perfusion. Protein and albumin values can be low as a result of loss within the peritoneal effusion or due to the underlying disease. Hypoglycemia is common in septic patients. Acid–base and electrolyte abnormalities are often detected.
Abdominal radiographs can show focal or diffuse loss of detail, often referred to as a ground-glass appearance, depending on the amount of free peritoneal fluid. In some cases, pneumoperitoneum may also be present (see below). The presence of organomegaly, mechanical GI obstruction, and GI radiopaque foreign body can also be identified on abdominal radiographs in some cases.
Abdominal ultrasound is the most commonly used imaging diagnostic tool to detect small amounts of free abdominal fluid or gas. Small pockets of fluid can be collected under ultrasound guidance. Furthermore, ultrasound can give information about the underlying cause of peritonitis.
Computed tomography (CT) has recently become widely used in veterinary medicine as an accurate screening test for differentiating surgical from nonsurgical acute abdominal conditions in dogs.[11]
Blind abdominocentesis can be used to collect free peritoneal fluid for cytological and biochemical evaluation. Single, four-quadrant, or peritoneal lavage can be used to collect peritoneal fluid. Septic peritoneal effusion is an exudate with protein concentration above 3.0 g/dL and nucleated cell counts above 7000 cells/μL. The presence of intra- or extracellular bacteria and toxic and degenerate neutrophils is diagnostic for septic peritonitis.
In one study, a blood-to-fluid glucose difference of more than 20 mg/dL was 100% sensitive and 100% specific for the diagnosis of septic peritoneal effusion in dogs and 86% sensitive and 100% specific in cats.[12] If a veterinary point-of-care glucometer is used, the plasma-to-fluid glucose cutoff value is greater than or equal to 38 mg/dL.[13] Also, blood-to-fluid lactate concentration can be used to aid in the diagnosis of septic peritonitis. A blood-to-fluid lactate difference of less than −2.0 mmol/L was 100% sensitive and 100% specific for the diagnosis of septic peritonitis in dogs.[12] Fluid cytology and nucleated cell count is more accurate than glucose or lactate measurements for the diagnosis of septic peritonitis in cats.

Treatment

Septic peritonitis is a surgical emergency. However, preoperative patient stabilization is paramount to improve the successful management of this critical condition.
The goals of surgical treatment include:

- Identification and treatment of the infection source via abdominal exploration.
- Reduction of the bacterial load and foreign material by abdominal lavage.
- Abdominal drainage (when indicated).
- Placement of a route for postoperative nutritional support.

Surgical technique

1. A ventral midline celiotomy approach is made (see Chapter 3).
   - Surgical swabs must be counted before and after the procedure, prior to abdominal closure.
   - The use of a surgical suction device with a Poole suction tip is required.
   - A sample of free peritoneal fluid and/or tissue coming from the infection source should be collected and submitted for aerobic and anaerobic bacterial culture and antimicrobial susceptibility testing.
2. The entire peritoneal cavity should be carefully explored in search of any source of infection.
   - All the intra-abdominal organs (GI and urogenital tracts, liver, gallbladder, pancreas, and abdominal lymph nodes) must be inspected and palpated.
   - In many cases, the omentum is adherent to the site of infection.
3. Once the source of infection has been identified, it is isolated with laparotomy swabs.

4. The most appropriate surgical treatment is performed, depending on the underlying infection source.
   - It should be taken into account that initial surgical plans can change depending on the intraoperative findings, and owners should be aware that they may need to be contacted during the procedure.
   - Leakage from the intestine is treated by enterectomy and omental wrapping or serosal patching (see Chapter 11).
   - Pancreatic and liver abscesses are treated accordingly (see Chapters 12 and 14).
   - Ruptured pyometra and prostatic abscess are treated by ovariohysterectomy and debridement and omentalization, respectively (see Chapter 20).
   - Splenic abscess is treated by splenectomy (see Chapter 12).
5. All resected tissue involved in the infection source should be submitted for histopathological examination.
6. Once the source of infection has been eliminated or corrected, abdominal lavage is performed with a warm (37°C–39°C) isotonic crystalloid solution (0.9% NaCl or lactated Ringer's). An initial minimum volume of 200–300 mL/kg of fluid is used or, alternatively, the amount of fluid necessary to obtain returning clear fluid. The effectiveness of lavage, the amount of fluid to use, and the ideal lavage solution are controversial.
7. Abdominal drainage should be considered if there is residual contamination or ongoing infection.
8. Surgical gloves and instrumentation should be changed for final abdominal lavage and abdominal closure. Surgical swabs should be counted before closure.
9. A nutritional support route may be placed under the same anesthetic episode. The authors' preferred route is an esophagostomy tube (see Chapter 5). However, safe use of gastrostomy tubes in cases of septic peritonitis has also been reported.[14]

Abdominal drainage

Postoperative retrieval of free abdominal fluid from persistent effusion or residual fluid lavage is beneficial to enhance the peritoneal defense mechanisms, improve the absorption of bacteria and endotoxins, and reduce intra-abdominal pressure. However, case selection is crucial due to the risk of ascending nosocomial infection and further protein and fluid loss. Abdominal closure without drainage is indicated in cases where definitive control of the infection source has been achieved with minimal or localized peritonitis. Abdominal drainage is indicated in cases of severe and generalized peritonitis, cases in which the infection source could not be controlled at first laparotomy, and if postoperative intensive care is available.

Different techniques of abdominal drainage have been described:

- open peritoneal drainage
- vacuum-assisted closure (VAC) drainage
- closed-suction abdominal drainage

Open peritoneal drainage consists of leaving a gap of 2–6 cm (depending on patient size) between the edges of the linea alba that has been partially closed with nonabsorbable suture in a loose simple continuous pattern. Alternatively, only the cranial-dependent portion of the abdomen is left open as described, whilst the caudal portion of the linea alba is closed routinely. In both scenarios the subcutaneous tissue and the skin are left open. A sterile absorbing bandage is applied and changed regularly with the animal sedated or anesthetized. Abdominal lavage could be performed daily with sterile saline before rebandaging. In dogs with septic peritonitis treated by this technique, the reported mortality rate is 48%.[15] The abdomen is normally closed within 3–5 days.

The vacuum-assisted drainage technique involves the use of a VAC device (Fig. 16.2; Video 16.1). The abdomen is left partially open, and a permeable layer is placed over the incision and covered with a polyurethane sponge followed by the VAC device. A recent study comparing open and VAC drainage showed no difference in survival or postoperative complications. However, vacuum-assisted drainage improved the local healing response on biopsy of abdominal tissue and eliminated the need for frequent bandage changes.[16] The VAC device is typically removed and the abdomen closed within 2–4 days.

The closed-suction abdominal drainage technique involves placing a fenestrated silicone drain inside the abdominal cavity connected by a nonfenestrated tube to an external suction reservoir (e.g., Jackson–Pratt drain). In dogs with septic peritonitis treated by this technique, the reported survival rate is 85%.[17] This is the authors' preferred technique of abdominal drainage. Compared to the other techniques described above, it demands less postoperative intensive care, the amount of fluid can be easily quantified and examined by cytological and biochemical analysis, there is no need for a second surgery to close the abdomen, and there is

Video 16.1. Negative-pressure system used for drainage in a dog diagnosed with septic peritonitis due to enteric wound dehiscence. Video courtesy of Matteo Rossanese.

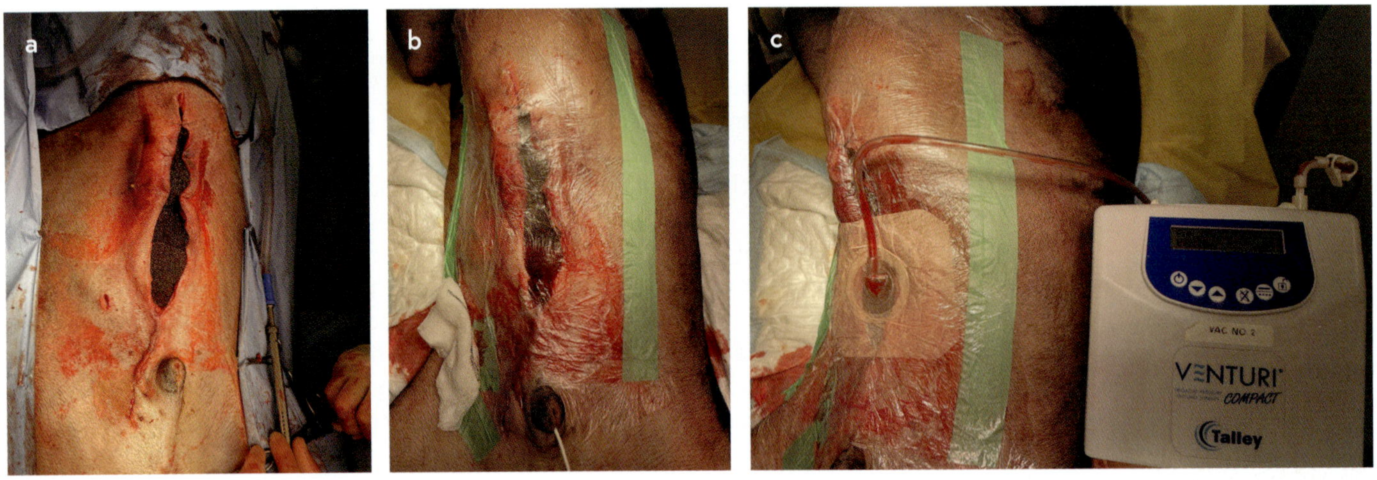

Figure 16.2 Vacuum-assisted drainage technique used in a dog diagnosed with septic peritonitis due to enteric wound dehiscence. (a) The abdominal organs were covered with omentum, the abdomen was left partially open, and a sterile foam was placed over the site. (b) The abdomen was sealed with an adhesive drape. (c) A negative-pressure system was maintained at –125 mmHg for the following 48 hours, before abdominal closure. Images courtesy of Matteo Rossanese.

a decreased risk of nosocomial bacterial infection and evisceration. The drain is left in place for 2–4 days and is generally removed with the animal awake.[17] Criteria for drain removal in patients with septic peritonitis managed with closed-suction drains is largely based on clinical judgement. Generally, the amount of fluid produced reduces progressively until a plateau is reached. It is worth remembering that normal fluid production in a body cavity with a drain in place can be up to 2 mL/kg/day. The macroscopic appearance of the drained fluid also changes over time, passing from turbid/serohemorrhagic to clear/serous. The predominant cells within the drained fluid remain neutrophils throughout abdominal drainage. However, the numbers of degenerate neutrophils and intracellular bacteria should decrease with time.
Hypoproteinemia (90% of cases), anemia (85% of cases), nosocomial infection, and edema (55% of cases) are the most common postoperative complications associated with these techniques.

Technique: Closed-suction abdominal drain placement (Fig. 16.3)

1. The Jackson–Pratt drain should be placed just before abdominal closure. The fenestrated part of the drain is placed between the diaphragm and the liver in the most dependent portion of the abdominal cavity.
2. A small paramedian skin incision is made, and a long, curved Rochester–Carmalt forceps is used to create a subcutaneous and muscular tunnel until reaching the peritoneum.
3. The extremity of the connecting tube is grasped and brought outside.
4. If the drain is provided with an introducer trocar, the trocar is inserted from inside (peritoneum) to outside (skin).
5. The connecting tube is secured to the skin with purse-string and finger-trap sutures.
6. Before connecting the nonfenestrated part to the "grenade" reservoir, a C-clamp may be placed.
7. The reservoir should be emptied every 4–6 hours until removal (see Chapter 5).
8. The drain can be removed pulling gently out the connecting tube with the animal either sedated or conscious.

Postoperative management

Intensive care is required for animals treated for septic peritonitis. Vital parameters (heart rate, respiratory rate, temperature, mucous membranes, direct/indirect blood pressure, pulse oximetry) should be recorded every hour. A multiparameter anesthesia monitor is helpful if available. To optimize postoperative care, central venous access, peripheral arterial access, and an indwelling urinary catheter may be placed. A central venous catheter is used to administer fluid, but also to measure central venous pressure and sample venous blood, as postoperative edema may make peripheral venous access challenging. An indwelling urinary catheter with a closed collection system is beneficial to reduce intra-abdominal pressure, facilitate nursing care, and monitor urine output, allowing accurate calculation of fluid balance.
Postoperative management of septic peritonitis includes intravenous fluid therapy, correction of electrolyte imbalances, monitoring and management of blood pressure, monitoring and management of hypoprotein-

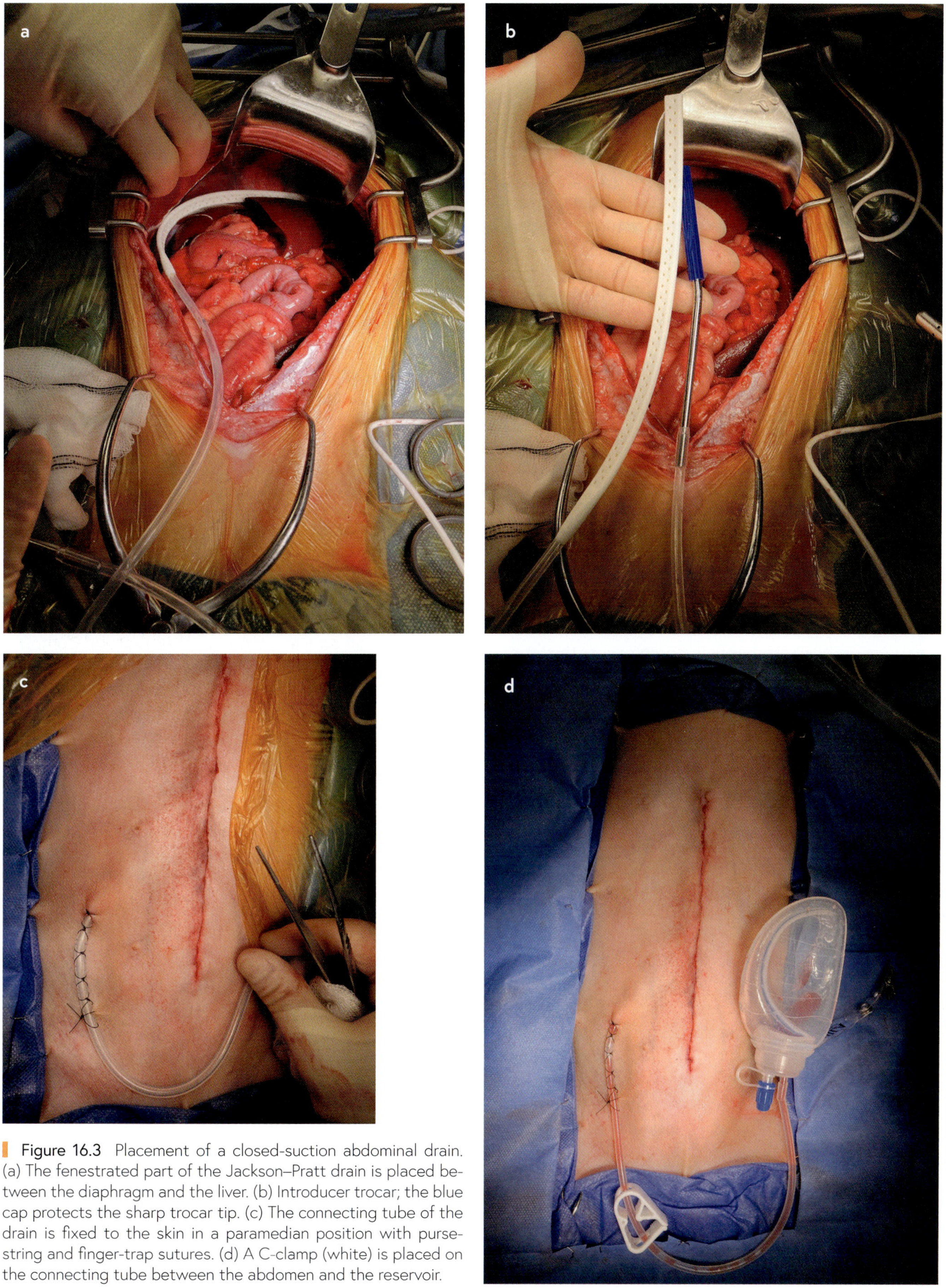

Figure 16.3 Placement of a closed-suction abdominal drain. (a) The fenestrated part of the Jackson–Pratt drain is placed between the diaphragm and the liver. (b) Introducer trocar; the blue cap protects the sharp trocar tip. (c) The connecting tube of the drain is fixed to the skin in a paramedian position with purse-string and finger-trap sutures. (d) A C-clamp (white) is placed on the connecting tube between the abdomen and the reservoir.

emia/hypoalbuminemia, nutritional support, analgesia, antibiotic therapy, and symptomatic treatment of GI clinical signs (e.g., antiemetics, prokinetics, antacids).
Body weight, blood pressure, and urine output are used to better calculate fluid therapy needs. Fluid replacement should also take into account the fluid drained from the abdomen, if drains are used, as well as ongoing losses (vomiting, diarrhea). Hypokalemia, hypoglycemia, hypocalcemia, and hypomagnesemia due to reduced nutrient intake and ongoing losses from vomiting or sepsis are common and should be monitored and corrected.
Intravenous fluid therapy alone may not be effective in maintaining adequate blood pressure. In these cases, vasopressors are indicated. Hypotension is defined as a systolic blood pressure below 100 mmHg and mean arterial blood pressure below 65 mmHg. The following are frequently used treatment targets to maintain:

- Mean arterial blood pressure ≥65 mmHg.
- Heart rate 80–140 bpm (dogs) or 180–220 bpm (cats).
- Good pulse quality.
- Capillary refill time 1–2 seconds.

Norepinephrine is the vasopressor of choice in cases of septic peritonitis. Generally, the lowest dose is started and is then titrated to effect. A second vasopressor (e.g., dobutamine) can be added if norepinephrine is not effective. Hypotension can be refractory to both fluid and vasopressor therapy; in some cases, this may be due to adrenal insufficiency (critical illness–related corticosteroid insufficiency), and low doses of dexamethasone (0.08 mg/kg) or hydrocortisone (1–2 mg/kg/day) can be used. Hypoproteinemia and hypoalbuminemia result in decreased plasma oncotic pressure, with life-threatening complications such as organ failure, coagulopathies, poor wound healing, and pulmonary edema. Synthetic colloids can be used in boluses of 5 mL/kg up to a maximum of 20 mL/kg (dog) or 15 mL/kg (cat). The administration of a large volume of plasma is required to increase albumin levels: 20 mL/kg of plasma is needed to increase serum albumin by 0.5 g/dL.[18] This is often cost prohibitive. Human serum albumin (25% diluted to 5%) has been successfully used in dogs with hypoalbuminemia and septic peritonitis.[19] However, dogs may develop acute adverse reactions to human serum albumin which can result in facial edema, fever, tachycardia, tachypnea, GI signs, acute death, and delayed type 3 hypersensitivity reactions. Administration of canine-specific albumin to dogs has been demonstrated to be effective in increasing serum albumin levels, which persisted for 24 hours. Moreover, adverse events were uncommonly observed.[20,21]
Nutritional support remains the most physiological way to provide proteins, energy, and other nutritional elements needed for recovery. Enteral nutrition is preferred over parenteral nutrition to maintain the integrity of the GI mucosa. Early (within 24 h from surgery) enteral feeding via a nasoesophageal/nasogastric, esophagostomy, or gastrostomy tube is encouraged, and it has been demonstrated that this reduces hospitalization times.[22]
Analgesic needs should be adapted to each case. Boluses or a constant-rate infusion of analgesic drugs can be administrated as required. Epidural analgesia is contraindicated in cases of sepsis and coagulopathy. Nonsteroidal anti-inflammatory drugs are not advised.
The choice of antibiotics should be based on bacterial culture and susceptibility testing results. However, an empirical broad-spectrum antibiotic should be started without delay as soon as the diagnosis is suspected or confirmed and appropriate samples have been obtained. A combination of antibiotics covering both aerobic and anaerobic bacteria should be considered. Metronidazole or ampicillin–sulbactam can be used for anaerobic bacteria in combination with a fluoroquinolone. A third-generation cephalosporin can be effective alone. Antibiotics should be continued for 2–4 weeks.

Outcome

The prognosis of animals treated for septic peritonitis varies greatly depending on the underlying cause, microbial pathogens involved in the infectious process, treatment, and species, among other factors. Comparison of treatments and techniques used is not possible. The survival rate for animals with primary peritonitis (excluding feline infectious peritonitis) is 40%–44%.[3] The overall survival rate for both dogs and cats with secondary peritonitis varies from 44% to 71%. The survival rate for dogs having recurrent peritonitis is 43.9%.[2] Development of respiratory disease, refractory hypotension, disseminated intravascular coagulation, and an admission plasma lactate concentration above 4 mmol/L are associated with a mortality of 73%, whilst the inability to normalize plasma lactate levels within 6 hours of admission has a 79% sensitivity and 100% specificity for nonsurvival.[23]

Bile peritonitis

Bile peritonitis is the result of direct contact of the peritoneum with bile. Bile salts, unconjugated bile acids, and other bile contents are cytotoxic, causing inflammation, hemolysis, changes in vascular permeability, and necrosis of vascular structures.[24–26] Leakage of sterile bile is normally responsible for chemical peritonitis. However, bile peritonitis can become septic due to altered peritoneal permeability allowing transmural migration of enteric organisms into the abdominal cavity and the bloodstream,[26] ascending GI contamination, or colonization by resident hepatic anaerobes.

Common causes of bile leakage are gallbladder disease, trauma, extrahepatic biliary obstruction, and complications of biliary surgery. Perforation of the duodenum or pylorus can also result in leakage of bile into the abdomen. The most common gallbladder diseases leading to rupture and leakage of bile are gallbladder mucocele and necrotizing cholecystitis.[24,27–29] Because of the poor vascularization of the gallbladder fundus, rupture usually occurs in this location. Blunt and penetrating trauma can cause rupture of the gallbladder or biliary ducts, and consequently bile leakage and peritonitis, in both dogs and cats.[30,31] Road traffic accidents, falls from a height, and, less commonly, gunshot injuries are causes of traumatic bile peritonitis.[30–32] The common bile duct is most commonly involved, but injuries (tear or avulsion) can also affect the cystic duct, hepatic ducts, or gallbladder.[28–33] The kinetic energy transferred from the blunt trauma to the body leads to a rapid cranial movement of the liver relative to the duodenum, causing avulsion of the common bile duct.[31]

Clinical presentation and diagnosis

In cases of blunt or penetrating trauma, clinical signs of bile peritonitis can develop a week or later after the initial trauma. The most common clinical signs associated with gallbladder disease or extrahepatic biliary obstruction include vomiting, diarrhea, weight loss, icterus, fever, and abdominal pain. However, acute signs of septic shock may be present in patients with septic bile peritonitis.

The diagnosis of bile peritonitis is based on the evaluation of free peritoneal fluid (Fig. 16.4). Cytological findings of bilious peritoneal effusion include increased number of macrophages and neutrophils and potential presence of bile pigments.[34] The absence of bile pigments in the fluid does not rule out bile peritonitis. A bilirubin concentration in the effusion at least two times higher than that in the serum is strongly supportive of bile peritonitis.[28] Intracellular bacteria may be seen in case of septic bile peritonitis, and this worsens the overall prognosis.

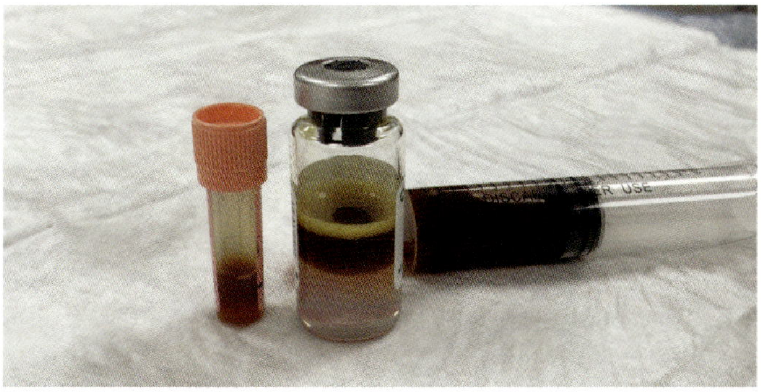

Figure 16.4 Bilious peritoneal effusion collected for cytology and bacteriology analysis.

Hematology, serum biochemistry, blood gas analysis, and urinalysis are recommended in case of suspected bile peritonitis. The findings are generally not specific, but they can help in the diagnosis of gallbladder disease and extrahepatic biliary obstruction. They include marked elevations in alkaline phosphatase, serum bilirubin, gamma-glutamyltransferase, alanine transferase, and mild to severe leukocytosis. An elevated concentration of serum lactate is expected in cases of biliary peritonitis, due to splanchnic ischemia, septic shock, and decreased lactate clearance by the liver.

Abdominal radiographic findings can be consistent with abdominal effusion (focal or diffuse loss of detail, ground-glass appearance, depending on the amount of free peritoneal fluid). In approximately 50% of dogs and up to 80% of cats, choleliths can be detected on plain radiographs.[28,35] Emphysematous cholecystitis can be suspected based on the presence of gas within the gallbladder.

Abdominal ultrasound is the most useful diagnostic imaging modality to investigate peritonitis and to evaluate the gallbladder and intra- and extrahepatic biliary tree. This technique has limited sensitivity but high specificity for gallbladder mucocele rupture.[36] Loss of gallbladder wall continuity, free fluid around the gallbladder, hyperechoic fat around the gallbladder wall, or striated echogenic material found outside the gallbladder are consistent with rupture of a gallbladder mucocele. Contrast-enhanced ultrasonography and CT have showed high sensitivity and specificity for detecting gallbladder mucocele rupture.[37,38]

Figure 16.7 shows an algorithm for the investigation and treatment of peritonitis.

Treatment

Treatment for biliary peritonitis includes exploratory laparotomy, resolution of the underlying cause, reestablishment of bile flow, removal of necrotic and infected tissue, and placement of a route for postoperative nutritional support. As for septic peritonitis, preoperative patient stabilization is crucial in the management of this surgical emergency.

Surgical technique

1. A ventral midline celiotomy approach is made (see Chapter 3). Surgical swabs must be counted before and after the procedure, prior to closure.
2. The cranial abdominal cavity should be carefully explored (Fig. 16.5). Generally, the omentum is adherent to the gallbladder and hepatic hilum.
3. Placing two stay sutures on the pyloric antrum and body of the stomach and applying traction caudally can help gain exposure to the gallbladder and extrahepatic biliary system.

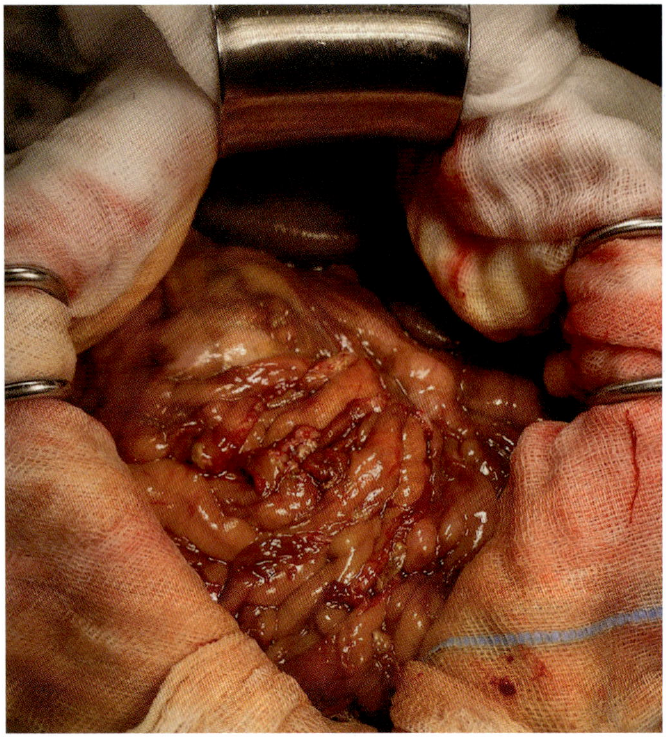

Figure 16.5 Bilious discoloration of the omentum and the serosal aspect of the abdominal organs of a dog with sterile bile peritonitis.

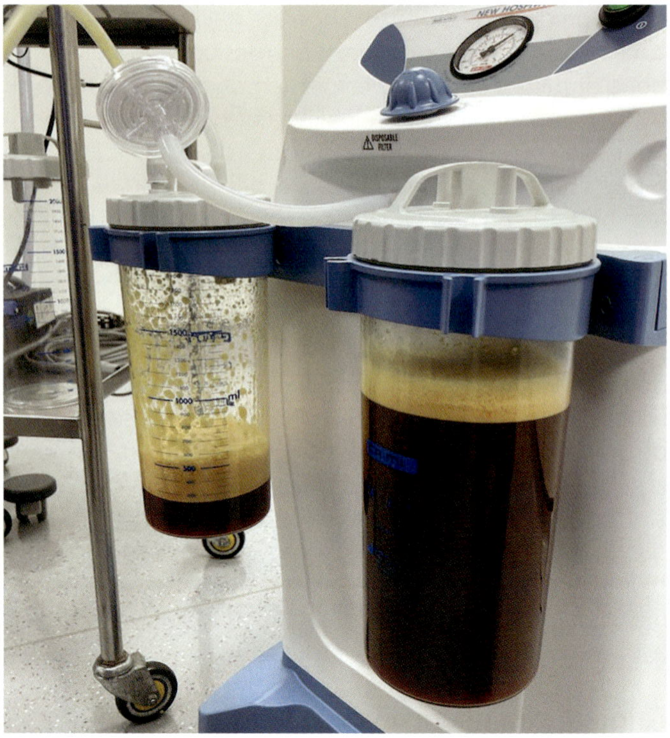

Figure 16.6 Bilious peritoneal effusion aspirated after abdominal approach.

4. The most appropriate surgical treatment is performed, depending on the underlying cause.
   - Gallbladder diseases are treated by cholecystectomy (see Chapter 13).
   - Cholelithiasis and choledocholithiasis are treated accordingly (see Chapter 13).
   - Cholecystectomy is performed in case of gallbladder rupture or avulsion of the gallbladder from the cystic duct.
   - Traumatic injuries to the hepatic ducts are treated by ligation on either side of the tear. The bile will be redirected through collateral ducts.
   - Traumatic longitudinal tears of the common bile duct can be primarily closed or ligated proximally to the tear and a cholecystoenterostomy performed (see Chapter 13).
   - Traumatic avulsions of the common bile duct from the duodenum are treated by cholecystoenterostomy.
5. All tissue removed should be submitted for histopathological and bacteriologic examination. Once the bile flow has been reestablished and the necrotic and infected tissue removed, abdominal lavage is performed (see above).
6. Abdominal drainage should be considered in patients with generalized bile peritonitis (Fig. 16.6) (see above).
7. Surgical gloves and instrumentation should be changed for final abdominal lavage and abdominal closure.
8. A nutritional support route is placed under the same anesthetic episode.

Postoperative management

Postoperative management of animals treated for bile peritonitis includes intravenous fluid therapy, correction of electrolyte imbalances, monitoring and management of blood pressure, monitoring and management of hypoproteinemia/hypoalbuminemia, nutritional support, analgesia, antibiotic therapy, and symptomatic treatment of GI clinical signs (e.g., antiemetics, prokinetics, antacids) (see above).

Outcome

Many variables, comorbidities and the septic status can affect the prognosis of bile peritonitis, and comparisons between different studies are challenging. The survival rate for dogs with septic bile peritonitis is between 4% and 23%, whereas survival rates of 87%–100% have been reported in sterile bile peritonitis.[27,28]

An increased level of serum lactate in dogs undergoing cholecystectomy has been associated with up to a 30% increase in mortality.[39] Other negative prognostic factors for cholecystectomy include elevated preoperative creatinine levels, postoperative hypotension, and prolonged prothrombin time.

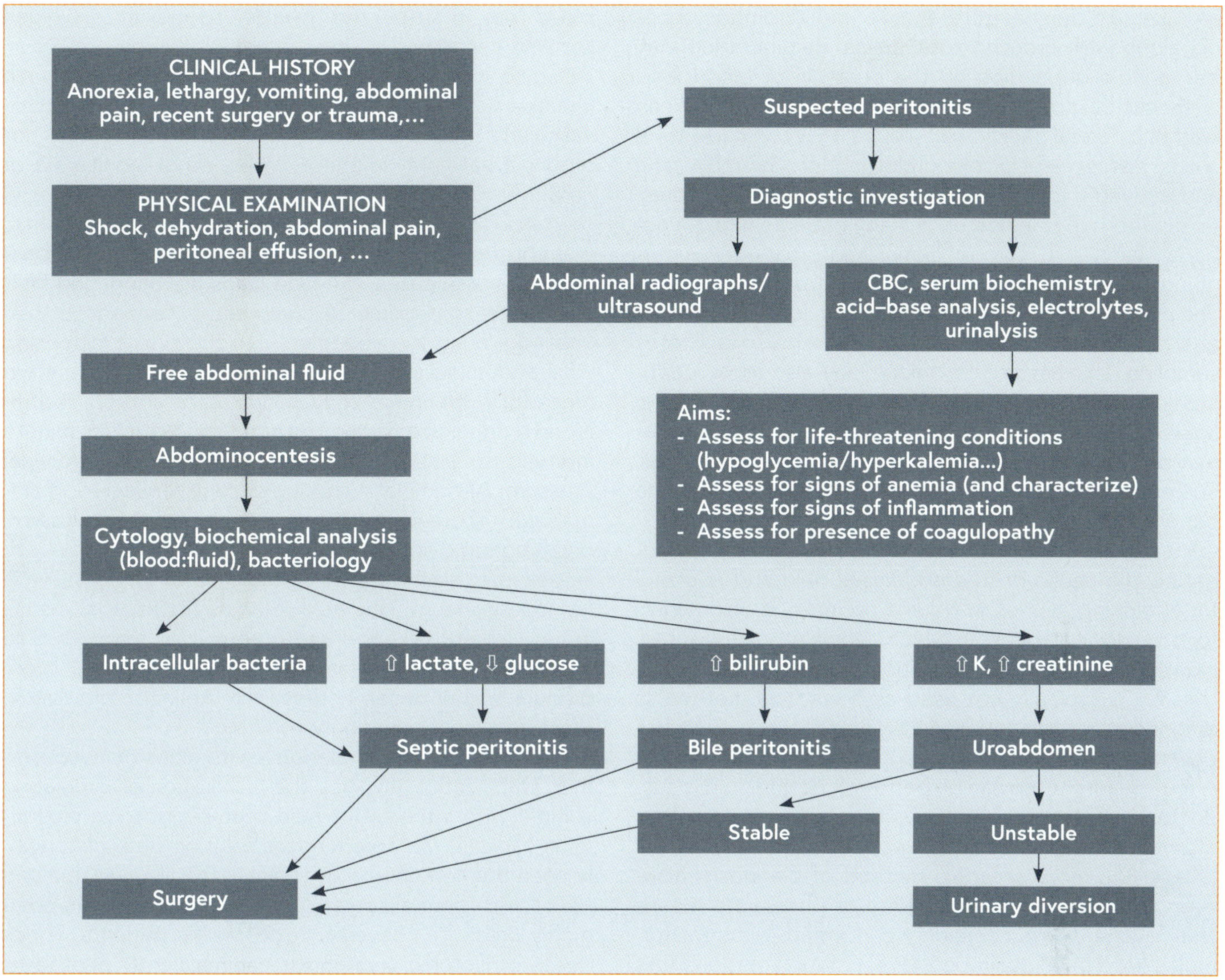

Figure 16.7 Algorithm for the investigation and treatment of peritonitis.

Hemoperitoneum

Hemoperitoneum, or hemoabdomen, is a common emergency presentation in dogs and may rapidly lead to life-threatening consequences. Malignant neoplasia is the most frequent etiology.[41] Hemangiosarcoma is the most commonly reported malignancy resulting in hemoabdomen, although numerous others have also been described.[42–46] However, preoperative diagnosis of malignancy continues to prove challenging in many cases.

Other causes of hemoperitoneum include blunt trauma, penetrating injuries, splenic torsion, liver lobe torsion, coagulopathies, peliosis hepatis, and iatrogenic causes.[42] In traumatic hemoperitoneum, splenic injury is the most common source of hemorrhage; however, laceration of the liver, kidneys, or vessels are also possible.[46]

Hemoperitoneum in cats is rare, but neoplasia is also usually implicated.[45]

Clinical presentation and diagnosis

Clinical signs of hemoperitoneum are predictable (albeit variable in severity), consistent with chronic or acute blood loss. Minor hemorrhage may result in minimal signs; however, anorexia, lethargy, collapse, pale mucous membranes, tachycardia, tachypnea, poor peripheral pulses, and cold extremities are seen with more severe blood loss. In addition, abdominal distension and periumbilical body wall bruising (Cullen's sign) may also be noted. A fluid thrill may be appreciated on abdominal ballottement.

Clinicopathological changes in patients with hemoperitoneum may be nonspecific depending on the amount and chronicity of blood loss. In animals with acute hemorrhage, serum biochemistry and hematology may initially be normal, although lactate levels may be elevated if significant hypovolemia is present. More chronic cases are likely to demonstrate anemia and thrombocytopenia along with reduced total solids. Regeneration may be variable depending on the duration of blood loss. It should be noted that initial splenic contraction can lead to a normal packed cell volume (PCV) with low total solids. Assessment of blood clotting (prothrombin time and activated partial thromboplastin time or viscoelastic monitoring) is indicated in many patients with hemoperitoneum (e.g., chronic hemorrhage, patients undergoing surgery, suspected rodenticide toxicity).

The presence of free abdominal fluid is confirmed preferably by abdominal ultrasonography, which also facilitates sampling. This imaging technique may also allow identification of the source of hemorrhage (e.g., mass lesions, splenic torsion). Radiography is relatively insensitive but may demonstrate loss of serosal detail and mass lesions. Survey radiographs are frequently indicated in trauma patients for documentation of concurrent injuries.

CT is an excellent method for detecting and investigating the cause of free abdominal fluid and is useful for assessing injuries in trauma patients. It also allows for staging of patients in which neoplasia is suspected. However, the need for sedation or anesthesia means that CT is typically not used as a first-line method of diagnosis, but it is rather delayed until the patient has been sufficiently stabilized.

A four-quadrant tap can be performed if free fluid is suspected but ultrasound is unavailable to assist sampling, although this may have a lower sensitivity. Peritoneal lavage is a more sensitive method of diagnosis; however, the widespread availability of ultrasound means that lavage is less commonly performed. Different formulas have been described for estimation of blood loss following peritoneal lavage; alternatively, a peritoneal lavage fluid PCV above 2%–5% is highly suggestive of intra-abdominal hemorrhage.[47]

Diagnosis of hemoperitoneum is confirmed by the identification of free blood within the abdominal cavity. This blood does not clot due to contact with the peritoneum. Blood which clots is therefore suggestive of inadvertent aspiration of a vascular organ such as the spleen or a blood vessel during sampling. The PCV of the fluid should be measured and compared with that of peripheral blood to confirm the diagnosis of hemoperitoneum. Fluid with a PCV above 5% will have a grossly hemorrhagic appearance. A yield of sanguineous fluid with a PCV of more than 25% of peripheral blood PCV and which does not clot is diagnostic for hemoperitoneum.

Treatment

The appropriate treatment is determined by the presenting status of the patient. Supplemental oxygen therapy is warranted in animals in which significant blood loss is suspected in order to maximize oxygen carrying capacity. This can be provided in several ways, including masks, nasal prongs or catheters, or oxygen chambers. Small volumes of hemoperitoneum in cardiovascularly stable patients (e.g., from trauma) may not require treatment. In these cases, serial monitoring of cardiovascular parameters and blood PCV is indicated to check for ongoing hemorrhage. Some patients may warrant the application of a compressive abdominal bandage. In these cases, the hind limbs are bandaged first, from distal to proximal. A compressive bandage is then applied around the abdomen with the aim of increasing intra-abdominal pressure. The bandage should be left in place for a maximum of 12 hours. Some authors recommend gradually removing the bandaging in 10–15-minute intervals to avoid sudden changes in intra-abdominal pressure. Abdominal wrapping is contraindicated in animals with thoracic compromise, such as pleural effusion, diaphragmatic hernia, or pulmonary contusions.[48]

Tranexamic acid may be beneficial for patients with hemoperitoneum. This acid reduces fibrinolysis, resulting in clot stabilization and greater clot strength. The recommended dosage is 10–20 mg/kg IV or PO every 8 hours; higher doses increase the likelihood of adverse reactions, most commonly vomiting.[49]

In unstable animals presenting with signs of hypovolemia, stabilization involves the restoration of circulating volume with intravenous fluid therapy. Isotonic crystalloids, typically lactated Ringer's solution, have historically been the first choice, as they are readily available and assist with normalization of the acidemia that is commonly present in severely hypovolemic patients. Shock doses of isotonic crystalloids are frequently quoted as 90 mL/kg in the dog and 60 mL/kg in the cat, but a more appropriate method may be to administer a 10 mL/kg bolus over 10–15 minutes followed by reassessment of cardiovascular parameters, with further boluses administered according to the desired effect. However, isotonic crystalloids rapidly move into the intracellular space, resulting in a short-term beneficial effect only and may contribute to tissue edema. Furthermore, aggressive (large-volume or normotensive) resuscitation may also cause dilution of coagulation factors and dislodgement of clots, exacerbating bleeding.[50] Colloid therapy theoretically helps improve the duration of volume resuscitation and the volume of fluids required, but their use is currently controversial. Potential side effects of colloids include coagulopathy, anaphylaxis, and acute renal injury; their use in critically ill humans is now considered contraindicated.[51] Hypertonic saline administration has been recommended, which reduces the need for large volumes of isotonic crystalloids by drawing fluid from the extravascular space; it is also reported to have immunomodulatory and anti-inflammatory effects.

However, appropriate isotonic crystalloid fluid therapy is required following administration to restore normal fluid balance to the intra- and extracellular space. Hypotensive or low-volume resuscitation aims to keep a mean blood pressure of 60–70 mmHg, with the rationale of maintaining perfusion of vital organs whilst reducing the detrimental effects of large-volume fluid therapy. Once definitive treatment has been carried out to resolve the source of hemorrhage, further resuscitation can be performed to normalize blood pressure. Early directed goals have been recommended in the treatment of hemorrhagic shock (Box 16.1).

Box 16.1. Suggested early directed goals for resuscitation of dogs and cats with hypovolemic shock

- Heart rate: 80–140 bpm (dog), 180–220 bpm (cat)
- Mucous membranes: Pink, capillary refill time 1–2 s
- Mean arterial blood pressure: 60–80 mmHg
- Systolic arterial pressure: 90–100 mmHg
- Peripheral oxygen saturation (SpO_2): >94%
- Partial pressure of oxygen in arterial blood (PaO_2): >80 mmHg
- Lactate: <2.5 mmol/L (monitor trend)
- Urine output: >1 mL/kg/h
- Packed cell volume: >25%

Blood transfusion may be indicated in patients with severe blood loss. Precise guidelines for when to transfuse are not available, but a PCV below 20% following resuscitation may be a prudent cutoff. Other guidelines include estimated blood loss of more than 20% of blood volume, persistent tachycardia, hypotension, and lethargy despite adequate volume resuscitation. The ideal transfusion product in case of acute hemorrhage is whole blood; however, this is rarely available. Packed red blood cells are readily available and are resuspended in isotonic saline prior to administration. Fresh frozen plasma can also be given to provide clotting factors and some degree of oncotic support in coagulopathic patients. Transfusion products should ideally be typed and crossmatched prior to administration to minimize the risk of reactions. Whilst this is not strictly required in the dog, provided previous transfusions have not been performed, it is always required in cats due to the presence of circulating alloantibodies. Autotransfusion can be useful in some patients undergoing surgery, particularly if allogenic transfusion is not available. Blood is aspirated directly into sterile syringes or, if available, cell-saver devices. If syringes are used, the blood should be filtered to minimize the potential for microthrombi delivery. Potential advantages of this option include lack of immune reactions and the relative ease with which this can be obtained in surgery. Possible complications of autotransfusion include microembolization, coagulopathy, sepsis, hemolysis, and/or electrolyte derangements. Autotransfusion in the presence of a ruptured neoplastic lesion is controversial due to the theoretical risk of tumor cell seeding. Leukocyte reduction filters, which may mitigate this risk, are commercially available.[52] Autotransfusion is contraindicated in patients with concurrent septic peritonitis.

Definitive treatment involves addressing the source of intra-abdominal bleeding. In patients with traumatic hemoperitoneum, a conservative approach is frequently successful.[46] Exploratory laparotomy is indicated if serial PCV measurements continue to decrease and if progressive signs of shock are noted. Exploration is also indicated for neoplastic causes of hemorrhage or when the cause of bleeding is associated with penetrating injury, diaphragmatic rupture, pneumoperitoneum, bile peritonitis, or septic peritonitis.

Surgical technique

1. A ventral midline celiotomy approach is made (Fig. 16.8). Making the abdominal incision from xiphoid to pubis is recommended if the source of hemorrhage is uncertain. This will allow for a more thorough exploration of the abdominal cavity.
2. Blood is suctioned from the abdomen to allow visualization of all structures. This can be performed with sterile syringes or a cell-saver device if autotransfusion is to be performed.
3. The abdominal wall is retracted to increase exposure.
4. If the hemorrhagic source is uncertain, a systematic exploratory laparotomy is performed. The spleen, liver, kidneys, and adrenal glands should be examined first because they are the most common

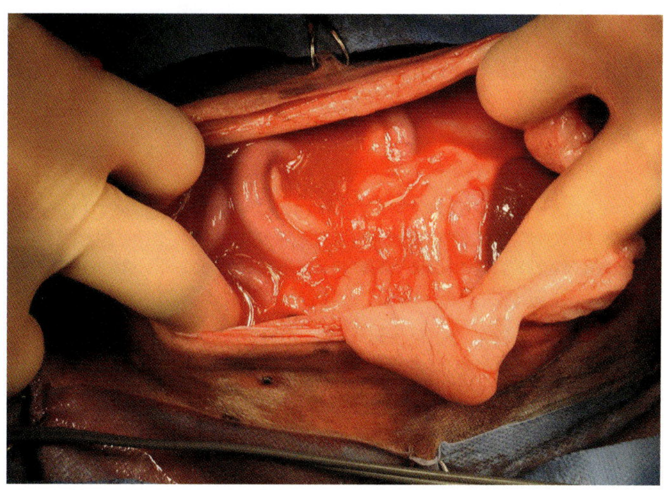

Figure 16.8 Ventral midline celiotomy approach showing intraperitoneal hemorrhage.

source of bleeding (Fig. 16.9). Localizing the source can be facilitated by packing the abdominal cavity with laparotomy pads once all the blood has been suctioned from the surgical field and removing them one by one whilst carefully assessing for bleeding.

5. Temporary hemostasis can be achieved by occlusion of the large abdominal vessels, if required (Table 16.1). This can be performed by use of atraumatic vascular clamps (e.g., Satinsky forceps, Cooley forceps), Rumel tourniquet, or digital occlusion.
    - The aorta can be occluded cranial to the cranial mesenteric artery (just craniomedial to the left adrenal gland).
    - The vena cava can be occluded permanently caudal to the renal veins,[53] while occlusion at the level of the adrenal glands is tolerated only for short periods of time.
    - The Pringle maneuver can be performed to slow bleeding from the liver. This involves carrying out a duodenal maneuver and then placing the index finger through the epiploic foramen along the ventral border of the caudal vena cava. The thumb is then used to compress all the vessels against the index finger. This does not completely prevent bleeding from the liver, as back bleeding can still occur via the hepatic veins. The Pringle maneuver can only be performed for short periods of time (10–20 min). Intermittent occlusion may help reduce the risk of reperfusion injury (Fig. 16.10).
6. The most appropriate surgical treatment is performed, depending on the source of hemorrhage:
    - Minor capsular laceration of organs can be managed by application of topical hemostatic agents or, potentially, by placement of small sutures within the organ capsule. If needed, topical hemostatic material can be used to form pledgets to reduce the likelihood of sutures tearing through.
    - Lacerations of the kidneys can be managed by performing a nephropexy to the body wall over the laceration or by wrapping the kidney in polyglactin mesh.
    - The most common source of spontaneous abdominal hemorrhage is splenic neoplasia and rupture. The spleen is exteriorized, if possible, and splenectomy is performed (see Chapter 12).
    - Neoplasia in other organs warrants removal of the affected organ or portion of the organ (see relevant chapter).

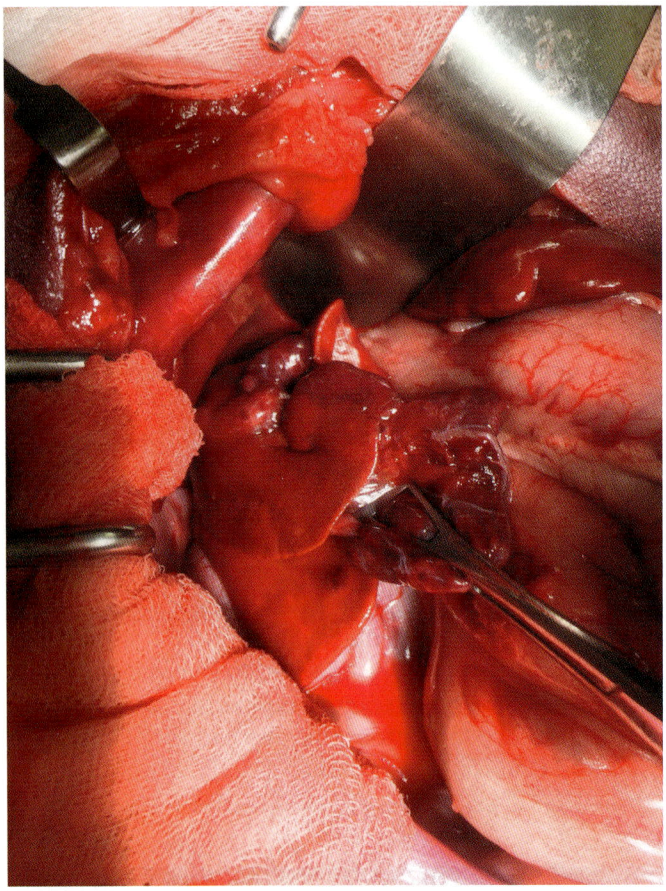

Figure 16.9 The source of hemorrhage from the previous figure was identified as a cavitated hepatic mass.

TABLE 16.1 - SUGGESTED TEMPORARY VESSEL OCCLUSION TIMES IN NORMOTHERMIC ANIMALS

Vessel	Suggested occlusion time (min)
Descending thoracic aorta	5–10
Abdominal aorta	30
Portal triad (Pringle maneuver), hepatic artery, portal vein, common bile duct	10–15
Hepatic artery	30
Splenic artery and vein	15–20
Renal artery and vein	30

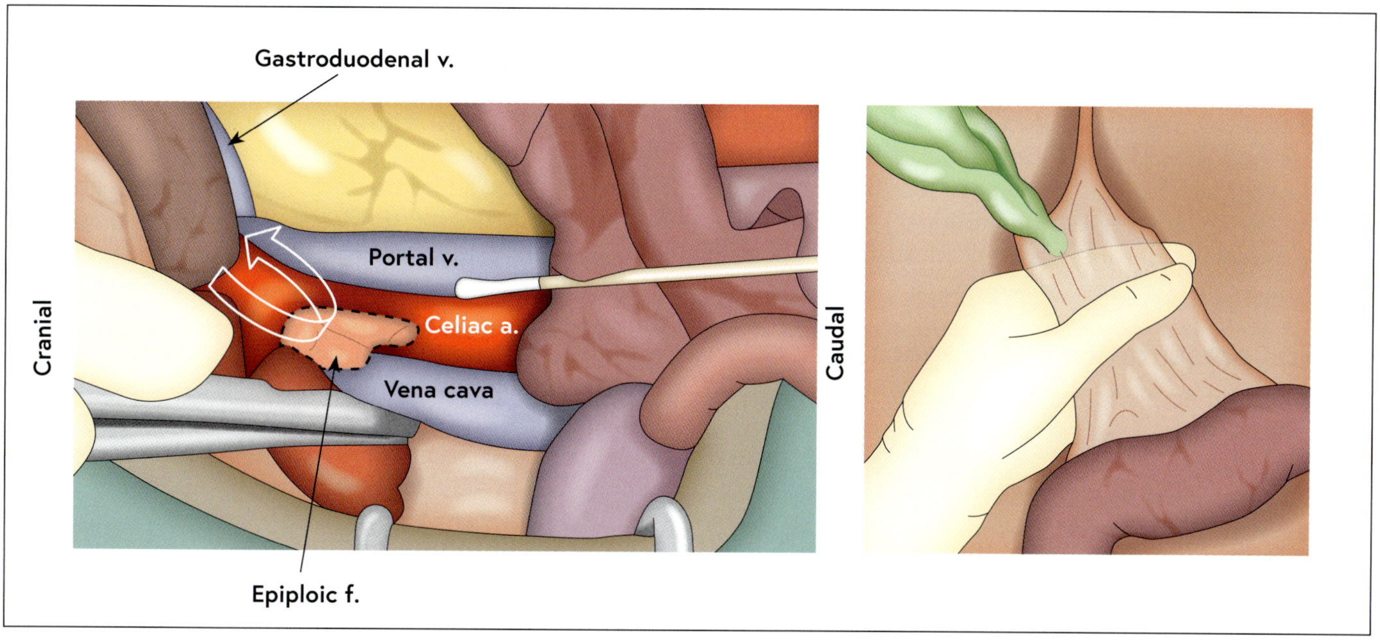

Figure 16.10 Pringle maneuver. More cranial finger placement (arrow) through the epiploic foramen prevents portal venous bleeding from the gastroduodenal vein.

Postoperative management

Postoperatively, patients should be checked for evidence of ongoing bleeding via serial monitoring of cardiovascular parameters and PCV. Any remaining fluid deficits should be corrected in the 12–24 hours following surgery. Some patients may benefit from monitoring of urine output to better assess fluid dynamics, allowing adjustment of inputs accordingly. Analgesia should be provided as needed, preferably adjusted based on pain scoring (e.g., modified Glasgow pain scoring index). Coagulopathic patients may benefit from further monitoring of coagulation status.

Outcome

Outcome depends on the inciting cause of hemoperitoneum. Spontaneous hemoperitoneum is more likely to have a malignant etiology (approximately 70%–75%, and most are splenic in origin).[54] Nevertheless, the short-term prognosis in these cases is good with appropriate management.[55] The long-term prognosis is ultimately dependent on final diagnosis, with hemangiosarcoma carrying a poor prognosis. Animals with benign causes of hemorrhage (e.g., trauma, splenic hematoma) are expected to have a good prognosis, provided that rapid cessation of bleeding can be achieved and appropriate support is given to maintain perfusion of vital organs. Histopathology is not 100% sensitive for malignant disease, with a recent study showing that 17% of patients with histopathologically benign splenic disease had an adverse outcome with premature death.[54] In contrast, dogs with bleeding liver tumors have been shown to have a more favorable prognosis, with over 60% being diagnosed with well-differentiated carcinoma or benign disease.[56] Protracted survival is therefore expected in these patients.

Pneumoperitoneum

Pneumoperitoneum (i.e., free gas within the peritoneal cavity) can arise from a variety of causes. In many spontaneous cases, this justifies immediate surgical exploration due to the potential of life-threatening pathology being present.

This condition can be classified as traumatic or spontaneous in origin. Pneumoperitoneum can remain for up to 34 days following surgery in dogs and, in isolation, does not require intervention. Nonsurgical trauma–induced pneumoperitoneum may be due to direct penetrating injuries, such as gunshot or bite wounds with injury to the GI tract, or secondary to blunt trauma. Blunt trauma may result in pneumothorax and air tracking into the abdomen, either via direct transfer across defects in the diaphragm or indirectly via the mediastinum through the crus or esophageal hiatus. Intestinal microperforations which subsequently seal have also been suggested as a potential route of air into the peritoneal cavity.[57] Other reported causes include endoscopy (biopsy, overdistension, perforation), gastrostomy tube placement, and positive-pressure ventilation.

Spontaneous pneumoperitoneum is typically associated with severe disease of abdominal viscera. Around 90% of cases result from perforation of the GI tract.[58,59]

This may be due to neoplasia, gastric dilatation and volvulus, intestinal ulceration, intestinal foreign bodies, drug induced, hepatic disease, uremia, inflammatory bowel disease, parasitic disease, polytrauma, hypotension, or endocrinopathies. Other abdominal diseases include ruptured splenic or hepatic abscesses, biliary tract disease,[39] and severe genitourinary tract disease (e.g., bladder or uterine rupture). Idiopathic pneumoperitoneum has also been reported.[60]

Clinical presentation and diagnosis

Initial presenting signs may be variable depending on the underlying disease process. They may, therefore, range from mild or absent signs to those of severe disease, such as lethargy, collapse, or signs of shock. Animals with pneumoperitoneum of traumatic etiology may present with numerous concurrent injuries. Similarly, clinical pathology findings are variable and reflect the inciting cause.

Abdominal radiography has been shown to have a sensitivity of 80% and accuracy of 85% for the diagnosis of pneumoperitoneum, although this was variable depending on experience.[61] In patients with small volumes of air, diagnosis may be challenging due to the superimposition of intraluminal gas within the GI tract.[58] In equivocal cases, horizontal-beam radiography may be helpful to highlight small volumes of gas. For this, the animal is placed in left lateral recumbency and horizontal-beam ventrodorsal projections are taken. However, standard left lateral projections may be as sensitive as horizontal-beam projections if evaluated by experienced radiologists (Fig. 16.11).[62] Horizontal-beam radiography with right lateral positioning may result in superimposition of the gastric fundus with the region of interest, resulting in the misinterpretation of fundic gas as free abdominal gas.[63] This projection is therefore not recommended. Other radiographic findings may relate to the underlying pathology, such as loss of serosal detail, intestinal foreign bodies, intestinal distension, or mass lesions.

Ultrasonography has also been shown to be a relatively sensitive method of detecting a volume of free abdominal gas above 0.2 mL (83% sensitivity, 89% specificity) in healthy experimental dogs.[64] The presence of free gas results in acoustic shadowing or an enhanced peritoneal stripe sign. However, this may be less consistent in animals with concurrent intra-abdominal pathology,[65] and the ultrasonographer's experience is also likely to affect results.[61] Nevertheless, ultrasonography may be a useful tool for the assessment of intra-abdominal pathology which may underlie pneumoperitoneum.

CT is highly sensitive for the detection of pneumoperitoneum, allowing visualization of free gas without superimposition of other structures.[61,66] In a study comparing diagnostic imaging findings in animals with GI ulceration, CT showed a 93% sensitivity for the detection of GI perforation with identification of the site of ulceration, intramural gas, free abdominal gas, and peritoneal fluid.

Treatment

In some instances of traumatic pneumoperitoneum, surgical intervention may not be required.[57,67] In animals in which blunt force trauma has been identified as the inciting cause and in which no evidence of abdominal visceral injury can be identified on imaging, a conservative approach may be justifiable.

Patients with a large volume of free abdominal air may develop signs of tension pneumoperitoneum. In this situation, abdominal hypertension develops and leads to decreased venous return and abdominal compartment syndrome, resulting in decreased perfusion of intra-abdominal viscera. The signs of this syndrome

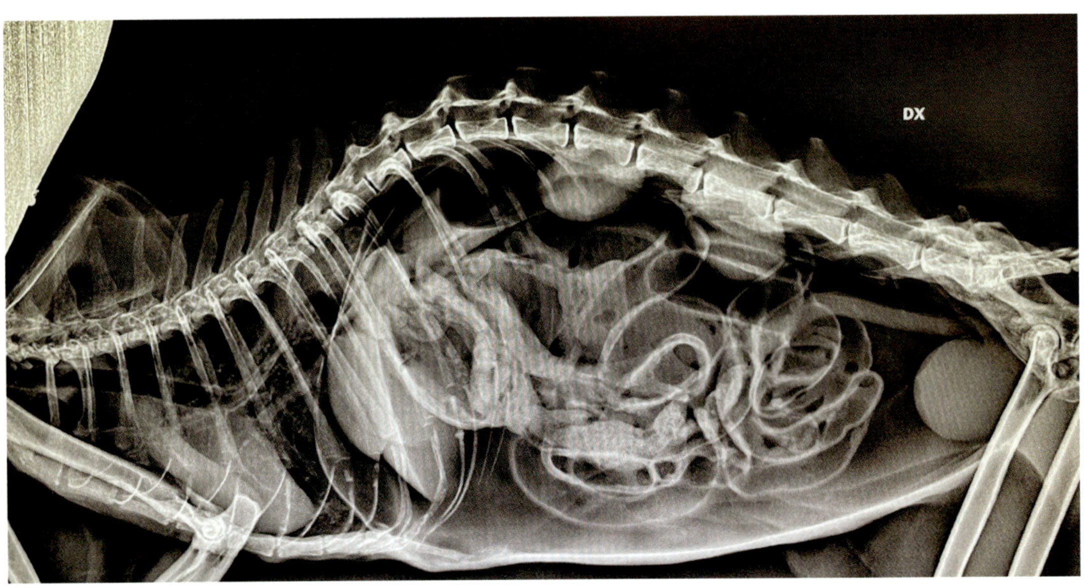

Figure 16.11 Radiograph of a 7-year-old cat with spontaneous pneumoperitoneum. Image courtesy of Filippo Cinti.

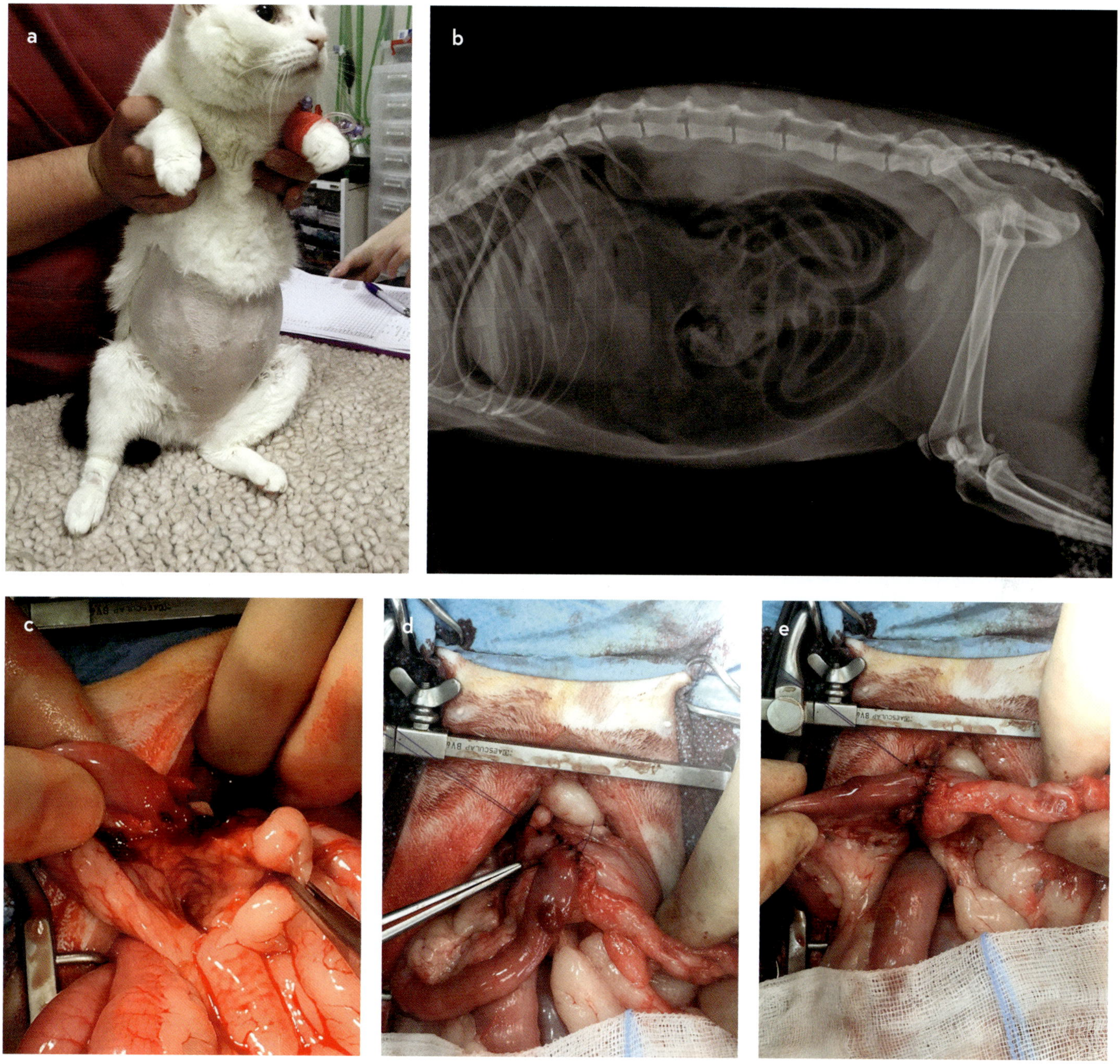

Figure 16.12 Traumatic pneumoperitoneum in a 5-year-old cat after gastrointestinal endoscopy and biopsy. (a) Clinical and (b) radiographic appearance showing abdominal distension. (c) Laceration and avulsion of the duodenum close to the pyloric area. (d,e) Surgical treatment with intestinal resection and anastomosis. Images courtesy of Filippo Cinti.

are similar to those of gastric dilatation and volvulus: progressive respiratory and cardiac compromise leading to severe shock. Treatment involves rapid needle decompression of the abdomen, which leads to immediate relief of clinical signs.

Most cases of spontaneous pneumoperitoneum warrant emergency exploratory laparotomy to identify and resolve the source of gas leakage. The reader is referred to the appropriate chapters on abdominal surgery for further details on specific case management (Fig. 16.12).

Outcome

Studies in which medical management was employed for spontaneous pneumoperitoneum have shown poor survival outcomes.[58,59] In contrast, surgically managed cases had much improved overall survival, with 65% of all causes of pneumoperitoneum surviving to discharge in one study[58] and 58% of spontaneous cases surviving to discharge in another.[59] Endoscopy-associated perforation and pneumoperitoneum carries a good prognosis.[65]

KEEP IN MIND

- Acute generalized secondary septic peritonitis is the most common form of peritonitis in small animal practice.
- Full-thickness perforation and leakage of bacteria from the gastrointestinal tract is the most common cause (60%–63%) of peritonitis in dogs and cats.
- Septic peritonitis is a surgical emergency that requires prompt abdominal exploration.
- Prognosis for septic peritonitis remains guarded and varies greatly depending on the underlying cause, microbial pathogens involved in the infectious process, treatment, and species, among other factors.
- A serum:effusion bilirubin concentration ratio above 2 is supportive of biliary peritonitis.
- The survival rate for dogs with septic bile peritonitis is 4%–23%, whereas survival rates of 87%–100% have been reported in case of sterile bile peritonitis.
- Hemoperitoneum is common dogs and is most frequently due to malignant neoplasia.
- Tranexamic acid administration may be beneficial in patients with hemoperitoneum.
- Spontaneous pneumoperitoneum is typically associated with severe disease of the gastrointestinal tract.
- CT imaging is the most sensitive tool for detection of peritoneal gas, and surgical exploration is justified in most cases of pneumoperitoneum.

References

1. Volk SW. Peritonitis. In: Silverstein DC, Hopper K (eds.). *Small Animal Critical Care Medicine*, 2nd ed. St. Louis, MO: Elsevier; 2015. pp. 643–648.
2. Barfield DM et al. Retrospective evaluation of recurrent secondary septic peritonitis in dogs (2000–2011): 41 cases. *J Vet Emerg Crit Care*. 2016; 26(2):281–287.
3. Culp WT, Zeldis TE, Reese MS, Drobatz KJ. Primary bacterial peritonitis in dogs and cats: 24 cases (1990–2006). *J Am Vet Med Assoc*. 2009; 234(7):906–913.
4. Laroche M, Harding G. Primary and secondary peritonitis: An update. *Eur J Clin Microbiol Infect Dis*. 1998; 17(8):542–550.
5. Ruthrauff CM, Smith J, Glerum L. Primary bacterial septic peritonitis in cats: 13 cases. *J Am Anim Hosp Assoc*. 2009; 45(6):268–276.
6. Hosgood G, Salisbury SK. Generalized peritonitis in dogs: 50 cases (1975–1986). *J Am Vet Med Assoc*. 1988; 193(11): 1448–1450.
7. Winkler KP, Greenfield CL. Potential prognostic indicators in diffuse peritonitis treated with open peritoneal drainage in the canine patient. *J Vet Emerg Crit Care*. 2000; 10:259–265.
8. Bentley AM, Mayhew PD, Culp WT, Otto CM. Alterations in the hemostatic profiles of dogs with naturally occurring septic peritonitis. *J Vet Emerg Crit Care*. 2013; 23(1):14–22.
9. Gilroy C, Raab O, Hanna P. Pathology in practice. *J Am Vet Med Assoc*. 2020; 257(2):161–164.
10. Costello MF, Drobatz KJ, Aronson LR, King LG. Underlying cause, pathophysiologic abnormalities, and response to treatment in cats with septic peritonitis: 51 cases (1990–2001). *J Am Vet Med Assoc*. 2004; 225(6):897–902.
11. Shanaman MM, Schwarz T, Gal A, O'Brien RT. Comparison between survey radiography, B-mode ultrasonography, contrast-enhanced ultrasonography and contrast-enhanced multi-detector computed tomography findings in dogs with acute abdominal signs. *Vet Radiol Ultrasound*. 2013; 54(6):591–604.
12. Bonczynski JJ et al. Comparison of peritoneal fluid and peripheral blood pH, bicarbonate, glucose, and lactate concentration as a diagnostic tool for septic peritonitis in dogs and cats. *Vet Surg*. 2003; 32(2):161–166.
13. Koenig A, Verlander LL. Usefulness of whole blood, plasma, peritoneal fluid, and peritoneal fluid supernatant glucose concentrations obtained by a veterinary point-of-care glucometer to identify septic peritonitis in dogs with peritoneal effusion. *J Am Vet Med Assoc*. 2015; 247(9):1027–1032.
14. Elmenhorst K, Pérez López P, Belch A, Demetriou JL. Retrospective study of complications associated with surgically-placed gastrostomy tubes in 43 dogs with septic peritonitis. *J Small Anim Pract*. 2020; 61(2):116–120.
15. Woolfson JM, Dulisch ML. Open abdominal drainage in the treatment of generalized peritonitis in 25 dogs and cats. *Vet Surg*. 1986; 15(1):27–32.
16. Spillebeen AL et al. Negative pressure therapy versus passive open abdominal drainage for the treatment of septic peritonitis in dogs: A randomized, prospective study. *Vet Surg*. 2017; 46(8):1086–1097.
17. Adams RJ, Doyle RS, Bray JP, Burton CA. Closed suction drainage for treatment of septic peritonitis of confirmed gastrointestinal origin in 20 dogs. *Vet Surg*. 2014; 43(7): 843–851.
18. Devey JJ. Crystalloid and colloid fluid therapy. In: Ettinger SJ, Feldman EC (eds.). *Textbook of Veterinary Internal Medicine*, 7th ed., vol. 1. St. Louis, MO: WB Saunders; 2010. pp. 487–496.
19. Horowitz FB, Read RL, Powell LL. A retrospective analysis of 25% human serum albumin supplementation in hypoalbuminemic dogs with septic peritonitis. *Can Vet J*. 2015; 56(6):591–597.
20. Craft EM, Powell LL. The use of canine-specific albumin in dogs with septic peritonitis. *J Vet Emerg Crit Care*. 2012; 22(6):631–639.
21. Sahagian MJ et al. Retrospective analysis of the use of canine-specific albumin in 125 critically ill dogs. *J Vet Emerg Crit Care*. 2023; 33(2):192–200.
22. Liu DT, Brown DC, Silverstein DC. Early nutritional support is associated with decreased length of hospitalization in dogs with septic peritonitis: A retrospective study of 45 cases (2000–2009). *J Vet Emerg Crit Care*. 2012; 22(4):453–459.
23. Cortellini S, Seth M, Kellett-Gregory LM. Plasma lactate concentrations in septic peritonitis: A retrospective study of 83 dogs (2007–2012). *J Vet Emerg Crit Care*. 2015; 25(3): 388–395.
24. Mayhew PD, Weisse C. Liver and biliary system. In: Tobias KM, Johnston SA (eds.). *Veterinary Surgery: Small Animal*. St. Louis, MO: Elsevier Saunders; 2012. pp. 1601–1623. eds 2. 2018. pp. 1828–1852.
25. Mehler SJ. Complications of the extrahepatic biliary surgery in companion animals. *Vet Clin North Am Small Anim Pract*. 2011; 41(5):949–967.

26. Center SA. Diseases of the gallbladder and biliary tree. *Vet Clin North Am Small Anim Pract.* 2009; 39(3):543–598.
27. Mehler SJ, Mayhew PD, Drobatz KJ, Holt DE. Variables associated with outcome in dogs undergoing extrahepatic biliary surgery: 60 cases (1988–2002). *Vet Surg.* 2004; 33(6):644–649.
28. Ludwig LL, McLoughlin MA, Graves TK, Crisp MS. Surgical treatment of bile peritonitis in 24 dogs and 2 cats: A retrospective study (1987–1994). *Vet Surg.* 1997; 26(2):90–98.
29. Church EM, Matthiesen DT. Surgical treatment of 23 dogs with necrotizing cholecystitis. *J Am Anim Hosp Assoc.* 1988; 24(3):305–310.
30. Murgia D. A case of combined bilothorax and bile peritonitis secondary to gunshot wounds in a cat. *J Feline Med Surg.* 2013; 15(6):513–516.
31. Parchman MB, Flanders JA. Extrahepatic biliary tract rupture: Evaluation of the relationship between the site of rupture and the cause of rupture in 15 dogs. *Cornell Vet.* 1990; 80(3):267–272.
32. Watkins PE, Pearson H, Denny HR. Traumatic rupture of the bile duct in the dog: A report of seven cases. *J Small Anim Pract.* 1983; 24:731–740.
33. Mehler SJ, Bennet RA. Canine extrahepatic biliary tract disease and surgery. *Compend Contin Educ Small Anim Vet.* 2006; 28:302–315.
34. Vörös K et al. Ultrasonography and surgery of canine biliary diseases. *Acta Vet Hung.* 2001; 49(2):141–154.
35. Kirpensteijn J et al. Cholelithiasis in dogs: 29 cases (1980–1990). *J Am Vet Med Assoc.* 1993; 202(7):1137–1142.
36. Eich CS, Ludwig LL. The surgical treatment of cholelithiasis in cats: A study of nine cases. *J Am Anim Hosp Assoc.* 2002; 38(3):290–296.
37. Jaffey JA et al. Gallbladder mucocele: Variables associated with outcome and the utility of ultrasonography to identify gallbladder rupture in 219 dogs (2007–2016). *J Vet Intern Med.* 2018; 32(1):195–200.
38. Bargellini P et al. Evaluation of contrast-enhanced ultrasonography as a method for detecting gallbladder necrosis or rupture in dogs. *Vet Radiol Ultrasound.* 2016; 57(6):611–620.
39. Cordella A et al. Multi-phase multidetector-row computed tomographic features and laboratory findings in dogs with gallbladder rupture. *Res Vet Sci.* 2022; 153:137–143.
40. Malek S et al. Clinical findings and prognostic factors for dogs undergoing cholecystectomy for gall bladder mucocele. *Vet Surg.* 2013; 42(4):418–426.
41. Aronsohn MG, Dubiel B, Roberts B, Powers BE. Prognosis for acute nontraumatic hemoperitoneum in the dog: A retrospective analysis of 60 cases (2003–2006). *J Am Anim Hosp Assoc.* 2009; 45(2):72–77.
42. Brockman DJ, Mongil CM, Aronson LR, Brown DC. A practical approach to hemoperitoneum in the dog and cat. *Vet Clin North Am Small Anim Pract.* 2000; 30(3):657–668.
43. Hammond TN, Pesillo-Crosby SA. Prevalence of hemangiosarcoma in anemic dogs with a splenic mass and hemoperitoneum requiring a transfusion: 71 cases (2003–2005). *J Am Vet Med Assoc.* 2008; 232(4):553–558.
44. Pintar J, Breitschwerdt EB, Hardie EM, Spaulding KA. Acute nontraumatic hemoabdomen in the dog: A retrospective analysis of 39 cases (1987–2001). *J Am Anim Hosp Assoc.* 2003; 39(6):518–522.
45. Culp WT et al. Spontaneous hemoperitoneum in cats: 65 cases (1994–2006). *J Am Vet Med Assoc.* 2010; 236(9):978–982.
46. Mongil CM, Drobatz KJ, Hendricks JC. Traumatic hemoperitoneum in 28 cases: A retrospective review. *J Am Anim Hosp Assoc.* 1995; 31(3):217–222.
47. Connally HE. Cytology and fluid analysis of the acute abdomen. *Clin Tech Small Anim Pract.* 2003; 18(1):39–44.
48. Pratschke K. Approach to haemoabdomen in small animal patients. *In Pract.* 2020; 42(1):5–19.
49. Kelmer E et al. Effects of intravenous administration of tranexamic acid on hematological, hemostatic, and thromboelastographic analytes in healthy adult dogs. *J Vet Emerg Crit Care.* 2015; 25(4):495–501.
50. Hammond TN, Holm JL, Sharp CR. A pilot comparison of limited versus large fluid volume resuscitation in canine spontaneous hemoperitoneum. *J Am Anim Hosp Assoc.* 2014; 50(3):159–166.
51. Cazzolli D, Prittie J. The crystalloid–colloid debate: Consequences of resuscitation fluid selection in veterinary critical care. *J Vet Emerg Crit Care.* 2015; 25(1):6–19.
52. Ciepluch BJ. The ability of a cell salvage system and leukocyte reduction filter to remove hemangiosarcoma cells from dog blood. Master's thesis, Texas A&M University, 2016. Available at https://hdl.handle.net/1969.1/156947.
53. Nesbit RM, Wear JB Jr. Ligation of the inferior vena cava above the renal veins. *Ann Surg.* 1961; 154(Suppl 6):332–344.
54. Millar SL, Curley TL, Monnet EL, Zersen KM. Premature death in dogs with nontraumatic hemoabdomen and splenectomy with benign histopathologic findings. *J Am Vet Med Assoc.* 2022; 260(S1):S9–S14.
55. Stewart SD, Ehrhart EJ, Davies R, Khanna C. Prospective observational study of dogs with splenic mass rupture suggests potentially lower risk of malignancy and more favourable perioperative outcomes. *Vet Comp Oncol.* 2020; 18(4):811–817.
56. Reist AM, Reagan JK, Fujita SK, Walny AM. Histopathologic findings and survival outcomes of dogs undergoing liver lobectomy as treatment for spontaneous hemoabdomen secondary to a ruptured liver mass: Retrospective analysis of 200 cases (2012–2020). *J Am Vet Med Assoc.* 2023; 261(2):237–245.
57. Philp HS, Hammond GJC. Nonsurgical management of traumatic pneumoperitoneum in a cat. *J Vet Emerg Crit Care.* 2018;28(6):591–595.
58. Saunders WB, Tobias KM. Pneumoperitoneum in dogs and cats: 39 cases (1983–2002). *J Am Vet Med Assoc.* 2003; 223(4):462–468.
59. Smelstoys JA et al. Outcome of and prognostic indicators for dogs and cats with pneumoperitoneum and no history of penetrating trauma: 54 cases (1988–2002). *J Am Vet Med Assoc.* 2004; 225(2):251–255.
60. Mehl ML et al. Idiopathic pneumoperitoneum in a dog. *J Am Anim Hosp Assoc.* 2001; 37(6):549–551.
61. Marwood R et al. Accuracy of radiographic diagnosis of pneumoperitoneum secondary to gastrointestinal perforation in dogs and cats. *Vet Rec.* 2022; 191(9):e2081.
62. Ng J et al. The left lateral projection is comparable to horizontal beam radiography for identifying experimental small volume pneumoperitoneum in the canine abdomen. *Vet Radiol Ultrasound.* 2020; 61(2):130–136.
63. Ferrell EA, Graham JP. Ultrasound corner—diagnosis of pneumoperitoneum. *Vet Radiol Ultrasound.* 2003; 44(3):307–308.
64. Kim SY, Park KT, Yeon SC, Lee HC. Accuracy of sonographic diagnosis of pneumoperitoneum using the enhanced peritoneal stripe sign in Beagle dogs. *J Vet Sci.* 2014; 15(2): 195–198.
65. Woolhead VL, Whittemore JC, Stewart SA. Multicenter retrospective evaluation of ileocecocolic perforations associated with diagnostic lower gastrointestinal endoscopy in dogs and cats. *J Vet Intern Med.* 2020; 34(2):684–690.
66. Fitzgerald E, Barfield D, Lee KC, Lamb CR. Clinical findings and results of diagnostic imaging in 82 dogs with gastrointestinal ulceration. *J Small Anim Pract.* 2017; 58(4):211–218.
67. Simmonds SL, Whelan MF, Basseches J. Nonsurgical pneumoperitoneum in a dog secondary to blunt force trauma to the chest. *J Vet Emerg Crit Care.* 2011; 21(5):552–557.

Chapter 17
Uroabdomen

Natalie Kovak, Christiana Fischer

Uroabdomen is defined as the collection of urine within the peritoneal and/or retroperitoneal space, and it results from rupture or leakage of any part of the urinary system. Uroperitoneum occurs due to rupture of the intra-abdominal urethra, bladder, and/or distal ureters. Uroretroperitoneum results from rupture of the proximal ureters or kidneys. The most common site of injury described in small animals is the bladder, followed by the proximal urethra, kidneys, and ureters.[1]

The predominant reported cause of uroabdomen in both dogs and cats is blunt force trauma secondary to vehicular trauma.[1,2] Other reported causes include pelvic fractures, urinary tract obstruction, neoplasia, penetrating trauma, and dehiscence following urinary surgery. A recent case report in a female dog indicated that obstipation and compressive urethral obstruction resulted in a uroabdomen.[3] Iatrogenic injury to the urethra during catheterization in an attempt to relieve a urethral obstruction has been a frequently reported cause of uroabdomen in male cats.[4] Additionally, decompressive cystocentesis to relieve bladder distension secondary to urethral obstruction may lead to leakage of urine into the abdomen.

Compared to females, male animals have a higher incidence of urinary tract rupture, which is likely attributable to their differences in urethral anatomy. Male urethras are narrower and fixed to surrounding bony structures, thus making them less adaptable to higher pressures and distension.[5] Regardless of cause, rapid diagnosis and treatment of uroabdomen is essential to reduce morbidity and mortality.

Clinical presentation

Patients may present with a wide variety of clinical signs depending on when the animal is evaluated. There may be a history of stranguria, hematuria, or recent trauma; however, evidence of urinary tract injury may not be clinically apparent early in presentation. Clinical signs may be vague, such as dehydration, vomiting, lethargy, and anorexia, or more severe in the face of metabolic derangements and any other injuries that may be present. Since trauma is the most common cause of uroabdomen in the veterinary patient,[2,6] it is important to perform a thorough physical examination as a means of accounting for all possible injuries and abnormalities. Physical examination findings may include signs of hypovolemic shock, tachyarrhythmias or bradyarrhythmias, abdominal pain, abdominal distension, and/or the presence of a fluid wave on abdominal palpation. Urine, which is hyperosmolar and rich in potassium, will draw extracellular fluid via osmotic forces as it accumulates in the peritoneal and/or retroperitoneal space. This third-spacing effect, combined with episodes of vomiting and decreased intake of fluids, leads to dehydration and possible signs of hypovolemic shock. A palpable urinary bladder does not rule out the possibility of uroperitoneum.[7] The presence of bruising and edema, specifically in the inguinal or perineal region, should raise concern for urinary tract rupture because extravasated urine into the subcutaneous tissue is extremely inflammatory. Additionally, concurrent pelvic fractures may be present in patients that have experienced trauma.

Initial patient stabilization

Initial evaluation should always include a full physical examination, with a focus on hemodynamic, respiratory, and cardiovascular stability. Patients presenting in circulatory shock should receive intravenous fluid resuscitation, with frequent reassessment of hemodynamic parameters including vital signs, pulse quality, capillary refill time, and blood pressure. A balanced isotonic crystalloid solution, such as lactated Ringer's solution or Normosol-R, should be administered as the first line for shock resuscitation with the goal to restore adequate perfusion.[8] Oxygen supplementation should also be provided if indicated. The patient's body surface should be assessed for external wounds, bruising, bleeding, or fractures of the pelvis, limbs, or ribs. These findings should raise suspicion for trauma and thus the potential for urinary tract injury. A focused assessment with sonography for trauma (FAST) should be performed to evaluate for peritoneal, pleural, or pericardial effusion. Visualization of the bladder on FAST does not rule out the possibility that a small, invisible rupture is present.[9] Alternatively, radiographs or ultrasound can be considered based on patient stability. If trauma to the thoracic cavity is also present, pneumothorax and/or pulmonary contusions should be ruled out. Depending on the timing and severity of the condition, peritoneal effusion may be accessible via abdominocentesis or peritoneal lavage for diagnostic purposes.

Full blood work including complete blood count, biochemistry, and electrolyte profiles should be evaluated. An emergency blood gas analysis may be sufficient for initial assessment and stabilization if hemodynamic compromise precludes drawing large volumes of blood. Laboratory findings may include leukocytosis characterized by neutrophilia (with or without left shift), hemoconcentration or anemia (secondary to hemorrhage), hyperkalemia, hyponatremia, hypochloremia, azotemia, hyperphosphatemia, and metabolic acidosis.[9] The presence of lactic acidosis on the blood gas panel may provide additional support of a compromised hemodynamic status.

Because the kidneys are responsible for excreting large amounts of potassium, free urine in the abdomen ultimately leads to hyperkalemia. Clinical manifestations of hyperkalemia may include generalized muscle weakness and cardiac arrhythmias. Thus, electrocardiographic assessment is warranted in all patients with suspected uroabdomen and may reveal the presence of cardiac arrhythmias including S–T segment depression, prolonged P–R intervals, widened QRS complexes, tall T waves, atrial standstill, ventricular fibrillation, or asystole. Initial treatment of arrhythmias should be aimed at cardioprotection and reduction of potassium concentration. Mild to moderate levels of hyperkalemia (>5.5 mmol/L, but <7.5 mmol/L) may not translate into electrocardiographic changes, and treatment with fluid therapy plus urinary diversion may be sufficient to reduce serum potassium levels.[1] Calcium gluconate administration acts to raise the threshold potential in cardiac myocytes, increasing the propagation of impulses in the sinoatrial and atrioventricular nodes, thus bringing the excitability of the cell back to normal. Additionally, drugs can be administered to promote intracellular flux of potassium. Regular insulin increases activity of the Na^+–K^+ ATPase pump, resulting in the movement of potassium intracellularly in exchange for sodium. Insulin should always be followed by administration of a 50% dextrose infusion to prevent hypoglycemia. Dextrose alone may be used, as it may stimulate endogenous insulin release. Similarly, terbutaline acts by stimulating beta-2 adrenergic receptors on cells, which also leads to increased activity of the Na^+–K^+ ATPase pump. An alternative to terbutaline administration is the use of nebulized albuterol. Finally, sodium bicarbonate administration increases blood pH, resulting in a shift of potassium from the extracellular space to the intracellular space in exchange for hydrogen ions.[2] This drug is considered a last-line therapy due to its possible deleterious side effects including paradoxical central nervous system acidosis and hyperosmolality. See Table 17.1 for common doses of the abovementioned emergency drugs. Ultimately, urinary diversion is necessary to prevent recurrence of hyperkalemia and provide definitive treatment for most patients.

Chemical peritonitis occurs from urine directly contacting the peritoneum, causing significant pain. Orthopedic or soft tissue injuries will also contribute to pain. Therefore, patients should be provided analgesia accordingly and serially monitored for adequate pain control. An appropriate first choice for analgesia is opioids, specifically pure μ-agonists, as these provide excellent pain relief and have minimal toxicity risks. Ketamine should be used with caution in uroabdomen patients, as side effects may include tachycardia. Additionally, ketamine is excreted via the kidneys and thus its use may result in a prolonged duration of action.

Diagnosis

Diagnosis of uroabdomen should be based on clinical history and physical examination findings and paired with imaging studies and clinicopathologic results. The severity of the changes noted on laboratory work will depend on several factors including the time elapsed

TABLE 17.1 - TREATMENT OF HYPERKALEMIA IN DOGS AND CATS[2,9]

Drug	Purpose	Suggested doses
Calcium gluconate 10% solution	Restores resting membrane excitability to prevent cardiotoxic effects	0.5–1.0 mL/kg IV over 10–15 minutes (with continuous electrocardiographic monitoring)
Regular insulin	Promotes intracellular flux of K^+ in exchange for Na^+	0.25–0.5 U/kg IV
50% dextrose	Increases endogenous insulin and prevents hypoglycemia	0.5 g/kg or 1–2 mL/kg
Terbutaline or albuterol	Promotes intracellular flux of K^+ in exchange for Na^+	0.01 mg/kg slow IV or SC, or 1–3 puffs
Sodium bicarbonate	Promotes intracellular flux of K^+ in exchange for H^+	1–2 mEq/kg slow IV

between rupture of the urinary system and diagnosis, comorbidities, and the inherent rate of diffusion of the molecules across the peritoneal membrane.[10] For example, the concentration of BUN/urea may be disproportionately higher than that of creatinine because urea is a small molecule that can freely diffuse across cell membranes.[11] Anemia may be present if there is significant hemorrhage associated with urinary tract rupture but may also be present secondary to other injuries.

The use of multiple imaging modalities may lead the clinician toward a diagnosis of uroabdomen, although the presence of abdominal effusion is a nonspecific finding. The diagnosis of abdominal effusion needs to be confirmed with abdominal radiographs, FAST, or ultrasound. These imaging modalities, particularly the latter two, can aid the clinician in sampling the effusion. If there is a suspicion of uroperitoneum or uroretroperitoneum, contrast radiographic studies can be helpful to locate the site of the tear within the urinary system.

If the rupture is believed to be within the urinary bladder or the urethra, positive-contrast cystography is recommended (Table 17.2). The patient will likely require sedation or general anesthesia along with the placement of a sterile urinary catheter in the most distal aspect of the urethra. This catheter should be used to empty the bladder and instill iodinated contrast, filling the urethra and bladder.[12] Orthogonal radiographs should be taken before instilling contrast to evaluate patient and urinary catheter position; it is important to include the entire lower urinary tract. Serial radiographs or fluoroscopy should be performed after instilling contrast (Fig. 17.1; Video 17.1). When infusing contrast, the bladder should be palpated to prevent overdistension. A recent prospective study in cadavers of dogs evaluated the use of microbubble contrast cystosonography for the diagnosis of ruptured bladders.[13] Agitated saline was infused into ruptured bladders through urethral catheters, and bladders were assessed sonographically. The study revealed a diagnostic sensitivity and specificity of 88.9% and 100%, respectively.

If the kidneys and/or ureters are thought to be ruptured, an excretory urogram, via injection of contrast media through an intravenous catheter, is the recommended contrast study. This procedure should be avoided in dehydrated or severely azotemic patients due to the risk of kidney injury.[12] A dose of 880 mL/kg of iodinated contrast is given as a rapid IV bolus and two orthogonal radiographs should be taken at 0, 5, 15, and 30 minutes after administration.[12] False-negative results may occur if insufficient volumes of contrast media are used or if not enough time elapses between administering the contrast and obtaining radiographs.[1]

Alternatively, positive-contrast nephropyelography is a

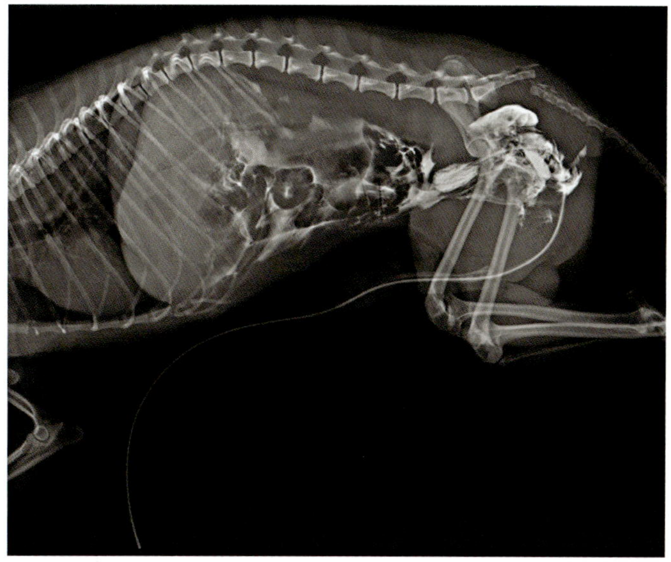

Figure 17.1 Positive-contrast cystourethrogram in a cat with rupture of the urinary bladder and urethra. There is contrast leakage at the site of urethral and bladder tear. Image courtesy of Filippo Cinti.

Video 17.1. Preoperative and postoperative positive-contrast urethrocystograms in a patient with uroabdomen due to a proximal urethral avulsion. In the former, note the accumulation of contrast dorsal to the bladder and the presence of an abdominal drain. In the latter, there is no evidence of contrast leakage and a cystostomy tube is present. Video courtesy of Matteo Rossanese.

TABLE 17.2 - INSTRUCTIONS FOR PERFORMING POSITIVE-CONTRAST CYSTOGRAPHY IN PATIENTS SUSPECTED OF HAVING TEARS WITHIN THE URINARY BLADDER AND/OR URETHRA[12]

	Typical bladder volume	Volume of iodinated contrast	Imaging techniques
Dog	5–10 mL/kg	5 mL/kg	Two orthogonal radiographs before and after contrast infusion
Cat	2–5 mL/kg	25 mL	Two orthogonal radiographs before and after contrast infusion

TABLE 17.3 - REPORTED CRITERIA FOR DIAGNOSIS OF UROABDOMEN BASED ON EFFUSION AND PERIPHERAL BLOOD CREATININE AND POTASSIUM CONCENTRATIONS[6,14,15]

	Fluid:blood creatinine ratio	Fluid:blood potassium ratio
Dog	>2:1 ≥1.25:1	>1.4:1
Cat	>2:1	>1.9:1

procedure that can be done if ureteral tear(s) is suspected. This procedure is technically challenging, requires general anesthesia, and ideally fluoroscopy would be utilized. The authors encourage the reader to defer to the reference for more information regarding performing nephropyelography.[12]

Abdominocentesis or peritoneal lavage with fluid analysis is recommended to confirm diagnosis of uroabdomen. A ratio of abdominal fluid creatinine concentration to peripheral blood creatinine concentration above 2:1 has been shown to be predictive of uroabdomen in dogs, with a specificity and sensitivity of 100% and 86%, respectively.[14] A ratio of abdominal fluid potassium concentration to peripheral blood potassium concentration above 1.4:1 was also predictive of uroabdomen in dogs, with a specificity and sensitivity of 100%.[14] A recent study aimed to evaluate additional effusion characteristics to better distinguish uroabdomen from other forms of ascites.[15] Results proved that fluid creatinine concentrations ≥2.1 mg/dL, a fluid creatinine:serum creatinine ratio ≥1.25, total protein concentrations <2.0 g/dL, and total nucleated cell counts >5000 cells/μL could be used as new criteria for the diagnosis of uroperitoneum in dogs. The authors of this study found that if an abdominal effusion met the aforementioned criteria, the accuracy for the laboratory diagnosis of uroperitoneum was 99.0%. Current recommendations for diagnosis of uroabdomen in cats are a ratio of effusion creatinine to blood creatinine above 2:1 and a ratio of effusion potassium to blood potassium above 1.9:1.[6] See Table 17.3 for a summary of the abovementioned criteria for diagnosis of uroabdomen in dogs and cats. Cytological evaluation of the effusion should be performed to check for the presence of intracellular bacteria, which would warrant the administration of parenteral antibiotics.

Treatment

Treatment of uroabdomen is twofold: urinary diversion followed by definitive repair. The goal of urinary diversion is to allow for urine drainage and management of electrolyte and biochemical derangements prior to general anesthesia and surgery. Figure 17.2 shows an algorithm summarizing the management of suspected urinary tract injury based on patient stability and site of presumed injury.

At a minimum, a urinary catheter should be placed to allow for the drainage of urine that is constantly being produced, assuming at least one kidney and ureter are intact. This helps to keep the urinary bladder decompressed and prevent further accumulation of urine within the abdomen. If there is a urethral tear, fluoroscopy can be used to aid in the placement of the catheter. Alternatively, percutaneous antegrade urethral catheterization can be attempted rather than repeated attempts at retrograde urethral catheterization in the face of a urethral tear.[16] Percutaneous antegrade urethral catheterization using fluoroscopy requires the patient to be positioned in lateral recumbency. The lateral abdomen is shaved and aseptically prepared. An IV catheter is placed transabdominally into the urinary bladder, toward the direction of the trigone. Then, a hydrophilic guidewire is inserted through the catheter, aimed toward the trigone, and passed anterogradely through the urethra. Once the wire exits out of the lower urinary tract, a well lubricated, appropriately sized urinary catheter can be passed retrogradely over the guidewire and directed into the urinary bladder. The wire and peripheral catheter are then removed. Alternatively, a temporary cystostomy tube may be considered in cases of urethral rupture (see Chapter 5).

Abdominal drainage of urine is also required to prevent ongoing electrolyte abnormalities, worsening azotemia, and urinary peritonitis. This can be achieved by single or repeated abdominocentesis, placement of an indwelling abdominal drain (e.g., locking-loop pigtail catheter), or placement of a peritoneal dialysis catheter (see Chapter 5). A peritoneal drainage system is imperative for patients with urinary tract rupture anywhere more proximal than the urethra (Fig. 17.3).

In animals with a urethral tear as their only source of urine leakage, an indwelling urinary catheter may be sufficient for full recovery, so long as the urethra can be catheterized and adequate peritoneal drainage of urine is achieved. Typical duration of indwelling transurethral catheterization for small punctures or longitudinal urethral tears is 10–14 days.[1] In a study of cats with urethral tearing, urethral catheters were removed 5–14 days after placement, with good outcomes.[17]

Surgical intervention is indicated in cases of large urethral tears that cannot be managed with indwelling catheterization or other urethral tears that have failed medical management. Surgery is also indicated for bladder rupture (Fig. 17.4) or urine leakage from the kidney and/or ureter. The type of surgery required will vary based on the location of the tear but may include nephrectomy, ureteronephrectomy, ureteral reimplantation, cystotomy, urethral anastomosis, perineal ure-

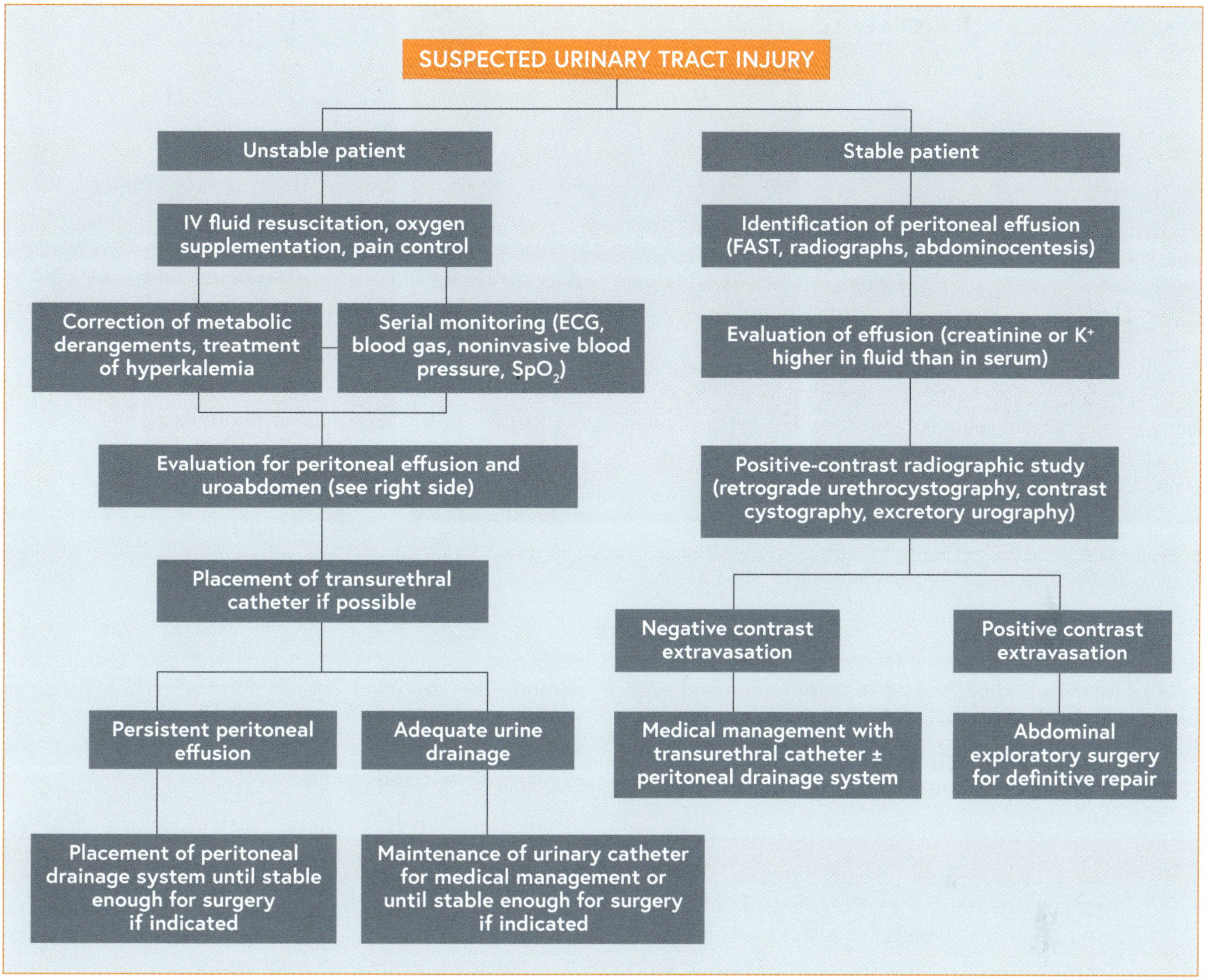

Figure 17.2 Algorithm for the management of suspected urinary tract injury based on patient stability and site of presumed injury.

throstomy, or a combination of these procedures.[1,6,18,19] Implants like urethral or ureteral stents or subcutaneous ureteral bypass may also be indicated, depending on the location and severity of the injury.[20,21] See Chapter 19 for a detailed description of these procedures.

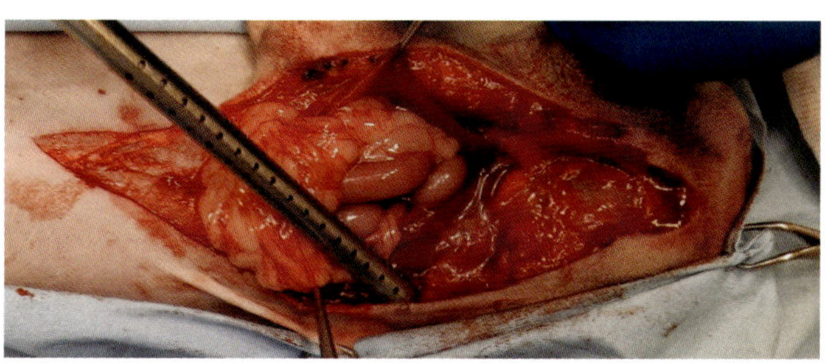

Figure 17.3 Intraoperative image of free abdominal fluid (uroabdomen). Image courtesy of Filippo Cinti.

Complications and outcomes

The development of uroabdomen can result in urinary peritonitis, which may also be septic if the urine is infected. Acute kidney injury can develop and may not be reversible depending on the type, cause, and severity of the urinary tract injury. Complications may also develop secondary to surgical intervention and include adhesion formation, strictures, ongoing urinary leakage, dehiscence, urinary incontinence, and urinary tract infections.[4,6,18,22]

Many studies agree that clinicopathologic features at presentation do not act as reliable prognostic indicators. In a study involving 22 dogs and 29 cats with urethral rupture, electrolyte disturbances, metabolic acidosis, and azotemia were not predictors of mortality.[4] In a more recent study evaluating 43 dogs with uroabdomen, serum creatinine concentrations at admission were not associated with survival.[22] Another

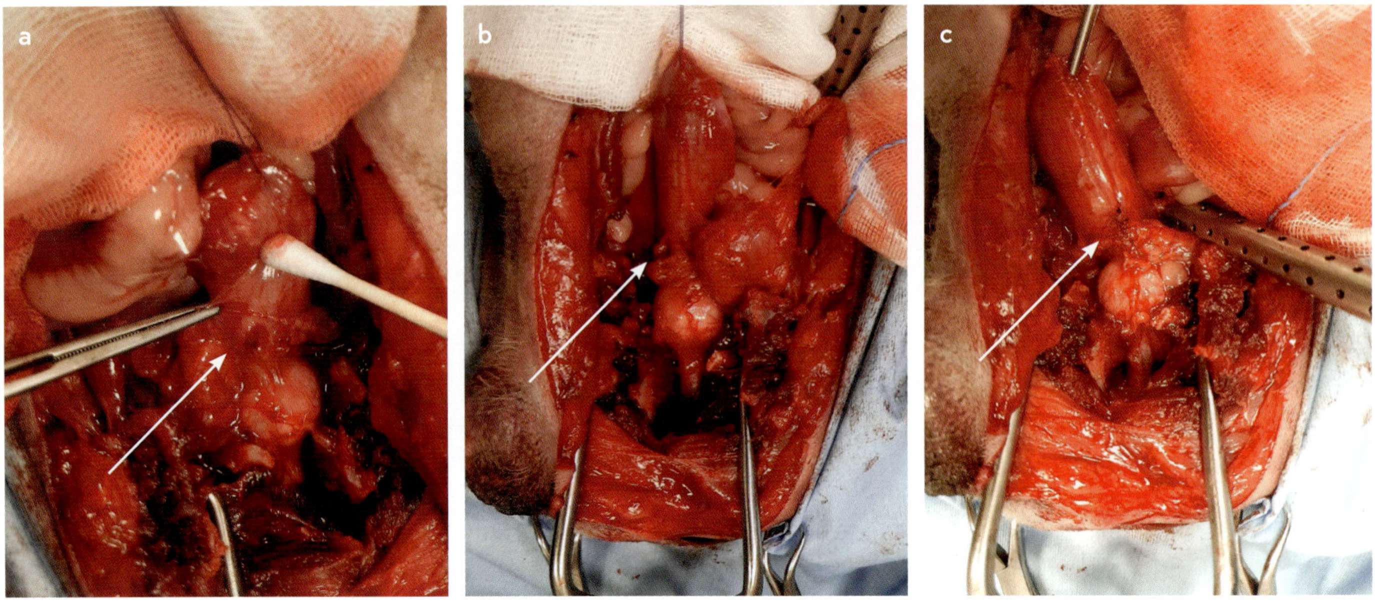

Figure 17.4 (a,b) Intraoperative images of a bladder neck tear (white arrow). (c) The lesion was sutured with simple interrupted sutures. Images courtesy of Filippo Cinti.

study evaluating 53 cats with uroabdomen concluded that potassium and packed cell volume at presentation were not predictors of survival.[19] However, this study found that elevations in creatinine were correlated with negative outcomes.

Prognosis seems similar for dogs and cats with uroabdomen. The reported overall survival to discharge is 78% and 74% in dogs[19] and cats,[22] respectively. In both species, the presence of multiple traumatic injuries is associated with reduced survival.[4,18]

KEEP IN MIND

- Trauma is the most common cause of uroabdomen in the veterinary patient, with the urinary bladder being the most common site of urine leakage.
- The presence of a palpable urinary bladder does not rule out the presence of uroabdomen.
- The most common clinicopathologic abnormalities include hyperkalemia, hyponatremia, hyperphosphatemia, azotemia, and metabolic acidosis.
- Rapid and appropriate correction of electrolyte abnormalities is imperative to improve patient stability.
- The diagnosis of uroabdomen can be confirmed based on imaging studies and fluid analysis. Specifically, potassium and creatinine concentrations in the fluid should be compared with those in the serum.
- Urinary diversion should be attempted in all patients with uroabdomen. This includes placement of an indwelling urinary catheter or cystostomy tube and drainage of abdominal effusion. Following urinary diversion, definitive surgery should be performed if indicated.

References

1. Colopy S, Townsend A, Bjorling D. Approach to the uroabdomen. In: Aronson L (ed.). *Small Animal Surgical Emergencies*, 2nd ed. Wiley Blackwell; 2022. pp. 285–296.
2. Stafford JR, Bartges JW. A clinical review of pathophysiology, diagnosis, and treatment of uroabdomen in the dog and cat. *J Vet Emerg Crit Care (San Antonio)*. 2013; 23(2):216–229.
3. Sherer TD, Brabson T. Obstipation leading to urethral obstruction and uroabdomen in a dog. *Vet Rec Case Rep*. 2020; 8(4).
4. Anderson RB, Aronson LR, Drobatz KJ, Atilla A. Prognostic factors for successful outcome following urethral rupture in dogs and cats. *J Am Anim Hosp Assoc*. 2006; 42(2):136–146.
5. Fossum T. Surgery of the bladder and urethra. In: Fossum T. *Small Animal Surgery*, 5th ed. Elsevier; 2019. pp. 678–719.
6. Aumann M, Worth LT, Drobatz KJ. Uroperitoneum in cats: 26 cases (1986–1995). *J Am Anim Hosp Assoc*. 1998; 34(4): 315–324.
7. Rieser TM. Urinary tract emergencies. *Vet Clin North Am Small Anim Pract*. 2005; 35(2):359–373.

1. Balakrishnan A, Silverstein D. Shock fluids and fluid challenge. In: Silverstein D, Hopper K (eds.). *Small Animal Critical Care Medicine*, 3rd ed. Elsevier; 2023. pp. 402–408.
2. Press S, Balakrishnan A. Uroabdomen. In: Drobatz K. *Textbook of Small Animal Emergency Medicine*. John Wiley & Sons; 2019. pp. 659–664.
3. Ross L, Labato M. Peritoneal dialysis. In: DiBartola S (ed.). *Fluid, Electrolyte, and Acid-Base Disorders*, 4th ed. Elsevier; 2012. pp. 665–679.
4. Wellman M, DiBartola S, Kohn C. Applied physiology of body fluids in dogs and cats. In: DiBartola S (ed.). *Fluid, Electrolyte, and Acid-Base Disorders*, 4th ed. Elsevier; 2012. pp. 4–29.
5. Wallack ST. *The Handbook of Veterinary Contrast Radiography*, 1st ed. San Diego Veterinary Imaging; 2003.
6. Muehlbauer E et al. The use of agitated saline as contrast agent in a contrast-enhanced cystosonography for detection of urinary bladder rupture in animal cadavers. *J Vet Emerg Crit Care (San Antonio)*. 2023; 33(3):327–331.
7. Schmiedt C, Tobias KM, Otto CM. Evaluation of abdominal fluid: peripheral blood creatinine and potassium ratios for diagnosis of uroperitoneum in dogs. *J Vet Emerg Crit Care*. 2001; 11(4):275–280.
8. Paes PRO et al. Laboratory diagnosis of canine uroperitoneum based on cellular and biochemical characteristics of serum and abdominal fluid. *Vet Clin Pathol*. 2022; 51(1):107–111.
9. Holmes ES, Weisse C, Berent AC. Use of fluoroscopically guided percutaneous antegrade urethral catheterization for the treatment of urethral obstruction in male cats: 9 cases (2000–2009). *J Am Vet Med Assoc*. 2012; 241(5):603–607.
10. Meige F, Sarrau S, Autefage A. Management of traumatic urethral rupture in 11 cats using primary alignment with a urethral catheter. *Vet Comp Orthop Traumatol*. 2008; 21(1):76–84.
11. Addison ES et al. A retrospective analysis of urethral rupture in 63 cats. *J Feline Med Surg*. 2014; 16(4):300–307.
12. Hornsey SJ et al. Factors affecting survival to discharge in 53 cats diagnosed with uroabdomen: A single-centre retrospective analysis. *J Feline Med Surg*. 2021; 23(2):115–120.
13. Milligan ML et al. Outcome of SUB placement for the treatment of benign ureteral obstruction in dogs: Nine dogs and 12 renal units (2013 to 2017). *J Small Anim Pract*. 2020; 61(7):428–435.
14. Berent AC, Weisse CW, Bagley DH, Lamb K. Use of a subcutaneous ureteral bypass device for treatment of benign ureteral obstruction in cats: 174 ureters in 134 cats (2009–2015). *J Am Vet Med Assoc*. 2018; 253(10):1309–1327.
15. Grimes JA, Fletcher JM, Schmiedt CW. Outcomes in dogs with uroabdomen: 43 cases (2006–2015). *J Am Vet Med Assoc*. 2018; 252(1):92–97.

Chapter 18
Trauma or prolapse of the urinary tract

Marie Burneko, Lillian R. Aronson

Renal and ureteral trauma

Renal injury

Clinical presentation and diagnosis

Trauma involving the kidney is uncommon in dogs and cats. Possible causes of renal injury include vehicular trauma, iatrogenic injury, bite wounds, and renal rupture (secondary to neoplasia or obstruction). Uroabdomen may be seen, but it most often develops from trauma to the distal ureters, bladder, or proximal urethra. Uroretroperitoneum is usually secondary to injury to one or both kidneys or to the proximal ureter without disruption of the peritoneum.[1] While with injury to the kidney alone uroabdomen generally does not develop, if there is avulsion of the ureter, uroabdomen may be present. If there is significant injury to the renal parenchyma or blood supply, hemoabdomen can occur. Animals may be anemic if a significant amount of blood has been lost. If only one kidney is affected and there is no underlying renal disease, azotemia is not usually present, and therefore unilateral renal injuries may be challenging to diagnose. In humans, avulsion or thrombosis of the renal artery is reported following blunt trauma, although this has been diagnosed infrequently in veterinary medicine. Most clinical signs in small animals are vague, but abdominal pain, retroperitoneal hematoma, hematuria, and hemoabdomen are reported in cases of renal trauma.[2]

Advanced imaging is necessary to diagnose most cases of renal injury. Intravenous pyelography (or excretory urography) is useful to evaluate the upper urinary tract. This can be accompanied by radiographs, fluoroscopy, and/or computed tomography (CT) and involves the renal angiographic phase/vascular phase (immediately after contrast injection), the nephrogram, and the excretory phase/pyelogram (contrast flows from the renal pelvis to the ureters and bladder).[3] Contrast-enhanced ultrasound is becoming a more frequently used tool to evaluate renal perfusion, but traditional Doppler flow ultrasonography can be very useful as well.[4,5] Contrast CT is useful to delineate renal injuries and evaluate the entire abdomen in cases of blunt abdominal trauma. Early and delayed CT of the kidney is necessary to evaluate both the nephrographic and excretory phase of the intravenous pyelogram to avoid missing any upper urinary tract abnormalities.[2]

Treatment

In humans, there is a trend toward conservative management of renal injuries, as many extensive injuries can be treated in this way. Life-threatening hemorrhage is described as the only absolute indication for surgical intervention, but if there is injury to the ureteropelvic junction or vascular pedicle, surgical exploration is generally recommended.[6,7] In dogs and cats, indications for surgery generally include uncontrollable hemorrhage, damage to the renal pedicle or necrosis of the kidney, and/or uroperitoneum/uroretroperitoneum.

Surgical technique: Kidney laceration repair

1. A routine midline celiotomy is performed (see Chapter 3).
2. The entire abdomen should be explored in case of blunt trauma. Close attention should be paid to the ureteropelvic junction to ensure there are no avulsions or lacerations.
3. The retroperitoneum should be opened and the kidney surface explored.
4. The renal capsule can be sutured with horizontal mattress sutures if the kidney is viable (4-0 to 3-0 absorbable monofilament suture) (Fig. 18.1). Omentum, the transversus abdominis muscle, and/or collagen sheeting can be used to buttress the renal capsule repair.
5. In case of kidney avulsion, nephropexy must be performed. This can be achieved by suturing the renal capsule to the abdominal body wall with simple interrupted sutures of 3-0 polypropylene.
6. The retroperitoneum and abdominal cavity are lavaged.

If the kidney is not viable, ureteronephrectomy is performed. Partial nephrectomy is not generally recommended, as it is uncommon that only one pole of the kidney is nonviable.

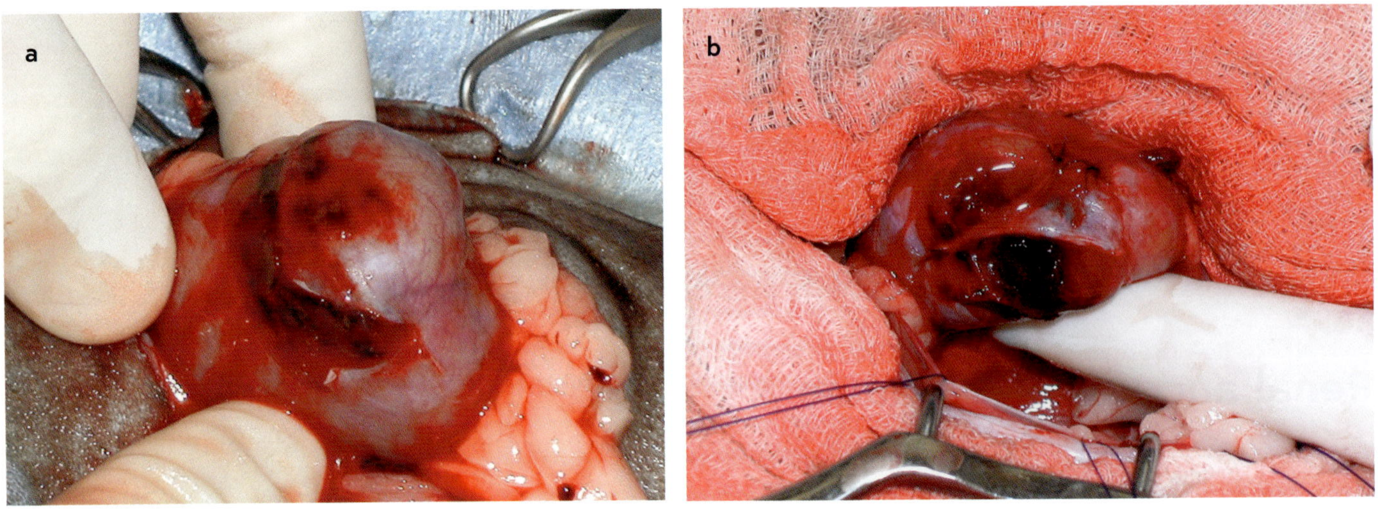

Figure 18.1 (a) Renal capsule laceration secondary to blunt force trauma. (b) Two horizontal mattress sutures have been placed to repair the renal capsule.

Surgical technique: Ureteronephrectomy

1. A routine midline celiotomy is performed (see Chapter 3).
2. The affected kidney is dissected free from its peritoneal attachments using a combination of electrocautery, bipolar vessel-sealing devices, cotton-tipped applicators, and blunt dissection.
3. The kidney may be flipped toward the midline to better expose the renal artery and vein, or these vessels can be dissected with the kidney in its normal position.
4. Two ligatures should be placed on the section of each vessel that will remain in the body, whereas one ligature can be placed on the section of vessel that will be removed with the kidney. The renal artery and vein are transected between the proximal and distal ligatures.
   - 2-0 or 3-0 absorbable or nonabsorbable mono- or multifilament suture may be used.
   - Bipolar vessel-sealing devices can be used if the blood vessels are <5 mm in diameter, but care should be taken if the artery and vein are sealed together, which has been proposed to potentially cause an arteriovenous fistula.
   - Hemoclips may be used, but the clip should be sized appropriately for the vessel.
5. The ureter is dissected to its junction with the bladder, and it is ligated at the level of the bladder with two ligatures placed on the ureteral stump. The ureter is then removed with the kidney.
6. Routine abdominal closure is performed.

Ureteral injury

Ureteral injury secondary to trauma is rare in dogs and cats, as injuries more commonly involve the bladder or urethra. In one study, only 0.01% of the overall hospital population was diagnosed with traumatic ureteral rupture, highlighting the rarity of this condition.[8] The majority of ureteral ruptures were located on the right side, but the study was small; no side predilection has been reported in humans. Iatrogenic injury to the ureters in small animals is seen most commonly in association with ovariohysterectomy, and it can include inadvertent ligation, laceration, or resection of ureteral tissue.

Clinical presentation and diagnosis

Clinical signs in animals with unilateral ureteral injury are generally vague, but abdominal pain, vomiting, lethargy, and hematuria are some of the most commonly encountered signs of potential ureteral injury. Uroabdomen may be present and will increase in volume the longer left untreated. If the contralateral kidney is normal, it is unlikely that acute azotemia will be detected at the time of ureteral injury. Inadvertent unilateral ureteral ligation may be challenging to diagnose, as there may be very general or no obvious clinical signs. In contrast, animals with bilateral ureteral ligation (with or without transection) usually present with severe electrolyte abnormalities, signs of shock, and potentially circulatory collapse.[9]

Signs of ureteral obstruction (e.g., from inadvertent ureteral ligation during ovariohysterectomy) can include the above listed signs as well as abnormalities in urination and persistent urinary tract infection (see Chapter 19).

A small subset of chronic traumatic ureteral ruptures have been reported where urine leakage into the retroperitoneal space results in a urinoma, a retroperitoneal accumulation of urine encased in a fibrous sac with no epithelial lining.[10–12] This has been more commonly reported in cats, and the majority of cases were diagnosed at least 10 days after the initial traumatic injury. Subtle, persistent clinical signs should prompt reevaluation of patients that have sustained trauma, and development of an abdominal mass following trauma can be an indicator of a paraureteral urinoma.

In an unstable patient, an abdominal ultrasound or intravenous pyelogram may be performed. Abdominal effusion consistent with uroabdomen combined with ultrasound findings of free retroperitoneal fluid should raise suspicion of a potential ureteral injury.[8] In cases of inadvertent ureteral ligation, common ultrasound findings include pyelectasia and ureteral dilation. The offending ligature may or may not be seen, but there is usually an abrupt taper to a more normal ureter distal to the ligation site (Fig. 18.2).[13] Intravenous pyelography alone can also diagnose ureteral rupture/laceration and obstruction, with a reported sensitivity of up to 100%.[14] Contrast CT may be useful in cases of blunt force trauma to evaluate for other injuries concurrently, and it may be more sensitive in locating small ruptures (Fig. 18.3).[3] Intravenous contrast should be administered with caution in animals with severe dehydration or azotemia, as prolonged excretion of the contrast medium can cause renal damage in humans.[3] Antegrade or retrograde contrast studies can also be used to aid in diagnosis, particularly if there is already an indication for exploratory surgery, as it may be easier and safer to perform these studies intraoperatively. Antegrade pyelography may also be performed percutaneously with the aid of ultrasound, fluoroscopy, and/or radiography, with a reported diagnostic rate of 94% in one study.[15] Diagnostic imaging findings in patients with a paraureteral urinoma can include a soft-tissue-opacity retroperitoneal mass on radiographs, a fluid-filled retroperitoneal sac with or without pyelectasia and ureteral dilation on ultrasound, and potentially evidence of urine leakage into the sac on contrast studies.[10,11] In one case report, ultrasound-guided aspiration of the sac contents yielded a diagnosis of urinoma based on the serum:fluid creatinine ratio.[12]

Treatment

In cases of suspected acute ureteral ligation, it is prudent to intervene quickly, as damage to the kidney will worsen over time. One study showed that glomerular filtration rate decreases permanently by 35% and 54% after 7 days and 14 days of complete ureteral obstruction, respectively.[16] Based on experimental studies, it is possible that removing the ligature alone may be successful if performed within a week of inadvertent ligation, although if there are any concerns regarding the viability of the ureter, more definitive interventions are necessary.[17] In case of chronic ureteral ligation, ureteronephrectomy is commonly performed (Fig. 18.4).

In general, treatment options for an injured ureter can be considered based on lesion location along the ureter, degree of ureteral length lost, functionality of the contralateral kidney, and patient stability. The ureter can be divided into the proximal third, mid-length, and dis-

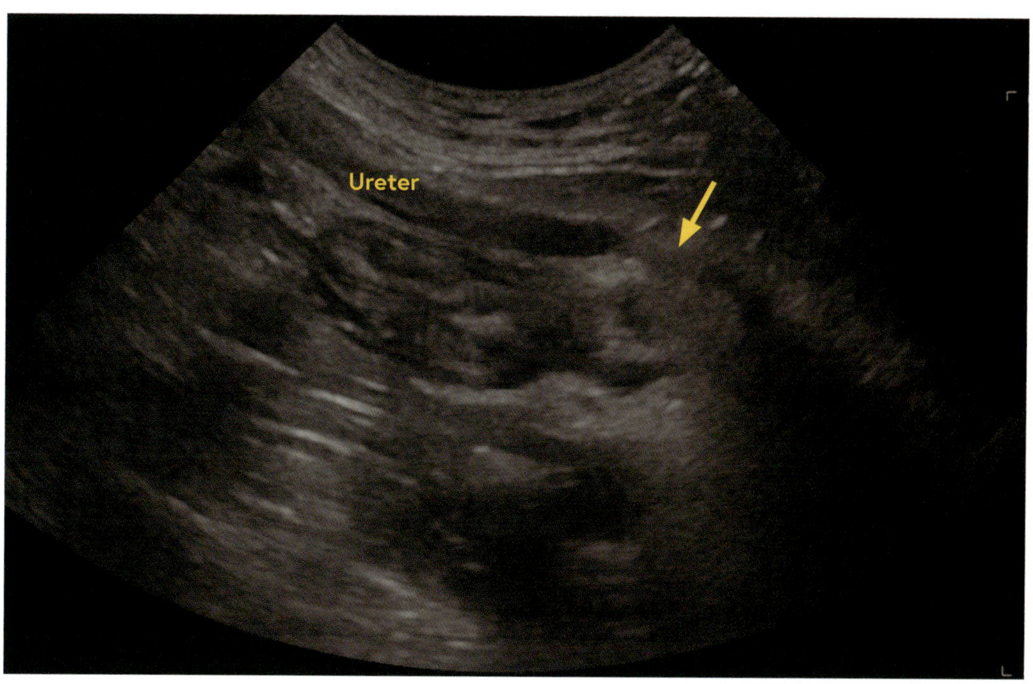

Figure 18.2 Ultrasound image of a ureteral obstruction secondary to inadvertent ureteral ligation in a dog. Note the dilated ureter proximal to the offending suture around the ureter (yellow arrow).

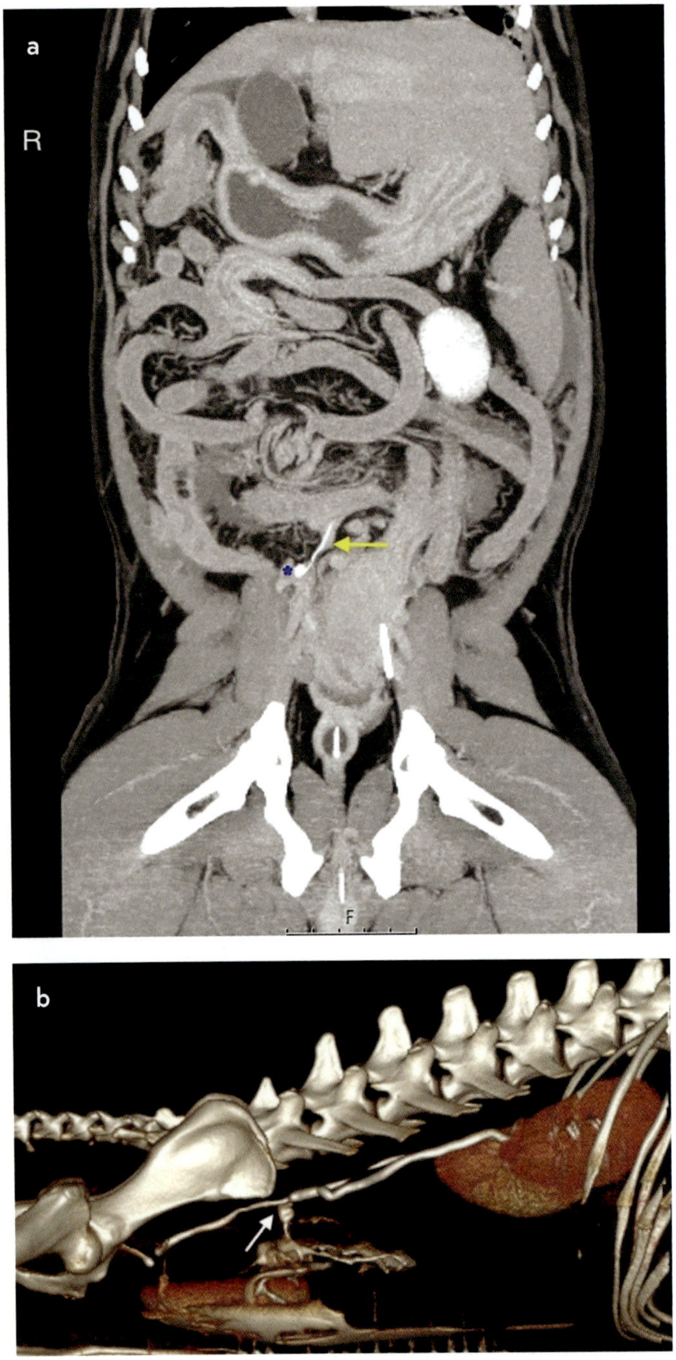

Figure 18.3 (a) Computed tomography image (dorsal reconstruction) of a dog with a right ureteral tear. The right ureter is indicated by the blue star. Note the leakage of contrast medium from the ureter (yellow arrow) following intravenous contrast administration. (b) 3D reconstruction of the computed tomography scan. The white arrow highlights leakage from the right ureter.

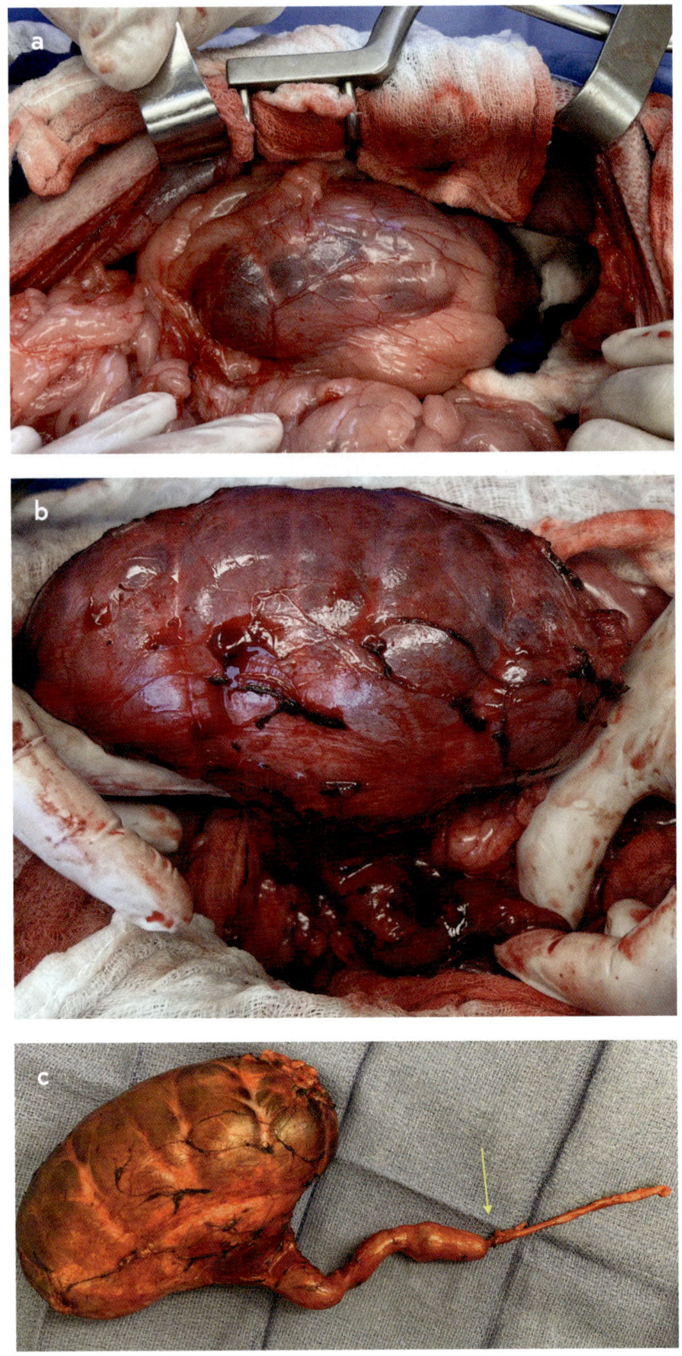

Figure 18.4 (a) Intraoperative image of a hydronephrotic right kidney secondary to suspected inadvertent ureteral ligation during prior ovariohysterectomy procedure. (b) Dissection of the right kidney and proximal ureter. Note the extreme hydronephrosis and ureteral dilation. The ureter, grasped by the surgeon's fingers, is proximally tortuous. (c) Right kidney following ureteronephrectomy. The yellow arrow points to the area of ureteral ligation.

tal third when considering surgical interventions. Surgical options generally include primary repair, ureteral resection and anastomosis, ureteral stenting or bypass, and ureteronephrectomy.[18] In the proximal ureter, primary ureteral repair, ureteral resection and anastomosis, subcutaneous ureteral bypass (SUB), and ureteral stenting are the most common surgical interventions employed. In the mid-ureter, more variability exists in terms of treatment options; all of the abovementioned interventions may be used, and ureteroneocystostomy may also be an option. An intra- or extravesicular technique may be used (see Chapter 19). If ureteral reim-

TABLE 18.1 - SUMMARY OF TENSION-RELIEVING TECHNIQUES THAT CAN BE EMPLOYED DURING URETERAL SURGERY	
Renal descensus	• Dissect kidney from peritoneal attachments • Suture kidney to body wall in more caudal location
Cystopexy	• Advance bladder cranially and suture to body wall or psoas muscle
Nephrocystopexy	• Suture bladder directly to kidney
Boari flap	• Create longitudinal flap of bladder tissue and suture to ureter via end-to-end or side-to-side anastomosis

plantation of the mid-ureter is pursued, it will likely be necessary to employ tension-relieving techniques to allow for healing of the reimplantation site (Table 18.1). Ureteral stenting can be a useful adjunct to ureteral anastomosis or reimplantation to decrease tension on the repair site and potentially decrease stricture formation. Inflammation of the ureter is common following trauma and surgical intervention; therefore, placement of a ureteral stent may also prevent ureteral obstruction secondary to ureteritis postoperatively.[13,19] In cases of distal ureteral injury, the most common surgical intervention is ureteral reimplantation, but the aforementioned techniques may potentially be considered as well.[19] If a large section of ureter is lost, ureteral anastomosis or reimplantation may not be feasible; in these cases, performing a Boari or modified Boari flap may be possible.[20] If there is extensive damage to the upper urinary tract, ureteronephrectomy may be considered as well.

Suture choice for ureteral repair, anastomosis, and reimplantation varies, but common choices include nylon and polyglycolic acid. Suture sizes generally range from 5-0 to 8-0. Continuous patterns result in the smoothest epithelial surface histologically, but they may increase the chance of ureteral stricture; interrupted sutures may be less likely to cause luminal narrowing.[18] Given the small diameter of canine and feline ureters, magnification of the operating field is necessary, either in the form of an operating microscope or surgical loupes.

Postoperative management

Any ureteral surgery may cause stricture or inflammation of the surgical site, which can result in partial or complete ureteral obstruction. The use of temporary ureteral stents is controversial, with some studies indicating a higher likelihood of fibrosis and potentially stricture formation. Recovery of renal function may be challenging to predict preoperatively, and owners should be counseled regarding the possibility that decreased renal function may be permanent. In any ureteral surgery, postoperative dehiscence is a potential complication, and the patient should be monitored for any increases in abdominal effusion or changes in attitude postoperatively. SUB devices and stents have the potential for unique postoperative complications such as persistent lower urinary tract signs, obstruction, recurrent urinary tract infection, and implant migration.[21–25] If the animal had a ureteral obstruction secondary to trauma (e.g., urinoma, blood clots, inflammation, acute ureteral ligation), postoperative dehydration and subsequent electrolyte abnormalities may be seen secondary to postobstructive diuresis. In these cases, body weight, renal and electrolyte values, perfusion parameters, and urine output should be monitored closely.

Outcome

The prognosis following ureteral injury is variable, depending on the severity of injury, the stability of the patient, other injuries sustained, the function of the contralateral kidney, and the development of postoperative complications. In general, intervention following inadvertent ureteral ligation or transection can result in a good prognosis. In one study, an excellent–good outcome was seen in 73% of cats and dogs with ureter injuries secondary to ovariohysterectomy complications following surgical intervention.[26] In another study evaluating ureteral rupture secondary to trauma, 50% of cases survived overall, with animals undergoing initial ureteronephrectomy having a good prognosis if the contralateral kidney had normal function.[8] However, since this study had very small case numbers, these results should be interpreted with caution. Another study evaluated a small subset of cats treated for ureteral obstruction with ureteroneocystostomy, with 92% having an acceptable long-term outcome.[27] Overall, owners should be counseled regarding the financial commitment, potential long-term management of chronic kidney disease, and potential risks of complications specific to the procedure performed when cases of ureteral injury are encountered.

Bladder trauma

Urinary bladder rupture is the most common cause of uroabdomen, and it can be secondary to blunt or penetrating trauma, urethral obstruction, bladder neoplasia, iatrogenic causes (e.g., catheterization, cystocentesis, bladder expression), trauma secondary to pelvic fractures, and as a complication of bladder surgery. Reported rates of bladder injury associated with pelvic fracture range from 1.6% to 7%.[28,29]

Clinical presentation and diagnosis

Clinical signs may be nonspecific and can include vomiting, anorexia, and lethargy. Physical examination findings may include a distended abdomen, abdominal pain, dehydration, cardiac arrhythmias, abdominal or inguinal bruising, and potentially signs of shock and hypoperfusion depending on the presence of other injuries.[30] Palpation of the bladder, ability to urinate, or visualization of the bladder on radiographs or ultrasound does not rule out the possibility of bladder rupture.[31]

Clinicopathologic findings associated with uroabdomen include azotemia, hyperkalemia, hyponatremia and hypochloremia, metabolic acidosis, hemoconcentration, neutrophilia, and hematuria. Abdominocentesis and fluid evaluation is an important diagnostic step in the diagnosis of uroabdomen. Abdominal fluid creatinine and potassium concentrations are elevated compared to peripheral blood values, and there are published ratios for diagnosis of uroabdomen. Cytology of the effusion may reveal intracellular bacteria, which confirms a diagnosis of septic uroabdomen.[30]

Diagnostic imaging is necessary to determine the location of the urinary tract injury, as stated previously. Plain radiographs may reveal loss of serosal detail and potentially a small or unobservable bladder, but otherwise they are not generally useful for localization of the injury. Positive-contrast retrograde or normograde cystograms are usually diagnostic for bladder rupture; however, false negatives can occur if the bladder is not filled adequately.[32] Diagnosis of bladder rupture is confirmed by extravasation of contrast medium from the bladder (Fig. 18.5). In trauma patients diagnosed with uroabdomen, contrast CT can be useful to identify concomitant injuries as well as bladder rupture. Intravenous contrast should be used with extreme caution in azotemic or dehydrated patients, as contrast-induced nephropathy has been reported in human and animal patients.[1]

Treatment

Uroabdomen is a medical emergency, and the patient should be stabilized in respect to renal function, electrolyte derangements, and cardiovascular status prior

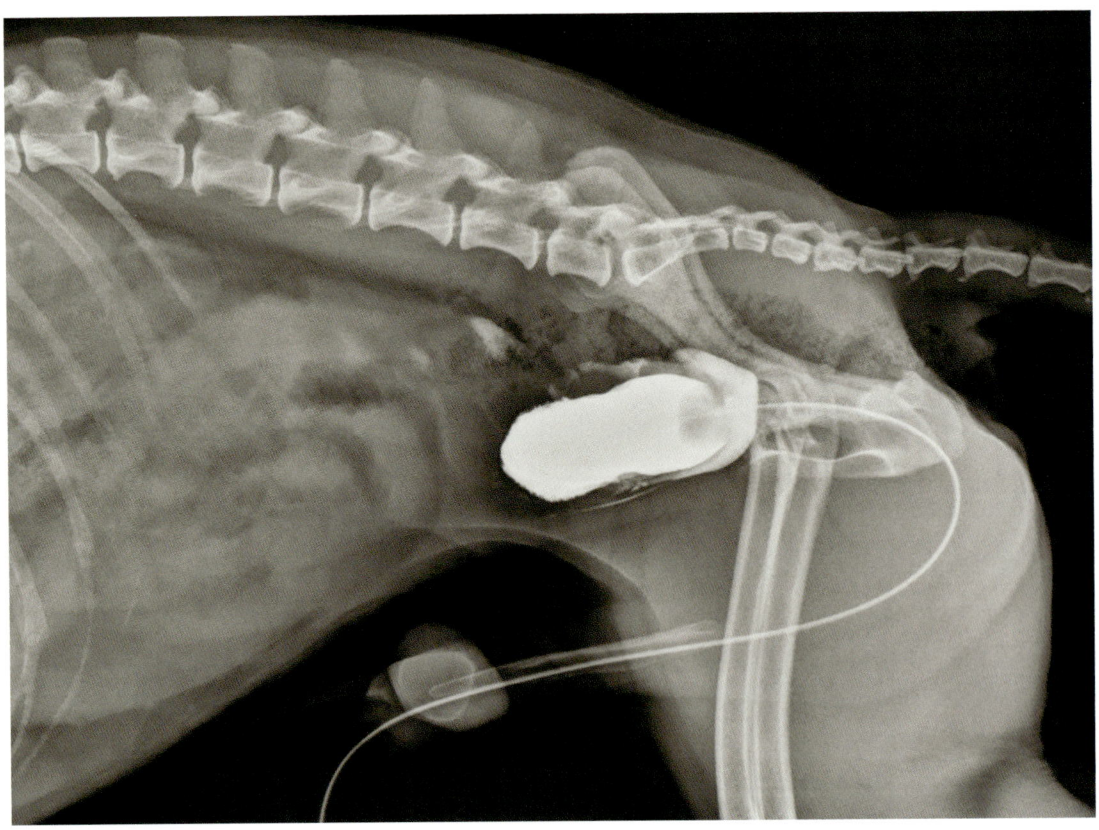

Figure 18.5 Retrograde contrast cystourethrogram in a dog with a bladder rupture. Note the contrast medium extravasation around the bladder.

to surgical treatment.[1] Urinary diversion in the form of an indwelling transurethral catheter and an abdominal drain or pigtail catheter may be necessary prior to definitive surgical treatment. Stabilization of patients diagnosed with uroabdomen is discussed in Chapter 17. Lacerations or ruptures of the bladder are surgically treated via debridement of the affected area, followed by one- or two-layer closure with a simple interrupted or continuous suture pattern. An absorbable monofilament suture material is generally chosen, such as polydioxanone, polyglycolic acid, or poliglecaprone 25. Nonabsorbable and braided suture materials have been implicated in the formation of uroliths and should therefore be avoided. Suture-associated calculi formation has also been associated with prolonged exposure of the suture to urine, thus it is recommended to avoid full-thickness bites (i.e., suture entering the bladder lumen) when possible.[33]

In humans, it has been reported that up to 75% of the urinary bladder may be resected without long-term changes to bladder function.[34] The exact amount of bladder that can be removed in small animals is unknown. It has been described that up to 70%–75% of the bladder may be removed without long-term incontinence, but persistent pollakiuria may occur.[35] It is important to preserve the trigone region, as regeneration of the bladder mucosa is secondary to the epithelium of the terminal ureters and urethra.[36]

Surgical technique: Partial cystectomy

1. A caudal abdominal incision is made from the umbilicus to the pubis. The abdomen is explored.
2. The bladder is exteriorized, isolated with moistened laparotomy swabs, and evaluated for necrosis, rupture, laceration, and other signs of trauma.
3. Placement of stay sutures, using 2-0 or 3-0 absorbable or nonabsorbable monofilament, can be helpful to manipulate the bladder.
4. Any necrotic or highly traumatized areas of the bladder should be trimmed with delicate scissors (e.g., Metzenbaum scissors) and removed.
5. Lacerations of the bladder should have the edges trimmed and reapposed.
6. The bladder is generally closed with a single-layer appositional pattern (simple interrupted or simple continuous) using 3-0 or 4-0 absorbable monofilament material. Include the submucosa in each suture bite.
   - If a large amount of bladder tissue has been resected, closure over a Foley catheter bulb can help ensure patency of the bladder lumen.
   - If the tissue at the suture line is questionable or if there is tension on the suture line, a serosal patch from the antimesenteric border of a loop of small intestine can be used. Alternatively, the area can be omentalized or buttressed with porcine small intestinal submucosa.
7. Urine and/or bladder tissue should be submitted for culture.
8. If a large amount of bladder has been removed, an indwelling urinary catheter can be maintained to monitor urine output and alleviate tension on the suture line.

Postoperative management and outcome

A urinary catheter is commonly placed after bladder repair to limit tension on the repair by keeping the bladder decompressed and is useful to monitor urine output following surgery. The bladder typically heals quickly compared to other organs, with 100% tissue strength present 14–21 days following injury.[31,37] Urine leakage following bladder surgery is rare, with one study reporting a 1.4% occurrence rate, but it is the most frequently reported postoperative complication. There has been no association found between bladder closure pattern and postoperative urine leakage, and an appositional single-layer closure pattern is safe and effective, with a minimal risk of urine leakage.[38] Inflammation of the lower urinary tract is common following bladder surgery, and signs such as pollakiuria, hematuria, and straining may be seen during the postoperative recovery period; these are typically self-limiting. Incontinence following partial cystectomy is extremely rare, but care should be taken to preserve the dorsal neurovascular pedicle of the bladder trigone to prevent this complication. Decreased bladder volume is possible following partial cystectomy, and is more likely after resection of >70% of the bladder or resection of the trigone.[35] Prognosis following a diagnosis of uroabdomen is largely dependent on the location of the urinary tract injury and concurrent injuries. Reported survival rates following a diagnosis of uroabdomen range from 62% to 79%.[31,39,40]

Urethral trauma

Urethral tears can occur secondary to many causes, including obstructive urethral calculi, blunt or penetrating trauma, iatrogenic causes (e.g., urethral catheter placement, inadvertent trauma during abdominal surgery, prescrotal castration, perineal herniorrhaphy), and obstruction or necrosis secondary to urethral neoplasia. In cats, the most common etiologies are vehicular trauma or iatrogenic damage to the urethra following attempted catheterization. The most common cause in dogs has been reported to be vehicular trauma, which may be associated with pelvic fractures.[41,42]

Clinical presentation and diagnosis

Clinical signs may include hematuria, dysuria, and anuria. There may be bruising in the abdominal or inguinal region. If there is a proximal urethral tear, uroabdomen may be present. In cases of pelvic or penile urethral injury, it is common for perineal, inguinal, and/or preputial bruising and swelling to occur. Some patients may be hemodynamically unstable, dehydrated, or azotemic, and electrolyte abnormalities may be present. In case of abdominal effusion, it should be analyzed, and a diagnosis of uroabdomen may be made by comparing the fluid creatinine and potassium concentrations with those of peripheral blood, as discussed earlier in this chapter.[43]

Positive-contrast studies are generally the diagnostic tool of choice for urethral tears. They may be performed with a normograde or retrograde contrast cystourethrogram, and either radiographs or fluoroscopy can aid in diagnosis. Gentle urethral catheterization can be attempted, and if this is possible, a portion of the urethra is likely intact, indicating partial rupture or laceration.[44] If performing a retrograde cystourethrogram, the urinary catheter should be backed out of the bladder and contrast should be injected as the urinary catheter is removed to facilitate evaluation of the entire urethra. Alternatively, if a radiological study is being performed, the entire contrast volume can be administered into the bladder, and a voiding cystogram can be performed with gentle bladder expression and serial radiographs. It is important to ensure that the penile urethra is imaged by pulling the hind limbs forward during the radiographic or fluoroscopic study. Extravasation of contrast medium from the urethra is diagnostic for a urethral tear (Fig. 18.6), but in cases of complete tearing of the urethra, contrast does not usually flow past the tear.[32] As discussed previously, contrast CT may be useful to evaluate the entire urinary tract as well as to assess for concurrent injuries in cases of trauma.

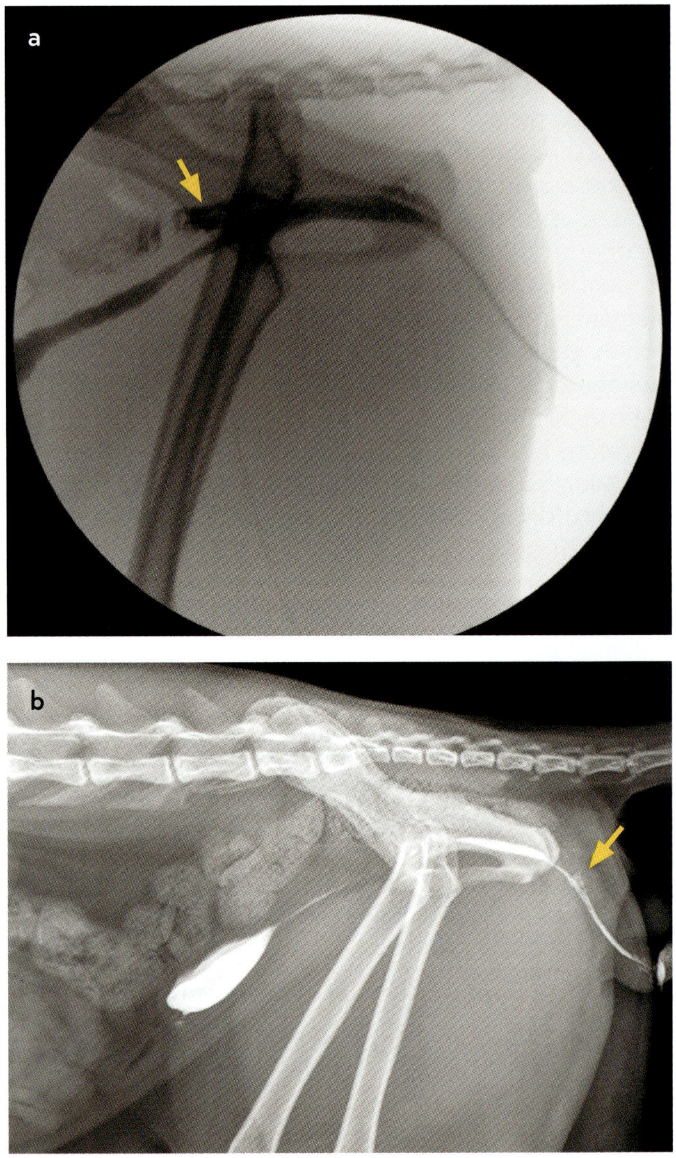

Figure 18.6 (a) Fluoroscopic retrograde contrast cystourethrogram in a dog with a mid-urethral tear. (b) Radiographic retrograde contrast cystourethrogram in a cat with a distal urethral tear. The yellow arrows highlight extravasation of contrast from the urethra.

Treatment

Urethral tears can be treated by conservative management with a transurethral catheter to achieve second-intention healing, by surgical repair, or by permanent urinary diversion. Treatment options should be considered based on the severity and location of the urethral injury. Permanent urinary diversion should be considered for irreparable injury to the distal urethra.

Conservative management can be considered in cases of partial rupture of the urethra. Temporary urinary diversion is necessary to prevent urine extravasation, which is toxic to the local tissues and can lead to necrosis. It is likely that temporary urinary diversion improves outcomes in patients with urethral injury, irrespective of which treatment option is chosen.[41] Urinary diversion may be implemented with placement of a transurethral catheter, a cystostomy tube or pigtail catheter, or both. The transurethral catheter may have advantages in alignment of the urethral mucosa and aid in mucosal healing.[43] Studies have shown that the urethral mucosa takes approximately 7 days to regenerate, and therefore at least 7 days of urinary diversion may be needed in cases of significant trauma to the urethra. However, the duration of urinary diversion is controversial, and studies have reported successful outcomes with urinary diversion times ranging from 3 to 21 days.[41,42,44] Prior to cessation of temporary urinary diversion, a contrast cystourethrogram should be performed, and it is likely prudent to repeat the study in 3–5 days following discontinuation of urinary diversion.[43]

If conservative management fails or if there is complete transection of the urethra, surgery is generally indicated. For primary repair or anastomosis of the urethra, the approach depends on the location of the tear, and pubic osteotomy may be required if the injury is in the pelvic canal. The ends of the urethra should be debrided and apposed and sutured with fine absorbable suture (usually 4-0 to 5-0 in dogs). The risk of stricture formation may be decreased if the anastomosis is performed over a urethral catheter.[45] An interrupted suture pattern is generally used to ensure appropriate alignment of the urethra, and each bite should include mucosa and submucosa. Tension at the repair or anastomosis site should be avoided, as dehiscence of the repair is more likely.

Permanent urinary diversion via urethrostomy bypasses the area of urethral injury, and the urethrostomy site depends on the location of the urethral injury. Scrotal urethrostomy is the treatment of choice in male dogs, as this is where the urethra is most superficial and wide.[46] Either a continuous or interrupted suture pattern may be used, ensuring bites are taken in the urethral mucosa and the skin. Fine absorbable suture material is generally used at the authors' institution. In male cats, perineal urethrostomy is most frequently performed. For more proximal defects, transpelvic and prepubic urethrostomy may be considered, with preference given to a transpelvic urethrostomy, as it is associated with a lower complication rate than prepubic osteotomy.[47] The specific surgical techniques for permanent urethrostomy and urethral resection and anastomosis are discussed in Chapter 19.

Postoperative management and outcome

Conservative management of urethral injuries with temporary urinary diversion has been reported to have a good prognosis, with success rates of up to 80% reported in the literature.[44] However, stricture formation and urinary tract infection have been associated with conservative management. It has been reported that a decrease in lumen size >60% may be necessary before clinical signs of stranguria develop; therefore, it is possible that stricture formation is more common than is reported.[45] Complications of urethral repair/anastomosis and urethrostomy include urinary tract infection, dehiscence, stricture, urine extravasation, and the development of lower urinary tract signs. The most common complication is urinary tract infection, which may occur during or after treatment. Success rates for perineal urethrostomy in cats are very good, with more recent studies reporting low major complication rates. Urinary tract infection following perineal urethrostomy in cats has been reported to occur in 22%–33% of cats, but most resolve after one course of targeted antibiotic therapy.[47,48] Studies have reported owner satisfaction rates of 88%–89% following perineal or transpelvic urethrostomy in cats, supporting the overall good prognosis for cats treated with these techniques.[49,50] Scrotal urethrostomy in dogs is also associated with a good long-term prognosis, with self-limiting postoperative hemorrhage being the most common short-term complication. Dehiscence, stricture, incisional infection, and incontinence have been suggested as potential complications but were extremely rare or not reported in two recent studies.[46,51]

Overall, outcomes for urethral injuries secondary to iatrogenic causes have a better prognosis than those caused by trauma. A good outcome is seen in 83%–91% of iatrogenic urethral injury and 50%–57% following traumatic urethral rupture.[41,43]

Urethral prolapse

Urethral prolapse is a term for the condition in which the urethral mucosa protrudes beyond the tip of the penis. It occurs most commonly in young, male, intact brachycephalic dogs and Yorkshire Terriers. The English Bulldog was the most commonly affected breed in one study and at the authors' institution.[52] The exact cause is unknown, but sexual excitement, uroliths, urinary tract infection, and developmental abnormalities have been suggested as contributing factors.

Clinical presentation and diagnosis

Many dogs with urethral prolapse present with mild to severe hemorrhage from the penis. A red or purple blister-like mass may be seen at the tip of the penis. Some dogs have hematuria or a history of self-trauma to the penis (Fig. 18.7).

Treatment

Treatment recommendations are generally surgical and can include urethral mucosal resection and anastomosis, urethropexy, or urethral mucosal reduction with purse-string suture placement. At the authors' institution, urethral resection and anastomosis is preferred, with or without urethropexy.

Surgical technique: Urethral resection and anastomosis

1. With the patient in dorsal recumbency, the penis is extruded and an appropriately sized red rubber catheter is placed in the urethra. A Penrose drain can be placed around the extruded penis and clamped with a hemostat to maintain penile extrusion.

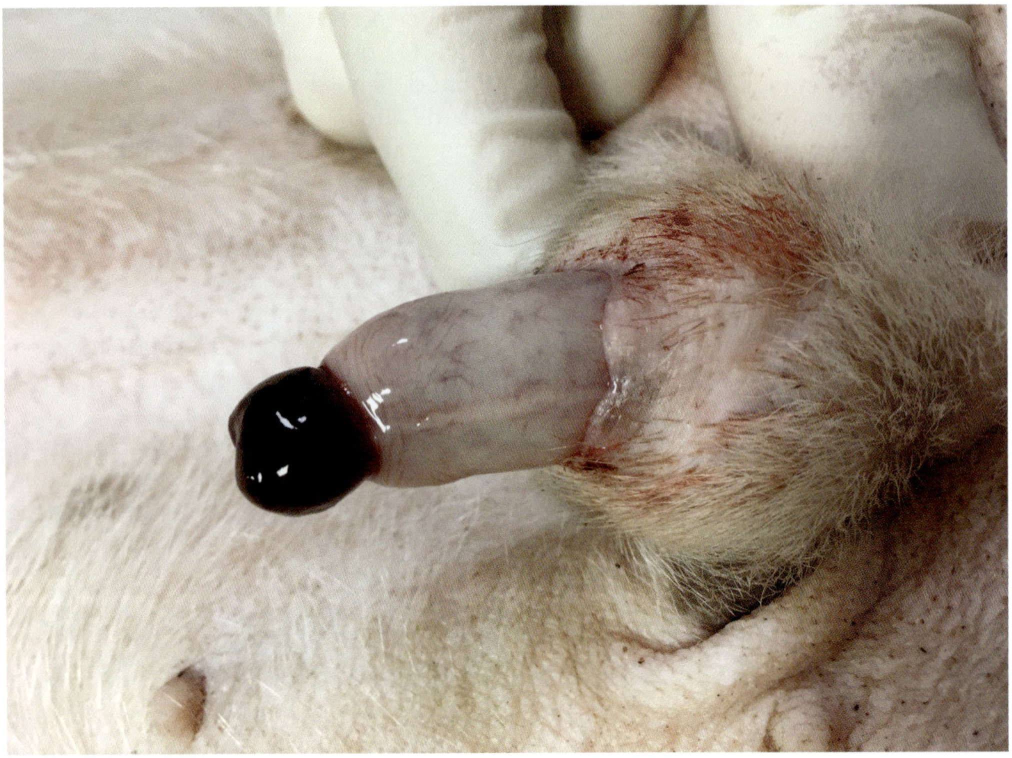

Figure 18.7 Urethral prolapse in a 7-year-old English Bulldog. Image courtesy of Filippo Cinti.

2. The prolapsed urethral tissue can be grasped with forceps, or stay sutures can be placed within it, to retract the tissue and allow for circumferential resection of the prolapsed urethral tissue.
3. The urethral mucosa should then be sutured to the penis using fine (4-0 to 6-0) absorbable monofilament in a simple continuous or interrupted pattern (placing the knot on the external surface).
4. Alternatively, transect one-third to one-half of the base of the prolapsed tissue around the circumference of the prolapse and start the anastomosis at one end of the transection. Once several sutures have been placed, continue to cut and suture the mucosa in stages until the entire circumference of prolapsed urethral mucosa is resected and anastomosed to the penile mucosa (Fig. 18.8).

Surgical technique: Urethropexy

1. With the patient in dorsal recumbency, the penis is extruded, and a grooved director is placed in the urethral orifice. If a previous resection and anastomosis has not been performed, the grooved director can help to reduce the prolapsed tissue.
2. At least two horizontal mattress sutures should be placed through the urethral mucosa and penile body to maintain reduction of the urethral tissue.
   a. A large-diameter taper-point needle (2-0 to 3-0 absorbable or nonabsorbable monofilament suture) should be passed from the external surface of the penis as far distal to the urethral orifice as the needle diameter allows.
   b. The needle is directed outwardly toward the urethral orifice and out through it. The grooved director helps prevent penetration of the opposite urethral mucosa.
   c. The needle is then passed back through the urethral orifice to the external surface of the penis, exiting at least 0.5 cm distal (toward the urethral orifice) from the initial suture bite through the penile body. The suture can then be tied, using caution not to tie this suture too tightly.
3. At least two sutures are placed equidistant to each other. The authors prefer to place four horizontal mattress sutures.
4. A urethral catheter of appropriate size should be passed to ensure that the urethral lumen is patent.

Postoperative management and outcome

Postoperative hemorrhage from the penis is the most commonly reported complication of surgical treatment of urethral prolapse and was reported in 39% of dogs in a recent study.[52] This study found that a continuous suture pattern for urethral resection and anastomosis was less likely to result in postoperative hemorrhage.

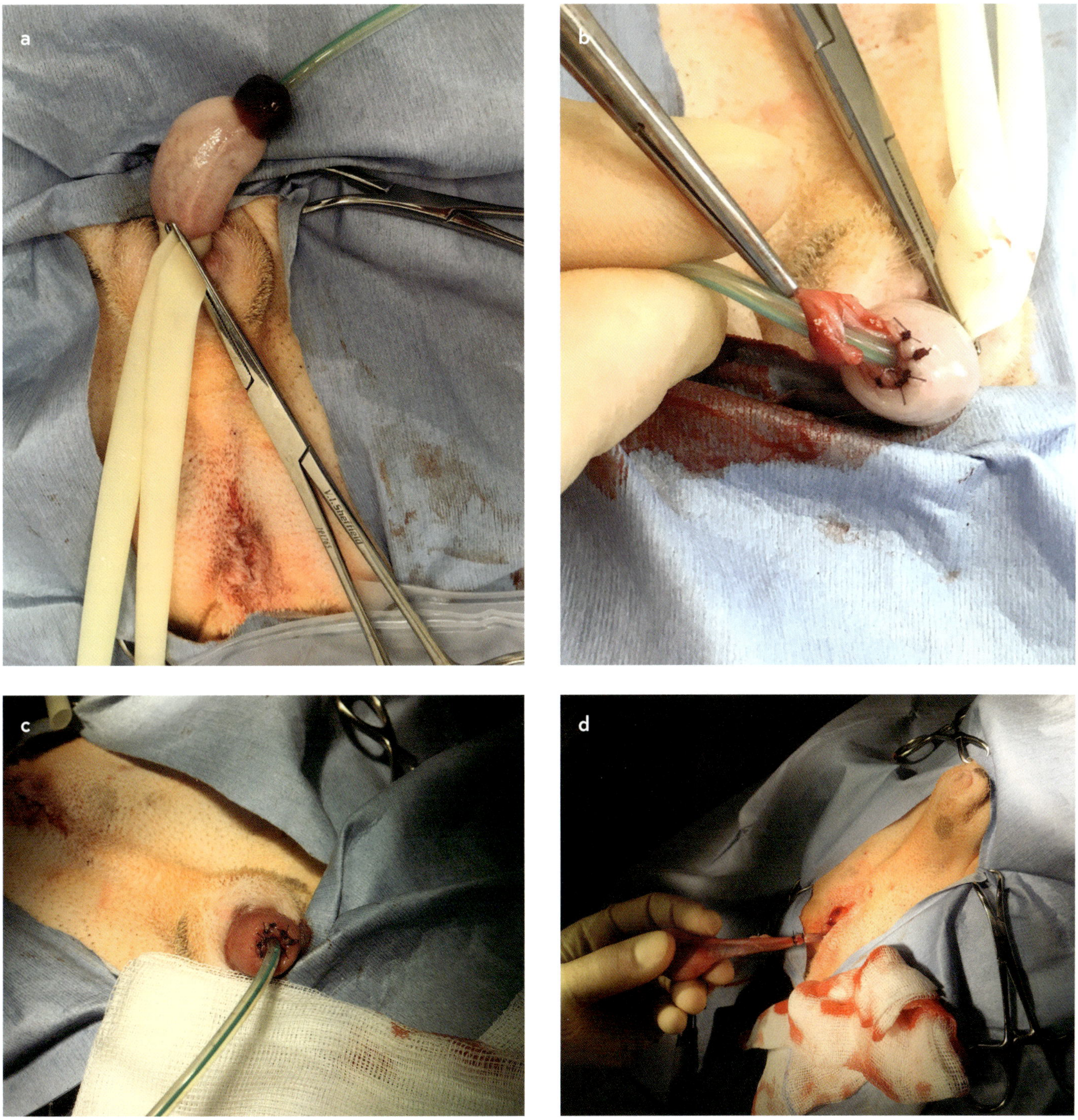

Figure 18.8 Urethral resection and anastomosis for treatment of a urethral prolapse. (a) The penis is extruded, a urinary catheter is placed in the urethra, and a Penrose drain is placed around the extruded penis. (b) Stages of resection and anastomosis are performed, with full-thickness simple interrupted sutures. (c) Final appearance after resection and anastomosis. (d) Prescrotal castration. Images courtesy of Filippo Cinti.

Recurrence of urethral prolapse is often reported and was seen in 57% of dogs in the same study. Recurrence was less frequent when sedatives were prescribed postoperatively, and they are routinely recommended at the authors' institution.[52] In a more recent study, recurrence was seen in up to 26.6% of cases, and was significantly higher in dogs that received a urethropexy alone for treatment (38.6% vs. 11% in dogs that received a urethral resection and anastomosis).[53] Routine castration is also recommended at the time of prolapse correction, although there is limited data on the impact of castration status on outcomes.

KEEP IN MIND

- Contrast cystography (normograde or retrograde) should be used to identify lower urinary tract trauma.
- Intravenous pyelography or contrast computed tomography should be used to identify upper urinary tract trauma. Abdominal ultrasound is useful in combination with both intravenous pyelography and cystourethrography.
- The most common site of urinary tract rupture causing uroabdomen in dogs and cats is the urinary bladder.
- Urinary diversion should be instituted, when possible, in cases of urinary tract injury in an unstable patient prior to general anesthesia and definitive surgery. This will make the patient a better anesthetic candidate and may decrease morbidity and/or mortality.
- Magnification or an operating microscope are invaluable when performing surgery on the upper urinary tract.

References

1. Stafford JR, Bartges JW. A clinical review of pathophysiology, diagnosis, and treatment of uroabdomen in the dog and cat. *J Vet Emerg Crit Care (San Antonio)*. 2013; 23(2):216–229.
2. Millward IR. Avulsion of the left renal artery following blunt abdominal trauma in a dog. *J Small Anim Pract*. 2009; 50(1):38–43.
3. Habing AM, Bryon JK. Imaging of the urinary tract. In: Weisse C, Berent A (eds.). *Veterinary Image-Guided Interventions*. Somerset, NJ: John Wiley & Sons; 2015. pp. 263–287.
4. Choi SY, Jeong WC, Lee YW, Choi HJ. Contrast enhanced ultrasonography of kidney in conscious and anesthetized beagle dogs. *J Vet Med Sci*. 2016; 78(2):239–244.
5. Dong Y et al. Quantitative evaluation of contrast-enhanced ultrasonography in the diagnosis of chronic ischemic renal disease in a dog model. *PLoS One*. 2013; 8(8):e70337.
6. Harris AC et al. CT findings in blunt renal trauma. *Radiographics*. 2001; 21(S1):S201–S214.
7. Goldman SM, Sandler CM. Urogenital trauma: Imaging upper GU trauma. *Eur J Radiol*. 2004; 50(1):84–95.
8. Weisse C, Aronson LR, Drobatz K. Traumatic rupture of the ureter: 10 cases. *J Am Anim Hosp Assoc*. 2002; 38(2):188–192.
9. Rosenblum ST, Aronson LR. Bilateral renal descensus and intravesicular ureteroneocystostomy for treatment of bilateral ureteral ligation and transection that occurred during ovariohysterectomy in two cats. *J Am Vet Med Assoc*. 2021; 260(1):100–109.
10. Dekerle B et al. Feline ureteral rupture with para-ureteral urinomas following blunt trauma: Clinical presentation and long-term outcome after treatment by urinary diversion for five cases from 2012 to 2019. *N Z Vet J*. 2023; 71(2):92–99.
11. Moores AP, Bell AM, Costello M. Urinoma (para-ureteral pseudocyst) as a consequence of trauma in a cat. *J Small Anim Pract*. 2002; 43(5):213–216.
12. Worth AJ, Tomlin SC. Post-traumatic paraureteral urinoma in a cat. *J Small Anim Pract*. 2004; 45(8):413–416.
13. Wormser C, Clarke DL, Aronson LR. End-to-end ureteral anastomosis and double-pigtail ureteral stent placement for treatment of iatrogenic ureteral trauma in two dogs. *J Am Vet Med Assoc*. 2015; 247(1):92–97.
14. Hamilton MH, Sissener TR, Baines SJ. Traumatic bilateral ureteric rupture in two dogs. *J Small Anim Pract*. 2006; 47(12):737–740.
15. Etedali NM, Reetz JA, Foster JD. Complications and clinical utility of ultrasonographically guided pyelocentesis and antegrade pyelography in cats and dogs: 49 cases (2007–2015). *J Am Vet Med Assoc*. 2019; 254(7):826–834.
16. Wen JG, Frøkiaer J, Jørgensen TM, Djurhuus JC. Obstructive nephropathy: An update of the experimental research. *Urol Res*. 1999; 27(1):29–39.
17. Brodsky SL, Zimskind PD, Dure-Smith P, Lewis PL. Effects of crush and devascularizing injuries to the proximal ureter. An experimental study. *Invest Urol*. 1977; 14(5):361–365.
18. Phillips H. Urinary tract trauma. In: Monnet E (ed.). *Small Animal Soft Tissue Surgery*. John Wiley & Sons; 2023. pp. 589–604.
19. Matthews K. Ureters. In: Johnston S, Tobias K (ed.). *Veterinary Surgery*, 2nd ed. St. Louis, MO: Elsevier; 2018. pp. 2202–2218.
20. Aronson LR, Cleroux A, Wormser C. Use of a modified Boari flap for the treatment of a proximal ureteral obstruction in a cat. *Vet Surg*. 2018; 47(4):578–585.
21. Nurra G et al. Clinical use and complications of percutaneous cystostomy pigtail catheters in 25 cats. *J Feline Med Surg*. 2022; 24(6):e28–e33.
22. Boullenger J et al. Transmural migration of a subcutaneous ureteral bypass into the intestine in three cats. *J Small Anim Pract*. 2022; 63(10):792–796.
23. Wuillemin F, Vachon C, Beauchamp G, Dunn M. Subcutaneous ureteral bypass device placement in 81 cats with benign ureteral obstruction (2013–2018). *J Vet Intern Med*. 2021; 35(6):2778–2786.
24. Kulendra NJ et al. Survival and complications in cats treated with subcutaneous ureteral bypass. *J Small Anim Pract*. 2021; 62(1):4–11.
25. Nicoli S et al. Double-J ureteral stenting in nine cats with ureteral obstruction. *Vet J*. 2012; 194(1):60–65.
26. Plater BL, Lipscomb VJ. Treatment and outcomes of ureter injuries due to ovariohysterectomy complications in cats and dogs. *J Small Anim Pract*. 2020; 61(3):170–176.
27. Lorange M, Monnet E. Postoperative outcomes of 12 cats with ureteral obstruction treated with ureteroneocystostomy. *Vet Surg*. 2020; 49(7):1418–1427.
28. Hoffberg JE, Koenigshof AM, Guiot LP. Retrospective evaluation of concurrent intra-abdominal injuries in dogs with traumatic pelvic fractures: 83 cases (2008–2013). *J Vet Emerg Crit Care (San Antonio)*. 2016; 26(2):288–294.
29. Selcer B. Urinary tract trauma associated with pelvic trauma. *J Am Anim Hosp Assoc*. 1982; 19:785–793.
30. Press S, Balakrishnan A. Uroabdomen. In: Drobatz KJ, Hopper K, Rozanski E, Silverstein DC (eds.). *Textbook of Small Animal Emergency Medicine*. John Wiley & Sons; 2018. pp. 659–664.

31. Aumann M, Worth LT, Drobatz KJ. Uroperitoneum in cats: 26 cases (1986–1995). *J Am Anim Hosp Assoc.* 1998; 34(4):315–324.
32. Bischoff MG. Radiographic techniques and interpretation of the acute abdomen. *Clin Tech Small Anim Pract.* 2003; 18(1):7–19.
33. Appel SL et al. Evaluation of risk factors associated with suture-nidus cystoliths in dogs and cats: 176 cases (1999–2006). *J Am Vet Med Assoc.* 2008; 233(12):1889–1895.
34. Peacock E. Healing and repair of peritoneum and viscera. In: Peacock E (ed.). *Wound Repair*, 3rd ed. Philadelphia, PA: Saunders; 1984. p. 438.
35. Stone EA, George TF, Gilson SD, Page RL. Partial cystectomy for urinary bladder neoplasia: Surgical technique and outcome in 11 dogs. *J Small Anim Pract.* 1996; 37(10):480–485.
36. Wishnow KI et al. Regeneration of the canine urinary bladder mucosa after complete surgical denudation. *J Urol.* 1989; 141(6):1476–1479.
37. Bellah JR. Wound healing in the urinary tract. *Semin Vet Med Surg Small Anim.* 1989; 4(4):294–303.
38. Thieman-Mankin KM, Ellison GW, Jeyapaul CJ, Glotfelty-Ortiz CS. Comparison of short-term complication rates between dogs and cats undergoing appositional single-layer or inverting double-layer cystotomy closure: 144 cases (1993–2010). *J Am Vet Med Assoc.* 2012; 240(1):65–68.
39. Grimes JA, Fletcher JM, Schmiedt CW. Outcomes in dogs with uroabdomen: 43 cases (2006–2015). *J Am Vet Med Assoc.* 2018; 252(1):92–97.
40. Hornsey SJ et al. Factors affecting survival to discharge in 53 cats diagnosed with uroabdomen: A single-centre retrospective analysis. *J Feline Med Surg.* 2021; 23(2):115–120.
41. Anderson RB, Aronson LR, Drobatz KJ, Atilla A. Prognostic factors for successful outcome following urethral rupture in dogs and cats. *J Am Anim Hosp Assoc.* 2006; 42(2):136–146.
42. Addison ES et al. A retrospective analysis of urethral rupture in 63 cats. *J Feline Med Surg.* 2014; 16(4):300–307.
43. Addison ES, Yool DA. Urethral trauma. In: Drobatz KJ, Hopper K, Rozanski E, Silverstein DC (eds.). *Textbook of Small Animal Emergency Medicine*. John Wiley & Sons; 2018. pp. 641–645.
44. Meige F, Sarrau S, Autefage A. Management of traumatic urethral rupture in 11 cats using primary alignment with a urethral catheter. *Vet Comp Orthop Traumatol.* 2008; 21(1):76–84.
45. Layton CE, Ferguson HR, Cook JE, Guffy MM. Intrapelvic urethral anastomosis. A comparison of three techniques. *Vet Surg.* 1987; 16(2):175–182.
46. Burrow RD, Gregory SP, Giejda AA, White RN. Penile amputation and scrotal urethrostomy in 18 dogs. *Vet Rec.* 2011; 169(25):657.
47. Sousa-Filho RP et al. Clinical outcomes of 28 cats 12–24 months after urethrostomy. *J Feline Med Surg.* 2020; 22(10):890–897.
48. Watson MT, Roca RY, Breiteneicher AH, Kalis RH. Evaluation of postoperative complication rates in cats undergoing perineal urethrostomy performed in dorsal recumbency. *J Feline Med Surg.* 2020; 22(4):399–403.
49. Ruda L, Heiene R. Short- and long-term outcome after perineal urethrostomy in 86 cats with feline lower urinary tract disease. *J Small Anim Pract.* 2012; 53(12):693–698.
50. Dumartinet C, Bernard F, Bernardé A. Outcomes and postoperative complications after transpelvic urethrostomy used as first-line surgery in 38 male cats with obstructive lower urinary tract disease. *J Feline Med Surg.* 2022; 24(6):558–564.
51. Newton JD, Smeak DD. Simple continuous closure of canine scrotal urethrostomy: Results in 20 cases. *J Am Anim Hosp Assoc.* 1996; 32(6):531–534.
52. Carr JG, Tobias KM, Smith L. Urethral prolapse in dogs: A retrospective study. *Vet Surg.* 2014; 43(5):574–580.
53. Healy D et al. Surgical treatment of canine urethral prolapse via urethropexy or resection and anastomosis. *J Small Anim 2024; 65(3):206–213.*
54. Paes PRO et al. Laboratory diagnosis of canine uroperitoneum based on cellular and biochemical characteristics of serum and abdominal fluid. *Vet Clin Pathol.* 2022; 51(1):107–111.

Chapter 19

Urinary tract obstruction

Lillian R. Aronson, Marie Burneko

Ureteral obstruction

Ureteral obstruction in companion animals may be congenital or acquired, benign or malignant, and it is a common indication for surgery in dogs and cats. Although urolithiasis is most common, other causes of obstruction encountered in our veterinary patients include congenital narrowing, dried solidified blood calculi, iatrogenic ureteral ligation, ureteritis, fibrosis, ureteral spasm, stricture, ureteral ectopia, retroperitoneal fibrosis following renal transplantation, and neoplasia.[1–6] The impact of any obstruction on renal hemodynamic variables and glomerular filtration rate, and ultimately the recovery of renal function, is influenced by the baseline condition of the kidneys, chronicity and degree of obstruction (unilateral or bilateral, partial or complete), concurrent use of nephrotoxic medications (e.g., nonsteroidal anti-inflammatory drugs), presence of infection, and whether or not the obstruction persists or has been relieved. Unfortunately, in many veterinary patients presenting with a unilateral ureteral obstruction, it is unclear if surgery will result in improvement of renal function, since the duration of the obstruction is often unknown.

Calcium oxalate (CaOx) is the predominant stone type identified in the ureter of cats. In one feline report, 98% of ureteral stones were composed of CaOx; 87% containing CaOx alone and 11% containing CaOx in addition to another mineral source.[7] These stones form in the renal pelvis and may subsequently migrate into the ureter, resulting in a partial or complete ureteral obstruction. Often in cats, a small, marginally functional and fibrotic, nonobstructed kidney is identified in conjunction with an enlarged, hydronephrotic obstructed contralateral kidney (often referred to as big kidney little kidney syndrome); however, both partial and complete bilaterally obstructed kidneys are also identified. Most cases presenting with a unilateral or bilateral obstruction secondary to urolithiasis also have underlying chronic renal disease from nonspecific interstitial nephritis and fibrosis. In a report evaluating the clinical, clinicopathologic, radiographic, and ultrasonographic abnormalities in cats with ureteral calculi, 76% (58/76) of cats that had a unilateral ureteral obstruction were azotemic and 55% (39/70) of cats had a small contralateral kidney.[7] In another report looking at the diagnosis and surgical management of obstructive ureteral calculi in cats, in 2 of 3 cats that had the glomerular filtration rate evaluated, the obstructed kidney contributed more than 75% to this rate.[1]

Limited information currently exists in the veterinary literature regarding the medical and surgical management of ureterolithiasis in dogs. In one report describing the surgical management of 16 cases, a similar proportion of struvite and CaOx stones were identified.[8] Unlike in cats, obstructive pyonephrosis secondary to ureterolithiasis is commonly identified in many of our canine patients.[8,9]

Although this section focuses on the clinical presentation and management of ureteral obstruction in dogs and cats secondary to urolithiasis, the surgical techniques described are universally used for many of the previously mentioned conditions that can result in obstruction.

Clinical presentation and diagnosis

Clinical presentation, as well as results of imaging studies, helps guide the clinician on the best approach for a given patient. Cats with uroliths affecting the ureter can present asymptomatic or with nonspecific clinical signs, including lethargy, weight loss, anorexia, vomiting, fever, polydipsia, and polyuria. Other signs of uremia, including oral ulcerations, may be observed. Hematuria may or may not be present. Patients may also show abdominal pain and splinting or renomegaly and a variable bladder size. Additionally, depending on the chronicity of the condition, cats may present unthrifty, with significant loss of muscle mass. Dogs more commonly present with signs of dysuria, stranguria, hematuria, polyuria, pollakiuria, incontinence, and signs of systemic illness often associated with pyelonephritis.

Diagnostic evaluation should include a complete physical examination, complete blood count and biochemical profile, and urinalysis and culture, as many affected patients are older and may have concurrent diseases. Additionally, a coagulation profile may be indicated for patients presenting with pyelonephritis and/or pyonephrosis if urosepsis is a concern. If pyelography is performed, a urine sample for culture should be collected from the renal pelvis, since in patients with complete ureteral obstruction, urine culture results from urine collected by cystocentesis may not be representative of urine collected from an obstructed kidney. For patients presenting with a heart murmur on auscultation, electrocardiography and echocardiography are indicated. Cardiac murmurs may be secondary to anemia, fluid overload, uremic toxins resulting in myocardial dysfunction, or primary heart disease.

Imaging including survey radiography and ultrasonography should be performed on all patients at the time of presentation. Plain abdominal radiography can be helpful with surgical planning by providing information on the number and location of radiopaque renal and/or ureteral calculi. Abdominal radiography has been shown to have 100% specificity, but only 66% sensitivity, for identifying ureteroliths in cats.[10] It is important to note that very small ureteroliths, radiolucent ureteroliths, or those overlying colonic contents or vertebral bodies are occasionally missed. In a retrospective study investigating the radiographic distribution of ureteral stones in 78 cats, 44% were identified in the proximal ureter, 41% were in the midureter, and 15% at the ureterovesicular junction. Additionally, larger stones were often lodged in a proximal location, and stones at the ureterovesicular junction were most commonly identified in male cats.[11]

Ultrasonography is often performed in conjunction with plain radiography and allows assessment of the degree of hydronephrosis and/or hydroureter, of the renal parenchyma, and for any evidence of perirenal inflammation or effusion. Uroliths are often identified as a hyperechoic, shadowing structure within the ureteral lumen. Dried solidified blood calculi are often either not identified at all on ultrasound or, occasionally, a small amount of mineralized, nonshadowing material may be seen. In a recent study on the diagnostic utility of ultrasonography for detecting the cause and location of obstruction, the sensitivity was 98% and 44% and the specificity was 96% and 98% for detection of ureteroliths and strictures, respectively.[12] A renal pelvic width greater than or equal to 13 mm has been shown to indicate obstruction in dogs and cats; however, it is important to note that pelvic dilation can be identified in other nonobstructive conditions, such as pyelonephritis.[13] Conversely, the absence of significant dilation does not rule out an obstruction, as minimal renal pelvic dilation (<4 mm) has been associated with obstruction in some cats.[14]

If the presence of obstruction is still in question based on ultrasound findings, antegrade pyelography can be performed to provide a more definitive diagnosis prior to making treatment recommendations. Other techniques that may be employed to help identify small ureteroliths as well as delineate the level of the obstruction include compression radiography, intravenous urography, computed tomography angiography, and magnetic resonance imaging. It is important to note that ureteral dilation identified using one of these modalities does not always extend to the level of the obstruction. If no recognizable cortical tissue is present, surgical correction of the ureteral obstruction will likely be of no value to the patient.

Treatment

Medical

Unfortunately, for patients presenting with CaOx urolithiasis, medical dissolution is not possible. Therefore, surgical intervention is often recommended if the stones are causing clinical disease. If intervention is necessary, it is not always clear when ureteral calculi should be addressed. If patients are clinically stable, an initial period of medical management may be attempted, including the parenteral administration of fluids alone or in combination with diuretic therapy (mannitol) to determine if passage of ureteral calculi will occur. Additional therapies with anecdotal efficacy include the administration of various smooth muscle relaxants, including prazosin, and anti-inflammatory corticosteroids (Table 19.1). Because of the concern for nephron damage/loss, previous recommendations included only a short

TABLE 19.1 - MEDICAL THERAPY FOR USE IN CONJUNCTION WITH PARENTERAL ADMINISTRATION OF FLUIDS TO INDUCE PASSAGE OF URETERAL CALCULI IN CATS

Drug	Mechanism of action	Dose in cats
Mannitol	Osmotic diuretic to increase urine flow	1 g/kg IV over 30 min, then 60–120 mg/kg/h CRI can be considered
Prazosin	Alpha-1 antagonist for ureteral smooth muscle relaxation	0.125–0.5 mg/cat PO every 12–24 h
Corticosteroids	Anti-inflammatory	Dexamethasone (can be given during hospitalization): 0.05–0.1 mg/kg IV every 24 h followed by 0.05 mg/kg IV every 24 h Prednisolone: 0.5 mg/kg/day PO

course (24–72 h) of medical management to promote stone passage prior to surgical intervention. In a recent publication describing a large cohort of cats treated medically for benign ureteral obstruction secondary to a number of causes, including urolithiasis, pyonephrosis, and stricture, a higher success rate of medical management was identified and the median time to a successful outcome was 16 days (range, 3–115 days).[15] This information is encouraging and offers a reasonable alternative for owners who decline surgical options for their cat. The author has observed some cats diagnosed with ureteral obstruction secondary to probable ureteritis responding successfully to the administration of anti-inflammatory doses of oral corticosteroids.

Because of the high incidence (>75%) of urinary tract infections in dogs presenting for ureteral obstruction, broad-spectrum antimicrobial therapy is indicated. In the author's experience, if medical management does not appear to be effective within 24–48 hours and a partial or complete ureteral obstruction is present, or if the ureterolith is associated with an infection that does not respond to medical therapy, minimally invasive ureteral stent placement with or without surgical intervention is recommended. Additionally, in patients that are unstable, immediate intervention may be recommended.

Surgical

Patient stabilization prior to anesthesia and surgery is essential for survival. Dehydration and hypovolemia should be addressed with fluid therapy; however, fluid overload is a significant concern in these patients and regular evaluation of body weight, urine output, packed cell volume/total protein, and left atrial to aortic ratio (LA:Ao) should be performed. All patients should have an electrocardiogram performed, and if arrhythmias are identified and associated with hyperkalemia they should be treated accordingly. Regarding antibiotic treatment, the true incidence of concurrent pyelonephritis in patients with a ureteral obstruction is unclear but tends to be a more common complication in dogs. In the critically ill uremic patient, if the uremia is associated with infection, aggressive treatment is recommended and should not be delayed until culture samples are collected. Antibiotic choice is often influenced by species, recent antimicrobial therapy, and overall renal function. In dogs, the combination of ampicillin (22 mg/kg IV every 8 h) and enrofloxacin (10–15 mg/kg IV every 24 h) provides broad-spectrum coverage and is a reasonable choice pending culture and sensitivity results. In cats, if there is concern regarding the ability to safely dose enrofloxacin in order to be efficacious, then a combination of clindamycin (10 mg/kg IV every 12 h) and cefotaxime (40 mg/kg IV every 6 h) is another feasible option. Correction of anemia with packed red cell or whole blood transfusions that are crossmatched compatible should be considered if the packed cell volume is less than 20% and/or the patient has developed clinical signs associated with the anemia, including lethargy and anorexia.

Ureteral obstruction in our veterinary patients can be challenging to treat surgically. The decision-making process regarding the optimal timing for the procedure and specific surgical recommendations can vary from patient to patient and are often determined by the clinical presentation, degree of azotemia, imaging results, and surgical findings. Like in human medicine, the author prefers the use of natural tissues to address an obstruction, as this avoids many complications inherent to implants, but all the options should be considered at the time of surgery. In some cases, a combination of techniques may be warranted. An important consideration for the surgeon is the availability of equipment as well as long-term equipment costs. The small size of the feline and canine ureter necessitates appropriate training in the use of magnification, which is critical to success in these cases. In cats and small dogs, the author recommends ×8–×10 magnification provided by an operating microscope. In larger dogs, surgical loupes providing ×2.5–×4.5 magnification may be adequate.

Surgical technique: Ureterotomy

When one or two stones are present, particularly in the proximal to midureter, ureterotomy is a reasonable treatment option.

1. A ventral midline abdominal approach is made (see Chapter 3).
2. The site of obstruction is identified. Stones may be visible on inspection of the urinary tract or may be palpable along the length of the ureter.
3. Once the stones are located, the affected ureteral segment is isolated using silastic material placed proximally and distally to the obstruction (Fig. 19.1).

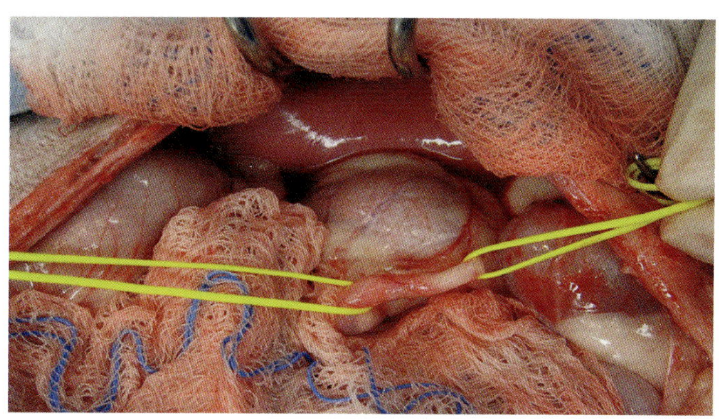

Figure 19.1 Isolation of the affected segment of ureter with silastic material placed proximally and distally to the ureteral obstruction.

In addition to maintaining the ureter in a fixed position for surgery, this prevents urine flow into the surgical field as well as the spontaneous retrograde movement of ureteroliths into the renal pelvis. Care should be taken when manipulating the ureter so as not to inadvertently traumatize it or disrupt its blood supply.

4. If the stone is mobile, a longitudinal incision is made in the dilated ureter just proximal to the obstruction, and the stone is removed using Jeweler's forceps. Occasionally, depending on the location, removal of multiple stones (>2) from the same ureterotomy incision may be possible.
5. In most cases, however, the stone is embedded within the wall of the ureter, and thus the incision must be made directly over the stone. For this, the author prefers a number 11 scalpel blade.
6. If the stone migrates into the renal pelvis during manipulation, a 22-gauge intravenous catheter can be inserted through the greater curvature of the kidney into the renal pelvis and flushing performed until the stone is expelled out of the ureterotomy site.
7. Prior to closure, a suture (3-0 to 5-0 prolene) can be placed distally through the ureterotomy site to prevent catching the back wall of the ureter during closure. The suture, which is acting as a stent, can be removed prior to the final suture being placed.
8. In cats and small dogs, closure of the ureterotomy site is completed using a full-thickness simple interrupted pattern with 8-0 or 9-0 nylon or polypropylene suture on a taper cut needle (Fig. 19.2). In medium- to large-sized dogs, 5-0 to 8-0 size suture may be more appropriate.
9. Following closure, the distal silastic is relieved first, followed by the proximal silastic, to reestablish urine flow. If an obvious leak is present, additional sutures can be placed.

Surgical technique: Ureteroneocystostomy

For stones lodged in the mid to distal ureter, a ureterotomy may be performed for urolith extraction, or the affected area of the ureter may be removed in toto and a ureteroneocystostomy performed. Both intravesicular and extravesicular techniques have been described and used successfully in both dogs and cats diagnosed with urolithiasis as well as cases of ureteral ectopia, congenital narrowing, trauma (including iatrogenic ureteral ligation), stricture, and neoplasia. Although previous literature recommends a ureteroneocystostomy for more distal obstructions, it is important to note that this procedure can be performed when only the proximal third of the ureter is available; however, tension-relieving techniques (e.g., renal descensus, cystopexy, cystonephropexy) may be necessary.

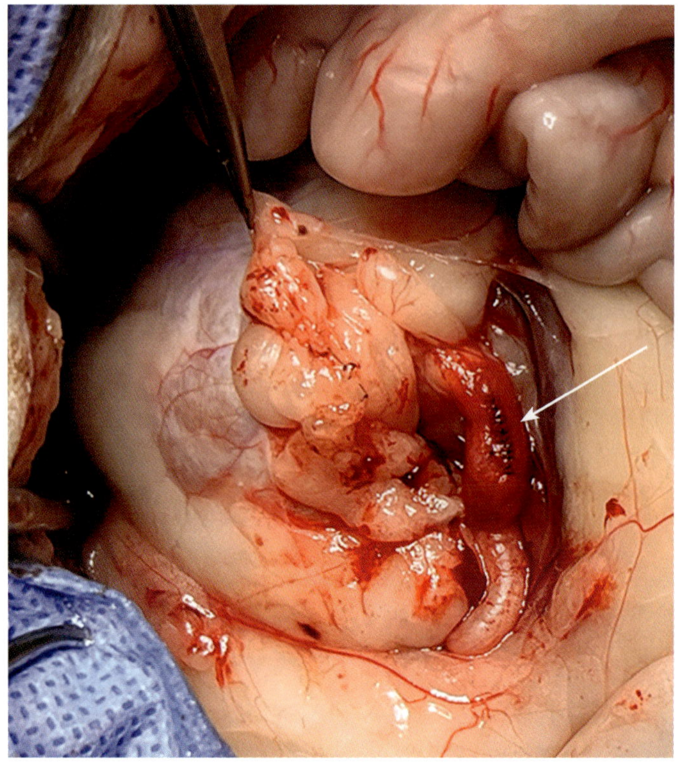

Figure 19.2 Ureterotomy closure (arrow) for a proximal ureteral obstruction in a cat using 8-0 nylon in a full-thickness simple interrupted pattern.

- To perform a renal descensus, the kidney is mobilized from its retroperitoneal attachments and moved caudally. The renal capsule is then sutured to an incision made in the adjacent body wall using four to six interrupted sutures of 4-0 polypropylene.
- For a cystopexy, the bladder is fixed cranially to the body wall or to the tendon of the psoas muscle using 3-0 to 4-0 absorbable or nonabsorbable sutures.
- When performing a cystonephropexy, additional sutures are placed between the bladder and the caudal pole of the kidney.

Intravesicular technique (Fig. 19.3)

1. A ventral midline cystotomy is performed.
2. Using a hemostat, the cut end of the ureter is brought directly into the bladder lumen through a hole created at the bladder apex.
3. The bladder is everted, the distal end of the ureter that was grasped with the hemostat is excised, the periureteral fat is removed, and the end of the ureter is spatulated for a distance of approximately 0.5–0.75 cm. If the ureter is very dilated, spatulation is not necessary.
4. The ureteral mucosa is sutured to the bladder mucosa using either absorbable or nonabsorbable monofilament material (5-0 to 9-0 depending on patient size and degree of ureteral dilation) in a simple inter-

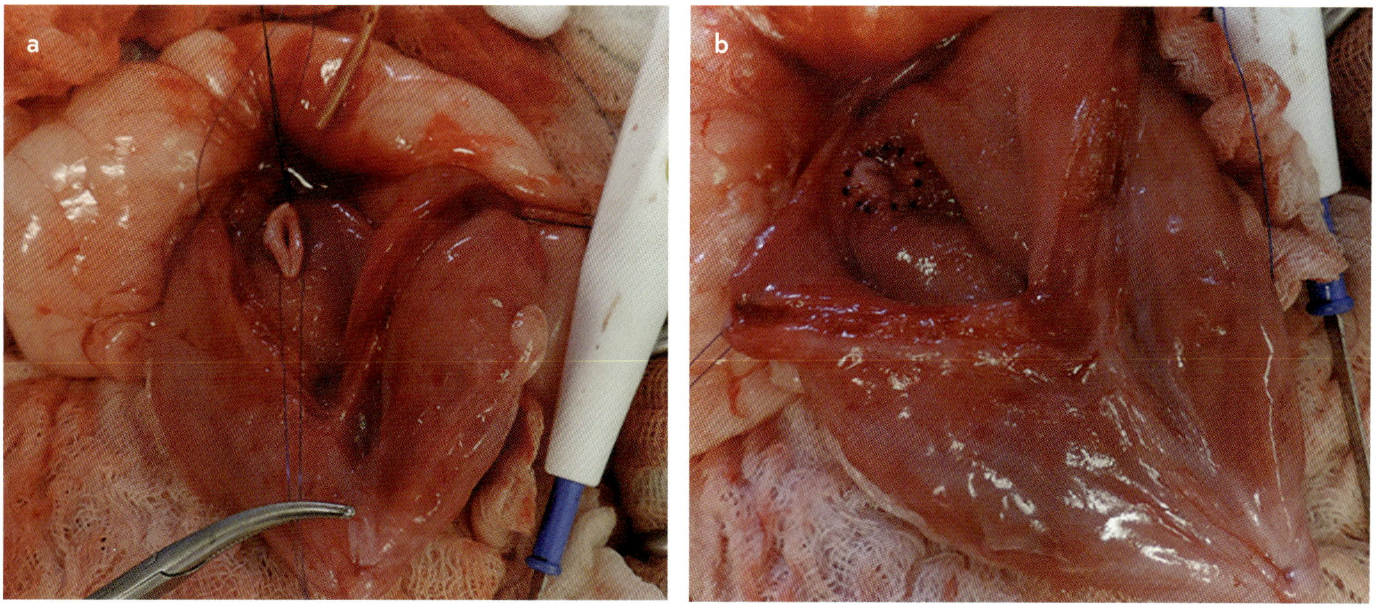

Figure 19.3 Intravesicular technique performed in a dog with a distal ureteral stricture. (a) The ureter is cut proximal to the area of pathology, which is resected, and the cut end of the ureter is brought directly into the bladder lumen through a hole created at the bladder apex using a hemostat. (b) The ureteral mucosa is sutured to the bladder mucosa using absorbable material (5-0 polydioxanone) in a simple interrupted pattern.

rupted pattern. Approximately eight to ten sutures are usually required.

5. To aid in stability of the anastomosis, a small bite of bladder wall can be incorporated with the mucosal bite at the crotch of spatulation and at the two other points of the triangle.
6. The ureter is examined to ensure ureteral patency by observing urine flow through the implantation site or by passing a suture retrogradely through the site into the distal ureter. Following completion of the anastomosis, the bladder is inverted and closed routinely.

Extravesicular technique (Fig. 19.4)

1. A 1 cm incision is made on the cranial ventral surface of the bladder, through the seromuscular layer, allowing the mucosa to bulge through the incision.
2. The end of the ureter is prepared for anastomosis as previously described for the intravesicular technique.

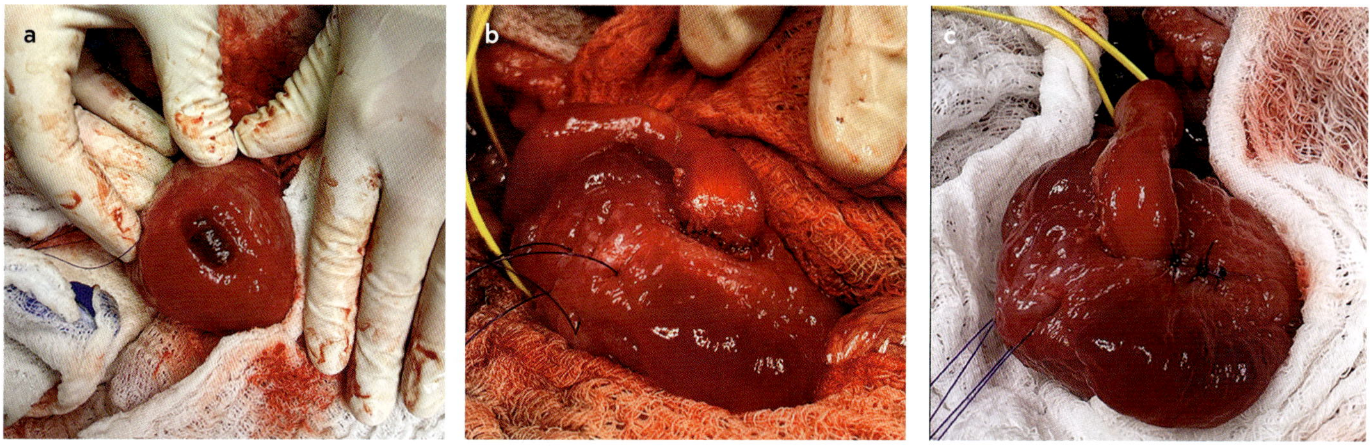

Figure 19.4 Extravesicular technique performed in a dog with an ectopic ureter. (a) An approximately 2 cm incision is made on the cranial ventral surface of the bladder, through the seromuscular layer, allowing the mucosa to bulge through the incision. An incision is made through the bladder mucosa at the caudal aspect of the incision to match the luminal size of the distal ureter. (b) Sutures are placed from the bladder mucosa to the ureteral wall to form a watertight seal. (c) The anastomotic site is depressed into the bladder lumen with the back end of a hemostat, and the seromuscular bladder incision is partially closed over the ureteral spatulation using three sutures of 3-0 polydioxanone. Images courtesy of Erin Gibson, University of Pennsylvania.

3. A 0.75 cm incision is made through the caudal portion of the bulging bladder mucosa. The size of the seromuscular and mucosal incision can vary depending on the size of the dilated ureter.
4. The first suture is preplaced (but not tied) between the cranialmost aspect of the bladder mucosal incision and the crotch of the ureteral spatulation. The next two sutures are preplaced to the left and right sides of the initial suture. A suture can be passed retrogradely in the ureteral lumen to ensure patency before tying these three sutures.
5. The distal corners of the ureter (the two other points of the triangle) are sutured to the caudal aspect of the bladder mucosal incision. The remaining portion of the spatulated ureter is sutured to the bladder mucosal incision to form a watertight seal.
6. The anastomotic site is depressed into the bladder lumen with the back end of a hemostat, and the seromuscular bladder incision is partially closed over the ureteral spatulation to provide additional support.
7. In patients presenting with ureteral obstruction secondary to fibrosis/stricture involving the proximal third of the ureter, successful treatment has been performed using either a modification of a Boari flap or a side-to-side anastomosis of the bladder to the proximal ureter using an extravesicular technique.[16,17]

Surgical technique: Ureteral anastomosis

Ureteral anastomosis is most commonly used for cases of trauma secondary to accidental ligation/transection, but it can be considered in patients with stricture or neoplasia resulting in obstruction.

1. The proximal and distal portions of the ureter are prepared for anastomosis by transecting the ends to remove any devitalized tissue. The vasculature should be preserved as much as possible.
2. To prevent stricture and leakage, an appropriately sized ureteral stent may be preplaced just prior to anastomosis (Fig. 19.5).
3. To perform the anastomosis, three simple interrupted absorbable or nonabsorbable sutures are placed 120 degrees apart (technique of triangulation) to appose the ureteral ends. The suture tags are left long to aid in manipulation of the ureteral ends. Simple interrupted sutures are placed between each third of the circumference until no gaps remain.
4. Stent removal, either cystoscopically or via a surgical approach, typically occurs approximately 1 month following placement.

Surgical technique: Ureteral stenting

Ureteral stenting is another option for the treatment of ureteral obstruction in dogs and cats and can be used as either the sole technique or in conjunction with other surgical and interventional procedures such as ureterotomy and extracorporeal shockwave lithotripsy. If ureteral integrity is of concern following a surgical procedure, a stent can be placed temporarily to divert urine during the healing process. Stent placement is also commonly performed in canine patients following a ureterotomy when the obstructive stone or inspissated material is associated with pyonephrosis. In addition to diverting urine, the stent allows for continued drainage of purulent material. In this situation, the stent should be removed once the ureterotomy is healed. If a stent is placed in conjunction with a ureterotomy, the ureterotomy incision is closed after the stent is in place. Ureteral stenting may also be indicated for patients with multiple ureteroliths located uni- or bilaterally with or without the presence of nephroliths. Additionally, stents have also been used

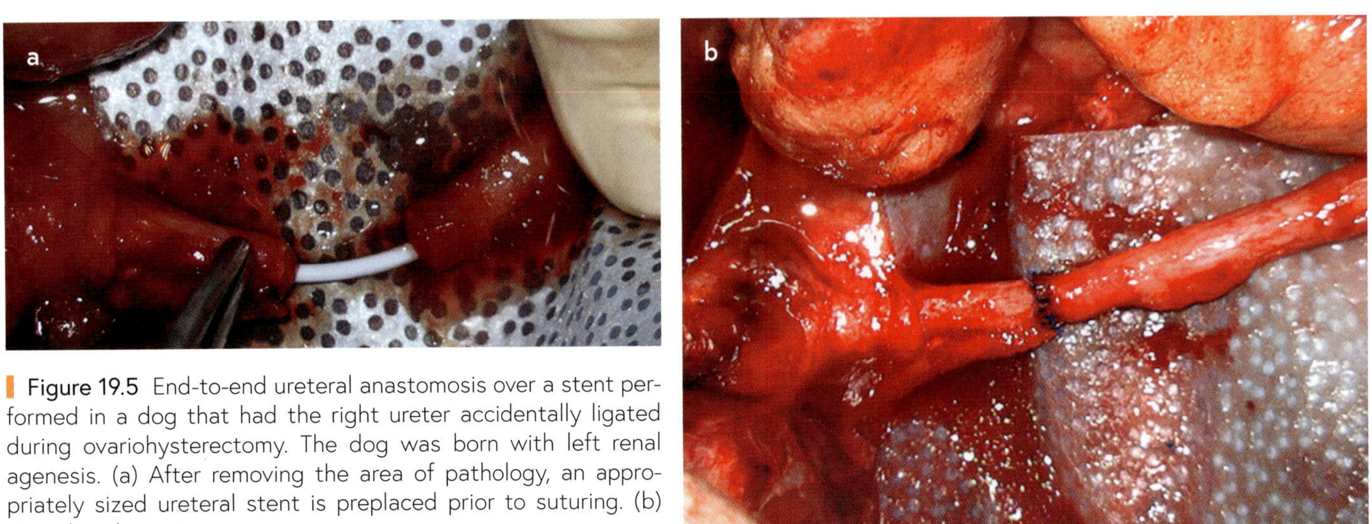

Figure 19.5 End-to-end ureteral anastomosis over a stent performed in a dog that had the right ureter accidentally ligated during ovariohysterectomy. The dog was born with left renal agenesis. (a) After removing the area of pathology, an appropriately sized ureteral stent is preplaced prior to suturing. (b) Completed anastomosis.

successfully to facilitate stone passage following extracorporeal shockwave lithotripsy and for treatment of malignant ureteral obstruction in dogs. Stents can be placed cystoscopically (most female dogs), cystoscopically in conjunction with a perineal approach (most male dogs), or surgically (all male cats, most female cats, dogs). Both antegrade and retrograde techniques have been described.[18] Regardless of the technique, intraoperative fluoroscopy should be available to aid in stent placement.

Retrograde technique (Fig. 19.6)

1. A ventral cystotomy is performed and the ureteral orifice of interest is located.
2. An angled hydrophilic guidewire is advanced through the ureterovesicular junction and into the distal ureter using fluoroscopy.
3. A ureteral catheter is advanced over the guidewire, the guidewire temporarily removed, and a ureteropyelogram performed.
4. The guidewire is then readvanced up the ureter into the renal pelvis, forming two loops of the guidewire.
5. The ureteral catheter is removed, and a double pigtail ureteral stent is passed over the guidewire until one curl is in the renal pelvis. The guidewire is removed. The other curl is left in the urinary bladder, and the cystotomy incision is closed.

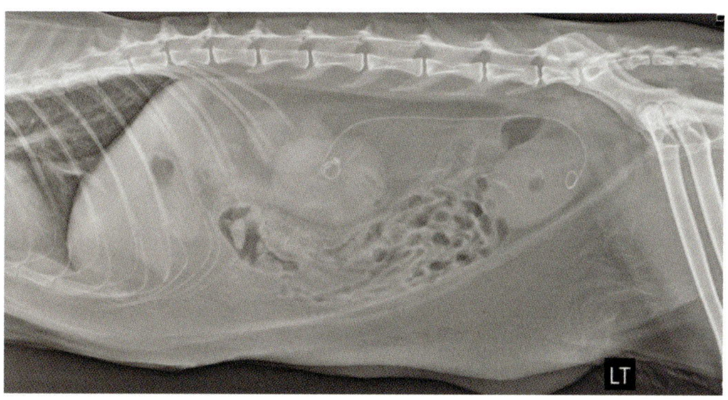

Figure 19.6 Radiograph following ureteral stent placement in a cat.

Antegrade technique

1. An appropriately sized intravenous catheter is used in conjunction with fluoroscopy to perform a surgical pyelocentesis through the greater curvature of the kidney.
2. A pyelogram is performed, and a hydrophilic guidewire is passed down the ureter into the urinary bladder.
3. A ureteral catheter is then placed antegradely or retrogradely over the guidewire to dilate the ureter.
4. The catheter is removed and an appropriately sized ureteral stent is passed retrogradely or antegradely over the guidewire.
5. If antegrade placement is performed, the guidewire exits a fenestration along the straight portion of the stent, allowing for the pigtail coil to remain outside of the kidney.
6. Through and through wire access is maintained as the stent is pulled distally into the bladder and allowing the coil to enter the renal pelvis. The guidewire is removed.

Subcutaneous ureteral bypass (SUB) systems

In human medicine, ureteral bypass devices were developed for patients with inoperable urinary obstructions secondary to end-stage genitourinary cancer as an alternative to permanent nephrostomy tubes. A similar device was developed for cats to treat ureteral obstruction as an alternative to ureteral stents. Since the introduction of the device in 2009, multiple versions have been developed to address complications associated with the device. In the most recent version of the device for companion animals (SUB 3.0, Norfolk Vet Products), the system is comprised of one or two locking-loop nephrostomy catheters, a multifenestrated cystostomy catheter, a subcutaneous port placed along the ventral body wall, and a connector junction for securing the catheters (Fig. 19.7). The reader is referred to the company website (https://norfolkvetproducts.com) for a detailed description of placement techniques.

Postoperative management

Postoperative care should be tailored to each individual patient but typically includes the administration of a balanced electrolyte solution (until the patient is eating and drinking and able to maintain their weight and hydration without additional fluid support), analgesic therapy, and potentially nutritional intervention. Placement of a multilumen jugular catheter facilitates the concurrent administration of intravenous fluids, blood products, analgesics, gastrointestinal protectants, antiemetics, and antibiotic therapy if indicated as well as blood sampling. Fluid diuresis is advocated after surgery of the urinary tract to prevent clot formation resulting in obstruction. Analgesia is usually provided by a combination of the local anesthetic (e.g., lidocaine, bupivacaine) placed at the time of surgical closure with systemic opioid administration (fentanyl constant-rate infusion, methadone, buprenorphine). For increased discomfort in SUB patients due to the need to perform a large amount of soft tissue dissection to place the port, the alpha-2 adrenergic agonist dexmedetomidine is often combined with local anesthetics and intermittent boluses of buprenorphine. Nasoesophageal or esophageal feeding tubes may be indicated for some patients in need of nutritional sup-

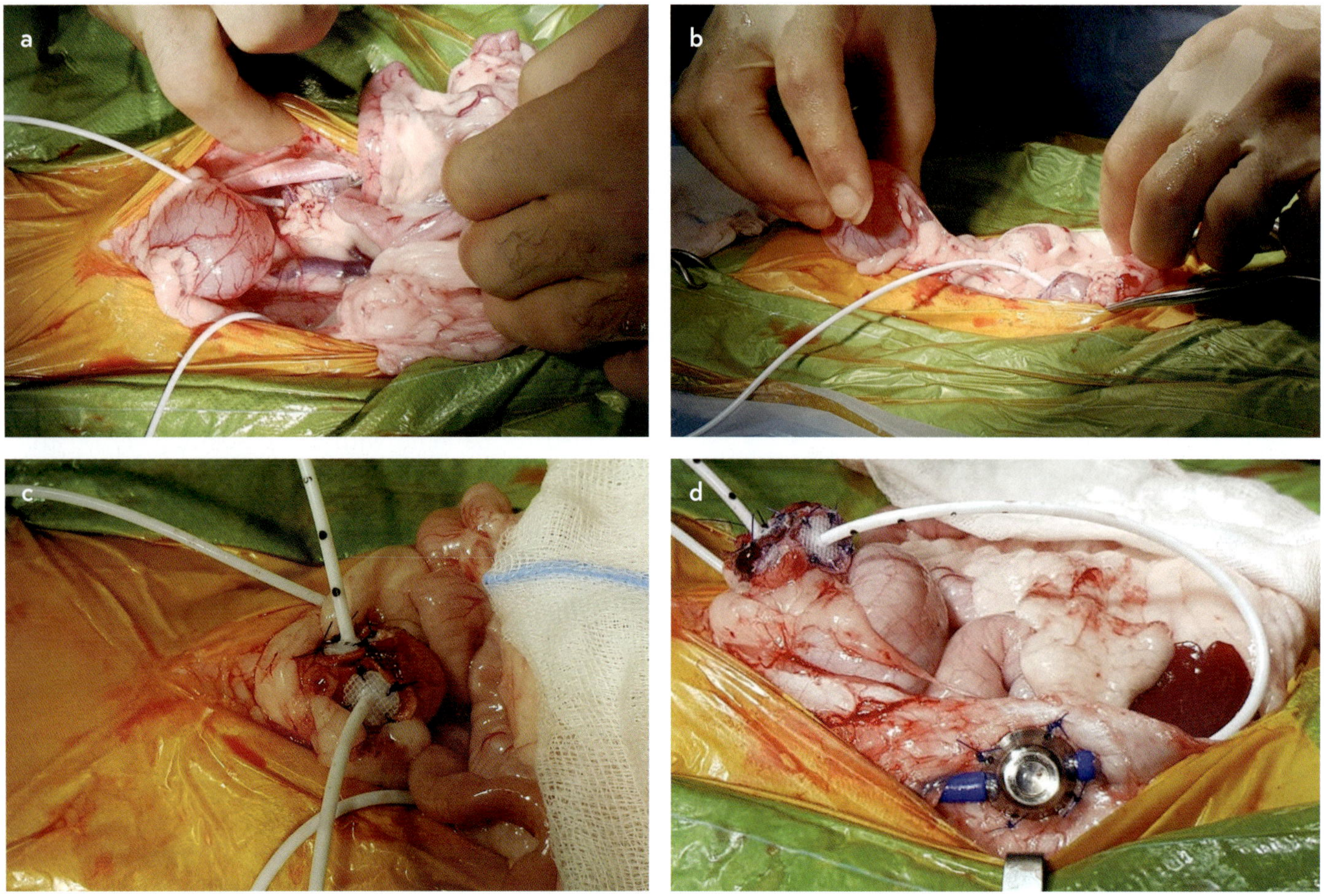

Figure 19.7 Intraoperative images of bilateral subcutaneous ureteral bypass placement in a 10-year-old cat. Placement of (a,b) the nephrostomy catheter, (c) multifenestrated cystotomy catheter, and (d) port. Images courtesy of Filippo Cinti and Tim Charlesworth (Veterinaria, n.2, 2021).

port as well as to allow for enteral water administration during the postoperative period. Urination should be carefully monitored for significant hematuria, and urine output quantified every 1–2 hours, particularly in the early postoperative period.

Antibiotic administration is based on urine culture and sensitivity results. For patients undergoing traditional techniques, including ureterotomy or neoureterostomy, if culture results are negative, only perioperative antibiotics are recommended. For patients with urinary implants, antibiotic therapy may be recommended for 2 weeks postoperatively, and if an infection is present, treatment based on culture and sensitivity results should be administered for 4–6 weeks. Additional urine cultures should be performed during the treatment period to make sure that appropriate antibiotics are being used and then following completion of antibiotic course.

Patients with a SUB device should have the device flushed at regular intervals based on clinician preference. Current published recommendations for postoperative management of the SUB device include flushing at 1 week, 1 month, and every 3 months thereafter following surgery.

Regardless of the procedure performed, regular follow-up medical management is recommended for this patient population because of their underlying renal disease.

Outcome

The most common complications associated with ureterotomy and neoureterostomy are leakage and stricture formation.[1,6] The small size of the feline ureter necessitates appropriate training in the use of magnification, which is critical to success in these cases. It has been the author's observation that complications including leakage and stricture are significantly reduced when appropriate magnification is used.

In a recent publication on ureteral surgery, 63 cats underwent a ureterotomy alone and 11 cats underwent a neoureterostomy alone. Intraoperative magnification was used for each technique. The incidence of perioperative complications for these cats was 3% (2/74). Survival to discharge was 92% and the median survival time was 1519 days.[6] In a large multicenter study with

89 cats (65 ureterotomy, 27 neoureterostomy, and 4 both), uroabdomen developed in 12% of cats that did not have a nephrostomy tube placed, and persistent ureteral obstruction was identified in 6% of cats, with the majority treated successfully with a revision surgery. The 6-, 12-, and 24-month survival rates following surgery in that study were 91%, 91%, and 88%, respectively.[1] In another study reporting on 12 cats requiring a neoureterostomy, 2/12 (17%) developed a uroabdomen requiring revision surgery and 11/12 (92%) were discharged from the hospital.[19] In a canine report describing a three-stitch neoureterostomy technique, 8/9 (89%) had an excellent long-term outcome.[20]

In a study evaluating postoperative mortality in 47 cats after ureterotomy, 3 patients (6%) developed a uroabdomen after the procedure. Perioperative mortality was reported at 21%; however, based on necropsy findings, the cause of death in approximately half of the cats was associated with progression of their chronic renal disease and not related to complications of the surgical procedure.[21]

In studies evaluating ureteral stenting in cats, the most common procedure-related complications included uroabdomen (8.7%–15%) and guidewire penetration (17%), and the most common short- and long-term complications included signs of sterile cystitis (11%–35%), urinary tract infection (8%–31%), encrustation (11%–26%), hematuria (18%–52%), and stent migration (6%–11%).[22–26] Perioperative mortality ranged from 7.5% to 18%, and stent exchange was necessary in 15%–27% of cats.[26] In a report of 43 cats that had ureteral stents alone placed, chronic lower urinary tract signs and confirmed infection were identified in 28% and 26% of cats with ureteral stents, respectively, while stent encrustation was identified in 2 cats (5%).[6]

In patients that have concurrent nephrolithiasis and ureterolithiasis, the nephroliths do have the potential to pass into a ureter that was recently unobstructed. The incidence of reobstruction has been reported in approximately 20%–22% of cases that have undergone a ureterotomy or ureteral stent placement. Recurrence of the obstruction was documented at a median of approximately 203 and 380 days in two separate studies.[1,6]

In a review of the current literature on SUB, 79%–94% of cats were discharged from the hospital and median survival times ranged from 274 to 827 days.[27–34] Some of the most frequent complications reported include device kinking (4.6%–10%), luminal mineralization (4%–25%), noninfectious cystitis (9%–38%), and urinary tract infection (20.8%–35.7%). Overall complication rates are reported as high as 88%, but more commonly around 48%–56%. Additionally, the need for revision surgery ranged from 8% to 27%, and in a recent multicenter report, transmural migration of 11 devices within the digestive tract also resulted in the need for a second surgical procedure.[35]

Urethral obstruction

Urethral obstruction in companion animals is a common reason for emergency presentation to the veterinarian. Obstruction most commonly results from urolithiasis, particularly cystoliths that migrate into the urethra from the urinary bladder or those that form in the urethra primarily. Other causes of urethral obstruction in dogs and cats include trauma, neoplasia, prostatic disease (male dogs), urethritis, crystalline-matrix urethral plugs, and caudal displacement of the bladder. Male cats often present on an emergency basis for clinical signs associated with feline lower urinary tract disease (FLUTD). The most common causes of FLUTD in cats include nonobstructive feline infectious cystitis, obstructive feline infectious cystitis resulting from crystalline-matrix urethral plugs (usually struvite), urolithiasis, and urinary tract infection. More recently, crystalline-matrix urethral plugs have been diagnosed in dogs, particularly male Pugs.[36] Although urethral obstruction resulting from many of the previously mentioned conditions occur in female dogs and cats, the narrow urethral lumen in males of both species predisposes them to complete obstruction more commonly from urolithiasis, neoplasia, urethrospasm, or swelling.

Clinical presentation

Many factors may contribute to the development of urolithiasis in dogs and cats, including breed predisposition, anatomic conformation, diet, water availability, and the presence of concurrent diseases or infections. Neutered male cats with higher body condition scores seem to be at increased risk for the development of urethral plugs resulting in obstruction. Clinical signs noted by the owner as well as on presentation often depend on the underlying cause and whether the obstruction is partial or complete, but they may include frequent licking of the prepuce, dysuria, pollakiuria, stranguria, hematuria, anuria, overflow incontinence, vocalization, repeated posturing to urinate, and discomfort when attempting to urinate. Anorexia, lethargy, and vomiting may also be noted.

Physical examination may reveal an enlarged, normal, or nonpalpable bladder, pain on abdominal palpation, and the presence of a fluid wave. Cardiac auscultation may be unremarkable or reveal bradycardia, tachycardia, or other arrhythmias. Rectal examination may identify calculi within the urethra. If obstruction is secondary to trauma and urine leakage occurs, clinical presentation will depend on the location of injury. Leakage of urine from the proximal urethra may result in a uroabdomen and abdominal bruising, whereas injury to the distal urethra may result in subcutaneous urine leakage with secondary bruising, oozing on the skin surface, and tissue devitalization in the perineal region. If the urethral obstruction is long-standing, causing severe azotemia, or in cases of urine leakage from rupture, patients may present depressed, obtunded, or comatose.

Initial stabilization

If urethral obstruction is suspected on initial presentation and physical examination, an intravenous catheter should be placed, retrograde urethral catheterization attempted, electrocardiogram placed, and stat blood work performed to determine if any metabolic derangements exist. If possible, initial blood work should include a venous blood gas analysis, packed cell volume/total solids, blood glucose, and a renal panel.

A focused assessment with sonography for trauma (FAST) scan can be performed to evaluate for the presence of abdominal effusion and/or confirm the presence of an enlarged obstructed bladder. If effusion is present, a sample should be submitted to evaluate creatinine and potassium levels, which should be compared to those of a peripheral blood sample taken concurrently. In dogs, a peritoneal potassium level 1.4 times that of serum and a creatinine level twice that of serum is highly suggestive of uroabdomen. In cats diagnosed with uroabdomen, the peritoneal to serum effusion ratios for potassium and creatinine are 1.9:1 and 2:1, respectively. The fluid rate and choice should be based on the hemodynamic status of the patient and any electrolyte and/or acid–base abnormalities. Patients that are hyperkalemic can present bradycardic, with ventricular arrhythmia and electrocardiographic changes including prolonged QRS complexes, widened P–R intervals, and spiked T waves. A balanced electrolyte solution (e.g., Plasmalyte) is often preferred over 0.9% NaCl since the amount of potassium in a balanced electrolyte solution will not contribute significantly to the hyperkalemia and is less acidic than 0.9% NaCl, thus not worsening the metabolic acidosis that is often present.

Successful retrograde urethral catheterization allows for temporary urinary diversion to further stabilize the patient until a definitive surgical procedure can be performed. Depending on the cause of obstruction, retrograde urohydropropulsion may be helpful if initial attempts at catheterization are unsuccessful.[37] If the bladder is already overdistended, a decompressive cystocentesis should be performed prior to performing the procedure.

Technique: Retrograde urohydropropulsion (Fig. 19.8)

1. The patient is placed in lateral recumbency under general anesthesia. Digital pressure is applied per rectum to the pelvic urethra.
2. A mixture of saline and lubricant is flushed retrogradely into the urethra while compressing the external urethral orifice, resulting in dilation of the urethral lumen.
3. Digital pressure on the pelvic urethra is released, propelling urethroliths into the bladder lumen.

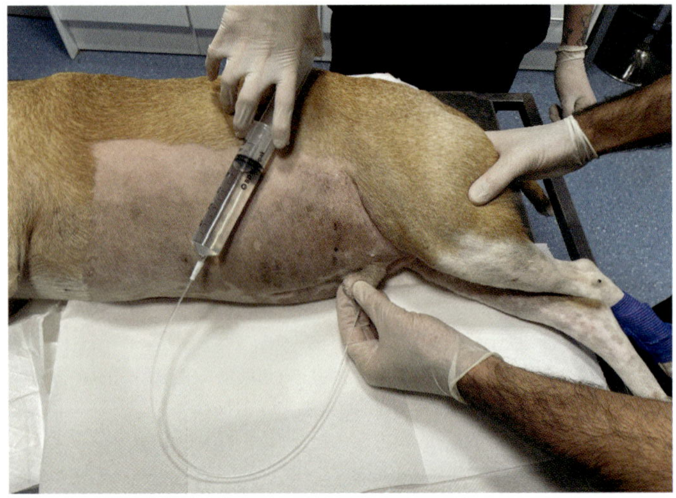

Figure 19.8 Retrograde urohydropropulsion in a male dog with a urethral obstruction. Note the digital pressure applied to the pelvic uretrha (per rectum) and around the external urethral orifice. Image courtesy of Filippo Cinti.

If catheterization is still unsuccessful, intermittent bladder decompression via cystocentesis, cystostomy tube placement, or normograde urethral catheterization are all potential options for stabilization until definitive surgical intervention can be performed. Both minimally invasive and open surgical options exist for cystostomy tube placement and the choice of technique often depends on equipment availability and comfort level of the clinician. For minimally invasive placement, a locking-loop pigtail catheter is placed using a Seldinger technique with the aid of ultrasound or fluoroscopy. Percutaneously placed tubes should remain in place for 2–4 weeks to allow adhesions to form between the body wall and urinary bladder.[38] Surgically placed cystostomy tubes (e.g., Pezzar, mushroom-tipped catheter, Foley, low-profile gastrostomy tubes) may be indicated for temporary or permanent diversion. See Chapter 5 for a description of surgical placement of a cystostomy tube as well as possible complications.

Diagnostic evaluation

Clinicopathological evaluation should include a complete blood count, biochemical profile, and urinalysis and culture of a sample obtained by cystocentesis. Any abdominal effusion should be submitted for creatinine and potassium level measurement, cytology, and culture. Creatinine and potassium levels should be compared to those from a concurrently drawn blood sample. Diagnostic imaging may include one or more of the following depending on the underlying cause of the obstruction: plain abdominal radiographs, positive-contrast retrograde urethrocystography, abdominal ultrasound, cystoscopy, and urethroscopy. If calculi are the cause of the obstruction, the number and correct location of the stones should be evaluated in all patients before surgery (via radiography, computed tomography, or ultrasound examination). If an underlying neoplastic process is thought to be causing the obstruction, a three-projection thoracic radiographic study should also be performed.

Treatment

Surgical technique: Cystotomy (Fig. 19.9; Video 19.1)

Uroliths within the urethra can often be retropropulsed into the urinary bladder, simplifying removal via a cystotomy.

1. A caudal ventral midline abdominal or paraprepucial approach is made.
2. Prior to isolating the bladder from the abdominal cavity with moistened laparotomy sponges, a urinary

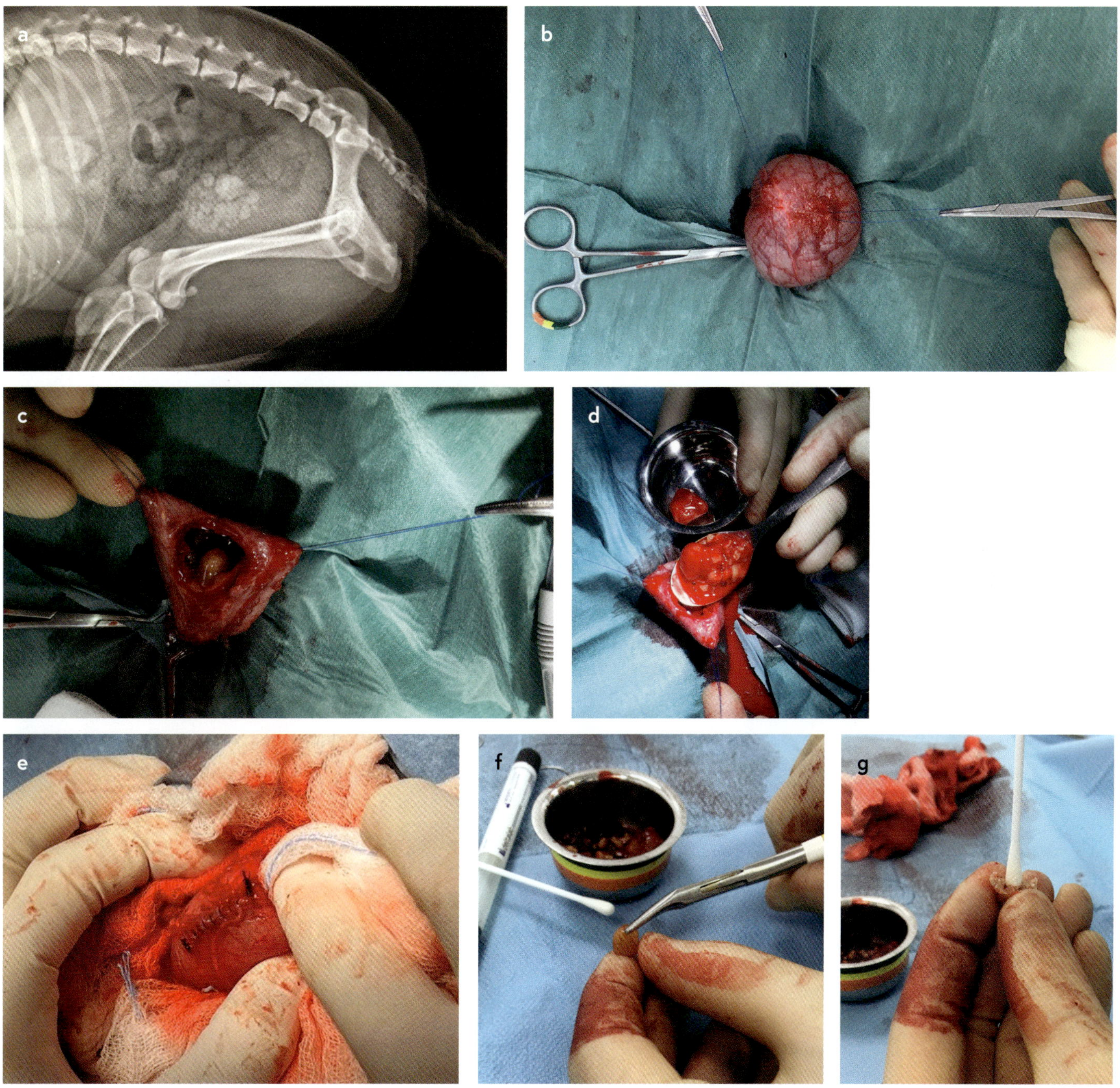

Figure 19.9 Cystotomy for urolith removal. (a) Preoperative radiograph. (b) Stay sutures to aid in exposure and manipulation. (c) Cystotomy. (d) Removal of calculi with a bladder spoon. (e) Closure of the bladder. (f) Intraoperative opening of a stone using rongeurs. (g) Swab from the core of the stone for culture. Images courtesy of Filippo Cinti.

Video 19.1. Cystotomy in an 8-year-old neutered male dog with bladder calculi. Video courtesy of Silvia Gatta.

catheter is placed to prevent uroliths from migrating into the urethra during manipulation of the bladder.

3. A stay suture is placed at the bladder apex, and a ventral midline cystotomy incision is performed in an avascular region if possible. Stay sutures can also be placed on either side of the cystotomy incision to aid in exposure.
4. Uroliths are removed with a bladder spoon, and retrograde flushing of the urethra is performed to dislodge and remove any remaining uroliths. If available, a flexible endoscope can be passed normogradely from the bladder to ensure removal of all uroliths prior to closure.
5. If needed, a full-thickness piece of the incision edge can be removed with scissors and submitted for culture and histology.
6. The cystotomy incision can be closed in a simple interrupted or simple continuous suture pattern with absorbable monofilament material such as 3-0 or 4-0 polydioxanone. The submucosa should be included in each suture bite.
7. Abdominal/pelvic radiographs can be performed following the procedure, prior to extubation, to ensure removal of all uroliths from the bladder and urethra.
8. The calculi can be sent for analysis. In some cases, a stone can be opened with rongeurs and a swab of culture performed from the core of the stone.

Surgical technique: Urethrotomy

Urethrotomy is indicated for (<3) obstructive, immovable uroliths in dogs that cannot be successfully flushed into the bladder via hydropropulsion. It is most commonly performed caudal to the os penis, in a prescrotal location; however, depending on the level of obstruction, the technique can be performed in a perineal prepubic or glans penis location.

Prescrotal urethrotomy (Fig. 19.10)

1. The patient is placed in dorsal recumbency with the pelvic limbs extended and abducted. Retrograde urethral catheterization is performed to facilitate identification of the urethra and location of the obstruction.
2. A skin incision (2–3 cm) is made on the midline, caudal to the os penis and cranial to the scrotum. Following subcutaneous tissue dissection, the retractor penis muscle is identified, isolated, and retracted laterally.

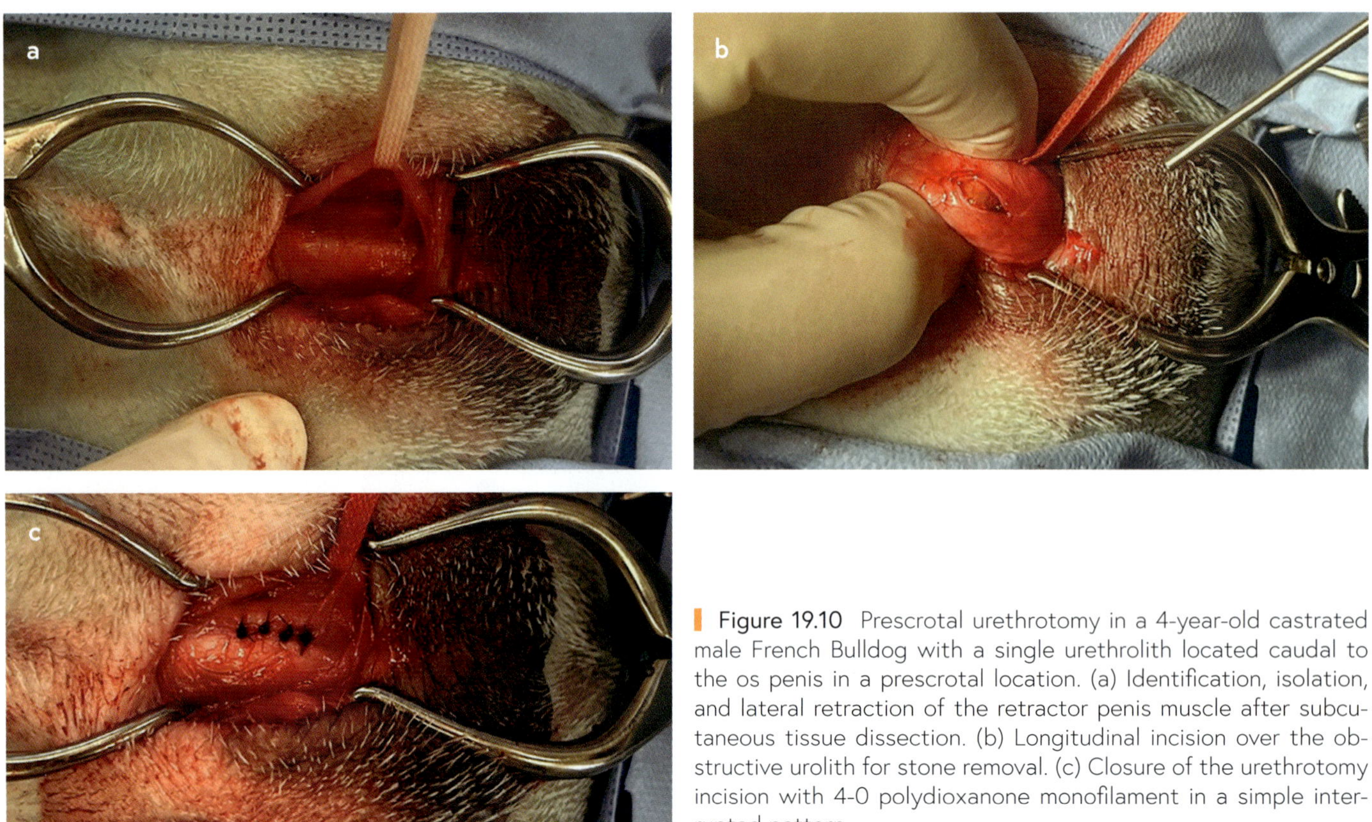

Figure 19.10 Prescrotal urethrotomy in a 4-year-old castrated male French Bulldog with a single urethrolith located caudal to the os penis in a prescrotal location. (a) Identification, isolation, and lateral retraction of the retractor penis muscle after subcutaneous tissue dissection. (b) Longitudinal incision over the obstructive urolith for stone removal. (c) Closure of the urethrotomy incision with 4-0 polydioxanone monofilament in a simple interrupted pattern.

3. The urethra, surrounded by cavernous tissue, is identified. A longitudinal incision is made over the obstructive urolith and the urolith removed with atraumatic forceps.
4. Hemorrhage is controlled with direct pressure to the area and as sutures are placed during closure.
5. The urethral catheter is advanced passed the urethrotomy site and into the bladder to confirm patency of the urethra and that no further obstructive uroliths remain. The technique can be performed in conjunction with a cystotomy if necessary to remove cystic calculi if present.

Potential complications of the technique include stricture, hematuria, stranguria, dysuria, pollakiuria, and urine leakage into the surrounding tissues.

Glans penis urethrotomy (Fig. 19.11)

A modification of the prescrotal technique is urethrotomy through the glans penis following retraction of the prepuce. This approach is used for calculi in the penile urethra along the ventral groove of the os penis when retrograde urohydropropulsion is unsuccessful and permanent urethrostomy can be avoided.

1. A piece of sterile gauze is tied around the base of the penis caudal to the bulbus glandis and pulled caudally to retract the prepuce during surgery.
2. A longitudinal incision is made along the ventral midline of the glans penis into the lumen of the urethra.
3. The calculi are removed and a urinary catheter placed into the bladder.
4. The urethral incision can be left to heal by second intention or sutured.

In a report of the technique, the procedure was associated with minimal hemorrhage and a low complication rate.[39]

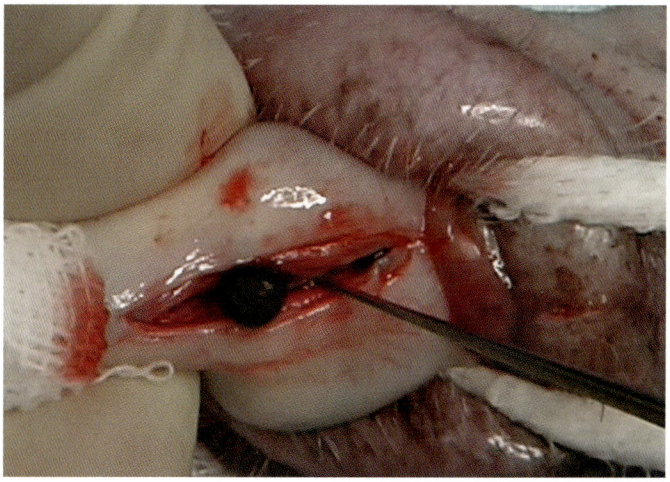

Figure 19.11 Ventral approach to the penile urethra and removal of urethral calculi. Image courtesy of Filippo Cinti and *Journal of Small Animal Practice*. 2015; 56:671–674.

Surgical technique: Urethrostomy

Permanent urethrostomy

Urethrostomy is most frequently performed in males to provide a permanent stoma to bypass an area of obstruction often resulting from urolithiasis in dogs and from obstructive FLUTD in cats. Other indications for permanent urethrostomy include hypospadias in dogs and obstruction due to stricture, trauma, or neoplasia involving the urethra, penile body, or prepuce. Additionally, the technique is also recommended for chronic stone formers that have experienced obstruction and are at risk for repeated obstruction.

Multiple sites have been described for permanent urethrostomy in male dogs, including prescrotal, scrotal, perineal, and prepubic locations. A transpelvic approach in a female dog as well as a modified preputial urethrostomy technique with preservation of local anatomy in four dogs have also recently been reported.[40,41] The scrotal location is the preferred site in male dogs because the urethra is superficial and wide at this location and surrounded by the least amount of cavernous tissue, resulting in less hemorrhage compared to other locations. In male cats, urethrostomy can be performed in a perineal, transpelvic, or prepubic location.

Scrotal urethrostomy

1. The patient is positioned in dorsal recumbency with the caudal abdomen and perineal region prepped for aseptic surgery. A transurethral catheter (largest possible) is placed retrogradely into the bladder to facilitate identification of the urethra.
2. If the dog is intact, an elliptical incision is made at the base of the scrotum, retaining as much skin as needed to prevent tension on the urethrostomy site, and a routine castration is performed. If the dog is already neutered, an elliptical incision can be made to remove remnants of the scrotal sac.
3. Following subcutaneous dissection, the retractor penis muscle is identified, isolated, and retracted laterally off of the penile body.
4. The penis is stabilized with the nondominant hand, and an approximately 4 cm incision is made with a number 11 scalpel blade directly over the urinary catheter, on the midline, into the urethral lumen. Some surgeons prefer to complete the incision with iris scissors.
5. The urethral mucosa is sutured to the skin using 4-0 or 5-0 nonabsorbable monofilament material in a simple continuous or simple interrupted pattern. Suture bites should be approximately 2–3 mm apart, and care should be taken when handling the mucosa. Absorbable suture material is not recommended due to the inconsistent rate of absorption when placed in this location.[42]

6. To help facilitate excellent apposition during closure, some surgeons advocate including the entire thickness of the urethra and only the dermis and epidermis of the skin.
7. The distal urethra can be closed down if needed by apposing the urethra on the dorsal midline to the distal skin incision with a single mattress suture.

An Elizabethan collar is critical during recovery and until suture removal to prevent self-trauma to the incision. Suture removal occurs approximately 10–14 days following surgery and may require sedation. The stoma will decrease in size by approximately 50% after healing is complete.

Complications associated with the technique include hemorrhage, bruising, intermittent urine scalding, recurrent urinary tract infections, and rarely stricture associated with self-trauma, incorporation of previously traumatized tissue, or poor surgical technique. Intermittent hemorrhage, which is the most common complication, is often self-limiting and can last for 3–5 days after the procedure. If hemorrhage persists for more than 10–14 days, revision of the urethrostomy site may be indicated.

Perineal urethrostomy (Fig. 19.12)

1. Perineal urethrostomy can be performed with the cat in either ventral or dorsal recumbency. Additionally, a modification of the technique, anastomosing the urethra to a remnant of the preputial mucosa, has also been described.[43] Studies comparing the ventral and dorsal techniques have concluded that positioning the patient in dorsal recumbency may improve visualization during tissue dissection and accuracy in tissue apposition during closure.[44,45]
   - For the ventral technique, the cat is positioned in ventral recumbency on a padded perineal stand or with the hindquarters padded and legs hanging off the end of a table that tilts forward. The tail is secured cranially so that it is not in the surgical field.
   - For the dorsal technique, the cat is positioned on his back with a folded towel beneath the cat's caudal end to elevate the perineum. The hind legs are pulled cranially to improve exposure of the perineal region. This positioning has the advantage of allowing simultaneous access to the bladder for patients requiring a cystotomy.
2. The surgeon should identify the dorsal surface of the urethra for the incision regardless of the recumbency of the patient. A purse-string suture is placed.
3. An elliptical incision is made around the prepuce and scrotum starting approximately 1 cm distal to the anus. If the cat is intact, he is neutered at this time.
4. The penis is freed from the surrounding subcutaneous tissues and ligamentous attachments using both sharp and blunt dissection, and dissection is continued cranially to identify the paired ischiocavernosus muscles and their attachments to the pelvis. An Allis tissue forceps can aid in retraction and orientation of the penis and prepuce during dissection.
5. A hemostat is then passed around the ischiocavernosus muscle, mid body, and this muscle is transected using bipolar cautery. Some surgeons prefer to ligate the muscle with 4-0 absorbable monofilament suture material prior to sharp transection. Hemorrhage, if it occurs, can be controlled with bipolar cautery.
6. Dissection is continued dorsally until the bulbourethral glands are identified.
7. The penis is retracted dorsally and any remaining ventral penile ligaments are divided. The retractor penis muscle is dissected from the dorsal surface of the penis and resected.
8. The distal penis is transversely incised proximal to the reflection of the prepuce, the urethral lumen identified, and a tomcat polypropylene catheter placed. The catheter can be cut short to prevent damage to the bladder apex as the catheter is advanced cranially.
9. The urethra is incised along its dorsal midline using a number 11 scalpel blade and the catheter advanced as the urethra is cut to help control hemorrhage. The incision continues to the level of the bulbourethral glands, where the urethral diameter is approximately 4–5 mm. The urethral stoma should be able to accommodate the tips of a pair of hemostat forceps to the level of the hinge.
10. The urethral mucosa is sutured to the skin using 4-0 to 5-0 absorbable or nonabsorbable monofilament material. The author preplaces five stay sutures at the apex of the incision (10, 11, 12, 1, and 2 o'clock) from the urethral lumen to the perineal skin to allow accurate apposition of the tissues. Once the crown sutures are tied, the distal penis is ligated with either an encircling or mattress suture and transected.
11. Placement of the remaining sutures is performed alternating bites on each side or with a continuous suture pattern down each side. The remaining ventral skin incision is closed routinely, and any remaining urethral mucosa to skin sutures placed.
12. The purse-string suture is removed and an Elizabethan collar placed prior to recovery from anesthesia to prevent self-mutilation of the urethrostomy site. Blood clots that form at the site following surgery should not be removed.

Complications during surgery are uncommon but may include the inability to pass a urinary catheter as a result of lodged uroliths as well as a significantly traumatized urethral mucosa. Additionally, hemorrhage can occur during surgery from an inflamed urethral mucosa or during dissection of the ischiocavernosus muscles from

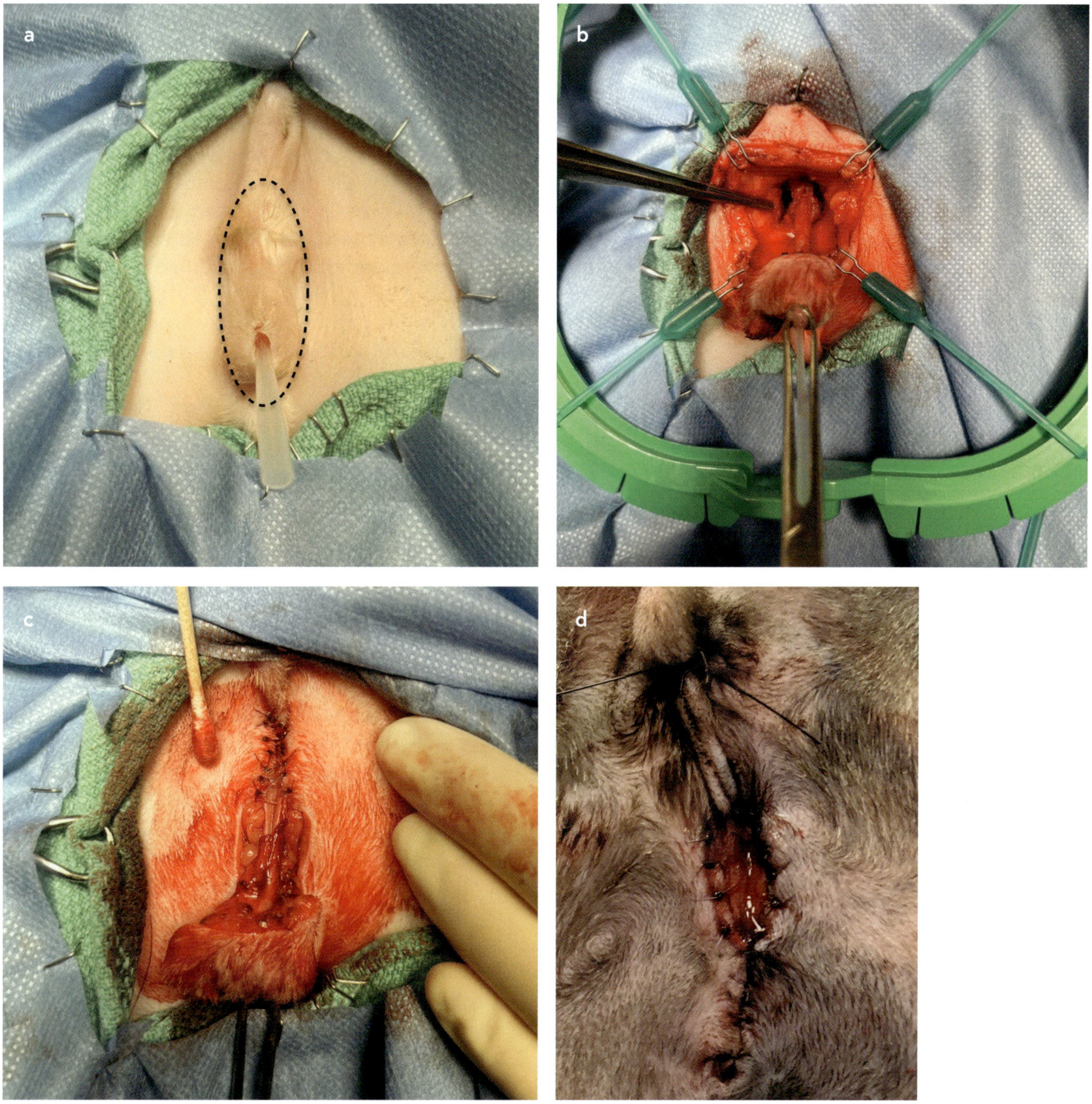

Figure 19.12 Perineal urethrostomy. (a) Elliptical incision around the prepuce and scrotum starting approximately 1 cm distal to the anus. (b) Dissection of the penis from surrounding subcutaneous tissues and ligamentous attachments, and transection of muscular attachments from the pelvis. (c) Suture placement to appose the urethral mucosa to the skin. The author preplaces five stay sutures at the apex of the incision first and places the remaining sutures alternating bites on each side. (d) Completed urethrostomy.

the pelvis. Early postoperative complications include hemorrhage, wound dehiscence, stricture formation, and urine extravasation. Stricture often results from improper surgical technique, including inadequate cranial dissection of the penis to the level of the bulbourethral glands, inaccurate apposition of the mucosa to the skin during suture placement, and self-induced trauma to the surgical site (Fig. 19.13).[46] Inaccurate mucosal apposition can also result in urine extravasation, significant inflammation, pain, and tissue necrosis. For patients that develop a stricture, revision is often feasible, since the cause is usually associated with incomplete cranial dissection of the penis. Urinary tract infections are the most common long-term complication identified and likely associated with the shortened urethral length and direct exposure of the urethral orifice.

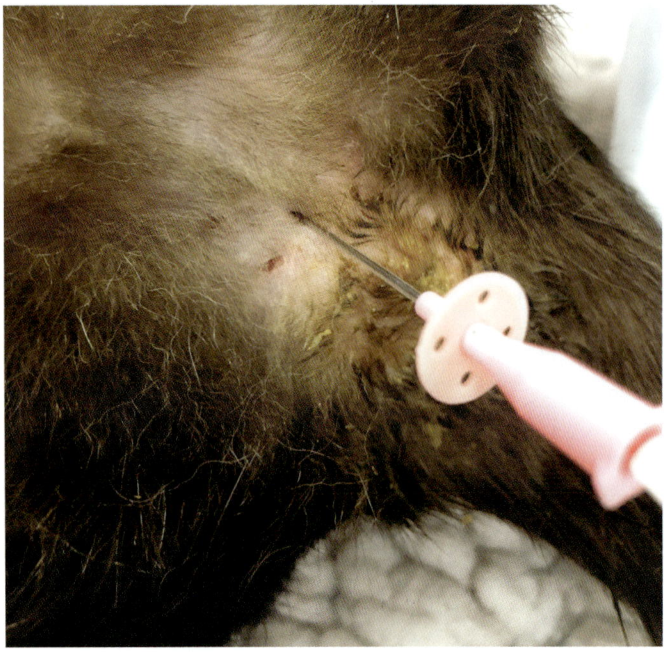

Figure 19.13 Stenosis of the perineal urethrostomy site requiring revision. Image courtesy of Filippo Cinti.

Transpelvic urethrostomy (Fig. 19.14)

Transpelvic urethrostomy has been used in cats as a primary procedure for the treatment of obstructive lower urinary tract disease or as a salvage procedure after perineal urethrostomy failures. Although the technique is most commonly reported in male cats, a recent report described its use in a female dog for the successful treatment of a congenital stricture involving the vagina and urethra.[40]

1. The cat is placed in dorsal recumbency, and an area including the abdominal and pelvic regions is clipped and aseptically prepared.
2. A urethral catheter is passed retrogradely into the urinary bladder. If this is not possible, a cystotomy is performed and a catheter passed normogradely to aid in identification of the pelvic urethra.
3. An elliptical incision is made around the penis and prepuce, and the penis is dissected free of the connective tissue attachments. The bulbourethral glands and ischiocavernosus and ischiourethralis muscles are identified.
4. A midline ventral incision is performed to identify the ventral aspect of the pubic symphysis and the median pelvic attachments of the adductor and gracilis muscles. These muscles are elevated laterally to expose the caudal margin of the ischium, and a 10 mm wide and 12 mm long area of bone is resected along the midline using bone rongeurs, with care taken to preserve the deeper soft tissues of the pelvis.
5. The ventral urethra and catheter are palpated, and a midline longitudinal incision is made over the catheter from the bulbourethral glands to a point 2–3 mm from the cranial margin of the ostectomy.
6. The urethra is sutured to the perineal skin using a simple interrupted pattern of 4-0 polypropylene. To limit tension on the anastomosis, it may be necessary to remove a small amount of subcutaneous fat. The distal penis is ligated and resected. If the bladder was approached, the laparotomy incision is closed routinely.[47]

Potential benefits of this technique compared to a standard perineal urethrostomy include a decreased risk of incontinence, since dissection around important neurovascular structures is not performed, and a reduced incidence of stricture. Reported complications include mild urinary incontinence, hematuria, dysuria, urinary tract infections, premature suture loosening, and hind limb urine staining.

Prepubic urethrostomy

Prepubic urethrostomy is a salvage procedure recommended for patients that have sustained significant damage to the intrapelvic and/or distal urethra resulting in insufficient urethral length available to perform a standard perineal or transpelvic urethrostomy. The technique can be performed in male and female dogs and cats.

1. A ventral midline caudal abdominal incision is made in cats and female dogs, and a paraprepucial incision is made in male dogs.
2. The proximal urethra is carefully dissected from the surrounding tissue as far distally into the pelvic canal as possible, taking care to avoid injury to associated innervation and blood supply.
3. The urethra is transected, and the end of the urethra is brought either through the abdominal incision or through a separate stab incision in the abdominal musculature 2 cm paramedian to the ventral midline. The site chosen should allow for a gentle arc of the urethra to avoid kinking.
4. If the urethrostomy site is placed along the ventral midline abdominal incision, a small gap is left in the linea alba to accommodate the distal urethra, and the rest of the linea is closed routinely.
5. A modification of the technique has also been described which creates a tunnel through the midbody of the rectus abdominis muscle in an attempt to avoid kinking and decrease tension at the urethrostomy site.[48]
6. Two interrupted sutures are placed using 4-0 to 5-0 absorbable material between the urethral adventitia and body wall at least 1–2 cm proximal to the cut end of the urethra to tack the urethra in place.

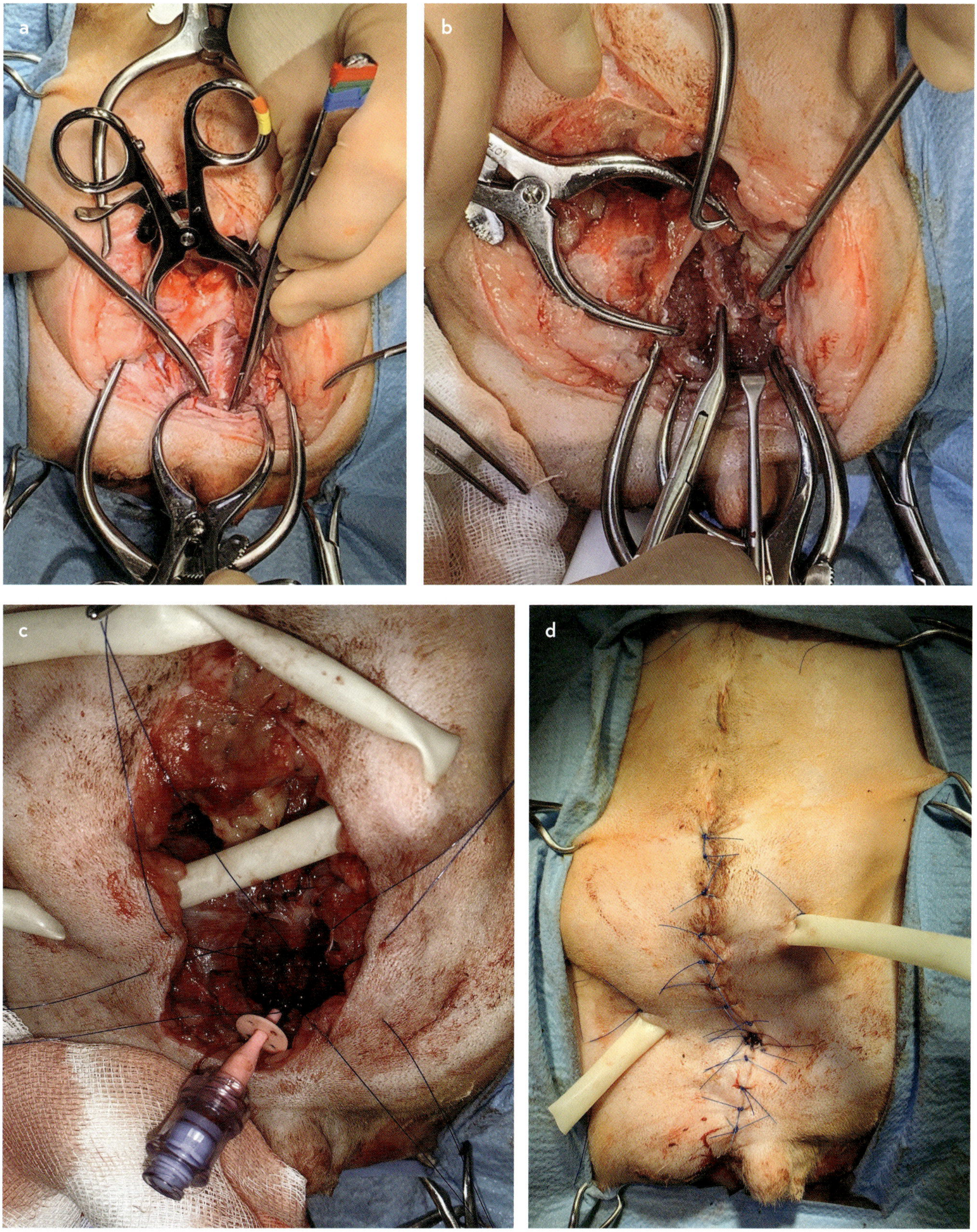

Figure 19.14 Transpelvic urethrostomy in an 8-year-old cat to treat stenosis, a complication following perineal urethrostomy. (a) Ventral midline incision to identify the ventral aspect of the pubic symphysis. (b) Resection of the ischium along the midline using bone rongeurs. (c) Identification and incision of the urethra. Application of a passive drain and partial removal of subcutaneous fat. (d) Suturing of the urethra to the perineal skin using a simple interrupted pattern. Images courtesy of Filippo Cinti and Tim Charlesworth.

7. The end of the urethra is spatulated (approx. 1 cm) using a "fish mouth" technique, and the urethral mucosa is sutured to the skin in a simple interrupted pattern using 3-0 or 4-0 absorbable monofilament material. The remainder of the skin wound is closed routinely.

Although patients learn to posture differently during urination, urine scalding and dermatitis can be a significant problem. Urinary incontinence has been reported in 17%–38% of cats undergoing this procedure and potentially could exacerbate urine scalding.[49] Careful dissection of the urethra to preserve innervation to the sphincter is important. In one report, long-term complications, including incontinence, were more common in cats undergoing prepubic urethrostomy compared to other locations.[50]

Other potential complications include urinary tract infections, urinary obstruction associated with stricture of the site or urethral kinking, and necrosis of surrounding skin.[49] Patients should wear an Elizabethan collar until suture removal to prevent self-trauma during the healing process.

KEEP IN MIND

- Urolithiasis is the most common cause of ureteral obstruction in veterinary patients.
- Calcium oxalate is the predominant stone type identified in the ureter of cats. In dogs, a similar proportion of calcium oxalate and struvite stones are identified, with many canine patients presenting with obstructive pyonephrosis.
- Surgical intervention is often recommended if the stones are causing clinical disease, and may involve ureterotomy, ureteroneocystostomy, ureteral stenting, or the placement of a subcutaneous ureteral bypass device.
- The scrotal location is preferred for permanent urethrostomy in male dogs, since the urethra is relatively wide and more superficial, resulting in less hemorrhage compared to other locations.
- In male cats, the perineal location is preferred for permanent urethrostomy and can be safely performed with the patient in ventral or dorsal recumbency.
- Although less frequently performed, transpelvic and prepubic urethrostomy have been described in both male and female dogs and cats for treating more proximal obstructions or salvaging a failed perineal urethrostomy.

References

1. Kyles AE et al. Management and outcome of cats with ureteral calculi: 153 cases (1984–2002). *J Am Vet Med Assoc*. 2005; 226(6):937–944.
2. Westropp JL et al. Dried solidified blood calculi in the urinary tract of cats. *J Vet Intern Med*. 2006; 20(4):828–834.
3. Zaid MS, Berent AC, Weisse C, Caceres A. Feline ureteral strictures: 10 cases (2007–2009). *J Vet Intern Med*. 2011; 25(2):222–229.
4. Cohen L et al. Bilateral ureteral obstruction in a cat due to a ureteral transitional cell carcinoma. *Can Vet J*. 2012; 53(5):535–538.
5. Wormser C, Phillips H, Aronson LR. Retroperitoneal fibrosis in feline renal transplant recipients: 29 cases (1998–2011). *J Am Vet Med Assoc*. 2013; 243(11):1580–1585.
6. Wormser C, Clarke DL, Aronson LR. Outcomes of ureteral surgery and ureteral stenting in cats: 117 cases (2006–2014). *J Am Vet Med Assoc*. 2016; 248(5):518–525.
7. Kyles AE et al. Clinical, clinicopathologic, radiographic, and ultrasonographic abnormalities in cats with ureteral calculi: 163 cases (1984–2002). *J Am Vet Med Assoc*. 2005; 226(6):932–936.
8. Snyder DM et al. Diagnosis and surgical management of ureteral calculi in dogs: 16 cases (1990–2003). *N Z Vet J*. 2005; 53(1):19–25.
9. Kuntz JA, Berent AC, Weisse CW, Bagley DH. Double pigtail ureteral stenting and renal pelvic lavage for renal-sparing treatment of obstructive pyonephrosis in dogs: 13 cases (2008–2012). *J Am Vet Med Assoc*. 2015; 246(2):216–225.
10. Lekcharoensuk C et al. Trends in the frequency of calcium oxalate uroliths in the upper urinary tract of cats. *J Am Anim Hosp Assoc*. 2005; 41(1):39–46.
11. Nesser VE, Reetz JA, Clarke DL, Aronson LR. Radiographic distribution of ureteral stones in 78 cats. *Vet Surg*. 2018; 47(7):895–901.
12. Wormser C, Reetz JA, Drobatz KJ, Aronson LR. Diagnostic utility of ultrasonography for detection of the cause and location of ureteral obstruction in cats: 71 cases (2010–2016). *J Am Vet Med Assoc*. 2019; 254(6):710–715.
13. D'Anjou MA, Bédard A, Dunn ME. Clinical significance of renal pelvic dilatation on ultrasound in dogs and cats. *Vet Radiol Ultrasound*. 2011; 52(1):88–94.
14. Lemieux C, Vachon C, Beauchamp G, Dunn ME. Minimal renal pelvis dilation in cats diagnosed with benign ureteral obstruction by antegrade pyelography: A retrospective study of 82 cases (2012–2018). *J Feline Med Surg*. 2021; 23(10):892–899.
15. Merindol I, Vachon C, Juette T, Dunn M. Benign ureteral obstruction in cats: Outcome with medical management. *J Vet Intern Med*. 2023; 37(3):1047–1058.

16. Aronson LR, Cleroux A, Wormser C. Use of a modified Boari flap for the treatment of a proximal ureteral obstruction in a cat. *Vet Surg*. 2018; 47(4):578–585.
17. Oyamada K et al. Extravesicular, two-layer, side-to-side ureteroneocystostomy combined with tension-relieving techniques for feline proximal ureteral obstruction: A retrospective study. *Vet Surg*. 2023; 52(7):972–982.
18. Berent AC. Ureteral obstructions in dogs and cats: A review of traditional and new interventional diagnostic and therapeutic options. *J Vet Emerg Crit Care (San Antonio)*. 2011; 21(2):86–103.
19. Lorange M, Monnet E. Postoperative outcomes of 12 cats with ureteral obstruction treated with ureteroneocystostomy. *Vet Surg*. 2020; 49(7):1418–1427.
20. Pratschke KM. Ureteral implantation using a three-stitch ureteroneocystostomy: Description of technique and outcome in nine dogs. *J Small Anim Pract*. 2015; 56(9):566–571.
21. Roberts SF, Aronson LR, Brown DC. Postoperative mortality in cats after ureterolithotomy. *Vet Surg*. 2011; 40(4):438–443.
22. Berent AC, Weisse CW, Todd K, Bagley DH. Technical and clinical outcomes of ureteral stenting in cats with benign ureteral obstruction: 69 cases (2006–2010). *J Am Vet Med Assoc*. 2014; 244(5):559–576.
23. Nicoli S et al. Double-J ureteral stenting in nine cats with ureteral obstruction. *Vet J*. 2012; 194(1):60–65.
24. Manassero M et al. Indwelling double pigtail ureteral stent combined or not with surgery for feline ureterolithiasis: Complications and outcome in 15 cases. *J Feline Med Surg*. 2014; 16(8):623–630.
25. Kulendra NJ, Syme H, Benigni L, Halfacree Z. Feline double pigtail ureteric stents for management of ureteric obstruction: Short- and long-term follow-up of 26 cats. *J Feline Med Surg*. 2014; 16(12):985–991.
26. Deroy C et al. Comparison between double-pigtail ureteral stents and ureteral bypass devices for treatment of ureterolithiasis in cats. *J Am Vet Med Assoc*. 2017; 251(4):429–437.
27. Berent AC, Weisse CW, Bagley DH, Lamb K. Use of a subcutaneous ureteral bypass device for treatment of benign ureteral obstruction in cats: 174 ureters in 134 cats (2009–2015). *J Am Vet Med Assoc*. 2018; 253(10):1309–1327.
28. Wuillemin F, Vachon C, Beauchamp G, Dunn M. Subcutaneous ureteral bypass device placement in 81 cats with benign ureteral obstruction (2013–2018). *J Vet Intern Med*. 2021; 35(6):2778–2786.
29. Livet V et al. Placement of subcutaneous ureteral bypasses without fluoroscopic guidance in cats with ureteral obstruction: 19 cases (2014–2016). *J Feline Med Surg*. 2017; 19(10):1030–1039.
30. Kulendra NJ et al. Survival and complications in cats treated with subcutaneous ureteral bypass. *J Small Anim Pract*. 2021; 62(1):4–11.
31. Pennington CE, Halfacree Z, Colville-Hyde C, Geddes RF. Factors associated with positive urine cultures in cats with subcutaneous ureteral bypass system implantation. *J Feline Med Surg*. 2021; 23(4):331–336.
32. Kopecny L et al. Risk factors for positive urine cultures in cats with subcutaneous ureteral bypass and ureteral stents (2010–2016). *J Vet Intern Med*. 2019; 33(1):178–183.
33. Vrijsen E et al. Complications and survival after subcutaneous ureteral bypass device placement in 24 cats: A retrospective study (2016–2019). *J Feline Med Surg*. 2021; 23(8):759–769.
34. Deprey J et al. Risk factors and clinical relevance of positive urine cultures in cats with subcutaneous ureteral bypass. *BMC Vet Res*. 2021; 17(1):199.
35. Véran E et al. Multicenter retrospective evaluation of transmural migration of subcutaneous ureteral bypass devices within the digestive tract in cats. *J Vet Intern Med*. 2022; 36(5):1677–1685.
36. Stiller AT, Lulich JP, Furrow E. Urethral plugs in dogs. *J Vet Intern Med*. 2014; 28(2):324–330.
37. Piermattei DK, Osborne CA. Urohydropulsion—non surgical removal of urethral calculi in male dogs. In: Kirk RW (ed.). *Current Veterinary Therapy VI: Small Animal Practice*. Philadelphia, PA: WB Saunders; 1977. pp. 1194–1196.
38. Berent A, Weisse C. Urinary diversion techniques. In: Monnet E (ed.). *Small Animal Soft Tissue Surgery*, 1 st ed. Oxford, United Kingdom: John Wiley & Sons; 2013. pp. 600–614.
39. Cinti F, Pisani G, Carusi U, Buracco P. Urethrotomy of the glans penis in three male dogs with urolithiasis. *J Small Anim Pract*. 2015; 56(11):671–674.
40. Chiaramonte A et al. Transpelvic urethrostomy in a female dog with congenital vestibulovaginal and urethral stenosis: A case report. *Vet Surg*. 2022; 51(4):706–712.
41. Giansetto T, Broux O, Bolen G, Claeys S. Preputial urethrostomy with preservation of the local anatomy in 4 dogs. *Vet Surg*. 2022; 51(8):1295–1303.
42. Bleedorn JA, Bjorling DE. Urethra. In: Tobias KM, Johnston SA (eds.). *Veterinary Surgery: Small Animal*, 1 st ed. St. Louis, MO: Elsevier Saunders; 2012. pp. 1993–2010.
43. Yeh LS, Chin SC. Modified perineal urethrostomy using preputial mucosa in cats. *J Am Vet Med Assoc*. 2000; 216(7):1092–1095.
44. Slunsky P et al. Effect of intraoperative positioning on postoperative neurological status in cats after perineal urethrostomy. *J Feline Med Surg*. 2019; 21(10):931–937.
45. Watson MT, Roca RY, Breiteneicher AH, Kalis RH. Evaluation of postoperative complication rates in cats undergoing perineal urethrostomy performed in dorsal recumbency. *J Feline Med Surg*. 2020; 22(4):399–403.
46. Phillips H, Holt DE. Surgical revision of the urethral stoma following perineal urethrostomy in 11 cats: (1998–2004). *J Am Anim Hosp Assoc*. 2006; 42(3):218–222.
47. Bernarde A, Viguier E. Transpelvic urethrostomy in 11 cats using an ischial ostectomy. *Vet Surg*. 2004; 33(3):246–252.
48. Bresciani L, Mosca A, Romussi S. Modified prepubic urethrostomy with body wall tunneling: Description of technique and long-term outcome in eight male cats. *Vet Surg*. 2022; 51(2):353–360.
49. Sousa-Filho RP et al. Clinical outcomes of 28 cats 12–24 months after urethrostomy. *J Feline Med Surg*. 2020; 22(10):890–897.
50. Seneviratne M, Stamenova P, Lee K. Comparison of surgical indications and short- and long-term complications in 56 cats undergoing perineal, transpelvic or prepubic urethrostomy. *J Feline Med Surg*. 2021; 23(6):477–486.

Chapter 20

Genital emergencies

Erin Gibson, Rachel Williams

Female genital emergencies

The ovary is a paired female gonadal organ that is positioned just caudal to the caudal pole of the kidney. It consists of an inner medulla, with blood vessels, nerves, lymphatics, smooth muscle, and connective tissue fibers, and an outer cortex containing follicles within connective tissue stroma.[1]

The uterine tube, which is predominantly composed of the infundibulum, leads from the ovary to the horn of the uterus. During ovulation, infundibular fimbriae within the ovarian bursa swell and prevent intraperitoneal passage of oocytes.

The uterus consists of a body and two horns. It has three layers: an outer serosal layer, a middle muscular layer (myometrium), and the thickest, innermost epithelial layer (endometrium).

The cervix is located between the uterine body and the vaginal vault. The vaginal mucosal stratified squamous epithelium is organized into longitudinal folds. The outer striated muscle of the urethra is confluent with the terminal third of the vagina. The vaginal canal terminates at the vestibule, which has a smoother darker red mucosal lining.

The uterine horns, uterine body, and ovaries are attached to the dorsolateral walls of the abdomen by the broad ligament. This structure is a folded layer of peritoneum that contains nerves and vessels that feed the attached structures and also contains fingerlike projections of fat. The broad ligament is divided into the mesovarium and mesosalpinx (ovary) and mesometrium (uterine horn and body, cervix, and cranial vagina).

The ovarian artery arises from the aorta and provides arterial blood supply to the ovary; this artery may also supply the capsule of the kidney and the uterine horn. The uterine artery arises from the vaginal artery and anastomoses with the uterine branch of the ovarian artery. The ovary is drained by the right and left renal veins, which connect to the vena cava and left renal vein, respectively. The uterine vein drains the majority of the uterine horn and body.[1]

Dystocia

Dystocia is a very uncommon (<5% of at risk females) condition characterized by difficult or obstructed labor leading to the failure of passing through the normal stages of parturition.[2,3] Causes of dystocia are divided into fetal and maternal, with maternal etiologies (primary uterine inertia) being predominantly responsible for feline and canine dystocia.[4,5]

Dystocia can be a life-threatening emergency for the mother, and for the neonates, and requires efficient and effective diagnosis and surgical treatment when indicated. It should be noted that most animals that present with this condition will require surgery. The surgical method and approach vary slightly from case to case depending on the cause of dystocia, the patient's needs, and the capabilities of the care team.

The option to perform ovariohysterectomy should be carefully discussed with owners. If the patient's intrinsic factors confer a moderate to high risk of dystocia, sterilization should be recommended to avoid complications for the animal in the future.

Very little is known about feline dystocia, but a similar approach to that of canine dystocia can be considered in cats.

Clinical presentation and diagnosis

Normal gestation in the dog is approximately 63 days (range, 56–72 days) from the date of first known breeding. The cat gestation period is 65 days (range, 52–74 days) from breeding to onset of parturition. Uniquely, female cats are induced ovulators and may allow multiple matings to enable superfecundation or kittens sired by different males.[6,7]

Stage 1 of parturition consists of uterine contractions that progress in effort as well as cervical dilation, and it can be difficult to detect. Stage 2 is characterized by active abdominal and uterine contractions culminating in fetal delivery. Stage 3 is the time period during which the fetus and placenta are expelled.[4,7,8]

In dystocic animals, identifying the etiology of dystocia is crucial to determine the most appropriate treatment strategies. Uterine inertia is the most common cause of dystocia in small animals. Primary uterine inertia is a failure to normally proceed through parturition despite adequate fetal and maternal size. Complete primary uterine inertia prevents the birth of any puppy or kitten, while partial primary uterine inertia results in the birth of some but not all offspring.[5] The cause of primary inertia may be different in each patient and, in many cases, is unknown. It has been associated with abnormal or low hormone levels (prostaglandins, oxytocin) and litters that are too large or too small, preventing normal stimulation. Electrolyte disorders (hypocalcemia, hypoglycemia) have been identified in dystocic animals, but this is rarely reported in the literature.[4,9]

Secondary uterine inertia is the exhaustion of the myometrium due to maternal or fetal factors leading to obstruction of the birth canal, including narrowed birth canal or fetal malposition. Importantly, this problem must be surgically managed and no attempts at medical management are advised, as this can prolong time until definitive care and worsen outcomes for the mother and fetuses. Other causes of dystocia beyond uterine inertia include birth canal obstruction (ie pelvic fractures), abnormal fetal presentation, and fetal–maternal mismatch.

In dogs, litter size and progressive age have been associated with an increased risk of dystocia.[10] Canine brachycephaly bears a high risk of dystocia, likely secondary to fetal–maternal mismatch due to the mother's relatively short pelvis and pelvic canal and narrow pelvic outlet.[11] Risk factors for feline dystocia are poorly reported, but similar factors may be associated.[4]

In cats and dogs presenting with dystocia, medical management may be attempted if indicated, although there appears to be a high rate of failure (2/3 of cats and >1/2 of dogs) to alleviate dystocia.[3–5]

If dystocia is suspected based on presentation, physical examination can be helpful in identifying the cause of dystocia (e.g., rectal exam, vaginal exam, abdominal palpation). It is important to keep in mind that anterior or posterior fetal presentation can be appropriate.[5] Common types of malposition include transverse and breech presentations. If fetal position cannot be digitally normalized in such cases, surgery is indicated.

Abdominal radiographs can help identify causes of dystocia as well as indicators of fetal viability. Typically, radiographic signs of loss of fetal viability occur at least 24 hours after death and can be less reliable compared to ultrasound findings. The presence of gas within or around the fetus, overlapping bones of the cranium, and tightly curled or collapsed fetal skeleton are all suggestive of nonviability.[12]

Ultrasound is helpful in detecting fetal heart beats, identifying uterine malposition or rupture, and guiding decision-making for caesarean section (C-section). Fetal stress is associated with reduced fetal heart rate and can be used in decision-making.[13]

Absolute indications for emergency C-section include failure to respond to medical management of primary uterine inertia, fetal distress, or stillbirths of previously viable fetuses. Other indications include dystocia due to secondary uterine inertia or evidence of uterine torsion or rupture, and unresolvable fetal malposition, fetal-maternal mismatch, or birth canal obstruction from soft tissue (vaginal stenosis) or pelvic (fracture) abnormalities. Duration of dystocia without resolution should be minimized as much as possible due to the risk of worsened fetal and maternal outcomes.[2,14]

Treatment

The patient should be stabilized as much as possible prior to the intervention if surgery is indicated and elected. Electrolyte abnormalities, dehydration, and hypoglycemia should be evaluated and corrected. Anemia or hypotension related to hemorrhage should be evaluated for and treated if noted.

A complete review of the medical management of dystocia is beyond the scope of this chapter. Briefly, calcium gluconate and oxytocin can be considered for cases of primary uterine inertia for their action in strengthening uterine contractions and increasing frequency of uterine contractions, respectively. Careful monitoring of maternal and fetal parameters is essential during attempted medical management.[14]

Regarding anesthesia, briefly, the primary goals are rapid time from induction to delivery of the neonates, maintenance of uterine blood flow, and minimization of anesthesia of the neonates to enable rapid wakefulness following delivery. Preoxygenation and medications to prevent emesis and aspiration should be provided (see Fig. 20.1a). Local blocks such as epidural or line blocks over the site of incision should be considered. Nonsteroidal anti-inflammatory drugs may be used effectively in the patient and are associated with a low excretion into breast milk, making them ideal for use in the postpartum period; however, they should be avoided in case of mastitis, as excretion in the milk is higher.[15] Injectable anesthetics such as alfaxalone and propofol could be considered, as well as maintenance with inhalation agents (isoflurane).[16] Standard monitoring is indicated for these cases.

Surgical technique (Fig. 20.1)

1. The patient is clipped and prepared for surgery before induction. The full abdomen should be clipped from xiphoid to pubis.
2. Following induction, the patient is placed in dorsal recumbency, final aseptic preparation is performed, and the patient is draped from xiphoid to pubis. Elevating the patient's cranial thorax/neck/head can be considered to support spontaneous ventilation.
3. A ventral midline incision is made from the midabdomen, cranial to the umbilicus, to just cranial to the pubis (see Chapter 3). It should be noted that since the linea alba will be stretched and thin in

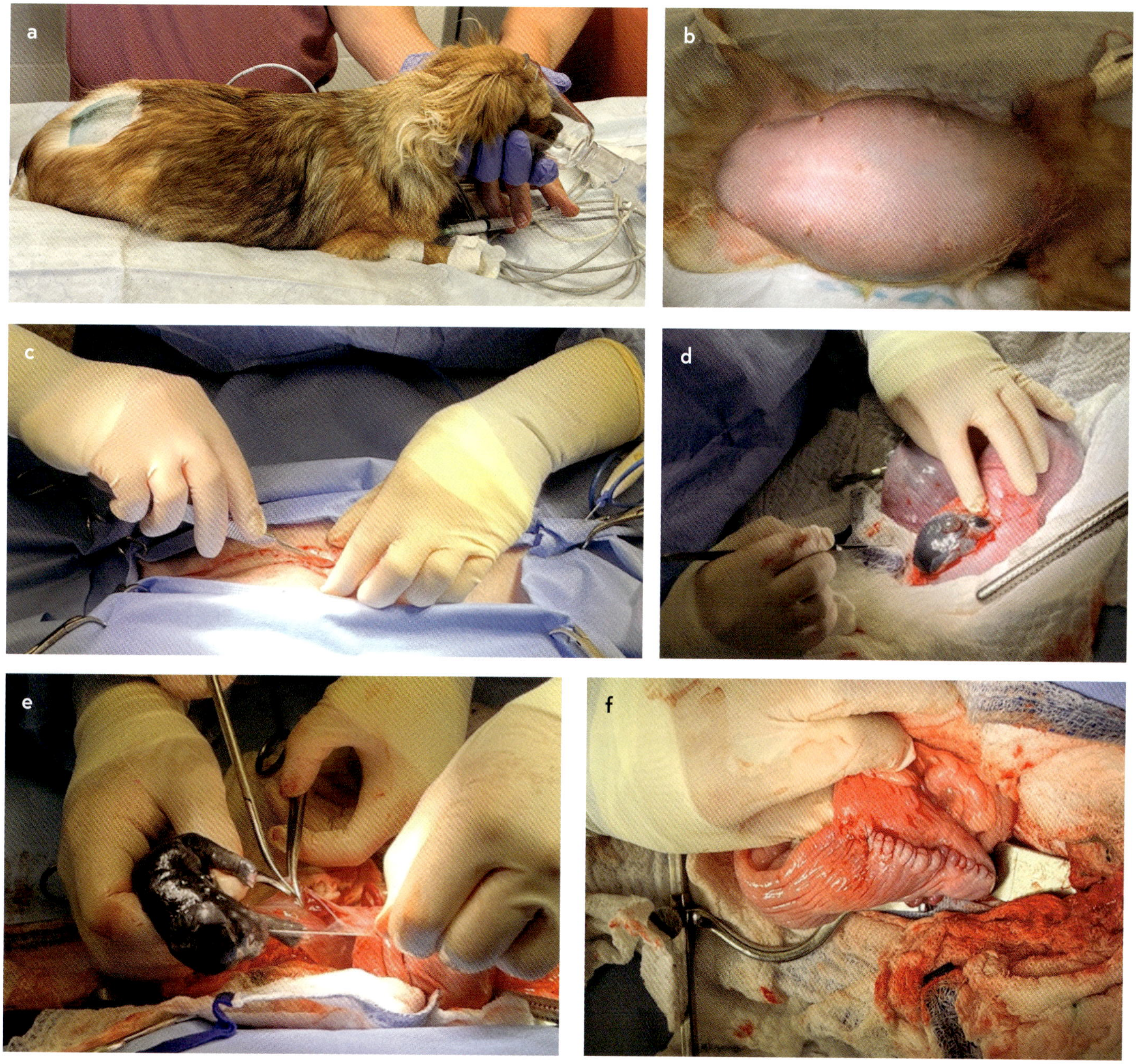

Figure 20.1 Cesarean section. (a) Preoxygenation of the mother prior to induction. The region of the epidural block is clipped and prepared as well. (b) The abdomen is clipped and the patient positioned for surgery immediately following induction. Clipping is typically performed before induction, if possible. (c) Ventral midline incision extending from the umbilicus, or cranial to the umbilicus, to the pubis. (d) Externalization of the uterus and full-thickness incision into the uterine body, being cautious of the depth of the incision. (e) Removal of the fetuses, disruption of the fetal membranes, and double clamping and transection of the umbilicus between the two clamps. (f) Closure of the uterine body with absorbable monofilament suture material in a simple continuous pattern.

these patients, inadvertent entry into the abdomen is possible. Lateral dissection of the mammary tissue should be avoided.

4. The incision is protected with moistened sponges, and the uterus is externalized. Care should be taken not to rupture the uterus or cause excessive trauma to the uterine ligaments, which can lead to excessive hemorrhage.
5. The uterine incision site should be planned to ensure rapid removal of the fetuses. It may be made more caudally if a fetus is lodged within the pelvic canal. Fetuses lodged more distally within the uterine horns may require separate incisions.
6. Following identification of a fetus and rupture of the amniotic sac, the fetal umbilicus is double clamped and transected between the clamps.

7. A neonate resuscitation team should be prepared to care for the newborns.
8. The next step varies depending on whether the uterus is to be preserved or removed:
   - If the uterus is to be preserved, the fetal membranes are usually removed from their placentation sites with gentle traction. These membranes can be tightly adhered and may bleed excessively when extracted; in these cases, they may be allowed to pass on their own to prevent excessive bleeding. The uterine incision is closed in one or two layers with 2-0 or 3-0 absorbable monofilament suture. A simple continuous pattern followed by an inverting pattern may be used.
   - If the uterus is to be removed, routine ovariohysterectomy is performed. Special attention should be paid to vascular ligations, as the blood supply to the uterus is expected to be robust.
9. The abdomen should be lavaged and suctioned, gloves and instruments exchanged, and closure initiated.
10. The linea alba, subcutaneous tissues, and skin are closed routinely. External sutures should be avoided to minimize the risk of the neonates suckling or irritating the incision.

En bloc removal of the uterus is reported, with neonatal survival rates comparable to those after standard C-section. It involves performing ovariohysterectomy prior to fetus removal, and subsequent passage of the entire uterus to assistants for removal of the neonates. This procedure could be considered if the female is to be spayed, if there are no viable fetuses, if there is infectious material that may contaminate the abdomen, or if the fetuses (when viable) are not in detectable distress.

En bloc uterine removal is less commonly performed and should only be considered by a surgeon with significant surgical experience to guarantee optimal outcomes for viable fetuses.

Postoperative management and outcome

Pain management should be provided and may include either an opioid or nonsteroidal anti-inflammatory drugs.[15,16] Following recovery, the female should be monitored, but, ultimately, prompt discharge after surgery is ideal to minimize maternal and fetal stress.

Among dystocic patients treated, the mortality rate is exceedingly low regardless of the procedure (C-section, with or without ovariohysterectomy, or en bloc removal of the uterus).[2,4,5,17] The neonatal death rate in pups and kittens born in dystocic environments ranges from 11% to 33%.[2,4,5,10]

Uterine torsion

Uterine torsion (i.e., twisting of a horn or the body of the uterus about the longitudinal axis) is a rare condition that has been identified in both pregnant and nonpregnant animals.[5,18–20] The uterus may be fully twisted, or one horn may be malpositioned in relation to the uterine body and contralateral horn. This condition may be related to broad ligament stretching, uterine wall weakness or flaccidity, increased physical activity, or pregnancy.[18–20] In the gravid uterus, this complication, even if affecting only one horn, frequently leads to poor fetal outcomes. This rare syndrome should be considered as a differential diagnosis in intact females with an acute abdomen. Preoperative diagnosis is exceedingly difficult, and definitive diagnosis may require exploratory laparotomy. Prompt surgical intervention is recommended if uterine torsion is diagnosed or highly suspected.

Clinical presentation and diagnosis

Clinical presentation may vary, but animals may be presented for lethargy, anorexia, abdominal distension, or abdominal pain, with or without a history of known pregnancy. In severe cases, uterine torsion can lead to significant illness, including peritonitis from bacterial translocation or uterine rupture. Physical examination may reveal a tube-like structure within the abdomen continuing into the caudal abdominal cavity. Anemia and/or alterations of leukocyte count may be noted. Uterine torsion is reported most commonly in pregnant animals, with or without dystocia. If it occurs in the nongravid uterus, uterine disorders such as pyometra, hematometra, or endometrial polyps have been implicated.[5,18–20]

Diagnosis may be suspected based on abdominal imaging, but exploration of the abdomen is often necessary to confirm diagnosis. Abdominal radiography may not identify a uterine torsion, but it can be used to confirm pregnancy. Ultrasound may reveal a fluid-filled viscus that may or may not be identifiable as the uterus.[12,18,20]

Treatment

The patient should be stabilized preoperatively, which may include red blood cell transfusion, intravenous fluid resuscitation, electrolyte derangement correction, and introduction of antibiotics.

Standard en bloc ovariohysterectomy should be performed. If surgery is carried out on a pregnant animal, C-section should be performed first. Derotating the uterus prior to removal should be avoided. Care should be taken to identify and avoid the ureters. In case of uterine rupture, abdominal lavage can be considered and broad-spectrum antibiotic coverage initiated if pyometra/infection is diagnosed or suspected.

Postoperative management and outcome

Postoperative care of the mother and viable fetuses should be performed as mentioned in the "Dystocia" section above, if relevant. Monitoring (e.g., vital signs, blood gas analysis) and intravenous supportive care until the animal is stabilized and discharged from hospital is appropriate.

If uterine torsion occurs in a pregnant animal, fetal viability may be compromised.[19] Regarding the mother, the severity of disease that she presents with will dictate prognosis. If stabilization and surgical intervention are prompt and effective, a good outcome for the mother is possible.

Uterine prolapse

Uterine prolapse is a rare condition that occurs most frequently as a complication of parturition and can occur within 48 hours of passage of the last fetus, although it has been reported in a nonpregnant cat.[21] It is the eversion of the uterus through the cervix into the vagina and exteriorization through the vulva. The prolapse can be complete, with both horns protruding through the cervix into the vaginal vault, or limited to the uterine body and one horn. Hemorrhage from tear of the ovarian or uterine arteries, uterine rupture, and/or contamination of the abdomen can lead to severe illness that requires rapid care.[21–23]

Animals presenting with this condition may be in various states of systemic compromise and should be treated as emergencies, with the goal of stabilization and prompt surgical intervention, as reduction is often not possible.

Clinical presentation and diagnosis

A tubular mass-like structure protruding from the vulva may be seen, as well as contamination of the structure, with or without hemorrhage (Fig. 20.2). Careful palpation should be made to ensure no other intra-abdominal contents (e.g., urinary bladder, small intestine) are present within the prolapsed uterus, and care should be taken to confirm no neonates remain intra-abdominally in pregnant animals.[22,24,25]

With ultrasound or abdominal radiographs, absence of the uterus within the abdomen may be noted. Free fluid in the abdomen may be indicative of tearing and subsequent hemorrhage of gonadal arteries, or uterine rupture. The tissue may be in various states of contamination, ischemia, or necrosis, which is important to note when considering treatment.[22,24]

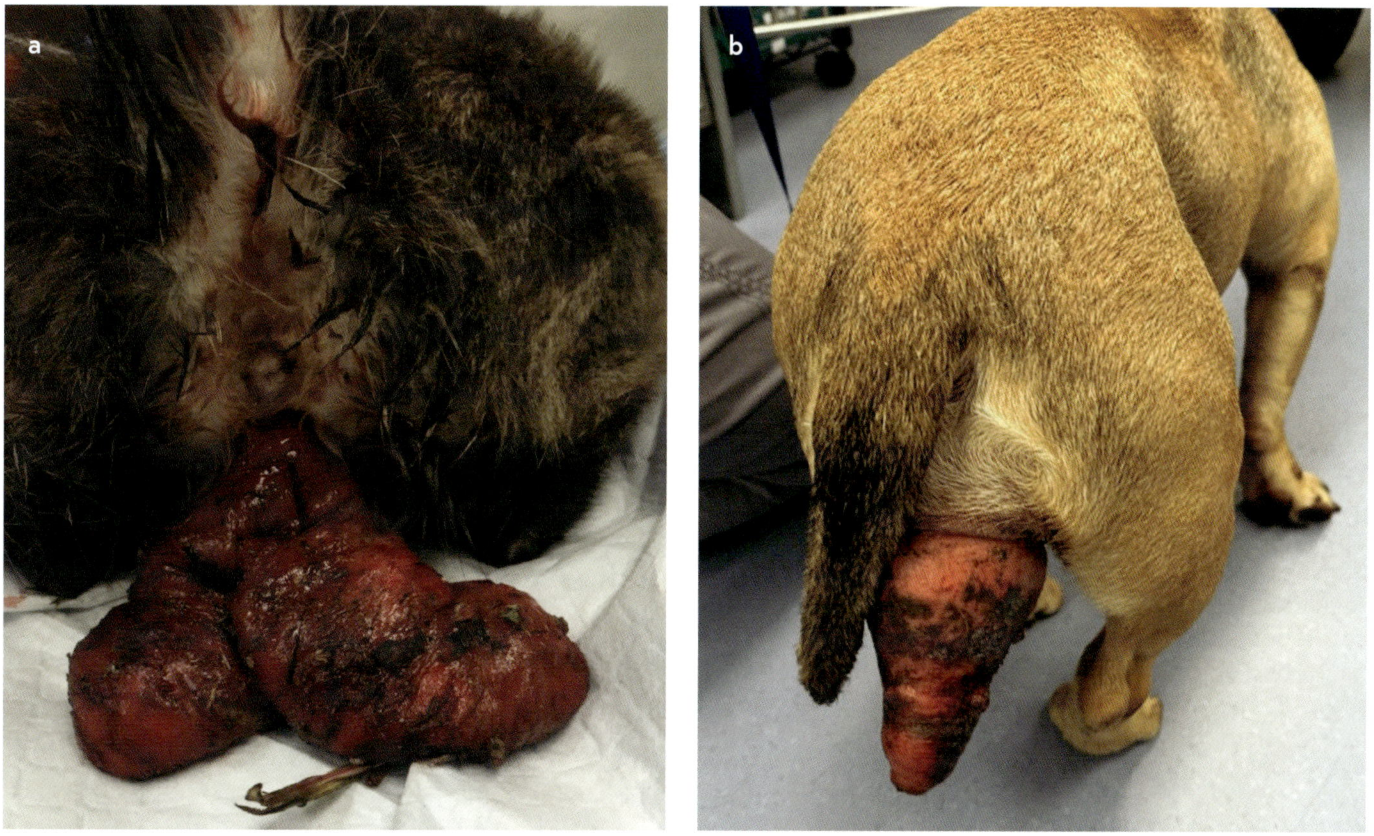

Figure 20.2 (a) Complete uterine prolapse in a cat, with moderate contamination and substantial congestion. (b) Single-horn (incomplete) uterine prolapse in a dog, with multifocal regions of necrosis. Image a courtesy of Philipp Mayhew; image b courtesy of William T. N. Culp.

Treatment

If manual reduction is attempted, general anesthesia is required. Decontamination of the prolapsed tissue should be performed prior to replacement. The prolapse can be lavaged with warm saline followed by a hyperosmotic solution to reduce edema and swelling. Water-soluble gel is used to lubricate the prolapsed uterus, and external pressure is applied. An episiotomy can be considered to assist in reduction.

Oxytocin (promotes uterine involution and cervix closure) may be administered following reduction, although the impact of this in dogs and cats has been incompletely evaluated.[24] Surgery should be performed if the uterine tissue is necrotic, if there is evidence of uterine rupture or substantial ongoing hemorrhage, or if the tissue is unable to be reduced. If the uterine tissue can be reduced, ovariectomy/ovariohysterectomy should be always considered to mitigate the risk of relapse. If nonreducible or too contaminated, urethral catheterization and amputation of the uterine horns and body from the site of prolapse, followed by laparotomy and ovariectomy, should be carried out. In the case of a fetus retained in one of the uterine horns, uterine reduction and C-section may be performed.[25]

Postoperative management and outcome

Ongoing monitoring and supportive care should be provided. Intravenous fluids, antibiotics, analgesics, and blood products may be considered depending on the degree of illness. Inflammation of the urethral papilla may lead to temporary obstruction or difficulty urinating, which should be monitored.[21–23,25] If this occurs, an indwelling urinary catheter can be placed temporarily, until inflammation resolves.

Outcomes in patients can be good overall if intervention is rapid and hemorrhage/contamination is resolved.

Vaginal prolapse

Vaginal prolapse is an exceptionally uncommon complication of the female reproductive tract. It is typically observed as the protrusion of doughnut-shaped tissue from the vulvar opening (Fig. 20.3). This condition has been associated with onset of dystocia, constipation, or forced separation during breeding. Due to the rarity of this condition, risk factors are difficult to ascertain, but a decrease in the progesterone levels or an increase in the estrogen levels paired with elevated intra-abdominal pressure in susceptible animals may allow this condition to occur.[26,27]

Clinical presentation and diagnosis

Vaginal prolapse has been graded by completeness, with type 3 considered complete prolapse, defined as the entire circumference of the vaginal wall presenting as a doughnut- or ring-shaped mass.[28]

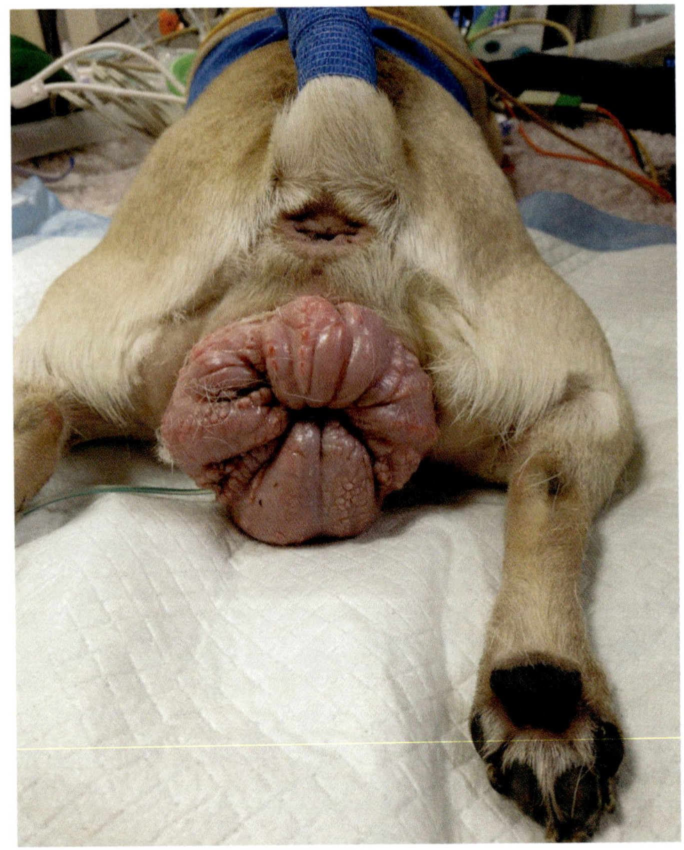

Figure 20.3 Vaginal prolapse, with the typical doughnut-shaped appearance. Image courtesy of Filippo Cinti and Tim Charlesworth.

If a mucosal mass-like structure everted from the vulvar opening is seen, differentiating between vaginal prolapse and vaginal edema/hyperplasia, clitoral hypertrophy, or vaginal/uterine tumors is important. Imaging of the prolapsed tissue and abdomen (ultrasound, abdominal radiographs) should be considered prior to any surgical intervention. Complete vaginal prolapse, arising from the floor of the vagina, is often accompanied by exteriorization of the urethral orifice, leading to the "doughnut" of protruding tissue, which can be helpful in distinguishing between hyperplasia/edema and prolapse (see Fig. 20.4).[26,27]

Treatment

If the tissue is viable, vaginal prolapse can be treated by replacement of the everted tissue following treatment of edema (as described for uterine prolapse). For this, general anesthesia is required. A purse-string or mattress sutures may be applied to the vulvar tissue to reduce the size of the vulvar opening and the risk of recurrence. Ovariohysterectomy may be considered to decrease cyclic exposure to estrogens and the risk of reprolapse.

If tissue viability is compromised or if the vagina cannot be completely reduced, cautious excision of the prolapsed tissue may be necessary, followed by ovariohysterectomy.

Surgical technique (Fig. 20.4)

1. The patient is placed under general anesthesia.
2. A urethral catheter should be placed preoperatively and remain in place throughout the procedure to avoid inadvertent damage to the urethral papilla.
3. If necessary, four full-thickness stay sutures are placed in healthy tissue, spaced 90 degrees apart. These sutures should include both layers of the prolapse.
4. One-third to one-half of the prolapsed tissue is resected 2–3 cm from the vulva, caudal to the stay sutures. Care should be taken not to damage the urethral papilla.
5. A single layer of full-thickness simple interrupted sutures, using 2-0 or 3-0 absorbable monofilament material, is used to create an anastomosis. The cut edges are sewn together.
6. The remaining tissue is cut and sewn in sections. The stay sutures are removed, and the everted vagina is manually reduced.
7. Cystopexy or colopexy may be necessary if additional organs are prolapsed.[26–28]

Postoperative management and outcome

Standard postoperative care is indicated. Special attention should be paid to the patient's ability to void or pass stool normally if other prolapsed organs (bladder, colon) have been surgically treated. Outcomes are generally good, but recurrence is possible, especially in intact female dogs.[28]

Pyometra

Pyometra (i.e., infection of the uterus) can be a life-threatening condition. In a Swedish study, the prevalence of pyometra in intact female dogs under 10 years of age was 24%.[29]

This disease has been associated with cystic endometrial hyperplasia (CEH), leading to a complex known as

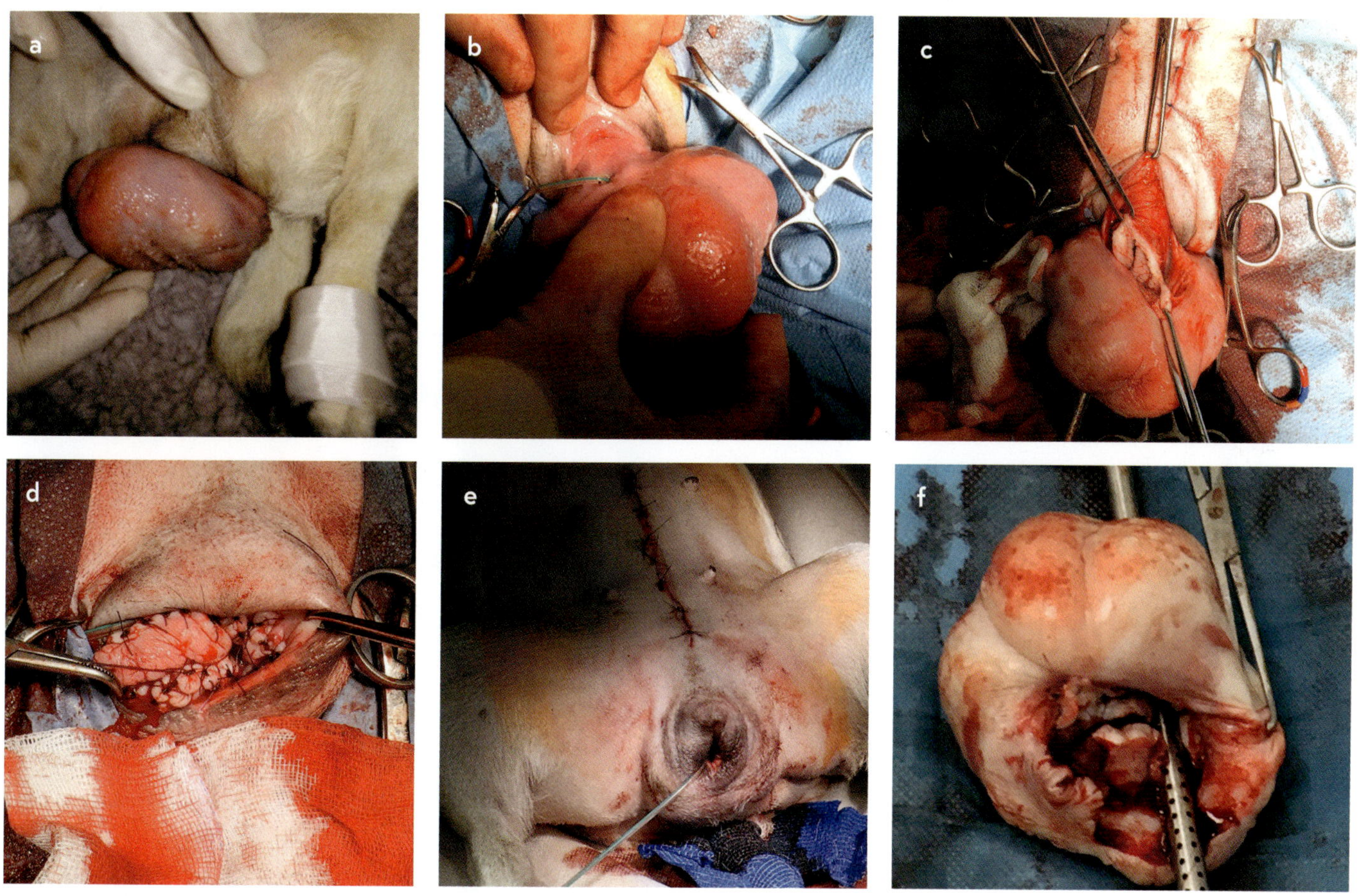

Figure 20.4 Resection and anastomosis of a vaginal prolapse in a female Pug. (a) Clinical presentation. (b) Urethral catheterization. (c) Resection of the prolapsed tissue 2–3 cm from the vulva, avoiding damage to the urethral papilla. (d) Anastomosis with a single layer of full-thickness simple interrupted sutures. (e) Reduction of the everted vagina, and ovariohysterectomy. (f) Vaginal prolapse after excision. Images courtesy of Filippo Cinti and Tim Charlesworth.

CEH-P. This complex appears to be primarily dependent on a high progesterone state, most commonly in diestrus, and is not seen in noncycling or sterilized animals.[30,31] Progesterone leads to endometrial proliferation, uterine glandular secretions, and decreased myometrial contractions, as well as leukocyte inhibition, which enables susceptibility to bacterial infection.[30] CEH-P appears to occur in female cats as well, although this type of hormonal cycling may be less predictable due to cats being induced ovulators and having shorter luteal phases.[32]

Clinical presentation and diagnosis

Clinical signs can be vague but include lethargy, vaginal discharge, dehydration, anorexia, and occasionally abdominal distension or abdominal pain. Vomiting, polydipsia/polyuria, and diarrhea may also be observed, while fever is uncommon on presentation.[33]

Alterations on blood work include mild to moderate normocytic, normochromic anemia, which may reflect chronicity. Leukopenia or profound leukocytosis may be discovered, although a normal leukogram may occur in up to 25% of cases.[34]

Elevations in urea or creatinine may be seen as well as hypoglycemia.[33] Azotemia is typically prerenal and may be accompanied by hyperproteinemia or hyperglobulinemia.[30,34] Hypoproteinemia may also be seen as a consequence of severe systemic inflammation and illness. Endotoxemia associated with *Escherichia coli* can decrease renal tubular sensitivity to antidiuretic hormone and lead to decreased urinary concentration, thereby causing isosthenuria, polydipsia, and polyuria.[34] Renal function alterations are often reversible with treatment. Concurrent urinary tract infection is possible. Cystocentesis should be performed cautiously and with ultrasound guidance if performed preoperatively, as there is substantial risk of entering the turgid uterine body.[30,34] Ultrasound is a useful tool in the diagnosis of pyometra in small animals.[35] It typically reveals enlarged uterine body and horns, with symmetric or segmental enlargement, echogenic contents, and a variable appearance of the uterine wall.[13] Uterine rupture may be suspected if free fluid is found in the abdomen.

Treatment

Dogs with closed pyometra (i.e., the infectious materials cannot drain because the cervix is closed) must be treated surgically on an emergency basis. Dogs with open pyometra (i.e., a partially or completely open cervix enables drainage) may be treated medically or surgically but must be evaluated on a case-by-case basis. Dogs who are stable and without evidence of systemic infection may be treated more conservatively. Regardless of the open or closed nature of pyometra, in case of failure to resolve infection with medical management or in patients who are critically ill or have signs of sepsis, surgical treatment must be applied.

Stabilization should be performed prior to any surgical intervention and should include prompt use of broad-spectrum antimicrobials. *E. coli* is the most common infective agent in pyometra, reaching the susceptible uterus via ascension through the vagina and cervix.[34,36] Peri- and postoperative administration of antibiotics for 7–14 days is typical. Uterine tissue and luminal fluid samples can be gathered at the time of ovariohysterectomy for culture in order to guide antibiotic therapy.

Generally, medical management is not recommended for pyometra but may be considered if the animal is intended for future breeding and has an open cervix to enable drainage. Promoting cervical relaxation, mitigating effects of progesterone, and inducing uterine contraction and emptying as well as managing bacterial infection are the goals of therapy, which typically includes the use of antibiotics and synthetic prostaglandins or antiprogesterone medications.[34,37] However, there is risk of uterine rupture or failure to resolve pyometra.

Surgical treatment consists of standard ovariohysterectomy. A full laparotomy incision may be necessary, especially if there is uterine rupture (Fig. 20.5). Care should be taken to identify and avoid damaging the ureters. The authors prefer to ligate the uterine artery and vein bundle with individual sutures around each, as well as

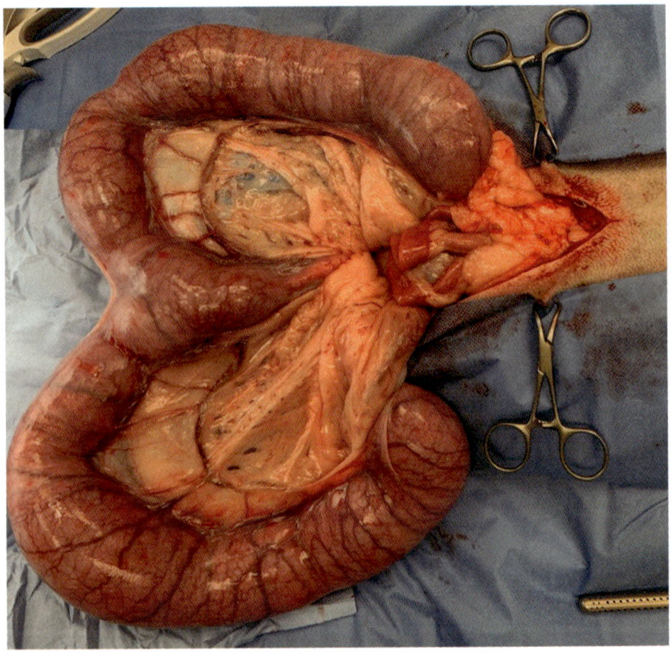

Figure 20.5 Moderately distended pyometra uterus fanned out after caudal abdominal incision. Image courtesy of Jennifer Huck.

to double ligate the uterine body. Following transection of the uterine body, the uterine stump should be copiously lavaged, and the remnant stump can be packed with omentum or oversewn in a continuous suture pattern with absorbable monofilament material. In case of uterine rupture or suspected peritonitis, extra care should be taken to flush extensively, and a drain may be placed and kept in place postoperatively.

Postoperative management and outcome

Intravenous fluid support, gastrointestinal support, antimicrobials, and correction of glucose or electrolyte derangements is required. Azotemia should be rechecked, and urine output and body weight change measured carefully. If an abdominal drain has been placed, fluid should be quantified and drain removal considered when fluid production reduces and plateaus (in any case, no longer than 3–5 days postoperatively) to minimize the risk of drain contamination. Antimicrobials should be modified according to culture results.

Female dogs treated with surgery have a high rate of survival, with a reported mortality rate in the nonspecialty setting of 3%–4%.[34,38,39] Feline survival is comparably good, with reported survival rates of 92%–100% in cats treated with ovariohysterectomy.[32,40] Animals presenting with uterine rupture, septic peritonitis, or shock may have a worse prognosis.

Male genital emergencies

The canine and feline male reproductive tract consists of the penis, testicles, and an accessory sex gland called the prostate. Cats also possess an additional accessory sex gland, the bulbourethral glands. The testes, or male gonads, are located in a haired scrotum and continue into the spermatic cord, which contains the vas deferens, testicular artery and vein, and cremaster muscle.

The prostate gland is found in close association with the bladder neck and most proximal portion of the pelvic urethra. Size of the prostate gland is known to be adrogen dependent, and castration may affect its size, even later in life. The prostate gland is divided into right and left lobes, which are further divided into lobules that contain many tubuloalveolar glands responsible for producing prostatic secretions. The tubuloalveolar glands empty into the prostatic urethra through many small communications along its length.[52]

The gland receives its blood supply from the prostatic artery, which arises from the internal pudendal artery. The prostate gland is drained by the prostatic and urethral veins, ultimately terminating in the internal iliac vein.[52]

Prostatic cysts and abscesses

Prostatic surgical emergencies are rare but can pose a serious and life-threatening problem. Prostatic disease in general has been reported in 2.5% of dogs and is even less frequent in cats.[41]

In dogs, prostatic cysts account for 5%–15% of prostatic disease cases and become infected in up to 42% of patients.[41–43] They may be sterile or nonsterile and extra- or intraparenchymal.[45,46] Intraparenchymal prostatic cysts (formerly called prostatic retention cysts) are suspected to occur secondary to an accumulation of prostatic secretions and may contain urine. The origin of extraparenchymal cysts is unknown. An important differentiating factor between these two types of prostatic cysts is that intraparenchymal cysts can be connected with the urethra, while extraparenchymal ones communicate with the prostatic capsule but not with the urinary system.[46]

Surgical treatment is generally recommended for prostatic cysts and may consist of partial or total resection with or without omentalization. Nonsurgical treatment has also been reported.[48,49]

Prostatic abscesses are less common than prostatic cysts, affecting 2%–7.7% of dogs with prostatic disease.[41,43] They are suspected to arise from an ascending infection of the urinary tract. *E. coli* is isolated most frequently, although *Staphylococcus* spp. and *Proteus* spp. are often implicated as well.[44] These abscesses can also result from hematogenous spread or from an infected cyst. Surgical treatment is recommended, as systemic antibiotic therapy, percutaneous drainage, and castration alone are potentially not sufficient to treat the underlying cause; however, nonsurgical management has also been described.[48]

Clinical presentation and diagnosis

Clinical signs associated with prostatic disease are frequently related to surrounding organs that are compressed secondary to the underlying disease process. Patients with prostatic cysts or abscesses may present with similar clinical signs, although the latter may be more systemically ill. Clinical signs that may be seen include dyschezia, hematuria, stranguria, constipation, and pain during defecation.[41,42] In severe cases, urinary obstruction can occur and may need to be relieved via catheterization or cystocentesis. Occasionally, patients will present with a wide-legged stance or will be stiff in their pelvic limbs.

On physical examination, abdominal pain may be detected, but signs are otherwise largely nonspecific. Rectal examination is often painful and may reveal an enlarged or asymmetric prostate gland. In case of a ruptured prostatic abscess, patients may be unstable and show signs consistent with septic shock. There may be fever and edema in the pelvic limbs and inguinal region due to interference with lymph drainage secondary to compression by the enlarged prostate gland.

A leukogram typically shows leukocytosis.[41] Biochemistry can reveal increases in alkaline phosphatase. In some patients, particularly in those that are septic, hypoglycemia and azotemia may be seen.[44] Microorganisms may be identified on urinalysis.

Radiographs may show prostatomegaly or a loss of serosal detail in the caudal abdomen. In case of a ruptured abscess, peritoneal effusion may be evident. Ultrasound is a more useful imaging modality for the prostate gland and can identify and better localize cystic structures and aid in sampling of any fluid that may be present. Aspiration of loculated structures in association with the prostate gland may reveal grossly purulent fluid, which increases suspicion for a prostatic abscess. Cytology and bacterial culture should be performed on any fluid that is obtained, and the presence of intracellular bacteria may be considered consistent with an abscess. Cytology and aerobic culture can also be performed on the third fraction of the ejaculate, prostatic wash, or urine (via urethral catheterization). However, urine and prostatic cultures may have a low level of concordance in 50% of cases, and a negative urine culture result does not mean that the prostate gland does not harbor infection.[47]

Treatment

Treatment of prostatic abscesses and cysts varies and there is limited consensus on the best therapy. Broadly, treatment can be divided into nonsurgical and open surgical treatment. Percutaneous ultrasound-guided drainage can be helpful diagnostically as well as therapeutically. When pursuing this treatment option, any fluid collected should be submitted for cytology as well as culture and susceptibility to rule out concurrent infection and tailor antimicrobial therapy if infection is present. To minimize the chances of leakage into the peritoneum, particularly in case of abscess, complete drainage of the prostatic fluid-filled structure with the patient under heavy sedation or general anesthesia is recommended. For many patients, multiple (one to four) drainage procedures are required over 6–64 weeks.[48,49] A moderate risk of recurrence has been reported after drainage.[50] Institutional limitations, such as availability of ultrasonographers capable of prostatic cyst/abscess drainage, should be considered prior to pursuing. Additionally, careful monitoring and multiple drainages should be anticipated. Other treatments that have been described in conjunction with drainage include alcoholization and instillation of platelet-rich plasma.[49]

Surgical treatment of prostatic abscesses centers around debridement and omentalization of the lesion. Debridement of the cyst/abscess may include partial or total resection while sparing the prostatic parenchyma. Most of these techniques are typically combined with castration to prevent recurrence, although medical management with antiandrogenic drugs and careful monitoring, to manage concurrent hyperplastic prostatic changes, could be considered in less critically ill patients.[51] While surgical treatment options historically included marsupialization, placement of passive drains, and partial prostatectomy, these are no longer recommended.[46]

Surgical technique (Figs. 20.6–20.8)

In general, patients with multiple regions of abscessation or septations that prevent effective percutaneous

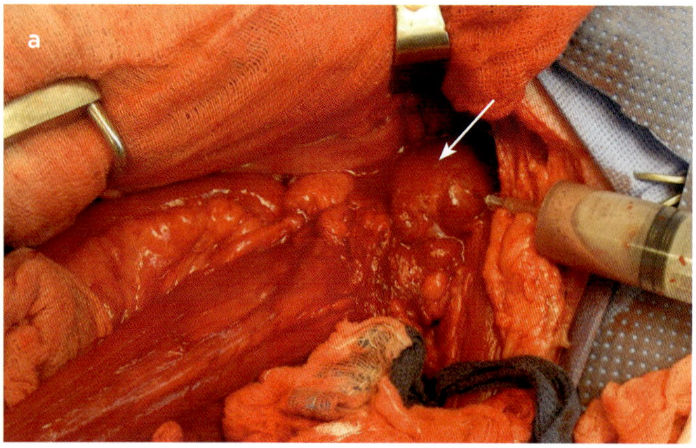

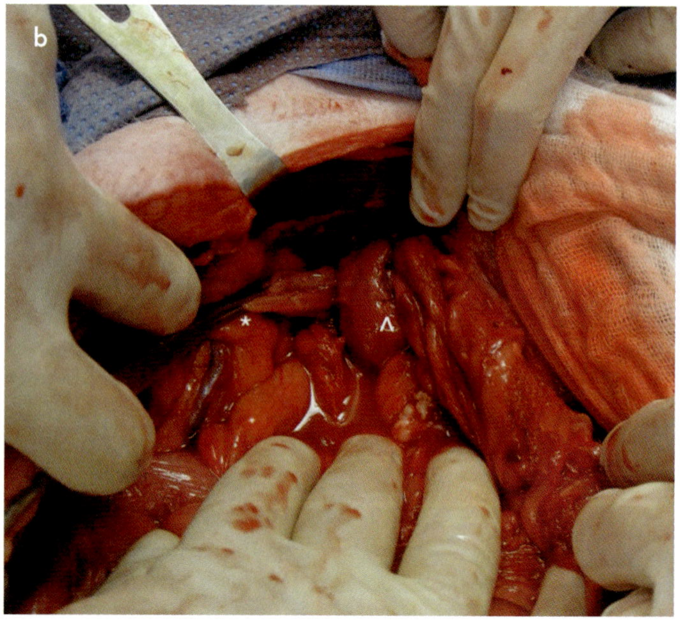

Figure 20.6 Surgical treatment of a prostatic abscess. (a) Intraoperative aspiration of the prostate gland (arrow), following caudal laparotomy, to confirm location of the abscessed loculations. (b) Fenestration of the prostate capsule (arrowhead) and subsequent passage of omentum through the prostate gland with a hemostat (asterisk). Images courtesy of Philipp Mayhew.

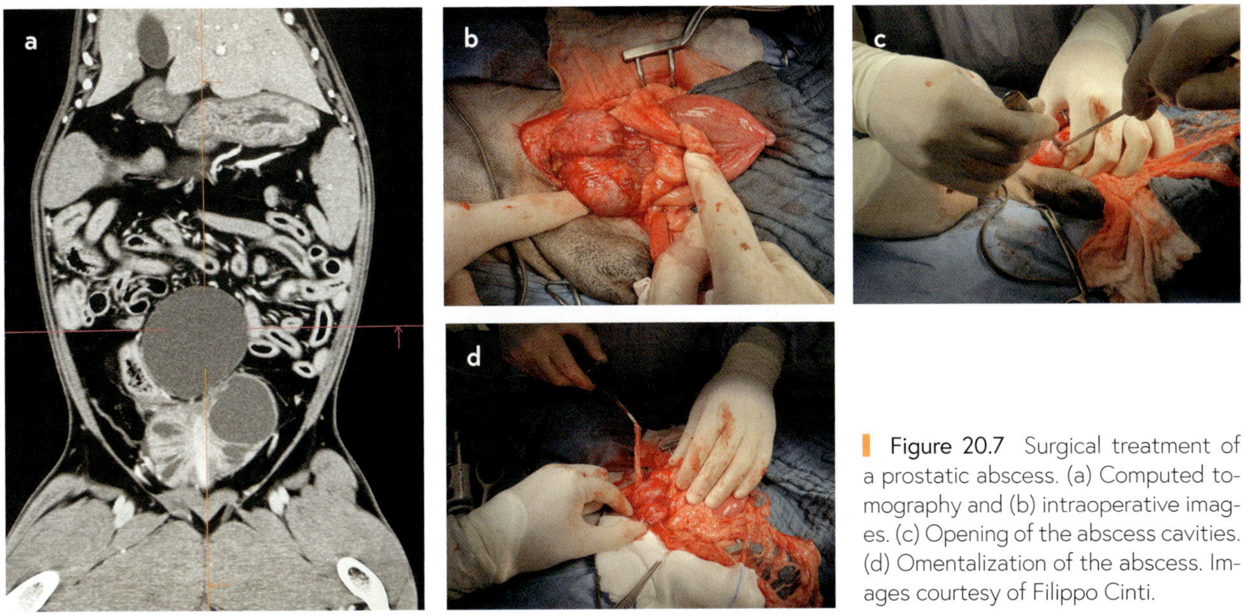

Figure 20.7 Surgical treatment of a prostatic abscess. (a) Computed tomography and (b) intraoperative images. (c) Opening of the abscess cavities. (d) Omentalization of the abscess. Images courtesy of Filippo Cinti.

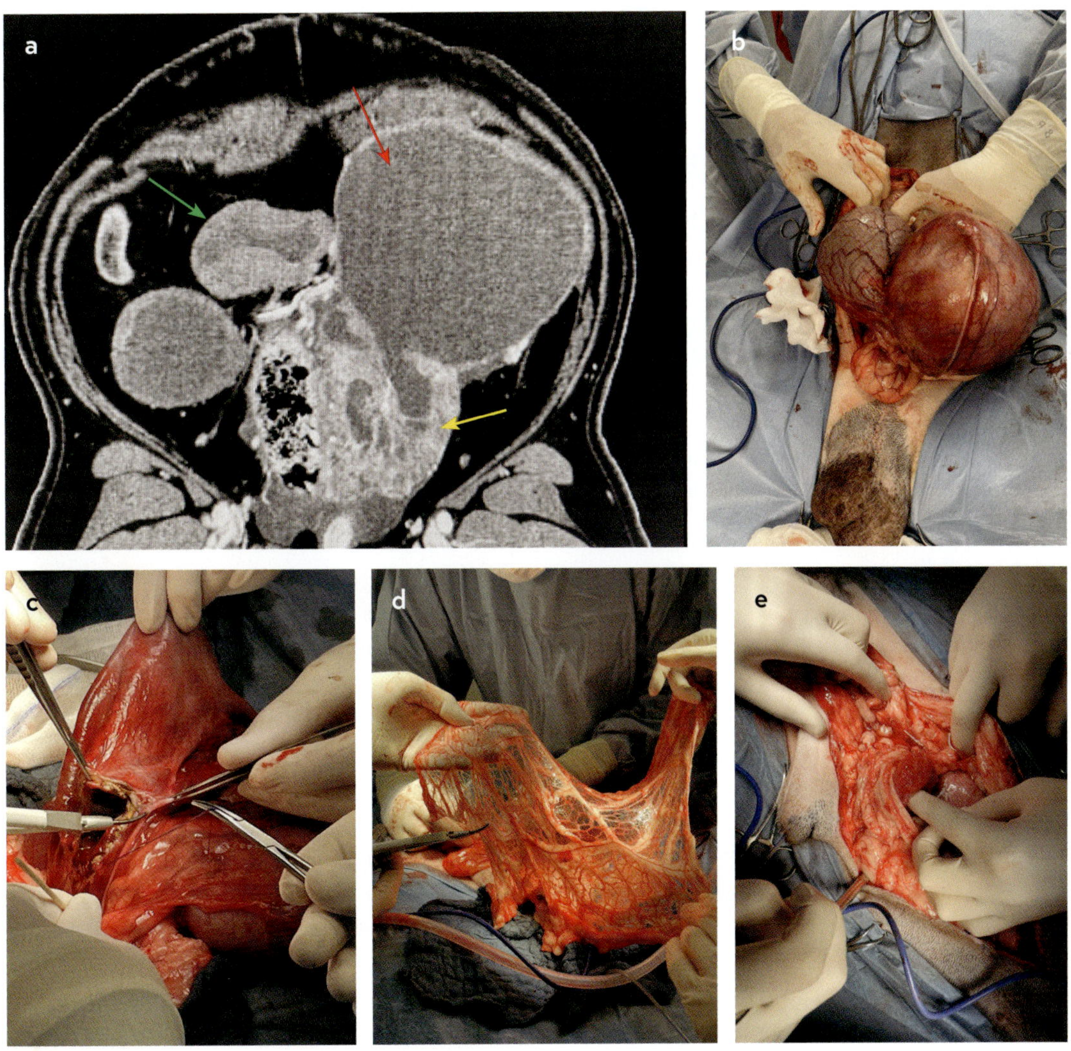

Figure 20.8 Surgical treatment of a large paraprostatic cyst. (a) Computed tomography (prostate gland, yellow arrow; bladder, green arrow; paraprostatic cyst, red arrow) and (b) intraoperative images. (c) Partial resection and (d,e) omentalization of the cyst. Images courtesy of Filippo Cinti.

drainage, patients with cysts that do not respond to medical management, or patients with septic peritonitis requiring abdominal drainage need surgery. The procedure of prostatic debridement and omentalization as originally described continues to be the authors' preferred method of treatment.[44]

1. The patient is placed in dorsal recumbency following aseptic preparation of the ventral abdomen, including the prescrotal skin to prepare for castration.
2. An appropriately sized urethral catheter should be placed to facilitate identification of the urethra.
3. Celiotomy should be made from the umbilicus to the pubis to enable exposure of the prostate gland (see Chapter 3). The incision should be extended if the gland remains intrapelvic and additional exposure is needed. In case of septic peritonitis, a larger celiotomy can be considered for adequate peritoneal lavage and decontamination.
4. The prostate gland should be packed off with laparotomy sponges. Stab incisions over the cyst/abscess into the lateral aspect of the gland can be performed to facilitate drainage. Prostatic loculations or septations should be carefully broken down digitally to develop a single intraprostatic cavity. Identification of the urethra is paramount to avoid iatrogenic damage.
5. Following the debridement/opening of prostatic abscess cavities, a hemostat is passed through one fenestration, transprostatically (while avoiding the urethra), and to the other side of the prostatic abscess. Omentum is grasped and drawn through the fenestrated prostate gland. Additional prostatic cavities are packed with omentum.
6. Prostatic cysts can be completely resected, or partially resected and omentalized as described above for prostatic abscesses. Following careful drainage to avoid intra-abdominal contamination, the cyst wall may be partially or totally resected using sharp dissection or electrocautery. Care must be taken around the bladder neck and prostate gland. Omentum may be packed into the remnant of the cyst and secured using monofilament suture.
7. Circumferential abscessation or cysts should be carefully opened to avoid trauma to the urethra.
8. In case of septic peritonitis, an abdominal drain should be considered and careful systemic management employed.
9. The abdomen is thoroughly lavaged and samples taken for culture and possibly histopathology.

Postoperative management

Postoperatively, an appropriate analgesic plan and intravenous fluid therapy should be established. Analgesics can include opioids given intermittently (methadone, hydromorphone) or by constant-rate infusion (fentanyl). If not otherwise contraindicated, a nonsteroidal anti-inflammatory drug can be administered. If an abscess or infection is suspected, broad-spectrum antibiotics are recommended. Culture and susceptibility testing results should be used to appropriately dictate antimicrobial therapy. It is recommended to select an antibiotic that is known to be efficacious in the prostate gland, such as a fluoroquinolone, a sulfonamide, a macrolide, or chloramphenicol.

As some patients with prostatic abscesses can be markedly unstable, blood pressure and heart rate should be monitored regularly, and pressor support provided as needed. Urinary incontinence or retention rarely occurs postoperatively and is often transient.[44,48,50] In rare cases, urinary retention develops likely as a result of

KEEP IN MIND

- Feline and canine dystocia often requires surgical treatment. Minimizing delay in surgical intervention, if indicated, will optimize maternal and fetal outcomes.
- Uterine torsion is rare and difficult to definitively diagnose preoperatively. If suspected or diagnosed, prompt surgical treatment is indicated.
- Vaginal and uterine prolapse are uncommon. Manual reduction or surgical amputation (ovariohysterectomy) can be considered. Patients should be thoroughly evaluated for concurrent prolapse of other abdominal organs prior to commencing treatment.
- In an open-cervix pyometra, medical management can be considered. However, emergency surgical care is necessary in pyometra patients with a closed cervix, with systemic illness, or if there is evidence of peritonitis, uterine torsion, or uterine rupture.
- Placing a urinary catheter during prostatic surgery is strongly recommended to aid in identification and protection of the prostatic urethra.
- Culture and susceptibility testing should always be performed on the fluid obtained from prostatic cysts/abscesses in order to appropriately determine the need for antimicrobial therapy.

aggressive dissection dorsal to the prostate gland.[44,45] In these cases, the administration of bethanechol may need to be considered.

Outcome

Overall, the outcome following surgery for a prostatic abscess or cyst is good to excellent, but it depends on the overall stability of the patient at the time of surgery. The postoperative complication rate is approximately 30%.[46] Major complications can include urine leakage into the peritoneum, urinary incontinence, and recurrence. Urinary incontinence occurs in 16%–27% of patients after surgery, but, as mentioned above, many times this is a transient complication.[45,46] Recurrence has been reported in approximately 5% of surgically treated patients.[44,46]

References

1. Evans HE, de Lahunta A. *Miller's Anatomy of the Dog*, 4th ed. Elsevier; 2013.
2. Traas AM. Surgical management of canine and feline dystocia. *Theriogenology*. 2008; 70(3):337–342.
3. Münnich A, Küchenmeister U. Dystocia in numbers—evidence-based parameters for intervention in the dog: Causes for dystocia and treatment recommendations. *Reprod Domest Anim*. 2009; 44 Suppl 2:141–147.
4. Bailin HG, Thomas L, Levy NA. Retrospective evaluation of feline dystocia: Clinicopathologic findings and neonatal outcomes in 35 cases (2009–2020). *J Feline Med Surg*. 2022; 24(4):344–350.
5. Darvelid AW, Linde-Forsberg C. Dystocia in the bitch: A retrospective study of 182 cases. *J Small Anim Pract*. 1994; 35(8):402–407.
6. Holst BS. Feline breeding and pregnancy management: What is normal and when to intervene. *J Feline Med Surg*. 2022; 24(3):221–231.
7. Smith FO. Guide to emergency interception during parturition in the dog and cat. *Vet Clin North Am Small Anim Pract*. 2012; 42(3):489–499.
8. Lamm CG, Makloski CL. Current advances in gestation and parturition in cats and dogs. *Vet Clin North Am Small Anim Pract*. 2012; 42(3):445–456.
9. Feldman EC, Nelson RW. *Canine and Feline Endocrinology and Reproduction*, 3rd ed. Saunders; 2015.
10. Cornelius AJ et al. Identifying risk factors for canine dystocia and stillbirths. *Theriogenology*. 2019; 128:201–206.
11. Dobak TP, Voorhout G, Vernooij JCM, Boroffka SAEB. Computed tomographic pelvimetry in English bulldogs. *Theriogenology*. 2018; 118:144–149.
12. Thrall DE. The uterus, ovaries and testes. In: *Textbook of Veterinary Diagnostic Radiology*, 7th ed. Saunders; 2018.
13. Mattoon JS, Nyland TG. Ovaries and uterus. In: *Small Animal Diagnostic Ultrasound*, 3rd ed. Saunders; 2015.
14. Davidson A, Cain J. Canine pregnancy, eutocia, and dystocia. *Vet Clin North Am Small Anim Pract*. 2023; 53(5):1099–1121.
15. Ferrari D et al. Concentration of carprofen in the milk of lactating bitches after cesarean section and during inflammatory conditions. *Theriogenology*. 2022; 181:59–68.
16. Robertson S. Anaesthetic management for caesarean sections in dogs and cats. *In Pract*. 2016; 38(7):327–339.
17. O'Neill DG et al. Canine dystocia in 50 UK first-opinion emergency care veterinary practices: Clinical management and outcomes. *Vet Rec*. 2019; 184(13):409.
18. De La Puerta B, McMahon LA, Moores A. Uterine horn torsion in a non-gravid cat. *J Feline Med Surg*. 2008; 10(4):395–397.
19. Kuroda K et al. Uterine torsion in a full-term pregnant cat. *JFMS Open Rep*. 2017; 3(2):2055116917726228.
20. Misumi K, Fujiki M, Miura N, Sakamoto H. Uterine horn torsion in two non-gravid bitches. *J Small Anim Pract*. 2000; 41(10):468–471.
21. Valentine MJ, Porter S, Chapwanya A, Callanan JJ. Uterine prolapse with endometrial eversion in association with an unusual diffuse, polypoid, fibrosing perimetritis and parametritis in a cat. *JFMS Open Rep*. 2016; 2(1):2055116915626166.
22. Deroy C, Bismuth C, Carozzo C. Management of a complete uterine prolapse in a cat. *JFMS Open Rep*. 2015; 1(1):2055116915579681.
23. Jadhao A et al. Uterine prolapse in a bitch: A case report. *J Entomol Zool Stud*. 2020; 8:1282–1284.
24. Biddle D, Macintire DK. Obstetrical emergencies. *Clin Tech Small Anim Pract*. 2000; 15(2):88–93.
25. Günay Uçmak Z, Uçmak M, Çetin AC, Tek Ç. Uterine prolapse in a pregnant cat. *Turk J Vet Anim Sci*. 2018; 42(5):500–502.
26. Sarrafzadeh-Rezaei F, Saifzadeh S, Mazaheri R, Behfar M. First report of vaginal prolapse in a bitch treated with oestrogen. *Anim Reprod Sci*. 2008; 106(1–2):194–199.
27. Ober CA et al. Vaginal prolapse with urinary bladder incarceration and consecutive irreducible rectal prolapse in a dog. *Acta Vet Scand*. 2016; 58(1):54.
28. Manothaiudom K, Johnston SD. Clinical approach to vaginal/vestibular masses in the bitch. *Vet Clin North Am Small Anim Pract*. 1991; 21(3):509–521.
29. Egenvall A et al. Breed risk of pyometra in insured dogs in Sweden. *J Vet Intern Med*. 2001; 15(6):530–538.
30. Smith FO. Canine pyometra. *Theriogenology*. 2006; 66(3):610–612.
31. Veiga GA et al. Cystic endometrial hyperplasia–pyometra syndrome in bitches: Identification of hemodynamic, inflammatory, and cell proliferation changes. *Biol Reprod*. 2017; 96(1):58–69.
32. Agudelo CF. Cystic endometrial hyperplasia-pyometra complex in cats. A review. *Vet Q*. 2005; 27(4):173–182.
33. Pailler S et al. Owner-reported long-term outcomes, quality of life, and longevity after hospital discharge following surgical treatment of pyometra in bitches and queens. *J Am Vet Med Assoc*. 2022; 260(S2):S57–S63.
34. Verstegen J, Dhaliwal G, Verstegen-Onclin K. Mucometra, cystic endometrial hyperplasia, and pyometra in the bitch: Advances in treatment and assessment of future reproductive success. *Theriogenology*. 2008; 70(3):364–374.
35. Bigliardi E et al. Ultrasonography and cystic hyperplasia–pyometra complex in the bitch. *Reprod Domest Anim*. 2004; 39(3):136–140.
36. Fransson B, Lagerstedt AS, Hellmen E, Jonsson P. Bacteriological findings, blood chemistry profile and plasma endotoxin levels in bitches with pyometra or other uterine diseases. *J Vet Med Ser A*. 1997; 44(1–10):417–426.
37. Melandri M et al. Fertility outcome after medically treated pyometra in dogs. *J Vet Sci*. 2019; 20(4):e39.
38. McCobb E et al. Surgery in a veterinary outpatient community medicine setting has a good outcome for dogs with pyometra. *J Am Vet Med Assoc*. 2022; 260(S2):S36–S41.
39. Pailler S et al. Findings and prognostic indicators of outcomes for bitches with pyometra treated surgically in a nonspecialized setting. *J Am Vet Med Assoc*. 2022; 260(S2):S49–S56.

40. Pailler S et al. Findings and prognostic indicators of outcomes for queens with pyometra treated surgically in a nonspecialized hospital setting. *J Am Vet Med Assoc*. 2022; 260(S2):S42–S48.
41. Krawiec DR, Heflin D. Study of prostatic disease in dogs: 177 cases (1981–1986). *J Am Vet Med Assoc*. 1992; 200(8): 1119–1122.
42. Polisca A et al. A retrospective study of canine prostatic diseases from 2002 to 2009 at the Alfort Veterinary College in France. *Theriogenology*. 2016; 85(5):835–840.
43. Black GM, Ling GV, Nyland TG, Baker T. Prevalence of prostatic cysts in adult, large-breed dogs. *J Am Anim Hosp Assoc*. 1998; 34(2):177–180.
44. White RA, Williams JM. Intracapsular prostatic omentalization: A new technique for management of prostatic abscesses in dogs. *Vet Surg*. 1995; 24(5):390–395.
45. Bray JP, White RA, Williams JM. Partial resection and omentalization: A new technique for management of prostatic retention cysts in dogs. *Vet Surg*. 1997; 26(3):202–209.
46. Del Magno S et al. Surgical treatment and outcome of sterile prostatic cysts in dogs. *Vet Surg*. 2021; 50(5):1009–1016.
47. Weese JS et al. International Society for Companion Animal Infectious Diseases (ISCAID) guidelines for the diagnosis and management of bacterial urinary tract infections in dogs and cats. *Vet J*. 2019; 247:8–25.
48. Boland LE, Hardie RJ, Gregory SP, Lamb CR. Ultrasound-guided percutaneous drainage as the primary treatment for prostatic abscesses and cysts in dogs. *J Am Anim Hosp Assoc*. 2003; 39(2):151–159.
49. Bigliardi E et al. Use of platelet-rich plasma for the treatment of prostatic cysts in dogs. *Can J Vet Res*. 2018; 82(4):264–270.
50. Lea C et al. Prostatitis and prostatic abscessation in dogs: Retrospective study of 82 cases. *Aust Vet J*. 2022; 100(6):223–229.
51. Christensen BW. Canine prostate disease. *Vet Clin North Am Small Anim Pract*. 2018; 48(4):701–719.
52. Evans HE, de Lahunta A. *Miller's Anatomy of the Dog*, 4th ed. Elsevier; 2013.

Chapter 21

Upper airway emergencies

Lynda Rutherford

Emergency stabilization of patients with upper airway disease

Treatment varies based on the underlying disease process, but the general emergency approach is similar in all patients with upper respiratory tract (URT) disease:

- The patient should be kept in a calm and cool environment, with minimal handling.
- Respiratory rate, pattern, and effort should be monitored.
- In hyperthermic patients, external cooling should be provided (e.g., fan, air conditioning).
- Oxygen supplementation is provided if needed (e.g., flow-by, oxygen cage, nasal prongs, nasal oxygen catheters, face masks).
- An intravenous catheter can be placed.
- The administration of anxiolytics and sedatives is considered. These agents can be administered intramuscularly if the patient is not stable enough to sustain the stress of a catheter placement. The dosage should be chosen based on the patient status, suspected disease, present condition, and route of administration (the lower and higher dosages are more appropriate for intravenous and intramuscular injection, respectively):
  - Trazodone 3–5 mg/kg orally or rectally.
  - Acepromazine 0.005–0.02 mg/kg IV or IM.
  - Medetomidine 0.001–0.01 mg/kg IV or IM.
  - Butorphanol 0.2–0.4 mg/kg IV or IM.
- In case of laryngeal or tracheal edema and swelling, short-acting corticosteroids can be used (dexamethasone 0.1–0.2 mg/kg IV).
- If sedation and oxygen therapy fail to stabilize the patient, intubation is indicated with rapid induction and minimal cardiopulmonary depression.
- If intubation with a regular endotracheal tube is not possible, emergency intubation can be achieved with a small rigid urinary catheter.
- If intraoral passage of a urinary catheter through the larynx is not possible, it can be passed into the trachea via a stab incision through the ventral neck into the cricoid/thyroid space or between the tracheal rings to provide oxygen until full airway access or tracheostomy is achieved.
- A temporary tracheostomy tube can be placed with the patient under total intravenous anesthesia and oxygen provided as detailed in the above two points.

Brachycephalic obstructive airway syndrome

Brachycephalic dog breeds, especially French Bulldogs and Pugs, have been becoming increasingly popular over the last 5–10 years. These breeds and their crosses have raised many challenging management issues for veterinarians, particularly as many owners fail to recognize that their pets are in a perpetual state of respiratory compromise. Extreme brachycephalic breeds, including Pugs, French Bulldogs, and English Bulldogs, have varying conformational URT abnormalities leading to brachycephalic obstructive airway syndrome (BOAS). Other breeds such as Staffordshire Bull Terriers, Cavalier King Charles Spaniels, Boston Terriers, Yorkshire Terriers, Chihuahuas, and Shar Peis can also be affected. BOAS is a multifactorial syndrome that has occurred due to foreshortening of the facial skeleton without corresponding reduction in soft tissues of the face. The primary components of BOAS are:

- increased nasal resistance as a result of stenotic nares (43%–85%) and aberrant or protruding turbinates;
- pharyngeal hypoplasia (redundant pharyngeal folds) with an elongated soft palate (86%–96%);
- tracheal hypoplasia, especially in the English Bulldog.

Secondary components, resulting from the chronic increased negative intra-airway pressure, include everted tonsils, everted laryngeal saccules (55%–59%), and laryngeal collapse (8%–70%).[1–7] Relative macroglossia has also been reported in extreme brachycephalic breeds, resulting in a reduction in URT volume.

BOAS will impact all aspects of veterinary care for these patients. They require careful management, as any increase in respiratory pressure, such as constant panting in an anxious dog, can really exacerbate their respiratory compromise, which could have potentially fatal consequences. These breeds are also affected by other breed/conformation-related health issues, such as dental disease, dermatological conditions (e.g., skin fold pyoderma), ocular disease due to increased globe exposure (leading to keratoconjunctivitis sicca, exposure keratitis, and corneal ulceration), neurological conditions due to hemivertebrae (leading to spinal cord compression), orthopedic disease (e.g., cranial cruciate ligament rupture, patellar luxation), and gastrointestinal dysfunction (e.g., regurgitation). These breeds are also at higher risk of aspiration pneumonia. All these factors need to be considered when treating these patients, and it is important to think of the whole patient and manage their health issues concurrently. Attempts should be made to reduce the number and length of anesthetic episodes. Also, great care must be taken when sedating these breeds. General anesthesia with intubation and a secure airway may pose less of a risk than heavy sedation.

It is important to be transparent with owners and discuss the increased risks posed to these breeds by hospitalization, sedation, or anesthesia. Reducing the time spent in the veterinary setting can be beneficial to reduce the patient's anxiety levels (e.g., admitting them as close to the surgery time as possible), and considering drugs such as trazodone as a pretreatment prior to a period of hospitalization can be helpful. Discussing that rapid collection may be necessary if the patient is becoming increasingly stressed is a helpful strategy.

Multiple studies have shown links between certain conformations and severity of BOAS. It would be helpful to assess for these traits in puppy checks or ideally discuss with potential owners before they purchase a puppy. The severity of nares stenosis is an indicator for BOAS severity in Pugs, English Bulldogs, and French Bulldogs. Risk factors for BOAS in English Bulldogs and French Bulldogs are similar and include being male, increased neck girth, and wider skull. Risk factors for Pugs are being female, increased distance between the eyes, and wider skull. Studies have shown that performing an exercise test increases the sensitivity of BOAS detection on a clinical examination. Exercising the dog with the owner for 3–5 minutes will often increase the respiratory noise and can be used to demonstrate to the owner that the dog is affected by BOAS. Stertor (nasal snorting) occurs due to nasal obstruction, whereas stridor (higher pitched laryngeal wheezing) occurs if there is an obstruction at the level of the larynx.

Clinical presentation and diagnosis

BOAS manifests clinically as increased respiratory noise (stertor or stridor), dyspnea, exercise intolerance, heat sensitivity, sleep disorders, cyanosis, collapse, and death. Patients with BOAS can present as an emergency, in respiratory crisis, and require careful management (see below). They may be collapsed, panting with severe stertor and stridor, or have had a collapsing episode. They usually have signs of URT obstruction, but since these breeds have an increased risk of aspiration pneumonia, they may also show associated signs such as depressed demeanor, lethargy, cough, and increased nasal discharge. Some patients with BOAS have ongoing upper gastrointestinal tract signs, such as regurgitation that is exacerbated with exercise or excitement.

Treatment

Emergency management

Sedation

Chemical sedation is helpful to reduce patient anxiety and facilitate management. The following sedatives can be used:

- Acepromazine 0.005–0.02 mg/kg IV or IM.
- Medetomidine 0.001–0.01 mg/kg IV or IM.
- Butorphanol 0.2–0.4 mg/kg IV or IM.

These drugs can be given in combination, and each individual drug at the above doses can be repeated once to help manage patients. The aim is to have the patient lying down, behaving calmly, and not panting. Once adequately sedated, one or two intravenous cannulas should be placed to provide intravenous access. A constant-rate infusion of medetomidine can be administered to keep the patient sedated (1–2 μg/kg/h).

Sedated patients with BOAS require very careful monitoring. They should still be conscious and able to walk or lift their heads when stimulated. The gag reflex should be present. Many of these patients will improve when adequately sedated (Video 21.1). Respiratory rate, effort, and pattern and mucous membrane color should be monitored. If the patient requires significant (subjective) effort for inspiration, induction of general anesthesia and intubation should be considered (see below).

Oxygen therapy

Oxygen can be provided via oxygen kennels or flow-by. Some patients will tolerate nasal cannulas when sedated.

Cooling

These breeds are susceptible to heat-related injury. Their body temperature should be checked and active cooling started if required (Table 21.1).

Video 21.1. Patient with severe stertor and dyspnea responding well to sedation and oxygen supplementation. Emergency intubation was not required. Video courtesy of Anna Frykfors von Hekkel.

TABLE 21.1 - VETCOMPASS CLINICAL GRADING TOOL FOR HEAT-RELATED ILLNESS IN DOGS			
Grade	**Clinical signs**	**Suggested treatment**	**Previous terminology used for presentation**
Mild	Continuous panting or respiratory effort unresolved following cessation of exercise or removal from hot environment. Lethargy, stiffness, or unwillingness to move.	Active cooling if hyperthermia is present. Rehydration (may be oral only). Supportive care for organ systems affected (e.g., oxygen for dyspnea). May be able to manage on the scene. Monitor for progression of clinical signs.	Heat stress
Moderate	Progression of stage 1 (mild)—no response to cooling and/or fluids. Hypersalivation, diarrhea, and/or vomiting (no blood present). A single seizure. Episodic collapse with spontaneous recovery (no impaired consciousness).	Active cooling if hyperthermia is present. Rehydration—may require intravenous fluids. Supportive care for organ systems affected (e.g., gastrointestinal support). Consider hospitalization to monitor progression of clinical signs.	Heat exhaustion
Severe	Progression of stage 2 (moderate). Any of the following: • Central nervous system impairment (ataxia, two or more seizures, profound depression, unresponsiveness, coma). • Liver or kidney dysfunction. • Gastrointestinal hemorrhage. • Petechiae/purpura.	Requires hospital care. Active cooling if hyperthermia is present. Coagulation assessment required. Supportive care for organ systems affected: • Neurological support (e.g., osmotic agents, seizure management). • Intravenous fluid therapy and blood glucose and electrolyte management. • Respiratory support (e.g., oxygen, intubation). • Circulatory support (e.g., vasopressors). • Gastrointestinal support (e.g., antiemetics, protectants, antibiotics). • Transfusion products.	Heat stroke

Source: Hall EJ et al. Proposing the VetCompass clinical grading tool for heat-related illness in dogs. *Sci Rep.* 2021; 11(1):6828.

Airway assessment

Airway assessment should be performed if anesthesia and intubation is necessary during the respiratory crisis or at a later stage if the patient responds well to emergency management. It includes grading the nares (mild, moderate, or severe stenosis) and intraoral structures (Box 21.1).

Box 21.1. Checklist for assessment of intraoral structures

- Tonsil size and eversion
- Pharyngeal edema
- Soft palate length and thickness
- Laryngeal collapse (grade I–III) and laryngeal edema/swelling (see below)
- Any other causes of upper respiratory tract obstruction such as intraoral or laryngeal masses (e.g., vocal fold granuloma; Fig. 21.1)

The next step in patient management will depend on individual patient factors as well as on the surgical capabilities of the veterinary staff and the practice setup for managing high-risk anesthetic patients. If oropharyngeal swelling and edema are present and seem to be significantly contributing to the URT obstruction, the patient may respond favorably to continued sedation and anti-inflammatory doses of corticosteroids (dexamethasone 0.1–0.15 mg/kg IV). If there is severe swelling as well as an overly long and thick soft palate, intubation and surgery or referral for surgery may be necessary. Some patients may require intubation for a period of time along with corticosteroid treatment (see below). It may be possible to extubate these patients after a few hours and consider surgery/referral at a later date. These patients should be carefully monitored after extubation and kept calm with medical sedation for several hours prior to discharge. Some patients will not tolerate extubation; in these circumstances surgery or referral for surgery should be performed.

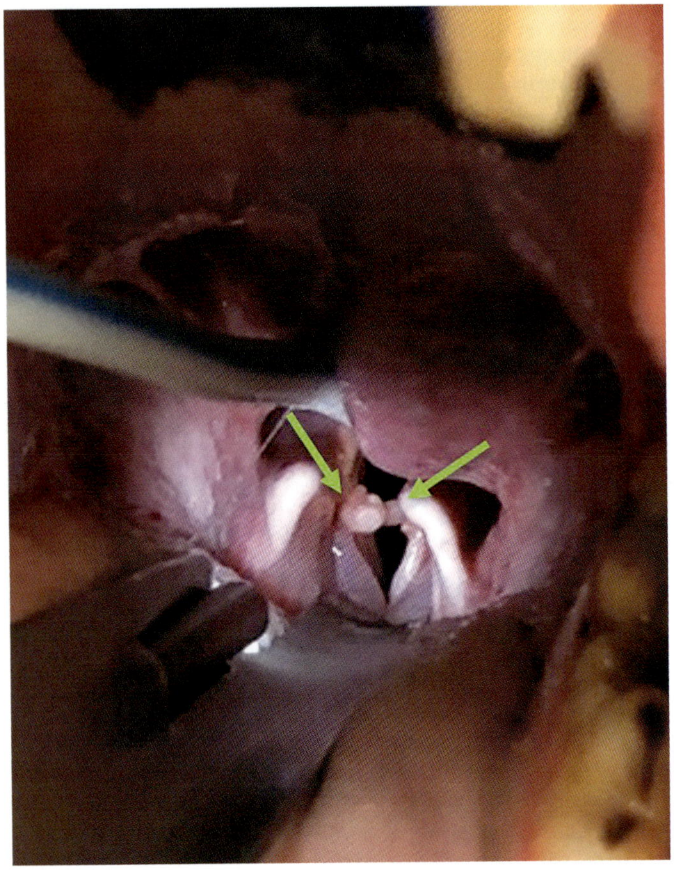

Figure 21.1 Bilateral vocal fold granuloma (green arrows) noted during airway examination for brachycephalic obstructive airway syndrome assessment. Both granulomas were sharply excised with a number 11 scalpel blade. Image courtesy of Matteo Rossanese.

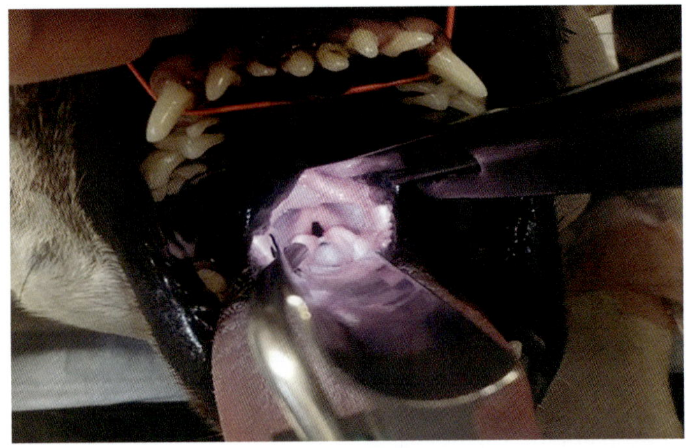

Figure 21.2 Intubation of a 1-year-old French Bulldog using two laryngoscopes. Note the everted saccules and medial deviation of the cuneiform processes (grade II laryngeal collapse).

Anesthetic management

Preanesthetic medication with a proton pump inhibitor, such as omeprazole or maropitant, may reduce postoperative regurgitation. This can be given once the respiratory crisis has been managed. Metoclopramide (1 mg/kg IV loading dose and 1 mg/kg/h CRI) whilst under anesthesia has been shown to reduce gastroesophageal reflux in anesthetized dogs. The constant-rate infusion can be continued at 1 mg/kg/day if the patient regurgitates frequently or regurgitates after general anesthesia.

The patient should be kept as calm as possible prior to general anesthesia. Preoxygenation prior to induction using flow-by should be used.

Anesthetic induction can be achieved using propofol or alfaxalone to effect via an intravenous cannula. It is important to have intravenous access in case reintubation is necessary during the recovery period.

Intubation can be facilitated by using two laryngoscopes (Fig. 21.2). One blade is used to depress the tongue (like for intubation of an unaffected dog), while the other is used to elevate the soft palate so the larynx can be clearly seen. The same technique can be used for oral and laryngeal examination. It is advisable to have a range of endotracheal tubes available.

Recovery from anesthesia is the highest risk time for these breeds, particularly if airway surgery has not been performed. The tissues in the oropharynx are relaxed, meaning the gag reflex could still be obliterated and respiratory obstruction is more likely. It is imperative that protocols are in place to manage the postoperative period. These breeds should be under constant supervision until they have completely recovered from general anesthesia. They should be extubated as late as possible (i.e., they should be fully conscious, sitting up, and able to swallow). These patients should be monitored for regurgitation. If regurgitation has occurred under general anesthesia, the esophagus should be lavaged with saline and suctioned as soon as possible. It is important to have a fully inflated endotracheal tube cuff whilst performing esophageal lavage.

A reintubation kit should be available in case respiratory obstruction/compromise occurs during recovery. It could include:

- an induction agent (already drawn up to the correct dose for body weight);
- laryngoscopes;
- a selection of endotracheal tubes, including two sizes smaller than the tube used for the first intubation to allow for laryngeal swelling;
- a urinary catheter to provide oxygen if the larynx is too swollen to allow intubation.

Respiratory compromise on recovery from general anesthesia can often be reduced by placing something in the mouth to keep it open. A roll of bandage material and pulling the tongue forward works well. Avoiding overheating during and on recovery from general anesthesia is important.

Surgical treatment

The main surgical procedures with the most impact for BOAS treatment are rhinoplasty, to increase the nares diameter, and partial staphylectomy, to reduce the length and thickness of the soft palate. There are numerous techniques described for both procedures. The two surgical techniques described below are applicable to first-opinion practice, as no special equipment is required.

Patient positioning

Although there are patient positioning aids, a method that is achievable without buying additional equipment is described below. The patient should be positioned in sternal recumbency. The head should be at the end of the operating table, away from the anesthetic machine if possible. A beanbag can be placed under the sternum. The head can be supported with the mouth open by suspending it between two drip stands using bandage material secured to the drip stands and canine teeth (Fig. 21.3). Care should be taken not to create a kink in the patient's neck, as this could decrease blood flow to the brain stem. The lower jaw can be taped to the operating table to create as large an operating field as possible. The patient should be positioned with the head straight. This open mouth position can be used for intraoral procedures such as partial staphylectomy, tonsillectomy, and laryngeal procedures including sacculectomy and partial cuneiformectomy.

Once the intraoral procedures have been performed, the upper jaw can be released and the nose positioned so it is lower than the rest of the head (Fig. 21.4). This allows bleeding from the nares to flow externally rather than internally, preventing blood aspiration.

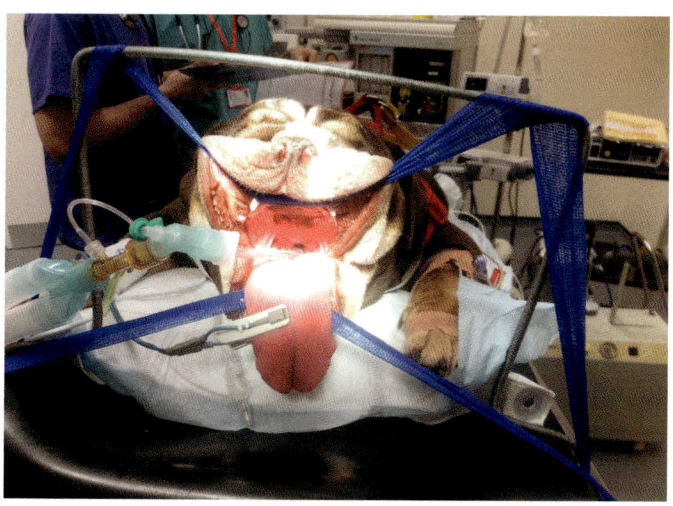

Figure 21.3 Patient positioning for intraoral procedures. A table stand has been used to elevate the upper jaw in this case; however, two drip stands can also be utilized for this purpose. A table that can be tilted to elevate the head allows the surgeon to stand when operating; if this is not possible, operating whilst seated may be helpful.

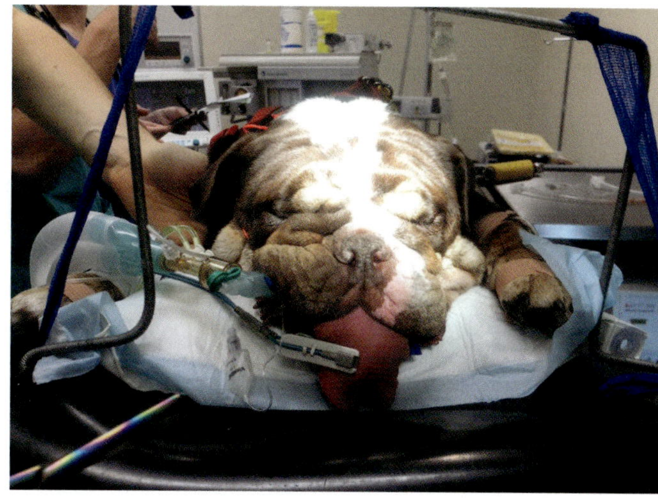

Figure 21.4 Patient positioning for rhinoplasty.

Surgical technique: Cut-and-sew partial staphylectomy (Fig. 21.5)

1. The patient is positioned as described above. The anesthetic depth is checked before starting; the patient should not be able to swallow. A swab is placed intraorally, caudal to the larynx, and the endotracheal tube cuff is ensured to be inflated, to reduce the risk of blood aspiration.
2. The soft palate incision should be planned with the aim to create an inverted U shape, with the lateral edges of the palate being longer than the central portion. The lateral aspect of the incision should be at the level of the caudal third of the tonsil, while the central aspect is more cranial, at the midtonsillar level.
3. The center of the free edge of the soft palate is grasped, firstly with DeBakey forceps, then transferred to Allis tissue forceps and pulled rostrally. Alternatively, a stay suture (4-0 monofilament) can be used.
4. Two lateral stay sutures (4-0 monofilament) are placed, one on each side, caudal to the section of palate that will be removed (i.e., at the level of the caudal pole of the tonsil). It is important to ensure that the suture is placed through the oral and nasal mucosa. These sutures will help to distinguish the two aspects of the mucosa when suturing.
5. Rostral traction is applied by securing these stay sutures with mosquito hemostats and hanging them from the mouth.
6. Long-handled Metzenbaum scissors are used to cut the palate. The scissor blades should be angled so the top blade is more caudal in the mouth and,

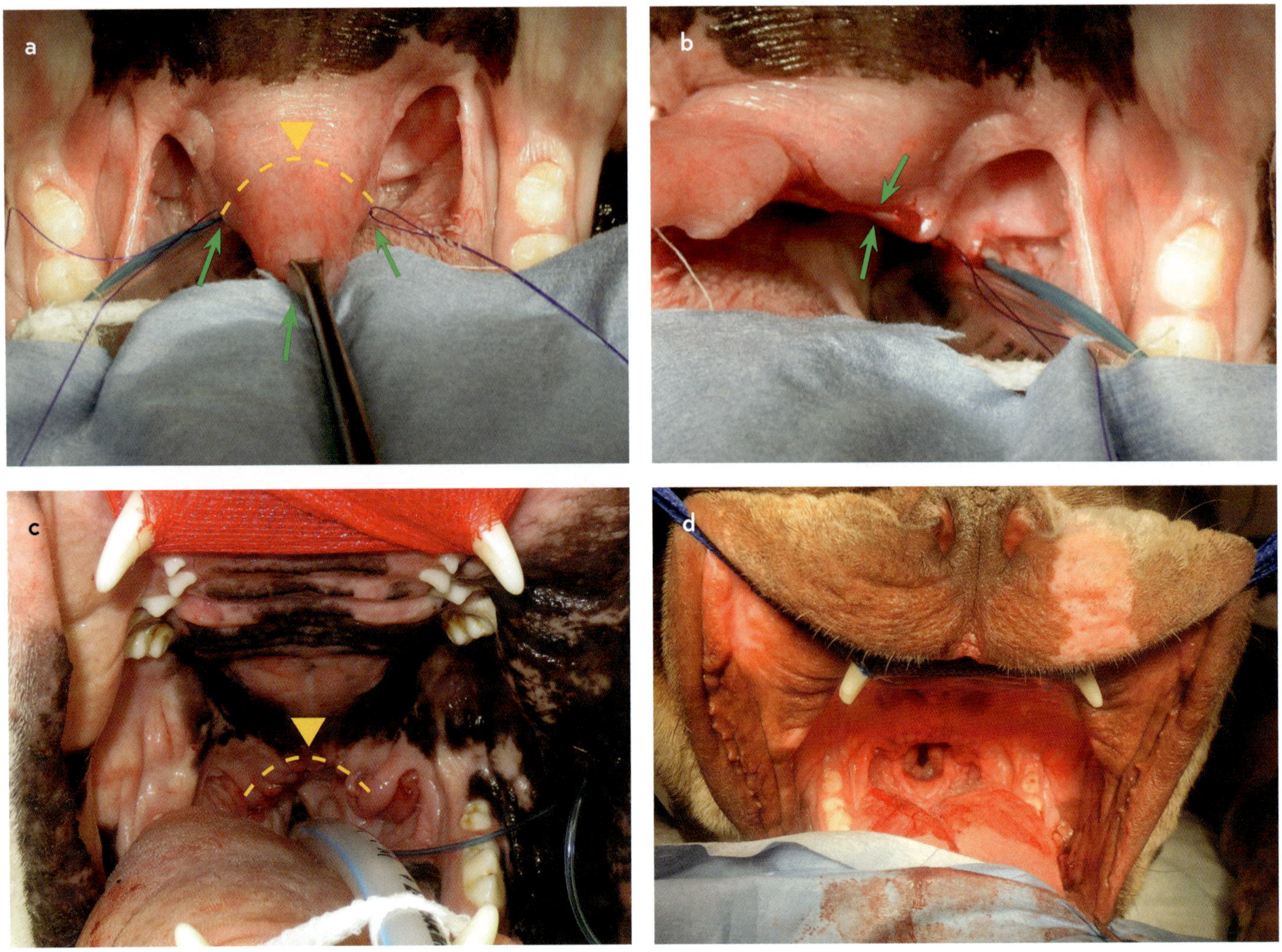

Figure 21.5 Cut-and-sew partial staphylectomy. (a) Intraoperative planning of the soft palate incision. The aim is to create an inverted U shape (dotted yellow line), with the lateral aspect of the incision at the level of the caudal third of the tonsil and the central aspect at midtonsil level (yellow arrowhead). Note the free edge of the soft palate pulled rostrally with Allis tissue forceps and two lateral stay sutures to delineate the start and end of the incision (green arrows). (b) The first half of the soft palate has been cut with a single stroke using Metzenbaum scissors. Note the oral and nasal mucosa (green arrows). (c,d) Intraoperative images after completion of staphylectomy. A curved free end of the soft palate with the rostral end overlapping the tip of the epiglottis is visible. Images courtesy of Matteo Rossanese and Lynda Rutherford.

therefore, more tissue remains on the nasal aspect of the palate—this also assists in closing the mucosal layers correctly.

7. The aim is to cut the palate with two smooth strokes, one closing the scissor blades from lateral to medial from the right side, and the other from the left side. The cuts should be angled so that more palate is removed centrally, creating an inverted U shape.
8. The nasal mucosa is sutured to the oral mucosa using 4-0 Vicryl Rapide or 4-0 Monocryl. If a simple interrupted pattern is used, suturing is started at the center and advanced laterally. If a simple continuous pattern is utilized, suturing is started at the beginning of the incision on the right side and advanced toward the left side. The sutures should be 3–5 mm apart, with a 5 mm bite of mucosa. It should be ensured that the nasal mucosa is included by manipulating the stay sutures and grasping the mucosa with DeBakey forceps if necessary. This process becomes easier once the first few sutures have been placed. The suture ends are cut short, 2–3 mm from the knot.
9. If bleeding occurs, it is usually from the palatine arteries that run laterally. Sutures placed in the lateral aspect of the stay sutures usually control any bleeding. If necessary, a swab can be used to apply direct pressure and left in situ while other procedures are performed; the swab should be removed prior to recovery from anesthesia. Bipolar diathermy can be judiciously applied directly to vessels.

10. The swab caudal to the larynx is removed after the intraoral procedures have been completed.

Serious complications of staphylectomy include death as a result of aspiration pneumonia, dyspnea and cyanosis requiring tracheostomy, and failure to recover from anesthesia. Less severe complications include coughing, noisy respiration, and gagging and retching. The prognosis of dogs after soft palate resection is good to excellent in 90% of cases, especially in dogs younger than 1–2 years of age.

Surgical technique: Modified vertical wedge resection rhinoplasty (Video 21.2)

The aim is to amputate the ventral portion of the dorsal and lateral nasal cartilage and associated epithelium. Starting with the left nostril is easier for a right-handed surgeon.

1. The ventromedial free edge of the nares is grasped with Adson tissue forceps and pulled medially.
2. A number 11 scalpel blade is used to remove a pyramidal wedge of nasal tissue. It is important to push the blade deep into the nasal tissue to ensure some of the alar cartilage is removed.
   a. The first incision is started at the dorsal aspect of the medial nares with the blade facing ventromedially (parallel to the medial aspect of the nares).
   b. A second incision starting from the same point is made in a ventrolateral direction (Fig. 21.6).
   c. A wedge-shaped section of nasal cartilage and associated epithelium is amputated by cutting the remaining ventromedial edge.
3. The bleeding is controlled with a cotton bud and direct pressure. This will stop once the sutures are placed.
4. The medial aspect of the nasal mucosa is sutured to the dorsolateral cut edge to achieve a larger nasal opening. The wound is closed by direct apposition using three simple interrupted sutures of 4-0 absorbable material (e.g., Monocryl, Vicryl): one on the ventral border, one on the dorsal aspect, and one in the deep tissue inside the nostril.
5. An attempt should be made to perform the technique in a similar way for the second nostril to help with symmetry and aesthetic appearance.

Video 21.2. Modified vertical wedge resection rhinoplasty of the left nostril in a French Bulldog. A number 11 scalpel blade is used to remove a pyramidal wedge of nasal tissue. Hemostasis is achieved by placement of three sutures (4-0 Vicryl). Video courtesy of Matteo Rossanese.

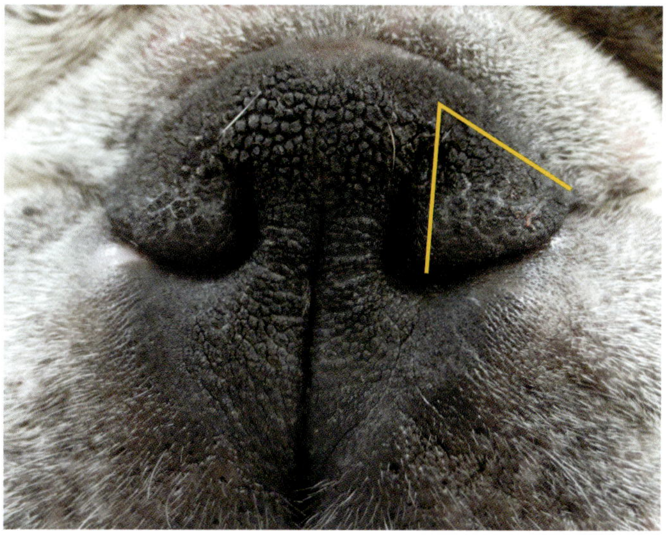

Figure 21.6 Intraoperative image demonstrating the position of the first two incisions (yellow lines) for modified vertical wedge resection rhinoplasty. Image courtesy of Matteo Rossanese.

Temporary emergency surgery for brachycephalic obstructive airway syndrome

Three different stages of laryngeal collapse are clinically recognized:

- Stage I: Laryngeal saccule eversion. This relatively mild stage is very common in brachycephalic dogs affected by BOAS.
- Stage II: Medial collapse of the cuneiform process of the arytenoid cartilage (see Fig. 21.2).
- Stage III: Collapse of the corniculate processes of the arytenoid cartilages, resulting in significant airway obstruction.[8]

Stage II and III laryngeal collapse have been reported in dogs as young as 4.5 months of age. Because laryngeal collapse represents a secondary condition, the initial treatment should be focused on surgical correction of the primary disease using lower-risk surgical procedures such as rhinoplasty for stenotic nares and partial staphylectomy for an elongated soft palate, although this is debated by specialist surgeons.[8]

Resection of everted laryngeal saccules is performed routinely by some surgeons but can lead to laryngeal webbing and severe postoperative complications. This procedure should be reserved for patients with subjectively large saccules or for those that have not improved as expected after rhinoplasty and partial staphylectomy. Patients that do not respond to staged surgical and medical management of airway disorders may require permanent tracheostomy. Alternatively, partial laser laryngectomy or laryngeal tie-back surgery may be attempted, but the effectiveness of these procedures for resolution of airway obstruction has not been extensively evaluated.[8]

Postoperative care

In general, after rhinoplasty and partial staphylectomy, the patient should be closely monitored and kept calm during recovery. Extubation should take place only when the animal is almost fully awake and consciously aware of the tube. The patient's pulse, body temperature, and respiratory rate and effort should be monitored frequently. Chemical sedation should be used to keep the dog calm and prevent panting. Food and water are only withheld until complete recovery. The animal should be monitored for any gagging, retching, vomiting, stridor, or development of dyspnea. After recovery, the dog is offered water and a small amount of soft food under supervision, and swallowing is carefully observed. If postoperative dyspnea occurs, either the patient can be heavily sedated (for 8–12 hours with an additional dose of corticosteroids administered) and reintubated with a small tube or a temporary tracheostomy can be performed.

If possible, the use of full opioid agonists should be avoided on recovery from general anesthesia due to the respiratory depressive effects. Partial agonists (buprenorphine) in combination with paracetamol or nonsteroidal anti-inflammatory drugs are often appropriate. Nonsteroidal anti-inflammatories should be avoided if a glucocorticoid was given. A 10-day oral course of omeprazole and 4-day course of oral maropitant may help reduce the incidence of regurgitation/esophagitis after general anesthesia. It is important to discuss with owners that often regurgitation is more frequent following general anesthesia but should be improving or have resolved in 3–5 days. The signs of aspiration pneumonia should be highlighted and the owners asked to monitor for them. Supervised feeding and drinking for 10 days postoperatively are prudent.

Outcome

Subjectively, when assessed via owner questionnaires the majority of brachycephalic dogs affected by BOAS improved after multilevel corrective URT surgery; however, approximately 70% continued to have clinical signs of airway obstruction.[4,6,7] Objective outcome measurements such as whole-body barometric plethysmography have supported this finding.[9] It has been concluded that the BOAS index decreased from 70% to 60% (where 100% is extremely severely affected by BOAS) after corrective airway surgery, corroborating the subjective findings of patients being improved but still affected.[10] Other studies have found that the resting respiratory rate, oxygen saturation, and distance walked are improved after airway surgery.[11] There is also evidence to support an improvement in gastrointestinal signs in these breeds after corrective airway surgery, most markedly in French Bulldogs.[4] It is important to treat each patient as an individual and try to tailor the surgical techniques performed to the individual's conformation. It should be discussed with owners that whilst their pet's breathing should improve after surgery, they will still be affected by airway obstruction and care should be taken to maintain lean body weight and avoid exercise when it is hot.

Laryngeal disease

The throat is a conduit for both the respiratory and digestive tracts and comprises the pharynx and larynx.[12] Dorsal to the soft palate, the nasopharynx is located between the choanae (end of nasal cavity) and the intrapharyngeal ostium. It connects the nasal cavity with the larynx and contains the pharyngeal opening of the auditory tubes. Caudally, the boundaries of the intrapharyngeal opening are the caudal edge of the soft palate and the palatopharyngeal arches. The oropharynx is the region between the soft palate and the base of the tongue, bounded laterally by the palatoglossal and palatopharyngeal arches and caudally by the tip of the epiglottis.[12] The soft palate forms the floor of the nasopharynx and the roof of the oropharynx. It is a mobile, valve-like partition that can be elevated to close off the proximal airway during swallowing or depressed to close off the oral cavity during nose breathing. During swallowing, it works with the epiglottis, which closes off the distal airway, to allow a bolus of ingesta to cross the respiratory tract. The laryngopharynx is the portion of the pharynx dorsal to the larynx, extending from the rostral border of the epiglottis to the caudal border of the cricoid cartilage.[12]

The larynx is a complex cartilaginous organ that, among its many functions, separates the respiratory and digestive tracts. It is formed by the cricoid, thyroid, and paired arytenoid cartilages and the epiglottis. The intrinsic and extrinsic muscles of the larynx interact under the control of the laryngeal neuromuscular system to move the larynx when swallowing and to open and close the vocal folds in order to protect the lower airways (coughing), to facilitate and regulate the respiratory airflow, and to vocalize.[12] A thorough understanding and knowledge of the local anatomy of the larynx is mandatory before initiating any surgical procedure in this region.

Severe or chronic pharyngeal or laryngeal disease can lead to weight loss and emaciation, inappetence, dyspnea, hypoxia, and aspiration pneumonia, which can all affect anesthesia protocols and wound healing. These factors should be addressed prior to surgery if possible.[12] Surgery of the pharynx or larynx may cause additional swelling in the airways and pooling of blood, saliva, and lavage fluid that may lead to aspiration. Intubation is indicated to protect the airways as well as to oxygenate the patient, but it may be complicated by swelling or tumors in the pharynx or larynx. A temporary tracheostomy may be indicated to bypass the oropharynx during surgery if normal endotracheal intubation is problematic or if the tube hinders visibility and surgical access.[13] Although prolonged intubation is an option after surgery, the animal must be kept sedated or anesthetized, requiring intensive monitoring. Furthermore, in a study of prolonged endotracheal intubation in dogs, laryngeal mucosal inflammation was observed after 24 hours, and after 1 week there was loss of mucosal architecture and inflammatory infiltrates were seen in the arytenoid cartilages.[14] Tracheostomy is more appropriate than prolonged endotracheal intubation when the pharyngolaryngeal airways are obstructed as a result of injury.[13] Therefore, if significant swelling or obstruction of the pharynx or larynx is expected in the immediate postoperative period, a temporary tracheostomy should be performed (see below).

In general, all patients undergoing pharyngolaryngeal surgery will benefit from preoxygenation before induction of anesthesia.[13] Preoxygenation is therefore imperative and may provide additional 3–5 minutes time for intubation of a difficult airway. This can be provided via a mask, nasal prongs, oxygen cage, or as flow-by until the airways are secured via endotracheal or per tracheostomy intubation. A preoperative anti-inflammatory dose of a corticosteroid (dexamethasone 0.1–0.15 mg/kg IV, IM, or SC) may reduce URT edema secondary to diagnostic or surgical manipulations and is routinely given for intralaryngeal and brachycephaly-related procedures, preferably before intubation.

Laryngeal surgery is most commonly performed for acquired laryngeal paralysis in older large- and giant-breed dogs, or for removal of laryngeal masses (via ventral laryngotomy or partial to complete laryngectomy). Partial or complete laryngectomy is rarely performed and is considered technically very demanding. These patients are best served by referral to a specialist surgeon. However, with proper anatomical knowledge, gentle tissue handling, use of appropriate instruments and technique, cautious use of anesthetics, and stringent perioperative care and monitoring, successful thyroid–arytenoid lateralization and ventral laryngotomy may be achievable in first-opinion practice.

Laryngeal paralysis

Idiopathic acquired laryngeal paralysis is the most common form of paralysis of the larynx encountered in veterinary practice. Large-breed dogs, such as Labrador and Golden Retrievers, Irish Setters, Leonbergers, and St. Bernards, are predisposed to idiopathic acquired laryngeal paralysis and may have an associated peripheral neuropathy resulting in pelvic limb dysfunction. Other cases of acquired paralysis of the larynx have been associated with endocrinopathies (e.g., hypothyroidism). Cranial mediastinal masses causing compression of the recurrent laryngeal nerve can also lead to laryngeal paralysis.

Congenital paralysis of the larynx has been reported in Bouviers des Flandres, Bull Terriers, Dalmatians, Rottweilers, and Huskies. It usually affects dogs around 1 year of age.

Clinical presentation and diagnosis

Patients with laryngeal paralysis can present as an emergency with URT obstruction, due to collapse, episodes of extreme dyspnea exacerbated by heat, and cyanosis. Most have a history of progressive exercise intolerance with increasing stridor (high pitched inspiratory noise) (Video 21.3). Other signs include dysphonation (change in voice/bark) and coughing/gagging after eating and drinking. On physical examination there may be signs consistent with aspiration pneumonia such as crackles/wheezes on thoracic auscultation. The clinical signs for congenital and acquired laryngeal paralysis are the same; however, the patient's age and signalment differ. Certain breeds (e.g., Rottweilers) affected by the congenital form present with generalized neurological signs, such as ataxia, paresis, tremors, and dyspnea.

Laryngeal paralysis is diagnosed by a laryngeal examination under a light plane of anesthesia; in affected animals the arytenoid cartilages are not able to abduct (Videos 21.4 and 21.5). It is helpful to have an assistant hold the patient's head in the position for endotracheal intu-

Video 21.3. Inspiratory stridor and dyspnea in a dog with laryngeal paralysis. Video courtesy of Filippo Cinti.

Video 21.4. Evaluation of laryngeal function in a cat without laryngeal pathology and in a dog with laryngeal paralysis. Both patients were placed under a light plane of anesthesia to ensure a reliable examination. In the cat, normal abduction of the arytenoid cartilages is observed during inspiration, while in the dog no movement is noted. Note the assistant indicating "in" during inspiration and "out" during expiration to rule out paradoxical laryngeal movement. Video courtesy of Matteo Rossanese.

Video 21.5. Laryngeal endoscopic examination of a dog with laryngeal paralysis. The arytenoid cartilages are not able to abduct. Video courtesy of Filippo Cinti.

bation for laryngeal examination, without compression under the neck. The assistant can say when the patient inspires to rule out paradoxical laryngeal movement (i.e., when the arytenoid cartilages are passively pulled medially during inspiration). Once diagnosed, the underlying causes listed above should be investigated.

Treatment

Emergency management

Like in patients with URT obstruction due to BOAS, keeping patients with suspected laryngeal paralysis calm is an essential step in managing the condition. With acute dyspnea, emergency medical treatment should be started with sedation, corticosteroids, supplemental oxygen, and cooling when necessary (see above for recommendations for BOAS that can be implemented in patients with suspected laryngeal paralysis). Many patients with URT obstruction become hyperthermic because they cannot regulate their body temperature with panting (see above for treatment of hyperthermia). Most cases can be stabilized medically. If the obstruction and/or mucosal swelling is severe, general anesthesia and intubation or a temporary tracheostomy should be performed.

Surgical treatment

Surgery is the definitive treatment for laryngeal paralysis; however, this is palliative, as it only addresses the URT obstruction, not the other neurological deficits or underlying causes. Dogs that are mildly affected or asymptomatic at rest may be managed with weight loss, stress reduction, exercise restriction, and care to prevent overheating. The aim of laryngeal surgery for paralysis of the larynx is to reduce airway resistance by increasing the lumen diameter. Many surgical techniques have been described, ranging from muscle–nerve pedicle transposition for reinnervation of the larynx to castellated laryngofissure and partial laryngectomy. Arytenoid lateralization procedures are recommended due to consistently good results with minimal complications. Both unilateral cricoid–arytenoid and unilateral thyroid–arytenoid lateralization procedures give reliable and comparable results and are equally effective in decreasing signs from a clinical point of view.[12]

Surgical technique: Cricoid–arytenoid lateralization (Videos 21.6 and 21.7)

Corticosteroids can be given during the induction of anesthesia to decrease postoperative mucosal swelling. The entire neck should be aseptically prepared for surgery. A lateral approach or a ventral paramedian approach can be used, depending on the surgeon's preference. The lateral approach is described below.

1. The animal is placed in right lateral recumbency (for a left cricoid–arytenoid lateralization), with a towel under the neck to elevate the laryngeal area.
2. A paramedian skin incision is made on the left side from the caudal angle of the mandible extending to 2 cm caudal to the larynx. The incision is ventral to the jugular groove.
3. The subcutaneous tissues and platysma muscle are then incised, and blunt dissection is performed lateral to the sternohyoid and sternocephalic muscles until the dorsal edge of the thyroid cartilage can be palpated and lifted.
4. Care should be taken to avoid the external jugular vein and its bifurcation; the incision should be ventral to this vein. Self-retaining retractors (e.g., blunt Gelpi retractors) may be useful to improve visualization.
5. An incision is made in the thyropharyngeal muscle along the dorsolateral edge of the thyroid cartilage. An atraumatic forceps can be placed on the thyroid cartilage lamina or stay sutures can be placed through the dorsal edge of the thyroid cartilage to retract and rotate the larynx laterally. Pulling the thyroid cartilage laterally also helps to demarcate the thyropharyngeal muscle (Fig. 21.7).
6. Medial to the thyropharyngeal muscle is a white membrane that is adherent to the thyroid cartilage.

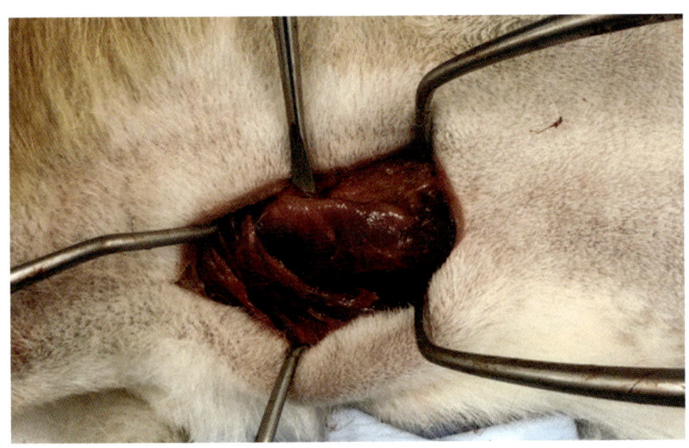

Figure 21.7 Intraoperative image of left-sided cricoid–arytenoid lateralization in a cadaver. Cranial is to the left of the image. A handheld retractor is placed medial to the dorsal edge of the thyroid cartilage and is pulling the thyroid cartilage laterally to demonstrate the thyropharyngeal muscle, which will then be transected.

Video 21.6. Laryngeal paralysis in an 8-year-old crossbreed dog. Cricoid–arytenoid lateralization technique (tie-back). Video courtesy of Filippo Cinti.

Video 21.7. A cat with right thyroid tumor and severe dyspnea and inspiratory stridor for laryngeal paralysis. After right thyroidectomy, left side tie back was performed. Video courtesy of Filippo Cinti.

It is the external surface of the mucosal lining of the laryngopharynx, and it should be cut with scissors to identify the dorsal cricoarytenoid muscle.

7. The muscular process of the arytenoid cartilage is identified by palpation and visualization. It is approximately 5 mm and is elevated on the dorsolateral aspect of the arytenoid cartilage.
8. The dorsal cricoarytenoid muscle is identified; it is triangular in shape and fans out dorsally from the muscular process of the arytenoid cartilage. It is often atrophied in patients with laryngeal paralysis. This muscle is transected at its insertion on the muscular process.
9. The cricoarytenoid joint is then disarticulated along the caudal edge using fine scissors. The opening should be large enough to see the joint surface and the medial aspect of the muscular process.
10. Excessive exposure and entering the laryngeal lumen should be avoided, if possible, as it may increase the risk of overabduction of the arytenoid cartilage.
11. The caudal aspect of the cricoid cartilage is palpated.
12. Two 2-0 nonabsorbable synthetic (polypropylene in large dogs) sutures are placed on the caudodorsal border of the cricoid cartilage, through the cricoid cartilage, and then through the medial aspect of the muscular process of the arytenoid cartilage (Figs. 21.8 and 21.9).
13. Both sutures are preplaced. The anesthetist or an unsterile assistant should deflate the endotracheal tube cuff and move the tube to ensure that the sutures have not accidentally caught part of the endotracheal tube.
14. A mosquito hemostat is used on the muscular process to pull the arytenoid into a more lateral and caudal position. Once positioned, the sutures are pulled and held before tying.
15. Abduction of the arytenoid cartilage is checked with the help of the anesthetist or unsterile assistant by intraoral visualization. Since this can be challenging with an endotracheal tube in place, extubation and reintubation may be necessary.
16. The rima glottis opening should not be larger than the size of the endotracheal tube in place. The epiglottis should still be able to cover the rima glottis to avoid the risk of aspiration during swallowing.
17. Both sutures are tied.

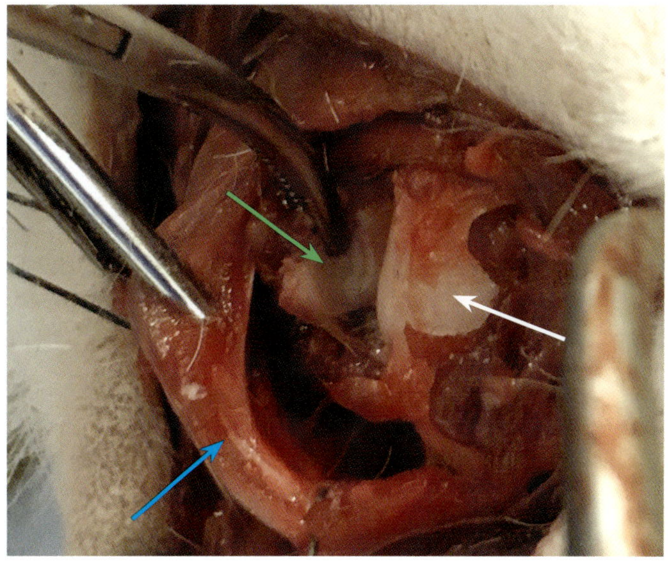

Figure 21.8 Intraoperative image of left-sided cricoid–arytenoid lateralization in a cadaver. Cranial is to the left of the image. The muscular process of the arytenoid cartilage has been grasped with a hemostat (this must be avoided in a live patient; the hemostat should be placed on the transected dorsal cricoarytenoid muscle on the lateral surface of the muscular process). The lateralization suture should penetrate the center of the muscular process medially and be passed through it to the lateral aspect. The blue arrow indicates the thyroid cartilage; the white arrow, the cricoid cartilage; and the green arrow, the medial aspect of the muscular process of the arytenoid cartilage (rotated laterally to show its medial aspect).

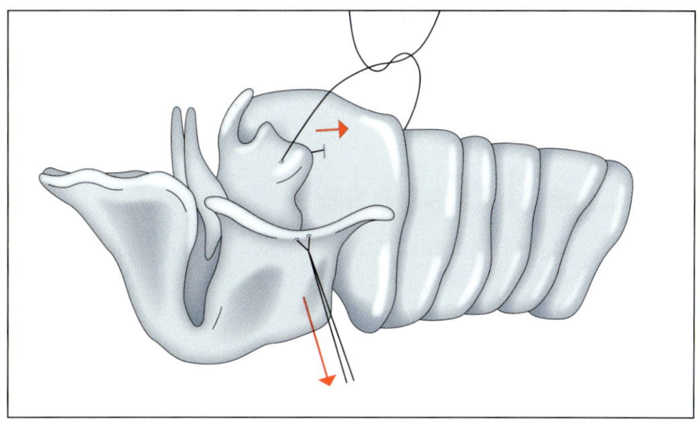

Figure 21.9 Suture placement for cricoid–arytenoid lateralization. One or two sutures are placed from the caudodorsal border of the cricoid cartilage to the muscular process of the arytenoid cartilage. Note the ventrolateral retraction of the thyroid cartilage with a stay suture.

18. The thyropharyngeal muscle is apposed with absorbable suture material in a simple continuous pattern.
19. The subcutaneous tissues and the skin are closed routinely.

Postoperative management

Patients benefit from close monitoring after surgery. Continued oxygen therapy may be indicated. Heavy sedation should be avoided; ideally the gag reflex should be present. It is essential to keep the patient calm and to avoid vocalization or panting. Food and water should be withheld until the patient has fully recovered. Some surgeons withhold food for 12–24 hours after anesthesia. Feeding should be supervised for a period of 7–10 days; soft food made into meatballs seems to be well tolerated. Fat-containing liquids (e.g., milk, gravy) should be avoided, as they are associated with severe aspiration pneumonia.

Outcome

Improvement in breathing has been reported in 90% of patients after arytenoid lateralization procedures, with 70% of dogs still being alive 5 years after surgery.[15] Complications of lateralization surgery are hematoma formation, suture avulsion, cartilage fracture, discomfort during swallowing, temporary glottic dysfunction, and coughing after eating or drinking, sometimes resulting in aspiration pneumonia.

Dogs with long-term laryngeal dysfunction have an on-going increased risk of aspiration pneumonia. Owners should monitor for this and seek veterinary guidance if the patient develops a soft cough, increased respiratory rate and effort, and/or signs of systemic disease.

Tracheal disease

The trachea receives and drains blood through the cranial and caudal thyroid arteries and veins, the bronchoesophageal arteries and veins, and the internal jugular veins. Tracheal innervation is supplied by the autonomic nervous system. Sympathetic fibers from the middle cervical ganglion and sympathetic trunk inhibit tracheal muscle contraction and glandular secretions, while parasympathetic fibers from the vagus and recurrent laryngeal nerves cause tracheal muscle contraction and glandular secretions.

Temporary tracheostomy

Temporary tracheostomy is indicated in patients with URT obstruction at the level of the nose, larynx, or cranial trachea. It is also used as an alternative route for endotracheal intubation in laryngeal surgery and as an ancillary procedure to prevent postoperative dyspnea after extensive surgical procedures on the pharynx or larynx. Temporary tracheostomy includes the introduction of a tracheal cannula that is left in place until the airways are patent. Tracheostomy tubes with two cannulas (human adult tracheostomy tubes) are the preferred option, as the internal cannula can be removed for cleaning whilst maintaining a patent airway. However, most brachycephalic dogs are too small to accommodate these tubes; therefore, human pediatric tracheostomy tubes can be used instead. As these tubes are small and flexible, patients require close monitoring to ensure the tube does not become kinked. Tracheostomy tubes with a tracheal cuff are also available. These tubes are useful for patients under general anesthesia or patients requiring on-going mechanical ventilation. However, they should not be used for long periods due to concerns over tracheal mucosal damage. Tracheostomy tubes should be approximately 40% of the tracheal diameter; this allows some space around the tube to help maintain a patent airway even if the tube lumen becomes obstructed. If purpose tracheostomy tubes are not available, an endotracheal tube can be trimmed to an appropriate length. Tracheal stoma stents are also available.[16]

Temporary tracheostomies require general anesthesia in all patients, including emergency cases. In patients requiring a tracheostomy tube urgently, it is best practice to intubate via the larynx, even with a small-diameter tube (e.g., urinary catheter), to provide oxygen. Anesthesia can then be induced and maintained using total intravenous anesthesia if necessary (e.g., patient with laryngeal trauma). This will allow thorough clipping and preparation of the ventral neck with a managed URT. True emergency tracheostomies without anesthesia and preparation should not occur.

It is useful to have an emergency kit with all the elements ready in case of such emergencies. It should include the following:

- Intravenous cannulas and T connectors
- Induction agent
- Intravenous needles and syringes
- Selection of tracheostomy tubes
- Some soft umbilical tape to secure the tube
- 3-0 polydioxanone suture
- 2-0 nylon or polypropylene suture

Surgical technique

1. The whole ventral neck should be clipped and aseptically prepared.
2. The patient is placed in dorsal recumbency, with the neck extended over a sandbag. Positioning is important; the patient should be straight and secured to the operating table with tape.
3. A midline skin incision of approximately 2 cm is made over the trachea at the midpoint between the larynx and the thoracic inlet (Fig. 21.10).

4. The subcutaneous fat and the left and right sternothyroid and sternohyoid muscles are divided in the midline by blunt dissection. Care should be taken not to damage the tracheal veins, which lie immediately lateral to the trachea on both sides.
5. A small self-retaining wound retractor is inserted to expose the trachea (Fig. 21.11).
6. Stay sutures (3-0 Ethilon or Prolene) are placed around two tracheal rings, above and below the area where the tracheal incision will be made, to help with tracheal manipulation (Video 21.8).
7. The ligament between two adjacent rings, at approximately ring number 5 when counting cranially to caudally, is incised with a number 11 scalpel blade. This incision should be approximately one-third (and less than half) of the circumference of the trachea (Fig. 21.12).
8. After temporarily discontinuing the inhalational agent, if used, the oropharyngeal endotracheal tube is removed and replaced by a tracheostomy tube, which is inserted through the tracheal window. Pulling the stay sutures apart facilitates tube placement. If the tracheostomy is performed prior to a more extensive procedure, an endotracheal tube should be used instead; the tracheostomy tube can be placed once the additional surgical procedure has been completed (Fig. 21.13).

Video 21.8. Placement of two tracheal stay sutures incorporating two tracheal rings each. Cranial is to the right of the video. Video courtesy of Matteo Rossanese.

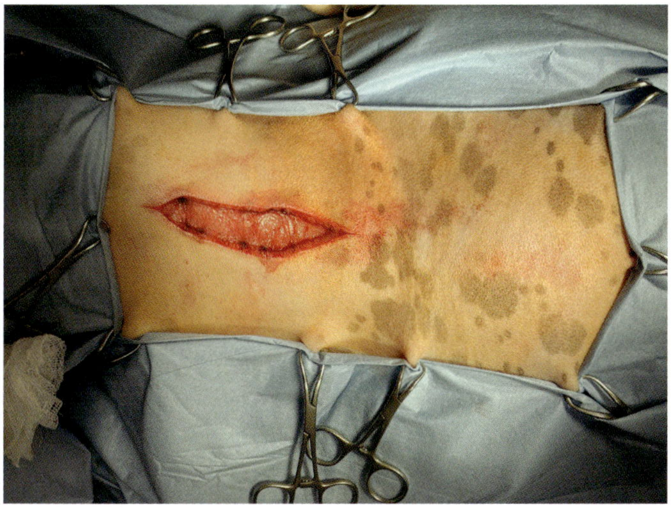

Figure 21.10 Ventral midline incision between the larynx and the thoracic inlet for temporary tracheostomy. Cranial is to the left of the image. Image courtesy of Anna Frykfors von Hekkel.

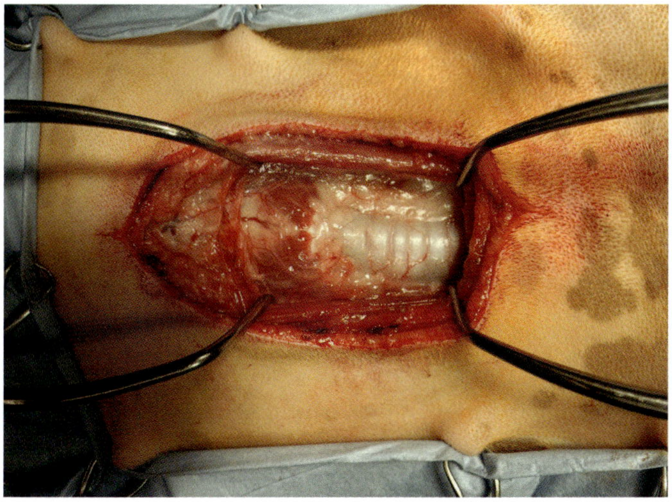

Figure 21.11 Exposure of the trachea with a retractor. Cranial is to the left of the image. Image courtesy of Anna Frykfors von Hekkel.

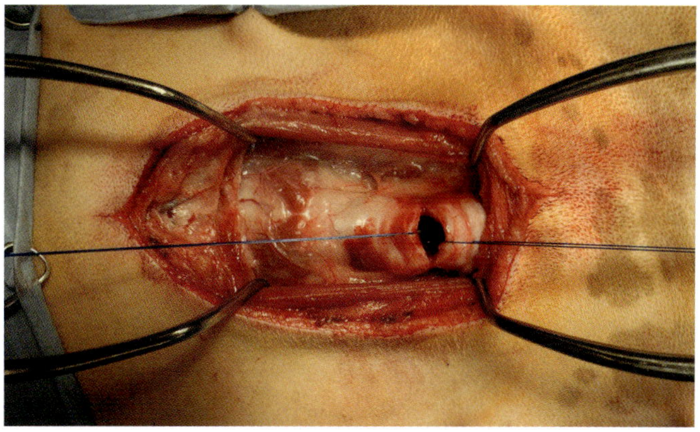

Figure 21.12 Placement of tracheal stay sutures and incision into the tracheal ligament. Cranial is to the left of the image. Image courtesy of Anna Frykfors von Hekkel.

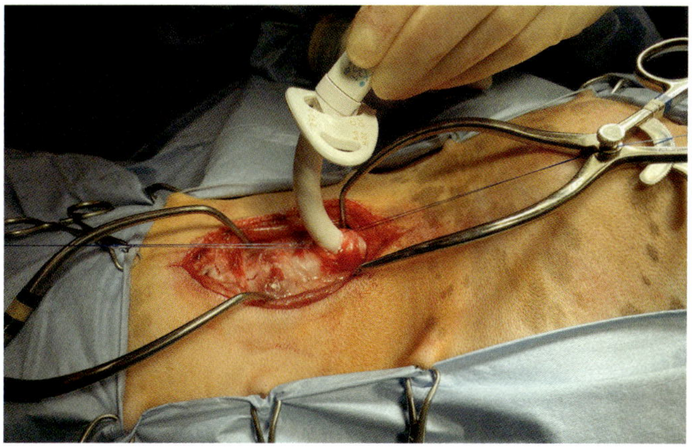

Figure 21.13 Insertion of a double-lumen tracheostomy tube, with the stay sutures in place. The skin incision will require skin sutures in the cranial aspect (to the left of the image). Image courtesy of Anna Frykfors von Hekkel.

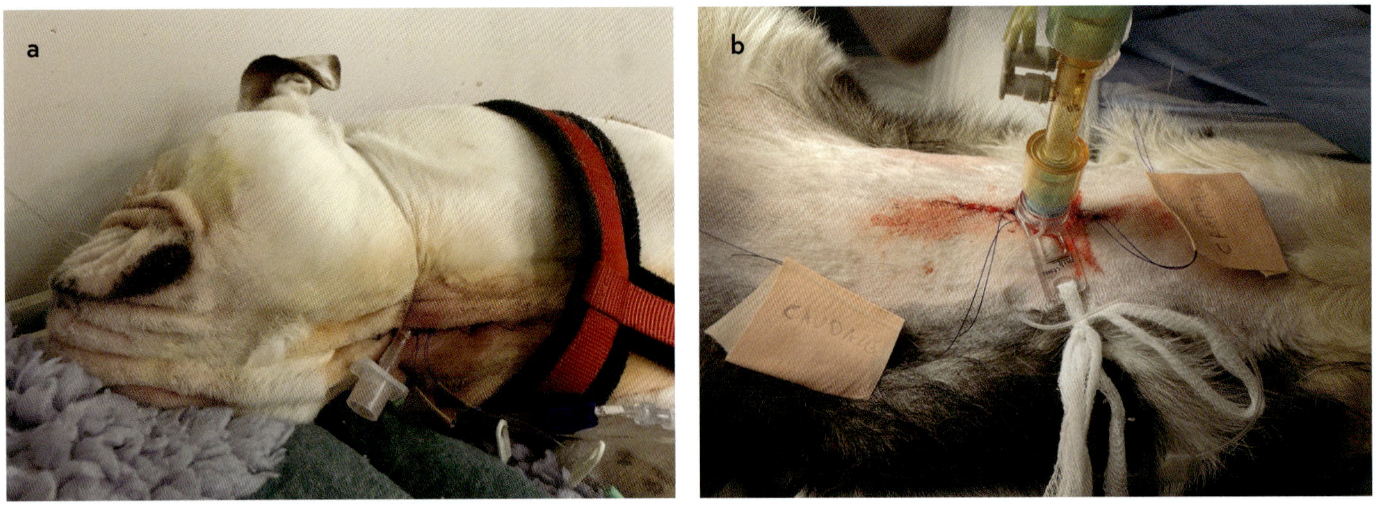

Figure 21.14 (a) English Bulldog with a temporary tracheostomy tube. In this case, a trimmed endotracheal tube was placed and secured using two sections of umbilical tape tied dorsally. Note that the stay sutures in the tracheal rings are still in place. (b) Close-up view of the temporary tracheostomy tube and the labeled cranial and caudal stay sutures in another patient. Image b courtesy of Filippo Cinti.

9. Two pieces of umbilical tape are attached to the wings of the tracheal cannula and tied around the neck. The cannula is left in place until the URT is patent.
10. If a large incision has been made, it can be partially closed by placing 3-0 polydioxanone in a simple continuous pattern in the muscles and 3-0 Ethilon skin sutures. It is important to not close the muscle and skin immediately adjacent to the tube but leave at least 2 cm of open incision cranial and caudal to the tube. This will help with tube maintenance, as the tube will need to be removed every 2–4 hours.
11. The long polydioxanone stay sutures placed around the tracheal rings should not be removed. After tying their two ends to form a long loop, the cranial and caudal sutures should be labeled (e.g., up/cranial and down/caudal, respectively). These sutures, which are useful if the tube needs to be replaced quickly, should remain in situ until the patient is ready to be discharged (Fig. 21.14).

Postoperative management

Any tracheal tube needs intensive nursing to avoid acute blockage of the stoma. Patients with tracheostomy tubes need to be monitored very closely, ideally in a position where they can be observed at all times because if they obstruct, they can die quickly.

Ideally, the inspired air should be kept moist by nebulization every 2–4 hours and the tube should be thoroughly cleaned every 2–4 hours, depending on individual tracheal mucus production. If there is an inner cannula, it should be removed and replaced after cleaning. Pediatric tubes need to be removed and replaced every time; two tubes should be available per patient. When cleaning, a fresh tube should be available for replacement in an emergency setting. At all times a kit with some induction agent, a new tracheostomy tube of the same or slightly smaller size, a laryngoscope, and an endotracheal tube should be next to the kennel in case of emergency. An intravenous cannula should be maintained throughout the entire hospitalization period. Stoma/wound care with bathing of the area twice daily and application of a barrier cream adjacent to the stoma can be helpful. In case of excessive secretions an absorbent sponge dressing can be placed between cannula and skin.

Outcome

Complications are reported to occur in 50%–95% of patients with a temporary tracheostomy. They include tube obstruction, inadvertent removal, gagging, coughing, vomiting, subcutaneous emphysema, pneumomediastinitis, pneumothorax, and infection.[17,18] The most common complication is obstruction by mucus plugs and inflammatory debris, which can be fatal (Fig. 21.15).[17] However, temporary tracheostomy was reported to have a successful outcome in 98% of patients in a study specifically looking at placement of temporary tracheostomy tubes in brachycephalic dogs after BOAS surgery.[18]

Temporary tracheostomy tube removal

Tracheostomy tubes are well tolerated and generally patients do not require on-going sedation unless they are anxious. The tube should remain in situ whilst the URT obstruction is still present (e.g., if placed for laryngeal edema, maintain the tube for at least 48 hours).

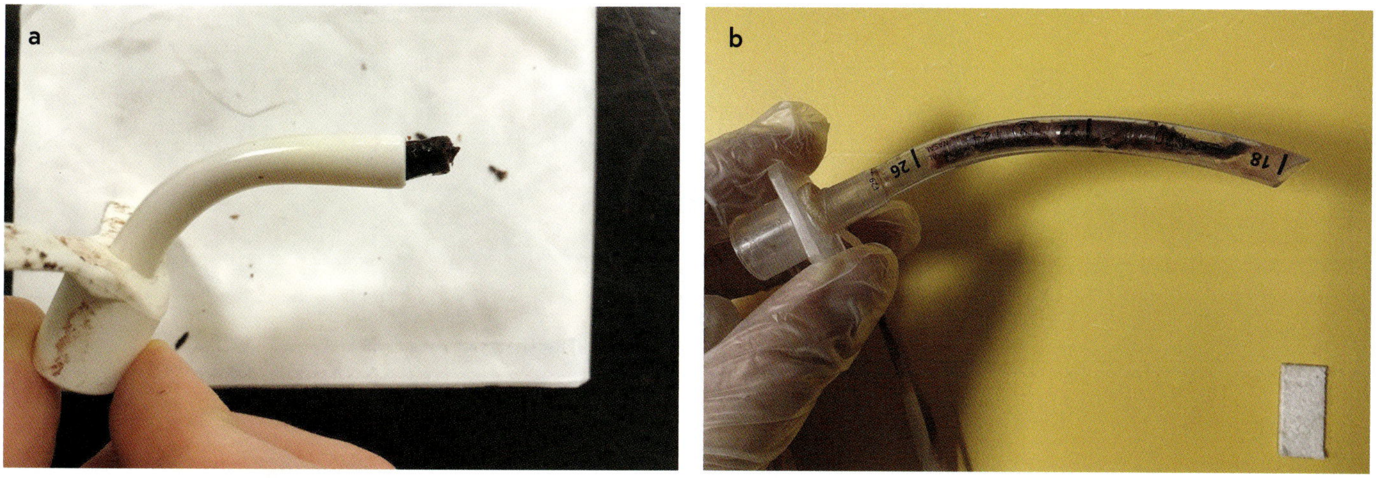

Figure 21.15 Two examples of tracheostomy tube obstruction. Both dogs showed an increased respiratory effort, and the tracheostomy tube was replaced. Full obstruction due to mucus, debris, and blood was noted. Images courtesy of Matteo Rossanese.

Video 21.9. Removal of a temporary tracheostomy tube from an 8-year-old Pug that presented with progressive dyspnea and grade-III laryngeal collapse. After partial cuneiformectomy, a tracheostomy tube was placed to aid recovery from anesthesia. Video courtesy of Anna Frykfors von Hekkel.

Some clinicians test if tracheostomy tube removal will be tolerated by occluding the tube; this can be useful but may not be representative of how the patient will fair without the tube in place. When the tube is removed, the animal should be observed for a period of at least 10 minutes. Ideally the patient should be allowed to walk around during this time (Video 21.9). If the patient exhibits an excessive increase in the respiratory rate or effort or becomes dyspneic, the tube should be replaced. Sedation or anesthesia induction may be necessary to ensure correct tube placement. An emergency intubation kit should be ready prior to tube removal (see above).
Once the tube has been removed and the animal is breathing well, patient discharge should be considered. It is prudent to observe the patient with the owner for a period of time, as often excitement can exacerbate any remaining URT obstruction. Mild sedation with oral trazodone or low-dose acepromazine/butorphanol can be useful for discharge. Acepromazine and butorphanol can be administered separately or administered together (coadministration) if required. The skin incision should be left open and usually heals quickly, in approximately 10–14 days, by second intention. The owner can perform stoma care by keeping the area adjacent to the stoma clean with water only. The owner should be instructed to only allow supervised access to water for 14 days and no swimming for at least this period to ensure the stoma has fully healed.

Permanent tracheostomy

A permanent tracheal stoma (tubeless tracheostomy) is sometimes the only solution when an obstructive disease of the URT is beyond treatment and a tracheal cannula has become a necessary condition for continuation of life. However, it should be borne in mind that homecare of a permanent tracheostomy is difficult and time-consuming.

Surgical technique

1. After induction of anesthesia, endotracheal intubation is performed via the oral route. Care should be taken that the cuff of the endotracheal tube is placed caudal to the planned site of the stoma and is adequately inflated.
2. The patient is placed in dorsal recumbency, with the neck extended over a sandbag. Positioning is important; the patient should be straight and secured to the operating table with tape.
3. The procedure starts with a ventral midline skin incision directed lengthwise over the cervical trachea for 8–10 cm. Unless there is a specific indication, the tracheostomy should be situated in the middle of the neck.
4. The underlying tissues are separated in the midline and the left and right sternohyoid muscles are separated over the entire length of the skin incision.
5. The ventral surface of the trachea is elevated by suturing the left and right sternohyoid muscles together dorsal to the trachea (Fig. 21.16).

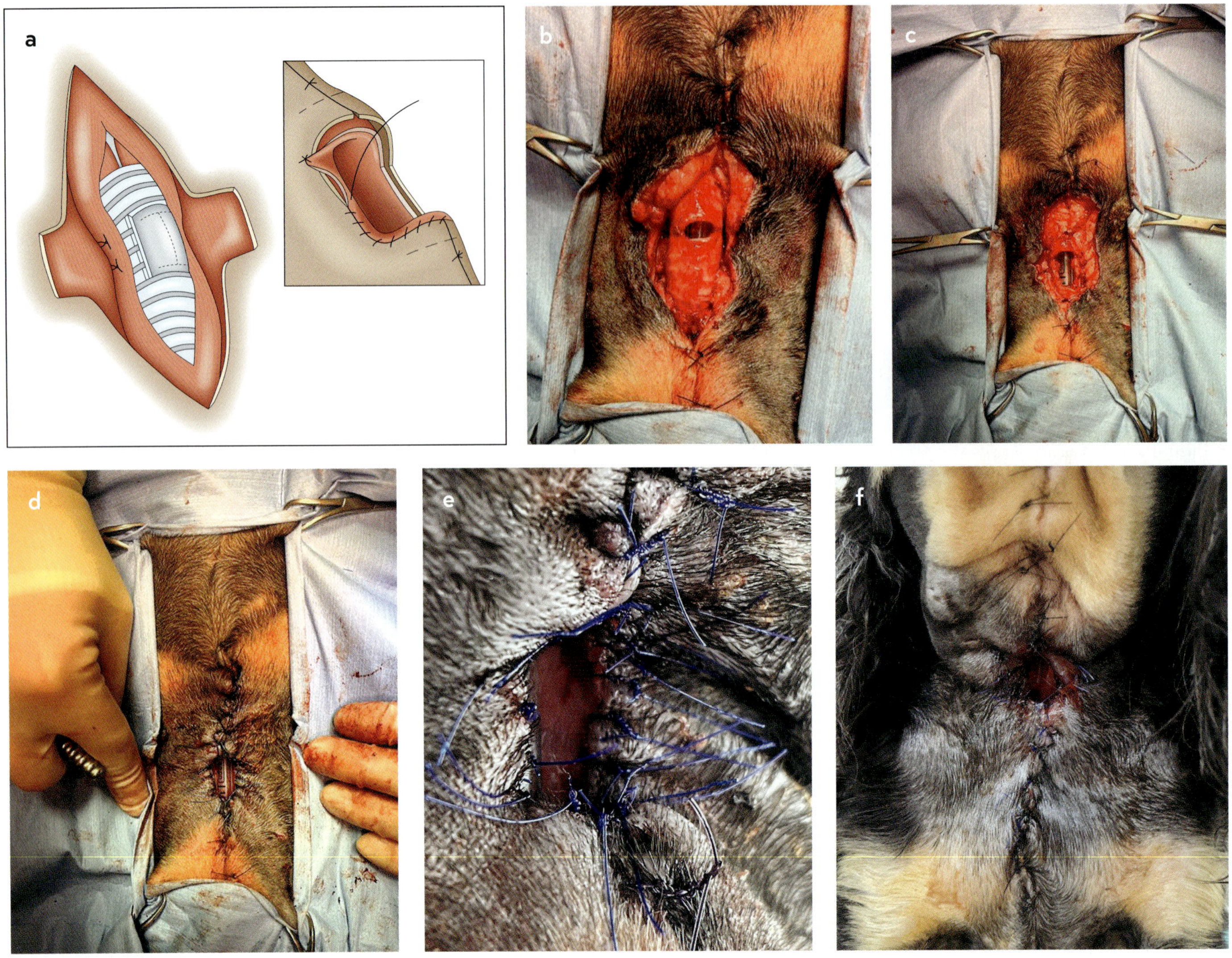

Figure 21.16 Permanent tracheostomy. (a) Schematic representation of the procedure. (b) The sternohyoid muscles are apposed dorsal to the trachea. (c) A segment of tracheal cartilage is removed (along three tracheal rings), and the perimucosal tracheal tissue is sutured to the dermis. (d) The tracheal mucosa is apposed to the skin using simple interrupted sutures. (e) Close-up view of the surgical site. (f) Appearance of the surgical site 24 hours after surgery. Note the tracheal secretions around the tracheostomy. Images courtesy of Matteo Rossanese.

6. The ventral half of the tracheal cartilage over three to four tracheal rings is excised in the center of the neck and skin incision.
7. The perimucosal tracheal tissue can be sutured to the dermis with 4-0 simple interrupted absorbable sutures.
8. A piece of skin the size of the stoma is then removed.
9. Apposition of tracheal mucosa and skin is vital. The cranial and caudal edges of the skin over the trachea are anchored to the trachea with one suture at each corner.
10. The most important part of the surgery then follows, being the apposition of the skin and the tracheal mucosa with multiple interrupted sutures at the edge of the stoma. The tracheal cartilage should be included in several of these sutures for reliable support. Simple interrupted sutures of 4-0 long-lasting absorbable monofilament or nonabsorbable material should be placed 2–3 mm apart (Fig. 21.16).
11. The subcutaneous tissue and the skin cranial and caudal to the stoma are then closed routinely.
12. If a neck skinfold is present, plastic skin surgery could be performed at each side of the stoma to avoid skinfold occlusion and stoma stenosis (Fig. 21.17).

Postoperative management

Initially, postoperative management is similar to that for temporary tracheostomy, with nebulization and suctioning. Aftercare consists of careful removal of the crusts around the stoma while the sutures are in place

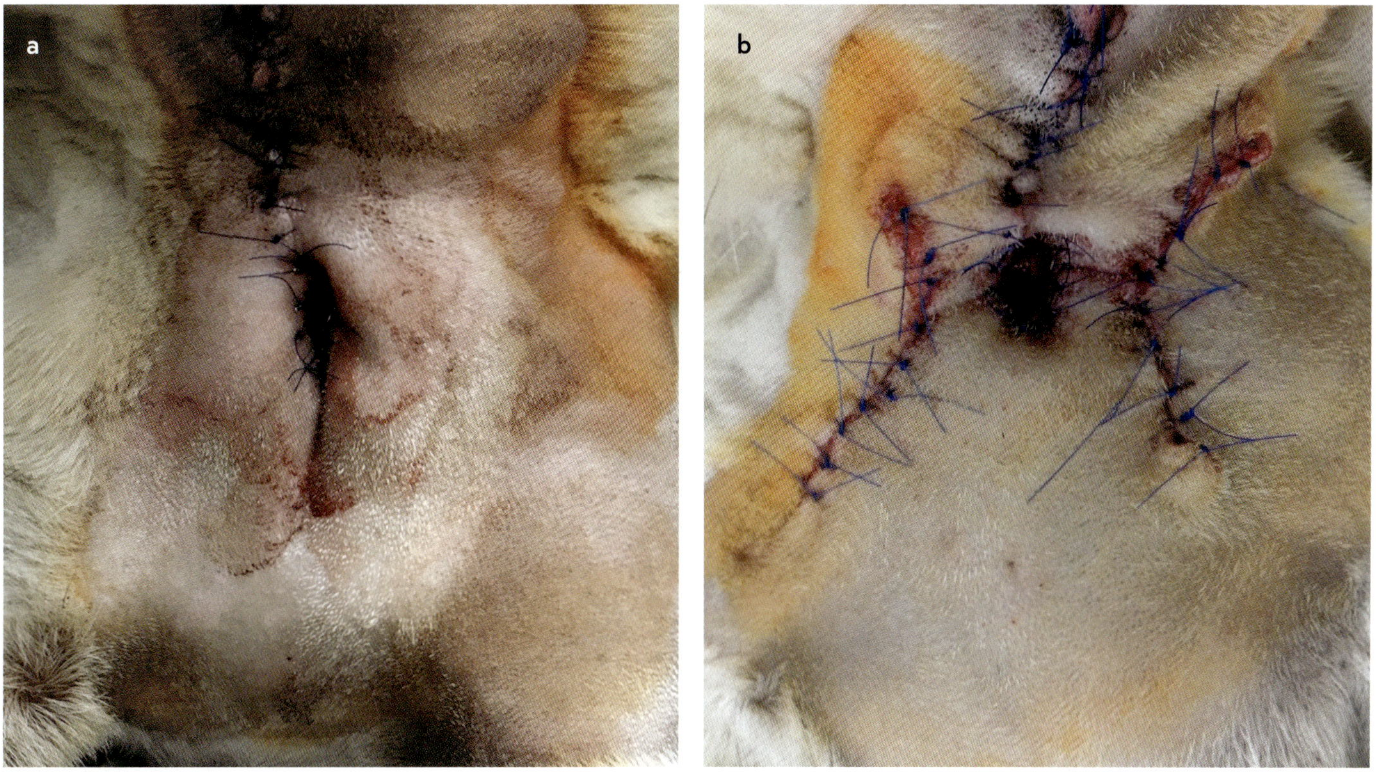

Figure 21.17 (a) Preoperative examination of skinfolds after permanent tracheostomy. (b) Skin fold surgery at each side of the stoma. Images courtesy of Filippo Cinti and Tim Charlesworth.

Video 21.10. Tracheostomy site cleaning 6 hours after permanent tracheostomy in a 10-year-old Cavalier King Charles Spaniel and evaluation 24 hours postoperatively. Video courtesy of Matteo Rossanese and Charlotte Banks.

(10–14 days) (Video 21.10). Cleaning should be gentle to avoid disrupting the stoma site. After this initial period of approximately 1 month, cleaning is needed less frequently, as excessive tracheal mucus production occurs during the healing phase. Instructions to the owner include regular clipping of the hair around the stoma, avoidance of contact with dust or airway irritants, and the lifelong prohibition of bathing and swimming. Collar and leads should be avoided; using a harness is recommended.

Outcome

Complications are similar to those of temporary tracheostomy tube placement. Major complications have been reported to occur in 50%–60% dogs, with aspiration pneumonia, skinfold occlusion, and stoma stenosis being most common.[19,20]

Stenosis of the stoma may not cause a functional problem for patients.[21] However, revision surgery was necessary in 35% of patients due to tracheal stenosis or skinfold occlusion.[20]

Other complications include tracheal collapse, surgical site swelling, wound dehiscence, and loss of normal vocalization.

A study reported that the overall median survival time after permanent tracheostomy was over 1000 days and concluded that it can be a viable treatment option for dogs with URT obstruction.[20]

Tracheal and laryngeal trauma

Traumatic lesions to the laryngeal cartilages can be treated by careful reapposition of the cartilage fragments if seen acutely after the traumatic incident. Long-lasting monofilament suture material (e.g., polydioxanone) can be used. If the laryngeal trauma is extensive, placement of a temporary tracheostomy tube is indicated. However, laryngeal trauma may not be detected at the time of injury and may result in stenosis. In this case, patients may present with dyspnea and exercise intolerance, and laryngeal stenosis/narrowing could be seen on laryngeal examination. Clinical signs may resolve with conservative treatment (anti-inflammatory medication) or may require surgical intervention, such as partial arytenoidectomy or cricoid–arytenoid lateralization.[22]

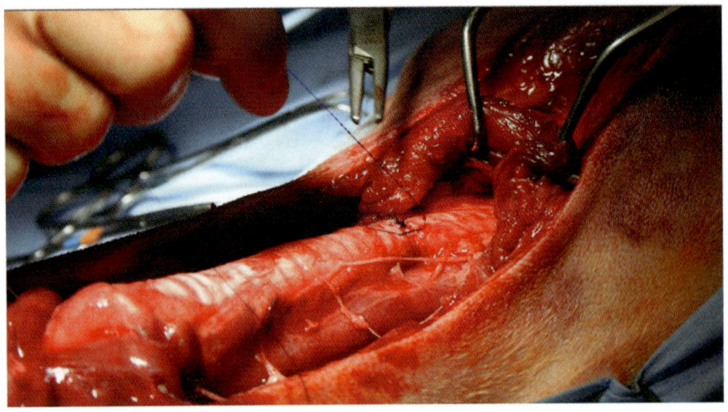

Figure 21.18 Intraoperative image of a 10-year-old Terrier that had received cervical bite injuries (cranial is to the left of the image). He presented with subcutaneous emphysema and pneumomediastinum; these signs increased the index of suspicion for a tracheal or esophageal injury. A tracheal injury was visualized during exploratory surgery. The image shows repair of the tracheal tear by placement of simple interrupted full thickness PDS sutures.

Surgical technique

1. A ventral midline approach is best for exploratory neck surgery.
2. Staying on the midline will help to avoid major blood vessels and nerves, which run lateral and dorsal to the trachea.
3. Stay sutures can be placed in the trachea so that the trachea can be gently retracted/rotated to allow visualization of the full circumference (Fig. 21.18).
4. Tracheal wounds can be closed with 4-0 or 3-0 full-thickness simple interrupted polydioxanone sutures (Fig. 21.19).
5. Care should be taken to identify and preserve the recurrent laryngeal nerves, which are very small and run along the lateral aspects of the trachea.

Video 21.11. Resection of the first two tracheal rings using a split-cartilage technique. Note the mobility of the trachea, allowing anastomosis without tension. Video courtesy of Matteo Rossanese.

Tracheal resection and anastomosis

Indications for tracheal resection and anastomosis[24] are tracheal tumors, stenosis, or trauma. While small tears in the tracheal wall (e.g., after minor trauma) can be closed primarily, in case of more extensive trauma or infected wounds part of the trachea may have to be resected. Approximately 20%–60% of the trachea may be resected and still allow for a tension-free anastomosis (Video 21.11). In adult animals, tracheal tissue is less elastic, so removal of a large section is better tolerated. When the tracheal tissue is more elastic in younger animals there is more tension on the repair, meaning that healing is impaired by the increased tension at the wound edges, increasing the risk of wound dehiscence. In puppies only 20%–25% of the trachea can be safely resected.[22] Excessive tension on the anastomosis site will cause healing by granulation tissue formation, which may lead to stenosis with clinical consequences.[21] With debridement or resection, the split-cartilage technique is preferred over other techniques, since it is easy to perform and results in a better anatomic alignment and less luminal stenosis. Tension-relieving sutures placed over several tracheal rings cranial and caudal to the anastomosis have been shown to reduce stenosis.[23]

Surgical technique (Figs. 21.20 and 21.21)

1. The cervical trachea is exposed using a ventral cervical midline incision from the larynx to the sternum.

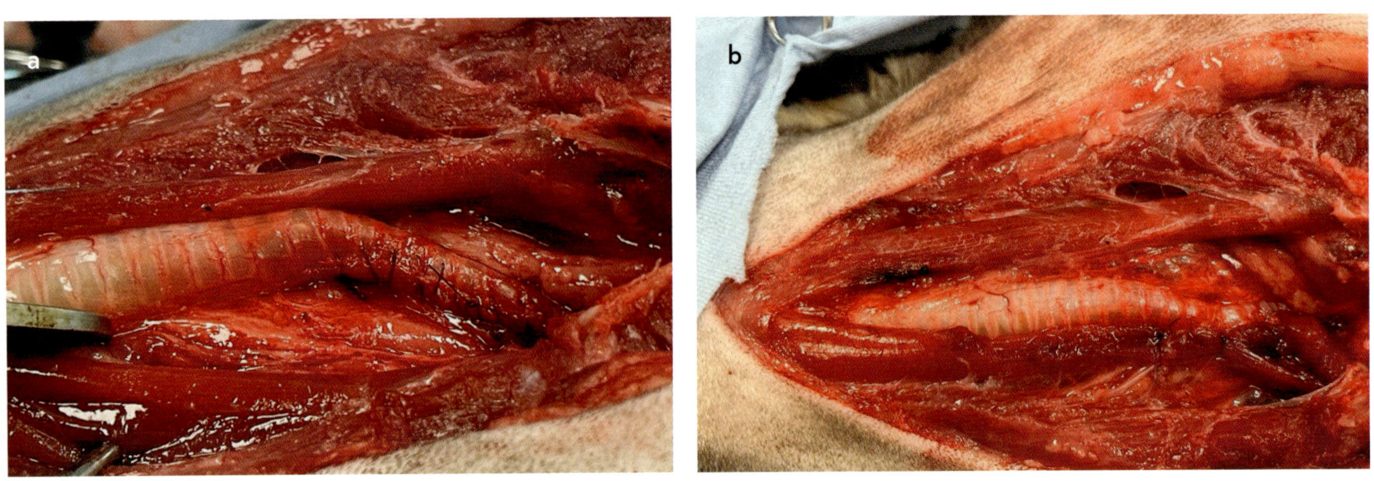

Figure 21.19 Intraoperative images of a 7-year-old cat with a large longitudinal tracheal laceration. A cranial sternotomy approach was performed to better visualize the tracheal tear at the thoracic inlet. (a) Suturing of the tracheal tear. (b) Muscle patch. Images courtesy of Filippo Cinti.

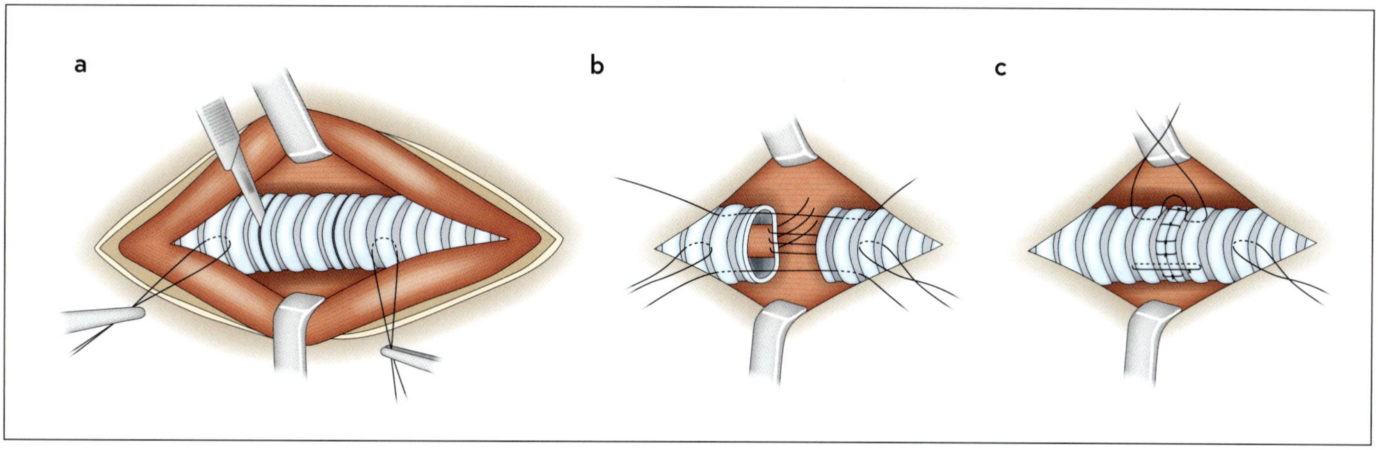

Figure 21.20 Schematic representation of the split-cartilage technique for tracheal resection and anastomosis. (a) Stay sutures are placed cranial and caudal to the area to be resected. (b) After resection, sutures are preplaced through the tracheal muscle and tracheal rings. (c) Tension-relieving sutures are placed around the cartilage rings cranial and caudal to the anastomosis site.

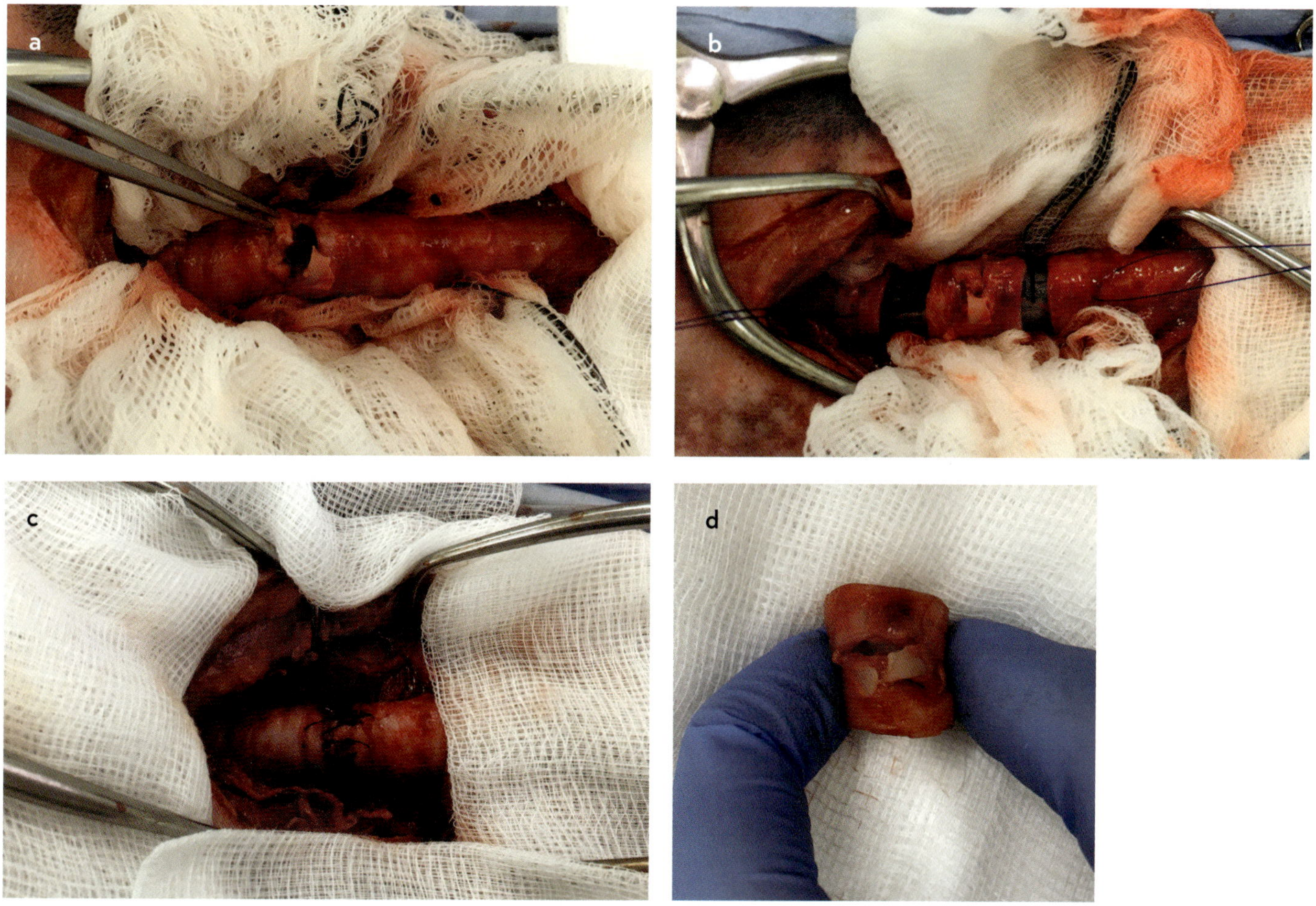

Figure 21.21 Tracheal resection and anastomosis in a 2-year-old Cocker Spaniel who had sustained cervical bite injuries and presented with subcutaneous emphysema and tracheal rupture, as demonstrated by tracheoscopy. (a) Intraoperative evidence of rupture of two tracheal rings in the midcervical region. (b) Resection of the ruptured rings. Note the placement of two stay sutures cranial and caudal to the resected trachea. (c) Tracheal anastomosis performed using simple interrupted 3-0 polydioxanone sutures. Note the placement of tension-relieving sutures around the cartilage rings cranial and caudal to the anastomosis site. (d) Resected tracheal segment, evidencing the two ruptured tracheal rings. Images courtesy of Matteo Rossanese.

For intrathoracic tracheal resections, a right lateral (paracostal) thoracotomy is preferred, unless indicated otherwise (e.g., by chest radiographs or because of left-sided thoracic trauma).

2. The trachea should be mobilized carefully. There should be enough space to allow an anastomosis without tension, but with preservation of the segmental blood and nerve supply.
3. Stay sutures should be placed around the tracheal rings cranial and caudal to the area of proposed resection.
4. The trachea is resected by splitting the cartilage circumferentially on each side of the proposed resection site.
5. After cutting the cartilage rings, the dorsal tracheal membrane is transected too, taking care not to perforate the endotracheal tube.
6. If placing the cuff of the endotracheal tube past the obstruction was not possible before resection, this resection must be performed quickly and the distal trachea has to be intubated rapidly and the tube cuffed, after which the anastomosis can be performed. The dorsal tracheal membrane is sutured first with three simple interrupted absorbable monofilament sutures. Then, the split cartilage rings are apposed with simple interrupted sutures spaced 2–3 mm apart.
7. If necessary, tension-relieving sutures are placed around the cartilage rings cranial and caudal to the anastomosis site.
8. Skin and muscular closure is routine.

Postoperative management

Patients require close monitoring, opioid analgesia, and oxygen support on recovery from anesthesia. A surgical drain may be placed depending on the nature and timing of the tracheal lesion.

Outcome

Short-term complications include surgical site infection and air leakage from the surgical site leading to subcutaneous emphysema, pneumomediastinum, or pneumothorax.[21] Long-term stricture formation can lead to clinical signs if the majority of the tracheal lumen is obliterated. This may require intervention such as balloon dilation or repeat resection and anastomosis. The latter may result in a downward spiral, as further resection will result in less trachea to suture, and stricture formation is more likely to occur if there is tension on the anastomosis site.

Tracheal collapse

Clinical signs in patients with tracheal collapse are characterized by a honking cough and progressive dyspnea. The defect is most commonly diagnosed in the Yorkshire Terrier and in other popular miniature breeds such as the Chihuahua, Pomeranian, Toy Poodle, Shih Tzu, and Lhasa Apso, but it has been reported in cats as well. This congenital defect affects the shape of the tracheal rings, making them wider in the laterolateral direction and flattened in the dorsoventral. Over time the rings may lose their ability to remain firm, and the dorsal membrane and tracheal muscle become lax. The dynamics of the collapsing trachea can best be observed by videofluoroscopy. Tracheobronchoscopy can demonstrate how the tracheal lumen collapses and allows assessment of the severity of inflammation and the presence of concurrent bronchitis and bronchial collapse. Samples may be obtained concurrent-

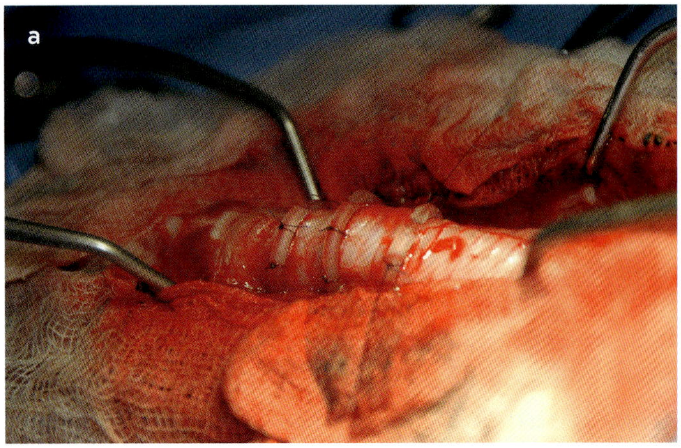

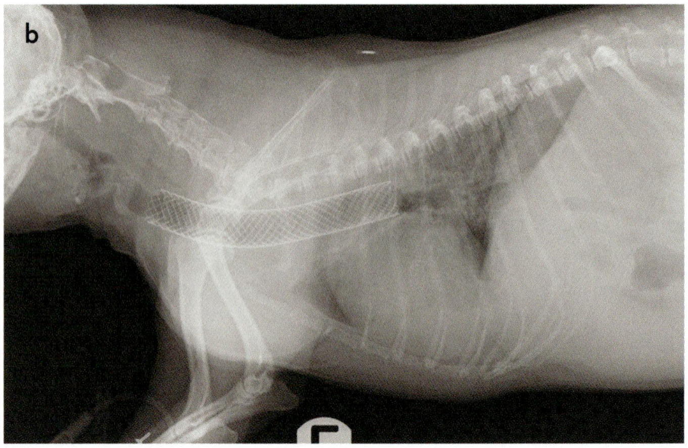

Figure 21.22 (a) Extraluminal tracheal ring prostheses in the cervical trachea. The rings were placed around the trachea with their opening on the ventral tracheal aspect and fixed in place with nonabsorbable monofilament sutures. (b) Intraluminal tracheal stenting performed under fluoroscopic guidance. Note how the stent spans the entire length of the trachea. Images courtesy of Dan Brockman and Matteo Rossanese.

ly for cytology and bacterial culture and sensitivity testing. A three-dimensional grading system has been described, where grades I to IV represent 25%, 50%, 75%, and 100% collapse, respectively.[25] Use of this grading system is only accurate when describing tracheobronchoscopic findings.

Treatment

Medical management is the mainstay of treatment and should be utilized until tracheal collapse is deemed to be life-threatening. Surgery should be reserved for cases refractory to medical management.[26] Whether extraluminal support or intraluminal stenting is pursued (Fig. 21.22), there is an approximately 40% chance of severe, possibly life-threatening, complications.[26]

Medical management

Exhausting medical management before intervention of any kind is recommended, as most dogs continue to require medications after surgery or stenting. Environmental modification and obesity management are important factors for treatment. A study described a 71% success rate with medical management for longer than 1 year in 100 cases, suggesting that intervention may be avoided altogether in selected patients.[27]

For acute exacerbation of tracheal collapse, medical management includes administration of sedatives, cough suppressants, and short-acting corticosteroids.[22] Affected animals often present in respiratory distress, and oxygen should be administered immediately. Often, mild intravenous sedation (acepromazine) can be helpful in easing respiration. Corticosteroids serve to treat airway swelling, which may be contributing to obstruction, and to reduce the inflammatory component of the disease. In the most severe, nonresponsive cases, endotracheal intubation may be necessary to secure the airway before intervention. Airway nebulization or humidification can be helpful in some dogs, and bronchodilators can be used to minimize small airway obstruction and reduce intrathoracic pressure, thereby decreasing the tendency of larger airways to collapse. If respiratory infection is suspected, a short course of antibiotics can be prescribed, with drug selection dictated by culture and sensitivity results.

For stable patients, additional measures that can be taken are control of body weight (weight loss is extremely important since it reduces the animal's oxygen demand) and the use of a harness around the chest rather than a collar or any device that restricts or compresses the neck. Smoke, dust, scented candles, carpet freshener, and any other potential irritants should be removed from the environment.

Video 21.12. Preoperative and postoperative (immediate, 24-hour, and 48-hour) evaluation of a 13-year-old Yorkshire Terrier with severe tracheal collapse (grade III–IV) who underwent tracheal stent placement. Video courtesy of Matteo Rossanese.

Tracheal stenting

Use of intraluminal stents can provide simultaneous support to the thoracic and cervical trachea while avoiding invasive procedures and potential nerve or vessel damage. The latest self-expanding stent designs are made of super elastic material, such as nitinol (an alloy of nickel and titanium). Advantages of intraluminal stenting include a shortened anesthetic time, immediate improvement in clinical signs related to tracheal collapse, and the ability to place the stent within the cervical and/or thoracic regions in a noninvasive manner.[26,28] Various stents are available, each with its own inherent strengths and weaknesses. Woven, reconstrainable, foreshortening stents are recommended. These stents are collapsed on a delivery system, can be recaptured after partial deployment (reconstrainable), and, because of their woven nature, undergo measurable shortening with placement as they reach maximum diameter (foreshortening).[22]

Measurement for stent size determination can be accomplished with radiography, fluoroscopy, tracheobronchoscopy, or a combination of these. The diameter of the trachea is measured at various levels on positive-pressure ventilation (15–20 cmH_2O), as is the length from the cricoid cartilage to the carina. A calibrated esophageal probe is used for reference. The dog is then subjected to tracheobronchoscopy to grade the degree of collapse and confirm the length of affected trachea. A stent is chosen that exceeds the widest measured diameter of the trachea on positive-pressure thoracic films by 10%–20%, or 2–3 mm.[28] It is preferable to span the entire length of the trachea, if possible, rather than simply the collapsed area, to account for the future collapse that invariably occurs.

Stent placement can be achieved with fluoroscopic guidance or direct visualization endoscopically.[28] After the procedure, the dog is recovered under direct observation in the intensive care unit, preferably in an oxygen cage (Video 21.12). Continued cough is expected after stent placement, and the patient should be discharged on antitussives, sedatives, and a tapering anti-inflammatory dose of corticosteroids. A 2-week course of antibiotics is also prescribed and should be altered based on the results of bronchoalveolar lavage sample analysis.

Repeat evaluation via physical examination and thoracic radiographs is recommended at regular intervals after stent placement. Survival to discharge is reported to be over 90%, with 95% of dogs experiencing immediate improvement in clinical signs (83%–89% of dogs for more than 1 year). Complications of endoluminal stenting are common (40%–47%) and can be severe.[26,28] Recorded complications include stent fracture, stent migration, tracheitis, collapse beyond the stented region, obstruction of the stent lumen with granulation tissue, and tracheal rupture.[26,28]

Surgical treatment

Surgery for tracheal collapse is only recommended for dogs that do not respond to medical therapy and have severe clinical signs as a result of a 50% or greater reduction of the tracheal lumen.[26,28] Generally only the cervical trachea and most proximal portion of the thoracic trachea are supported, even in cases with both cervical and thoracic tracheal collapse.[26,28] Many techniques have been reported; tracheoplasty using individual ring prostheses is described below.

Patients should be observed closely during the entire pre- and postoperative period. If necessary, they should be supported with oxygen and receive antibiotic treatment and corticosteroids.

Surgical technique

1. The animal is placed in dorsal recumbency, with the neck extended. A cervical midline approach to the trachea is performed.
2. The first tracheal prosthesis (commercial prosthetic ring or made from polypropylene syringe cases) should be placed one or two rings distal to the larynx.
3. Dissection around the trachea should only be performed in the area immediately around the trachea where the prosthetic ring is going to be placed. This is to preserve the recurrent laryngeal nerves and tracheal blood supply.
4. A tunnel is created immediately adjacent to the trachea using gentle dissection and passing of forceps. A ring is placed around the trachea with its opening on the ventral tracheal aspect.
5. The prosthetic ring is then fixed in place with non-absorbable monofilament sutures placed through the preplaced holes in the prosthesis and through the cartilage and/or dorsal tracheal membrane.
6. Four to six rings are placed this way 5–8 mm apart, with one or two rings at the thoracic inlet.
7. Closure is routine.

Survival to discharge is reported[26] to be over 90%, with an immediate improvement in clinical signs reported in the majority of dogs and 65% of patients not requiring additional medical management. Complications of extraluminal tracheal rings (35%–42%) include laryngeal paralysis, tracheal necrosis, collapse progression beyond tracheal rings, ring migration, tearing of the tracheal muscle during suture placement, and pneumomediastinum/pneumothorax.

KEEP IN MIND

- Brachycephalic breeds are at highest risk during anesthesia recovery. Close monitoring and calm recovery are vital, with extubation when fully awake. Clinicians should be ready to reintubate the dog and place a tracheostomy tube if necessary due to postoperative airway swelling (<5% of patients). Brachycephalic dogs are also highly sensitive to heat-related illness.
- Unilateral cricoid–arytenoid or thyroid–arytenoid lateralization procedures are effective in decreasing clinical signs in dogs with laryngeal paralysis. The ongoing risk of aspiration pneumonia is a long-term concern.
- Complications in patients with temporary tracheostomy tubes are common but manageable with correct intensive nursing.
- Careful owner education and patient habit adjustments are needed after permanent tracheostomy.
- Intraluminal tracheal stents provide support to the thoracic and cervical trachea while minimizing nerve or vessel damage, but complications are frequent and patients require ongoing medical management after stent placement.

References

1. Ladlow J, Liu NC, Kalmar L, Sargan D. Brachycephalic obstructive airway syndrome. *Vet Rec.* 2018; 182(13):375–378.
2. Poncet CM et al. Prevalence of gastrointestinal tract lesions in 73 brachycephalic dogs with upper respiratory syndrome. *J Small Anim Pract.* 2005; 46(6):273–279.
3. Riecks TW, Birchard SJ, Stephens JA. Surgical correction of brachycephalic syndrome in dogs: 62 cases (1991–2004). *J Am Vet Med Assoc.* 2007; 230(9):1324–1328.
4. Kaye BM, Boroffka SA, Haagsman AN, Ter Haar G. Computed tomographic, radiographic, and endoscopic tracheal dimensions in English Bulldogs with grade 1 clinical signs of brachycephalic airway syndrome. *Vet Radiol Ultrasound.* 2015; 56(6):609–616.
5. Oechtering GU. Brachycephalic syndrome—new information on an old congenital disease. *Veterinary Focus.* 2010; 20(2):2–9.
6. Fasanella FJ, Shivley JM, Wardlaw JL, Givaruangsawat S. Brachycephalic airway obstructive syndrome in dogs: 90 cases (1991–2008). *J Am Vet Med Assoc.* 2010; 237(9): 1048–1051.
7. Torrez CV, Hunt GB. Results of surgical correction of abnormalities associated with brachycephalic airway obstruction syndrome in dogs in Australia. *J Small Anim Pract.* 2006; 47(3):150–154.
8. Monnet E, Tobias KM. Larynx. In: Tobias KM, Johnston SA (eds.). *Veterinary Surgery: Small Animal.* St. Louis, MO: Elsevier Saunders; 2017. pp. 1718–1733.
9. Liu NC et al. Whole-body barometric plethysmography characterizes upper airway obstruction in 3 brachycephalic breeds of dogs. *J Vet Intern Med.* 2016; 30(3):853–865.
10. Liu NC et al. Outcomes and prognostic factors of surgical treatments for brachycephalic obstructive airway syndrome in 3 breeds. *Vet Surg.* 2017; 46(2):271–280.
11. Villedieu E, Rutherford L, Ter Haar G. Brachycephalic obstructive airway surgery outcome assessment using the 6-minute walk test: A pilot study. *J Small Anim Pract.* 2019; 60(2):132–135.
12. Ter Haar G. Throat anatomy and physiology. In: Harvey RG, Ter Haar G (eds.). *Ear, Nose and Throat Diseases of the Dog and Cat,* 1st ed. London: CRC Press; 2016. pp. 345–356.
13. Brainard BM, Hofmeister EH. Anesthesia principles and monitoring. In: Tobias KM, Johnston SA (eds.). *Veterinary Surgery: Small Animal.* St. Louis, MO: Elsevier Saunders; 2012. pp. 248–291.
14. Bishop MJ et al. Laryngeal injury in a dog model of prolonged endotracheal intubation. *Anesthesiology.* 1985; 62 (6):770–773.
15. MacPhail CM, Monnet E. Outcome of and postoperative complications in dogs undergoing surgical treatment of laryngeal paralysis: 140 cases (1985–1998). *J Am Vet Med Assoc.* 2001; 218(12):1949–1956.
16. Trinterud T, Nelissen P, White RA. Use of silicone tracheal stoma stents for temporary tracheostomy in dogs with upper airway obstruction. *J Small Anim Pract.* 2014; 55(11):551–559.
17. Nicholson I, Baines S. Complications associated with temporary tracheostomy tubes in 42 dogs (1998 to 2007). *J Small Anim Pract.* 2012; 53(2):108–114.
18. Stordalen MB, Silveira F, Fenner JVH, Demetriou JL. Outcome of temporary tracheostomy tube-placement following surgery for brachycephalic obstructive airway syndrome in 42 dogs. *J Small Anim Pract.* 2020; 61(5):292–299.
19. Occhipinti LL, Hauptman JG. Long-term outcome of permanent tracheostomies in dogs: 21 cases (2000–2012). *Can Vet J.* 2014; 55(4):357–360.
20. Grimes JA et al. Long-term outcome and risk factors associated with death or the need for revision surgery in dogs with permanent tracheostomies. *J Am Vet Med Assoc.* 2019; 254(9):1086–1093.
21. Hedlund CS. Tracheal resection and reconstruction. *Probl Vet Med.* 1991; 3(2):210–228.
22. Haynes AM, Seibert R, Sura PA. Trachea and bronchi. In: Tobias KM, Johnston SA, (eds.). *Veterinary Surgery: Small Animal.* St. Louis, MO: Elsevier Saunders; 2017. pp. 1718–1733.
23. Jordan CJ, Halfacree ZJ, Tivers MS. Airway injury associated with cervical bite wounds in dogs and cats: 56 cases. *Vet Comp Orthop Traumatol.* 2013; 26(2):89–93.
24. Lau RE, Schwartz A, Buergelt CD. Tracheal resection and anastomosis in dogs. *J Am Vet Med Assoc.* 1980; 176(2):134–139.
25. Tangner CH, Hobson HP. A retrospective study of 20 surgically managed cases of collapsed trachea. *Vet Surg.* 1982; 11(4):146–149.
26. Tinga S, Thieman Mankin KM, Peycke LE, Cohen ND. Comparison of outcome after use of extra-luminal rings and intra-luminal stents for treatment of tracheal collapse in dogs. *Vet Surg.* 2015; 44(7):858–865.
27. White RAS, Williams JM. Tracheal collapse in the dog—is there really a role for surgery? A survey of 100 cases. *J Small Anim Pract.* 1994; 35(4):191–196.
28. Weisse C. Insights in tracheobronchial stenting and a theory of bronchial compression. *J Small Anim Pract.* 2014; 55(4):181–184.

Chapter 22

Thoracic emergencies

Ben Mielke, Matteo Rossanese

The thoracic or pleural cavity is a potential space between the lungs, mediastinum, diaphragm, and thoracic wall, lined by the pleural membrane. A small volume of fluid (0.1 mL/kg in dogs, 0.3 mL/kg in cats) is normally present within the pleural cavity; this fluid lubricates the surface of the lungs to facilitate motion during breathing. Any disruption to the integrity of the chest wall can cause an increase in fluid or air accumulation in this space that can result in significant respiratory and cardiovascular consequences due to lung collapse and changes in venous return. The resultant restrictive breathing pattern, associated with the reduction in pulmonary expansion, is rapid and shallow (Video 22.1). It is important to remember that, if fluid accumulation is slow, the pleural cavity can accommodate large volumes of fluid (50–60 mL/kg in dogs, 20 mL/kg in cats) without causing signs of respiratory compromise.

In severe cases, paradoxical or discordant breathing can be present, characterized by the opposite movements of the thoracic and abdominal walls during the breathing cycle. That is, the thoracic wall contracts and the abdominal wall expands during inhalation, and the thoracic wall expands and the abdominal wall contracts during exhalation. This is often seen in case of severe pleural disease, impairment of the muscles that control thoracic wall movement, or significant thoracic injuries.

Sampling of pleural effusion via diagnostic thoracocentesis is indicated to classify the fluid (and this technique is therapeutic in patients with clinical signs of effusion or pneumothorax). This should be performed before any other diagnostic test in unstable or dyspneic patients. Fluid analysis should include cytology, nucleated and total red blood cells counts, specific gravity, aerobic and anaerobic bacterial culture, and biochemical evaluation (total protein, triglyceride, and cholesterol concentrations). Pleural fluid is generally classified into three categories (transudate, modified transudate, and exudate) based on protein concentration and cell count (Table 22.1); cell type and fluid specific gravity may also be considered. Clinically, classification includes pure transudate, serosanguineous, sanguineous (hemorrhagic), inflammatory, chylous, and neoplastic.

Video 22.1. Dog with rapid, shallow breathing associated with reduced pulmonary expansion due to pleural effusion. Oxygen flow-by is provided. Video courtesy of Stefano Cortellini.

Emergency stabilization of patients with lower airway and pleural disease

Treatment varies based on the underlying disease process, but the general emergency approach is similar in patients with lower airway or pleural space disease:

- A detailed patient history should be obtained, including information about the onset of clinical signs and preexisting medical conditions.
- The patients should be kept in a calm and cool environment, with minimal handling.
- Initial observational respiratory triage is done, including patient's posture, respiratory rate and effort, and breathing pattern. Whenever possible, a thorough physical examination is performed, including thoracic auscultation.
- Oxygen supplementation is provided at the point of triage and during handling. The method of choice

TABLE 22.1 - CLASSIFICATION AND CHARACTERISTICS OF PLEURAL EFFUSIONS

Fluid type	Total protein (g/dL)	Total nucleated cell count (cells/μL)	Specific gravity
Pure transudate	<2.5	<1500	<1.015
Modified transudate	2.5–7.5	>1500 – <7000	>1.015 – <1.025
Exudate	>3.0	>7000	>1.025

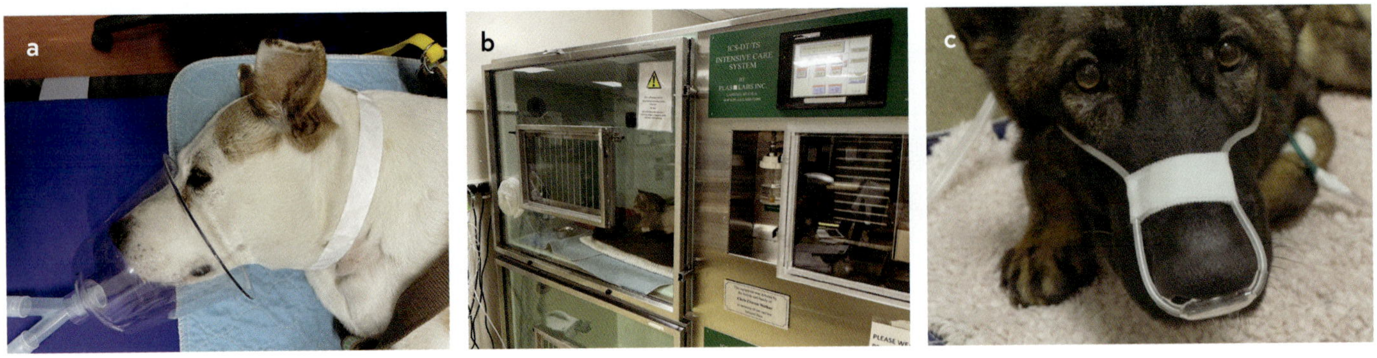

Figure 22.1 Oxygen supplementation. (a) Face mask with flow-by oxygen. (b) Oxygen cage with a cat receiving 60% oxygen. (c) Nasal prongs.

Video 22.2. Use of continuous suction thoracic drainage and oxygen supplementation with nasal prongs in a dog with spontaneous pneumothorax.

Video 22.3. Placement of a nasal cannula in a dog.

should be well tolerated by the patient (e.g., flow-by, oxygen cage, nasal prongs, nasal oxygen catheters, face masks) (Fig. 22.1; Videos 22.2 and 22.3).

- Rapid venous assessment with smooth and rapid intravenous catheterization.
- The administration of anxiolytics and sedatives is considered. These agents can be administered intramuscularly if the patient is not stable enough to sustain the stress of a catheter placement. The dosage should be chosen based on the patient status, suspected disease, present condition, and route of administration (the lower and higher dosages are more appropriate for intravenous and intramuscular injection, respectively):
    - Trazodone 3–5 mg/kg orally or rectally.
    - Acepromazine 0.005–0.02 mg/kg IV or IM.
    - Medetomidine 0.001–0.01 mg/kg IV or IM.
    - Butorphanol 0.2–0.4 mg/kg IV or IM.
- Analgesia is administered to ensure patient's comfort.
- If sedation and oxygen therapy fail to stabilize the patient, intubation is indicated with rapid induction and minimal cardiopulmonary depression. In some cases, positive-pressure ventilation is necessary for adequate respiratory stabilization.
- Point-of-care ultrasound is used to assess the presence of pulmonary changes or air or fluid in the pleural space. Thoracic radiographs or other diagnostics should be delayed until the patient is sufficiently stable.
- Thoracic drainage of air or fluid is performed by thoracocentesis. The inability to effectively evacuate the pleural space may warrant placement of a thoracostomy tube.
- Pleural fluid is submitted for analysis/cytology and aerobic and anaerobic bacterial culture.
- Assessment of the adequacy of oxygenation includes pulse oximeter and arterial blood gas sampling.
- When the patient is stable, the underlying disease can be addressed.

General techniques

Thoracocentesis (Fig. 22.2; Video 22.4)

1. The patient is placed in sternal recumbency. Oxygen is provided by flow-by, oxygen mask, or nasal prongs.
2. Sedation should be considered in stressed patients (e.g., butorphanol 0.2–0.4 mg/kg IV or IM; acepromazine 0.01–0.02 mg/kg IV or IM). Local anesthesia (e.g., lidocaine 0.25–1 mg/kg) is provided at the proposed thoracocentesis site by subcutaneous injection.
3. A wide area centered at the 7th to 9th intercostal space is clipped and aseptically prepared.
4. A 14–20-gauge needle, over-the-needle catheter, or butterfly catheter is connected to an extension set, three-way tap, and syringe.
5. Thoracocentesis is performed at the middorsal thorax between the 7th and 9th intercostal spaces. Ultrasound guidance should be used to locate the ideal area for thoracocentesis and to avoid any iatrogenic injury.
6. The needle is inserted in the middle of the intercostal space and advanced into the pleural space with its bevel perpendicular to the body wall. Slight negative pressure is applied to the syringe during insertion to confirm entry into the thorax. Needle insertion caudal to the rib should be avoided to prevent injuries to the intercostal vessels.

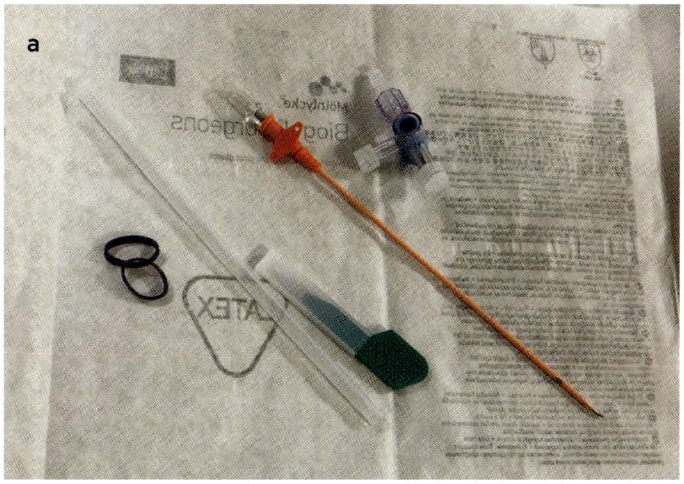

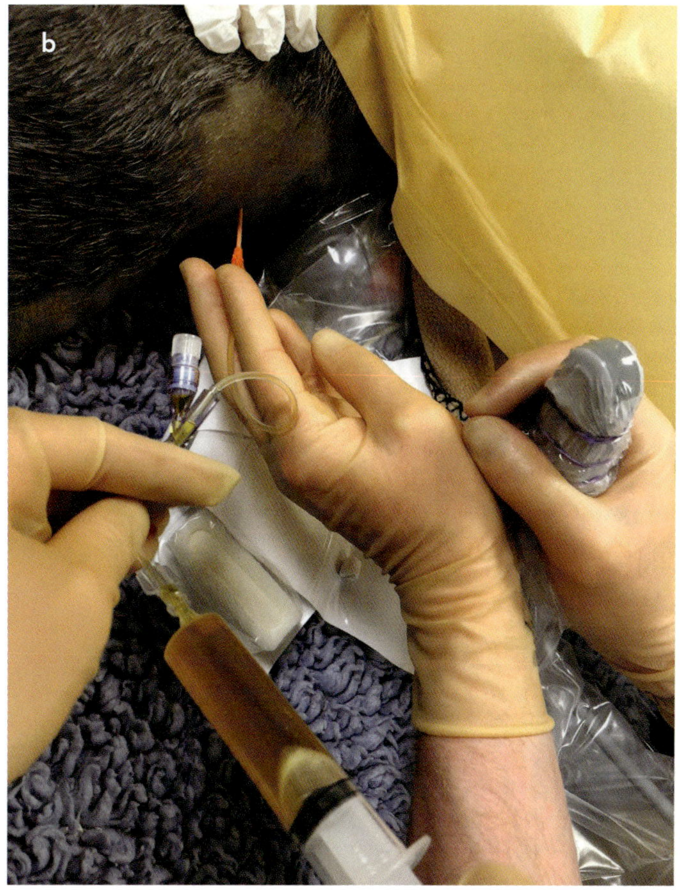

Figure 22.2 Thoracocentesis. (a) Centesis catheter. (b) The catheter was connected to a closed system and inserted at the middorsal thorax of the 7th intercostal space with the animal in sternal recumbency. Images courtesy of Simon Cook.

Video 22.4. Thoracocentesis performed in a dog using a butterfly needle connected to a closed system. Video courtesy of Simon Cook.

7. The needle is then redirected toward the inner thoracic wall at a 45-degree angle to avoid pulmonary injuries.
8. Fluid or air is slowly withdrawn until negative pressure is achieved. Ultrasound should be used to monitor the position of the needle and the reduction of fluids pockets.

Complications associated with needle thoracocentesis include lung laceration, hemorrhage, and reexpansion pulmonary edema. In case of rapid accumulation of fluid or air into the pleural cavity, placement of a thoracostomy tube should be considered (see Chapter 5). Criteria for thoracostomy tube placement can be found in Box 22.1.

Box 22.1. Criteria for placement of a thoracostomy tube

- Ineffective thoracocentesis.
- Presence of a large volume of fluid or air.
- Presence of tension pneumothorax.
- Repeated thoracic drainage required.
- Continuous or recurrent fluid or air accumulation.
- Post-thoracic surgery.
- Medical management of pyothorax.

Partial lung lobectomy

Partial lung lobectomy can be used for diagnostic biopsy or removal of localized pathology including abscesses, cysts, bullae, blebs, and lacerations.

1. This procedure can be performed through an intercostal thoracotomy, a median sternotomy, or a transdiaphragmatic approach.
2. The area to be excised is located and the lung lobe isolated with moistened swabs.
3. Two different techniques can be used for partial lung lobectomy:
   - Stapling technique (Fig. 22.3):
     a. An automatic stapling device is placed across the lobe, proximal to the lesion. The authors prefer to use a TA 30 with either a white (V3, 2.5 mm) or blue (3.5 mm) cartridge, or an Endo GIA with a purple (3.0–4.0 mm) cartridge.
     b. The device is used accordingly (see Chapter 6).
     c. The lung tissue is transected distal to the stapler with a pair of Metzenbaum scissors or a number 11 scalpel blade.
   - Suture ligation technique (Fig. 22.4):
     a. Two pairs of crushing forceps are placed across the lobe at the level of the desired transection point.

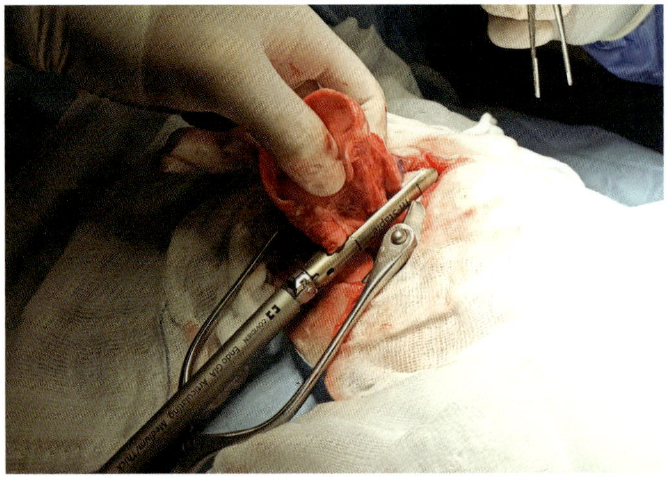

Figure 22.3 Partial lung lobectomy using an Endo GIA (45 mm length, purple cartridge) in a dog with a lung lobe abscess. Image courtesy of Filippo Cinti.

Video 22.5. After filling the thoracic cavity with sterile saline, the lung lobes are gently held below the surface of the saline while the lungs are inflated. Air bubbles can be seen, indicating an active air leak within the intrathoracic respiratory tract. Video courtesy of Karla Lee.

   b. One or two rows of a continuous overlapping hemostatic–pneumostatic suture using 3-0 or 4-0 absorbable material are placed 5–10 mm proximal to the crushing forceps.
   c. The lung tissue is transected proximal to the crushing forceps with a pair of Metzenbaum scissors or a number 11 scalpel blade.
4. Small air leaks and hemorrhages are usually self-limiting; otherwise, the surgical site can be oversewn using a simple continuous pattern of 4-0 or 5-0 absorbable or nonabsorbable monofilament material.
5. The surgical site is tested for leakage by filling the thoracic cavity with warm sterile saline and inflating the lungs (positive-pressure ventilation, maximum 12 cmH_2O in cats and 16 cmH_2O in dogs). Bubbling from the surgical site indicates air leakage (Video 22.5).

Total lung lobectomy (Video 22.6)

Total lung lobectomy can be used for removal of abscesses, cysts, bullae, blebs, lacerations, or neoplasia.
1. This procedure can be performed through an intercostal thoracotomy or a median sternotomy.
2. Moistened laparotomy swabs are used to isolate the affected lung lobe and to pack the surrounding lung lobes away.

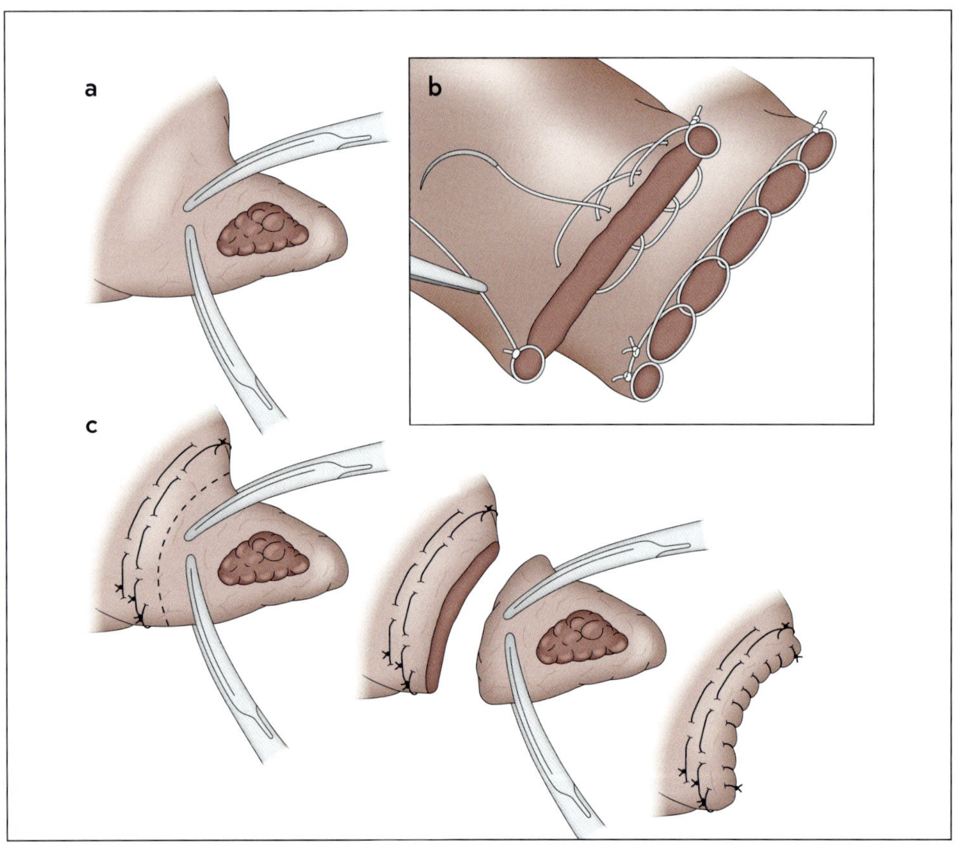

Figure 22.4 Schematic representation of partial lung lobectomy using the suture ligation technique. (a) Two pairs of crushing forceps are placed at the level of the transection point. (b) Two rows of a continuous overlapping hemostatic–pneumostatic suture are placed proximal to the crushing forceps. (c) The tissue is excised and the surgical site is oversewn.

Video 22.6. Total lung lobectomy of the right middle lobe using a TA 30V stapler in a patient with lung lobe torsion.

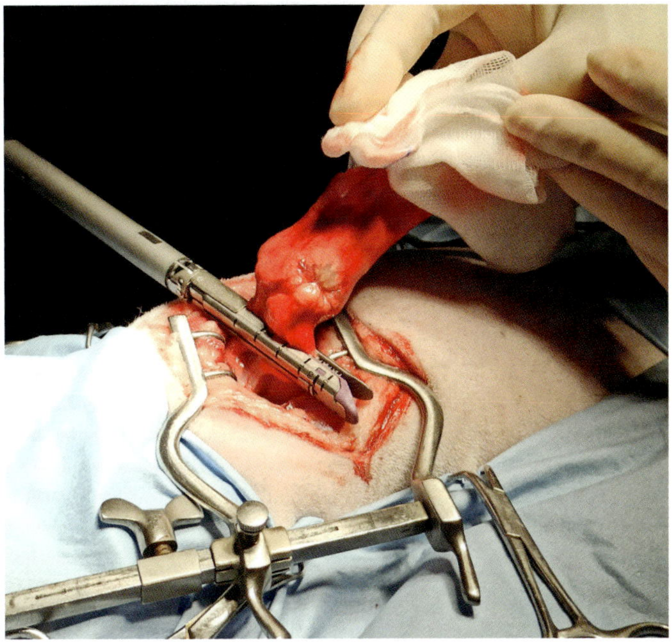

Figure 22.5 Total lung lobe lobectomy using an Endo GIA (45 mm length, purple cartridge) in a cat with pulmonary neoplasia. Image courtesy of Filippo Cinti.

3. To isolate the caudal lung lobes, the pulmonary ligament extending from the caudal edge of the pleura of the hilus to the mediastinal pleura is transected. This can be performed by using Metzenbaum scissors or a diathermy device.
4. The pulmonary vessels and lobar bronchus are identified and isolated.
5. Two different techniques can be used for total lung lobectomy:
   - Stapling technique (Fig. 22.5):
     a. An automatic stapling device (TA V3 white cartridge, TA 30 blue cartridge, or Endo GIA 45/60 mm purple medium/thick) is placed across the hilus or pedicle.
     b. The device is used accordingly (see Chapter 6).
     c. The lung lobe is transected distal to the stapler with a pair of Metzenbaum scissors or a number 11 scalpel blade.
   - Suture ligation technique (Fig. 22.6):
     a. The pulmonary artery is isolated by blunt dissection and triple ligated (two encircling proximally and distally and one transfixing in between) using 3-0 or 4-0 absorbable or nonabsorbable monofilament suture material. The artery is then transected between the two distal sutures (transfixing and encircling).
     b. The pulmonary vein (caudal to the bronchus) is bluntly dissected and double ligated using two encircling ligatures with 3-0 or 4-0

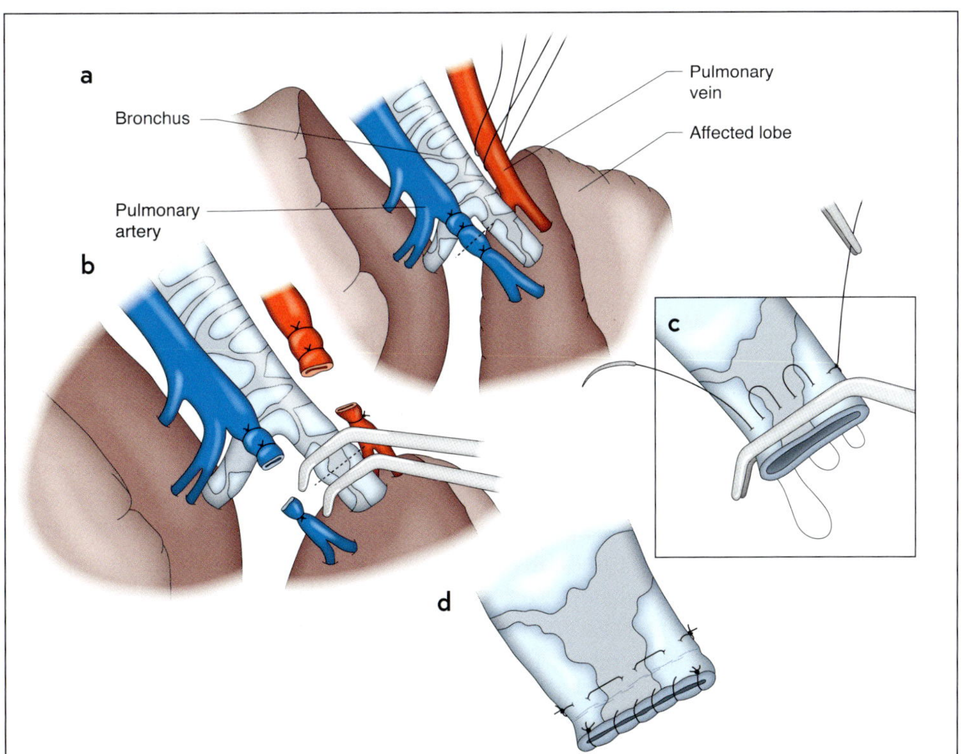

Figure 22.6 Schematic representation of total lung lobectomy using the suture ligation technique. (a) Encircling ligatures (two proximally and one distally) are placed in the pulmonary artery and vein. (b) The pulmonary artery and vein are transected, and the main bronchus is cross-clamped with two pairs of noncrushing forceps. (c) The main bronchus is transected and collapsed using interrupted horizontal mattress sutures. (d) The distal edge of the bronchus is oversewn.

absorbable or nonabsorbable monofilament suture material. The vein is then transected between the two ligatures.
c. The main bronchus is bluntly dissected, cross-clamped with two pairs of noncrushing forceps, and transected. The lung lobe is then removed.
d. The pedicle is cross-clamped with two pairs of noncrushing forceps at the level of the desired transection point.
e. The bronchus is collapsed with 3-0 to 4-0 absorbable or nonabsorbable monofilament suture material in an interrupted horizontal mattress pattern.
f. The distal edge of the bronchus is oversewn with 3-0 to 4-0 absorbable or nonabsorbable monofilament suture material in a simple continuous pattern.

6. The pedicle is released and inspected for bleeding or air leakage. Little bleeding or air leakage should seal spontaneously; otherwise, a suture can be placed (4-0 or 5-0 absorbable or nonabsorbable material) in a simple interrupted, cruciate mattress, or horizontal mattress pattern.
7. To detect air leaks, the thoracic cavity is filled with warm sterile saline while the ventilatory pressure is increased to about 20–25 cmH_2O (Video 22.5).
8. Before closure, a thoracostomy tube should be placed (see Chapter 5).

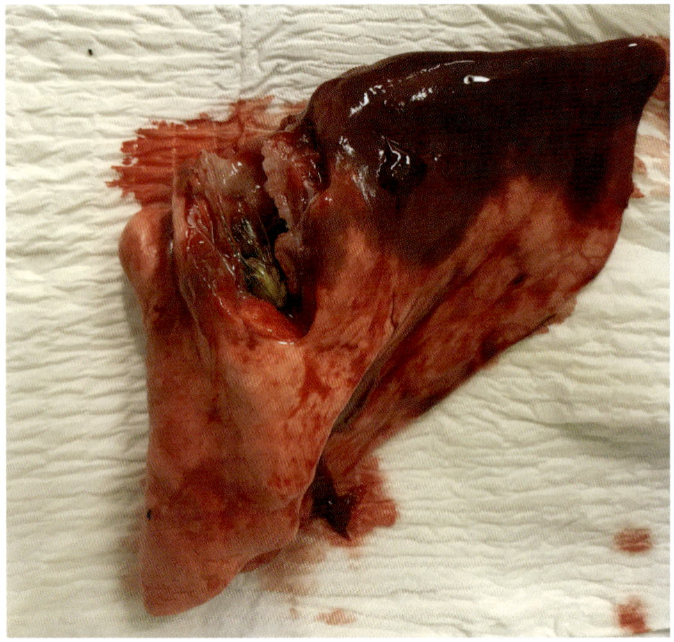

Figure 22.7 Grass awn in the main stem bronchus in a dog extracted via median sternotomy and lung lobectomy.

Pyothorax

Pyothorax, also known as thoracic or pleural empyema, is characterized by the accumulation of purulent fluid (exudate) within the pleural space. No data exist on the incidence of this disease in dogs and cats. The most common underlying cause is an infectious agent, such as bacteria (e.g., *Mycoplasma* spp.) or fungi, but identification of an underlying cause is reported in only 2%–22% of dogs and 35%–67% of cats.[1–3] Although the route of infection often remains unknown, the most frequent route in dogs is a migrating foreign body, such as plant material. A grass awn can enter the mouth or nose, migrate through the respiratory tract and lungs (Fig. 22.7), and penetrate into the pleural space or progress through the diaphragm and lodge into the sublumbar muscles. As this grass awn can carry oral bacteria into the lower respiratory tract, infection can occur.

Other reported causes of pyothorax in dogs derive from extension from adjacent structures (e.g., bronchopneumonia, esophageal perforation, mediastinitis, discospondylitis, thoracic neoplasia with abscessation), hematogenous spread, or direct inoculation (e.g., trauma, foreign bodies, parasitic migration, bite wounds, iatrogenic—from thoracocentesis, thoracostomy tube placement, or recent thoracic surgery). In cats, parapneumonic spread or bacteria inoculation by bite wounds is believed to be implicated. Other causes of pyothorax in cats are foreign body migration, hematogenous, or penetrating thoracic wounds. Pyothorax as a postoperative complication is reported in 6.5% of dogs undergoing thoracic surgery.[3] No clear breed predisposition has been identified, but hunting breed dogs and domestic shorthair and longhair cats are frequently reported. Young dogs (<5 years) and cats (4–6 years) are commonly affected.[5–7]

Clinical presentation and diagnosis

Clinical signs are commonly respiratory in nature, with a restrictive breathing pattern, dyspnea, and tachypnea being common. Other nonspecific clinical signs include lethargy, anorexia, cough, and pyrexia. Sepsis is also a common presentation in cats with underlying pyothorax. On physical examination, abnormalities on thoracic auscultation can be present, such as absence or reduction in normal lung sounds and muffled heart sounds. Evidence of thoracic trauma or wound should be ruled out. Animals are rarely examined during the acute phase of infection, and clinical signs are typically the result of chronic disease.

Diagnosis of pyothorax is based on a combination of thoracic imaging and pleural fluid analysis (cytological examination and fungal, aerobic, and anaerobic bacterial cultures). Pleural fluid can appear grossly turbid to opaque with flocculent material; a malodorous smell can also be present. Fluid analysis typically reveals an exudate (neutrophilic inflammation) with extra- or intracellular bacteria. Mixed bacterial populations (obligate anaerobes with or without facultative aerobic bacteria) are common, and identification of long filamentous bacteria, suggestive of *Actinomyces* or *Nocardia* species, has been linked to grass awn migration. If the patient has already received antibiotic therapy, bacteria may not be identified. Aerobic and anaerobic cultures typically reveal mixed populations, with *Pasteurella* spp., *Escherichia coli*, *Enterobacteriaceae*, anaerobes, and *Actinomyces*/*Nocardia* spp. being common in dogs and *Clostridium* spp. and *Pasteurella* spp. being frequent in cats. Hematology and serum biochemistry could reveal anemia, an inflammatory leukogram with a left shift or toxic neutrophils, and abnormalities compatible with organ dysfunction and systemic inflammatory response syndrome.

Thoracic imaging can include radiographs, ultrasound, or, preferably, computed tomography (CT). In patients with respiratory distress due to the volume of effusion, thoracocentesis should be considered before diagnostic imaging. Thoracic imaging aims to detect the cause of pyothorax. Foreign bodies, soft tissue tracts, or thoracic wall lesions can be detected. However, findings are often vague, including pleural thickening with associated effusion, pneumothorax, or regional lymphadenopathy or lymphadenomegaly. Thoracic radiographs could demonstrate interstitial to alveolar opacity and signs of pleural effusion such as interlobar fissure lines, loss of cardiac silhouette, and retraction of lung borders from the thoracic wall. Causes of pyothorax like focal pulmonary opacity, foreign bodies, or mass lesions can be detected. CT will show the abovementioned abnormalities more accurately and detect paths of migrating foreign bodies. Thoracic ultrasonography is an easy test to document pleural effusion and assist during fluid sampling. With pyothorax, fluid is echogenic and contains fibrin strands. Foreign bodies and abscessations can also be detected with ultrasonography.

Treatment

Clear treatment guidelines are available for the management of this condition in humans, but similar guidelines have not been established in dogs and cats.[4] Initial patient stabilization with oxygen supplementation, intravenous fluid therapy, and thoracocentesis is often necessary. Pyothorax can be treated medically or surgically. Medical management, typically used in cats, involves appropriate antimicrobial therapy, pleural drainage, and lavage through bilateral thoracostomy tube placement.

Surgical management is typically used in dogs or in animals in which a primary cause is identified, medical management fails, or pleural effusion persists beyond 3–7 days. It is important to note that in case of evidence of pulmonary or mediastinal abscessation or foreign body migration, surgery is advisable. Exploratory thoracotomy should be performed through a median sternotomy, as pyothorax is usually evident bilaterally, and simultaneous exposure of both pleural cavities may be preferable. Surgery involves drainage of the purulent material, removal of the primary cause, breakdown of any adhesions causing fluid pocketing, and appropriate antimicrobial therapy. It should be noted that currently there is no consensus on the appropriate therapy of canine pyothorax.

Technique: Thoracic lavage

1. The thoracic cavity should be completely drained through the thoracostomy tubes (see Chapter 5 for a description of thoracostomy tube placement).
2. Pleural lavage is started by slowly infusing warm sterile isotonic crystalloid fluids at an initial dose of 10–20 mL/kg every 6–8 hours. The solution is left in situ for 15–30 minutes and retrieved.
3. If well tolerated, for the following lavages, the fluid is infused at 20 mL/kg and left in situ for 60 minutes.
4. After instillation, the patient should be allowed to move around so that the fluid lavages the entire cavity.
5. It is important to calculate the amount of fluid instilled and retrieved. If less fluid is retrieved than was infused, tube complications, hypovolemia, and dehydration should be investigated.

Surgical technique (Figs. 22.8–22.10; Video 22.7)

1. A median sternotomy is performed (see Chapter 4).
2. Invasive positive-pressure ventilation is essential and can be performed manually or using a mechanical ventilator.

Video 22.7. Surgical management of pyothorax in a dog. After median sternotomy, the mediastinal attachments to the sternum are excised to improve visualization and allow placement of a retractor, and the pleural cavity is drained. The cranial and caudal mediastinum is debrided (mediastinectomy) with a vessel-sealing device, and all the lung lobes are carefully examined. The thoracic cavity is then copiously lavaged.

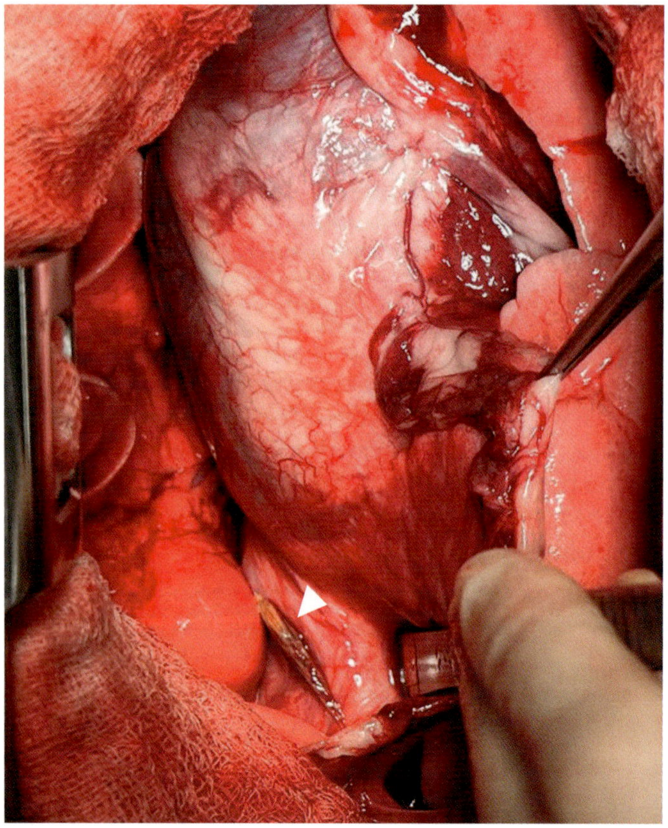

Figure 22.8 Mediastinectomy after median sternotomy in a dog with pyothorax. A foreign body (grass awn) was found within the thoracic cavity (arrowhead).

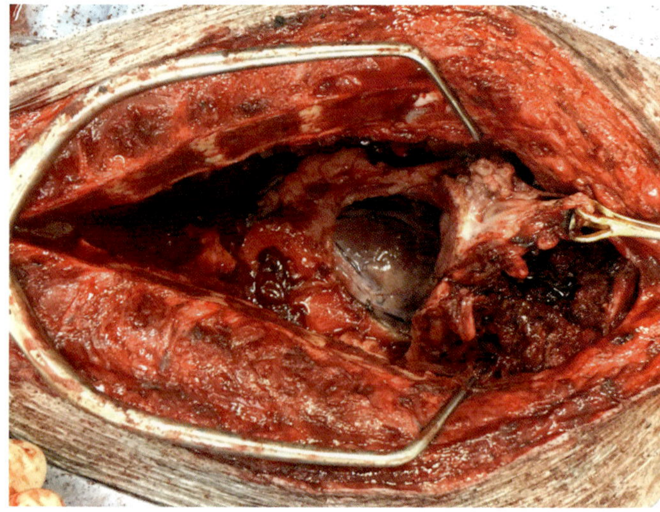

Figure 22.9 Mediastinectomy in a dog with a caudal mediastinum abscess. Pericardiectomy and partial excision of the diaphragm were also performed due to the severe adhesion to the mediastinum.

3. The mediastinal attachments to the sternum should be removed to improve exposure.
4. Finochietto retractors are placed to allow visualization of intrathoracic structures.
5. Ligation/cauterization of the internal thoracic artery and vein may be required to access the cranial thoracic cavity.

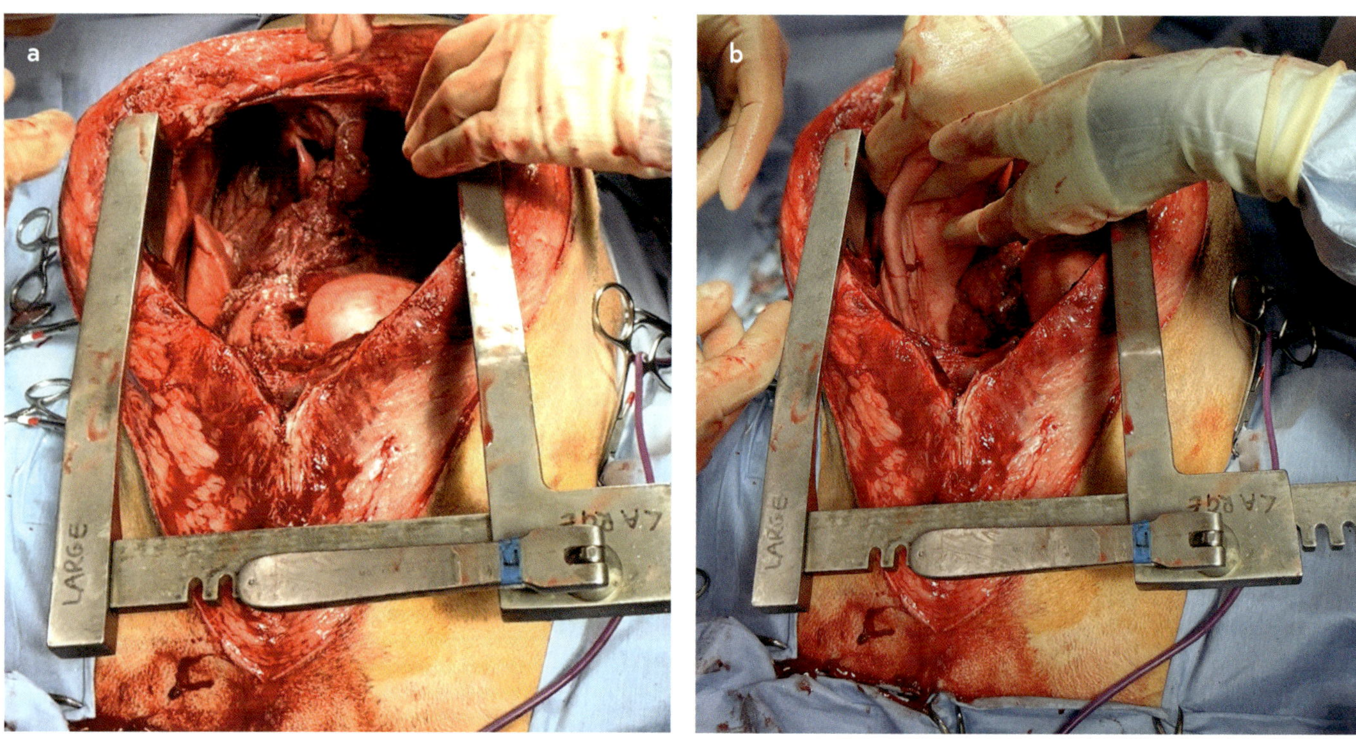

Figure 22.10 Exploratory thoracotomy in a dog with pyothorax. (a) Note the inflamed and thick caudal mediastinum and pericardium covering and collapsing the caudal lung lobes. (b) After mediastinectomy, all the surfaces of the lung lobes are evaluated.

6. Complete debridement of the cranial and caudal mediastinum (mediastinectomy) using a vessel-sealing device is required for accurate exploration. This should be submitted for histopathologic examination and culture and sensitivity testing. Note that, since the mediastinum is continuous with the pericardium, pericardiectomy may be required in some instances.
7. Every lung lobe should be carefully examined, including the accessory lung lobe located dorsal to the caudal vena cava and medial to the plica vena cava.
8. If a lesion is found in a lung lobe or a lobe fails to inflate, lung lobectomy should be performed using a TA 30V stapler. Any other intrathoracic lesions should be resected.
9. In chronic cases, mature adhesions can be present between the lung lobes and between the lung lobes and the pleura/thoracic wall. Careful dissection is needed, as the lung lobe can be easily damaged, in which case lobectomy is required.
10. The pleural surface of the diaphragm is evaluated. A large malleable retractor is used on the diaphragm to indirectly push the abdominal organs, especially the liver, caudally and allow evaluation of the most dorsocaudal aspect of the pleural cavity.
11. Unilateral or bilateral thoracostomy tube placement is performed. If thick purulent material is present, large-bore tubes are preferable.
12. The thoracic cavity should be thoroughly lavaged with warm saline until the fluid is clear in appearance.
13. In case of lung lobectomy, the surgical site is checked for air leakage and bleeding by filling the thoracic cavity with warm sterile saline and providing positive-pressure ventilation. Bubbling from the surgical site indicates air leakage.
14. Sternotomy closure is routine (see Chapter 4).

Postoperative management

Following sternotomy, the patient should be closely monitored for signs of pain, alteration in ventilation, ongoing pleural effusion, and residual pneumothorax. Vital parameters, including heart rate, blood pressure, respiratory pattern, and temperature, as well as urine production and electrolytes must be checked for the first 24–48 hours. Mechanical ventilation should be continued if necessary. Oxygen supplementation should be given to patients with oxygen saturation below 95%. The thoracostomy tube may be used to administer local anesthesia (bupivacaine 0.5%, up to 1.5 mg/kg) whilst it remains in place. Instillation of bupivacaine is painful and the animal could react; therefore, diluting the bupivacaine with sterile saline (50:50) is suggested. The local anesthetic is distributed by gravity and provides analgesia for up to 12 hours. This dose has minimal cardiovascular effects and can be used safely even in patients that have undergone pericardiectomy.

Removal of the thoracostomy tube should be considered when fluid production decreases (<2–3 mL/kg/day) and fluid appearance is serosanguineous. Clinical improvement should be noted. Cytological fluid analysis should demonstrate senile and nondegenerate neutrophils with no toxic changes, and no bacteria should be detected. Median duration of the thoracostomy tube is 5–8 days in patients undergoing medical management. Antibiotics should be administered intravenously and continued orally for a minimum of 6–8 weeks based on culture and sensitivity testing results. Mean duration of ongoing antibiotic therapy is 4–6 weeks.

Exercise should be restricted for at least 2 weeks after surgery, with 10–15-minute slow on-leash walks allowed 2–3 times daily. Exercise can be gradually increased after the first 2 weeks. The surgical site should be rechecked 10–14 days postoperatively.

Outcome

Complications may include thoracostomy tube complications, abdominal effusion, disseminated intravascular coagulopathy, and death. The recurrence rate in dogs and cats ranges from 0% to 14%, with a median disease-free interval of 50 and above 400 days in dogs treated medically and surgically, respectively. The prognosis for canine and feline pyothorax can be good with appropriate treatment. The overall survival rate for dogs and cats with pyothorax is 83% (range, 29%–100%) and 62% (range, 8%–100%), respectively.[5–11] In dogs, differences in survival among treatments have been reported, including 29% for dogs undergoing thoracocentesis only, 77% for dogs undergoing pleural lavage and drainage and antibiotic therapy, and 92% for dogs undergoing surgical management.[1,2,5,12,13] A high mortality rate (67%) has been reported in dogs developing pyothorax as a complication after thoracic surgery.[8] There is currently no evidence regarding characteristics that can predict patient outcome or long-term survival at initial presentation; however, recurrence in dogs has been associated with a high mortality rate. Early diagnosis and intervention are essential to improve the chance of successful outcome in dogs and cats with pyothorax.

Pneumothorax

Pneumothorax is a potentially life-threatening condition characterized by the presence of air within the pleural space, requiring prompt recognition and treatment. Air can enter the pleural space from various sources, including the airways (trachea, bronchi, lungs), esophagus, or thoracic wall. Pneumothorax impairs both ventilation and oxygenation, leading to increased intrathoracic pressure and lung collapse. This results in a significant decrease in tidal volume, ventilation/perfusion mismatch, and hypoxemia, followed by decreased venous return and cardiac output and subsequent tachypnea, tachycardia, shock, and death. Tension pneumothorax is a severe form of pneumothorax that occurs when a one-way valve effect allows air to enter the pleural space without possibility to escape, causing increased intrapleural pressure.

This condition is primarily classified based on etiology as acquired or spontaneous. Acquired pneumothorax can occur secondary to trauma (e.g., blunt force trauma, penetrating trauma) or be iatrogenic (e.g., thoracocentesis, thoracostomy tube placement, thoracic surgery, bronchoscopy/esophagoscopy, nasogastric tube placement, mechanical ventilation, tracheal intubation) (Figs. 22.11 and 22.12).

The most common cause of pneumothorax is leakage from thoracic wall penetration by blunt thoracic trauma; however, penetrating trauma (e.g., dog bites, gunshots, arrows, porcupine quills, stab wound, foreign body penetration) has been reported.[14–17] Traumatic pneumothorax can be classified as either open or closed. Open pneumothorax occurs when the pleural space communicates directly with the atmosphere. Some penetrating injuries are called "sucking chest wound" due to a large defect in the thoracic wall that allows air to enter the pleural cavity during breathing, collapsing the lungs and reducing ventilation.

Spontaneous pneumothorax is diagnosed in the absence of a traumatic or iatrogenic cause. This condition is relatively rare and may occur without (primary) or with (secondary) pulmonary disease. Primary spontaneous pneumothorax is caused by the rupture of pulmonary blebs or bullae and is the most common cause of spontaneous pneumothorax in dogs (36%–68% of cases), while it has not been reported in cats.[14–20] It is most frequently diagnosed in healthy, young to middle-aged, large-breed or deep-chested dogs with no underlying pulmonary disease, and Siberian Huskies are overrepresented, but it can occur in any breed and at any age. Blebs and bullae usually appear on the edges of the lung parenchyma, and the exact reason for development is not completely understood. Blebs form when air becomes trapped between the internal and external layers of the pulmonary visceral pleura (Fig. 22.13). Bullae are subpleural air-filled spaces arising following destruction, dilation, and confluence of adjacent alveoli within the lung parenchyma and can vary substantially in size (Fig. 22.14). Both conditions produce the same clinical signs, and distinguishing between them may not be clinically relevant.

Secondary spontaneous pneumothorax has been observed in case of pulmonary neoplasia (11% of dogs and 14% of cats), pleuritis, secondary to migrating grass

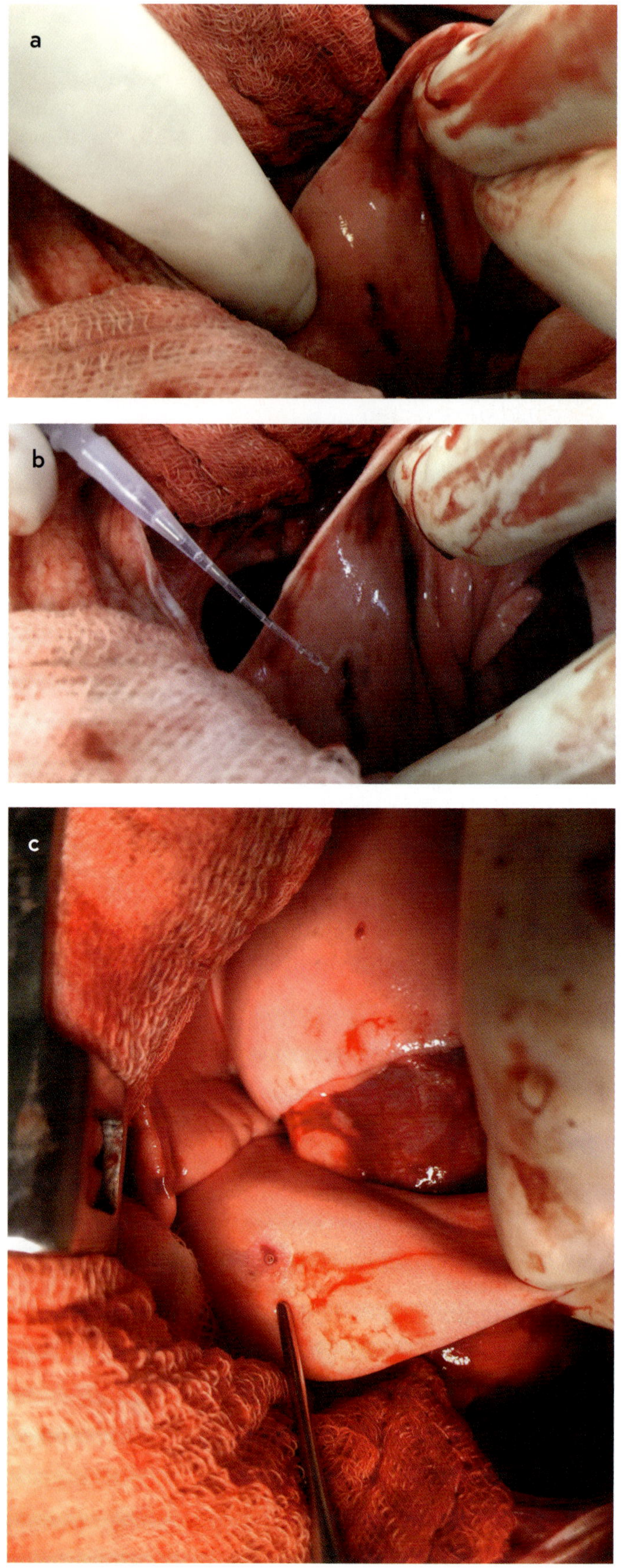

Figure 22.11 (a) Superficial laceration in a lung lobe causing pneumothorax. (b) Sealing of the laceration using cyanoacrylate. (c) Evidence of the seal. The lung lobe was therefore preserved.

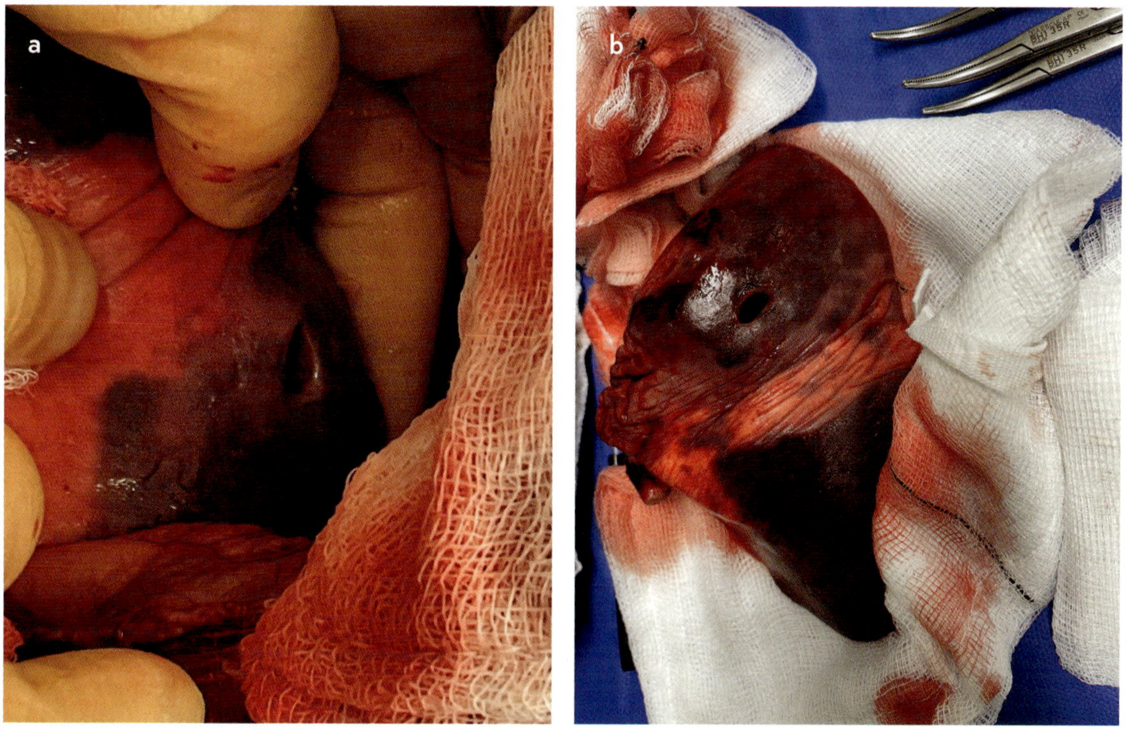

Figure 22.12 Deep pulmonary laceration. Lung lobectomy was needed.

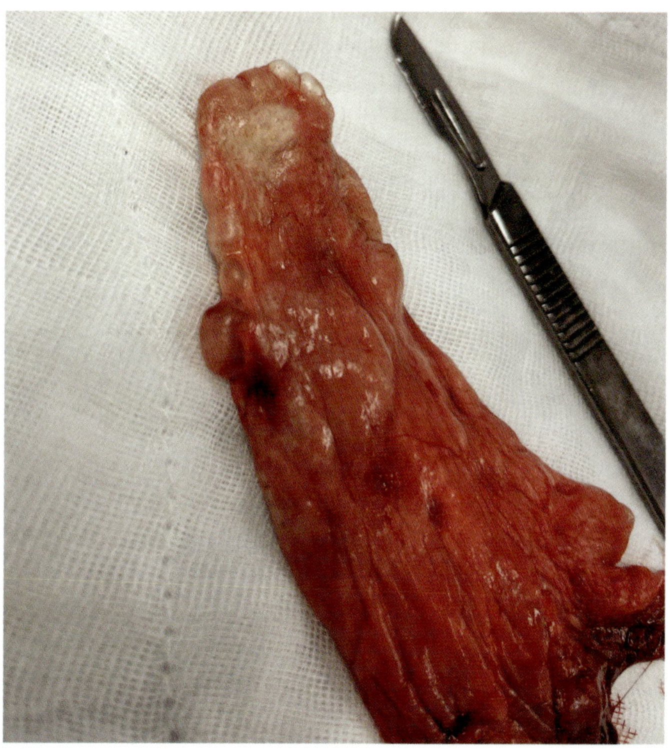

Figure 22.13 Typical appearance of pulmonary blebs at the tip of a lung following lung lobectomy in a dog with spontaneous pneumothorax.

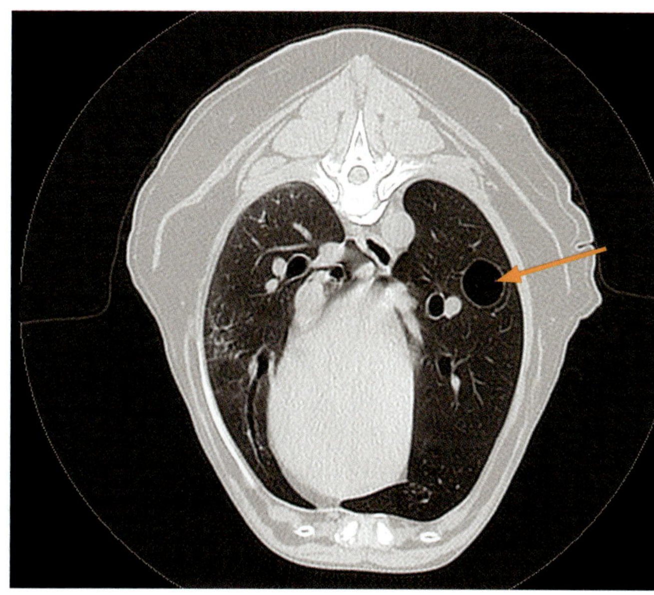

Figure 22.14 Transverse thoracic computed tomography image of a dog with pulmonary bullae (arrow). This is a common incidental finding on computed tomography.

awns, and, most common in cats, secondary to feline asthma or inflammatory airway disease. A typical signalment has not been reported, but this is the only type that has been described in cats.[14–17]

Clinical presentation and diagnosis

Prompt diagnosis and appropriate management are crucial to ensure optimal outcomes for affected patients. Based on the severity and duration of pneumothorax, animals show varying degrees of respiratory difficulty or distress. Patients commonly present with a restrictive breathing pattern (increased respiratory rate and shallow inspirations) often accompanied by a paradoxical

abdominal motion (thorax and abdomen moving in opposite directions) suggestive of pleural space disease.
On clinical assessment, animals may show signs of outward trauma, paradoxical movement of the chest wall, increased abdominal effort, or open-mouthed breathing. Decreased lung sounds are present dorsally, and percussion of the thorax reveals increased resonance, with tympanic sounds in case of tension pneumothorax. Tachycardia can be present as a compensatory mechanism due to reduced venous return to the heart and subsequently diminished cardiac output. Tension pneumothorax should be suspected in animals that appear "air hungry", tachycardic, tachypneic, and, in severe cases, cyanotic. Intrapleural volumes of air up to 45 mL/kg cause no clinical signs in healthy dogs and reabsorb spontaneously in approximately 2 weeks.
Investigations should be performed with caution in patients in respiratory distress, as their condition can rapidly deteriorate due to the stress associated with restraint and positioning. Animals should be initially stabilized. Sedation can be provided using low doses of acepromazine and/or butorphanol to reduce stress while avoiding respiratory depression. Oxygen supplementation can be provided via an oxygen cage, mask, or by flow-by. Pulse oximetry is used to verify the need of oxygen (oxygen saturation <95%). Thoracocentesis should be performed in dyspneic patients suspected of having pneumothorax. Open chest wounds should be covered immediately with an occlusive sterile dressing and wound debridement and closure delayed until the patient is stable.
Diagnosis is based on thoracic radiography. The ideal projection is somewhat controversial; however, in general, pneumothorax is more apparent in lateral thoracic projections. Common radiographic findings in animals with pneumothorax are reported in Box 22.2. Radiographic findings in case of tension pneumothorax include severe pulmonary atelectasis, flattening or tenting of the diaphragm, and barrel-shaped thorax on dorsoventral projections. Pneumomediastinum is present in animals with tracheal and/or esophageal tears.

Box 22.2. Radiographic signs of pneumothorax in dogs and cats

- Retraction of the lungs from the thoracic wall, with focal or generalized interposed radiolucency.
- Dorsal displacement of the cardiac silhouette (lateral projections).*
- Increased opacity and diffuse interstitial pattern of atelectatic lung lobes.
- Mediastinal shift (unilateral pneumothorax).

*Elevation of the cardiac silhouette may also be present in case of microcardia, fat accumulation, or overinflation of lungs in deep-chested dogs.

Although thoracic radiographs are very helpful for the identification of pneumothorax, they are poor at identifying the underlying cause, particularly in the case of pulmonary bullae or blebs. If an underlying cause is not detected on thoracic radiographs, the cause is highly likely to be blebs or bullae.
In patients with respiratory compromise, ultrasound can be performed in sternal recumbency or with the animal standing.[21,22] Serial examination can identify pneumothorax progression and help with the decision for intervention. Ultrasound findings in patients with pneumothorax include the absence of a glide sign (rhythmic sliding of hyperechoic lines between visceral and pleural surfaces) and an abnormal curtain sign (vertical edge separating the lungs from the abdominal contents).[21,22]
CT is considered the gold standard for diagnosis of pneumothorax because of its ability to detect small volumes of air that could be missed on radiographs. It is frequently used for the detection of the underlying cause and for surgical planning.[23–25] However, it is often performed after the diagnosis of pneumothorax and with the patient adequately stabilized. Prior to a CT scan, free air should be evacuated (via thoracocentesis or a thoracostomy tube) and the lungs expanded to improve the detection of any underlying pulmonary cause (Fig. 22.15).
The sensitivity of CT for detection of pulmonary bullae is low (42%–57%). Acquiring images with the patient in sternal and dorsal recumbency may improve identification of blebs and bullae.[23–25] Other causes of pneumothorax (e.g., neoplasia, migrating foreign bodies) are readily identified, hence CT is still recommended. In

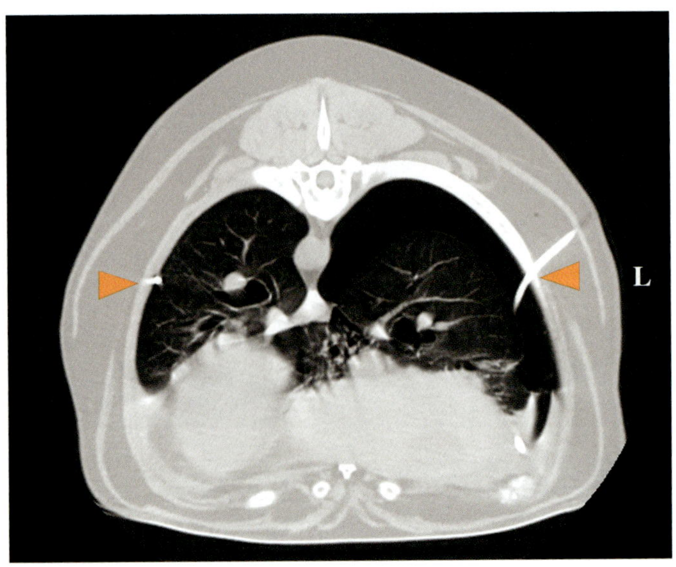

Figure 22.15 Transverse thoracic computed tomography image of a dog with spontaneous pneumothorax secondary to ruptured pulmonary blebs. Bilateral Mila chest drains (arrowheads) were placed to stabilize the patient prior to investigation. Note the residual pneumothorax on the left side of the thorax.

animals with traumatic pneumothorax, it is important to look for any concurrent injuries (e.g., fractured ribs, pulmonary contusions, pleural effusion). In case of lung pathology, a definitive diagnosis should be obtained to guide treatment.

In the absence of a nonsurgical disease (e.g., pneumonia, pulmonary metastatic disease), exploratory thoracotomy through median sternotomy should be performed regardless of the imaging results.

Treatment

Effective management of pneumothorax requires accurate diagnosis, prompt intervention, and appropriate treatment of any underlying cause. The aim is to relieve respiratory distress, restore lung function, and optimize the patient's cardiovascular status.

Patient stabilization should be performed with thoracocentesis following diagnosis of pneumothorax or if there is a clinical suspicion in an animal showing signs of respiratory difficulty. Specific treatment depends on the source of the pneumothorax: open thoracic wounds should be immediately covered and definitive closure pursued once the patient is stable; minor external wounds, blunt trauma, or lung injury due to thoracocentesis or thoracostomy tube placement can be treated conservatively, but close monitoring is mandatory.

If ventilation is severely impaired, immediate intubation and manual ventilation is required. Care should be taken to assess for the presence of tension pneumothorax prior to ventilation, as this may exacerbate underlying cardiorespiratory compromise. In these situations, placement of a thoracostomy tube is strongly recommended to remove air and reestablish negative pressure in the pleural space.

Thoracocentesis is used in case of large accumulations of air or if the animal shows clinical signs. Thoracostomy tubes allow for ongoing drainage without subsequent trauma and patient discomfort associated with thoracocentesis. These tubes are placed in case of tension pneumothorax, rapid and continuous accumulation of air, need to drain the chest more than twice in 24 hours, and after any thoracic surgery (see Chapter 5 for a description of thoracostomy tube placement). Thoracostomy tube drainage can be intermittent or continuous. Intermittent drainage of the thorax by manual syringe aspiration should be performed every 1–6 hours based on the rate of air accumulation. Continuous drainage can be used in animals with severe fluid accumulation or when negative pressure cannot be achieved. This allows for better ventilation and healing of small leaks by enabling pleural adhesion formation. However, the specific equipment and close patient monitoring required makes this rarely practical in general practice settings. The use of a three-chambered water seal suction apparatus is thus recommended, which relies on a water seal between the suction pump and the thoracostomy tube to avoid air entry into the thorax. Active drainage should be maintained at 5–10 cmH_2O. Continuous suction may be required for several days (Fig. 22.16).

Strict conservative management of spontaneous pneumothorax in dogs is often unsuccessful, and surgical exploration of the thorax is indicated in animals with continued air accumulation for more than 2–5 days or if the cause is identified (e.g., pulmonary abscess or foreign body, bullae, blebs, esophageal foreign body, pulmonary mass). Closed traumatic pneumothorax with no evidence of esophageal or airway perforation is often self-limiting, and conservative management successful.

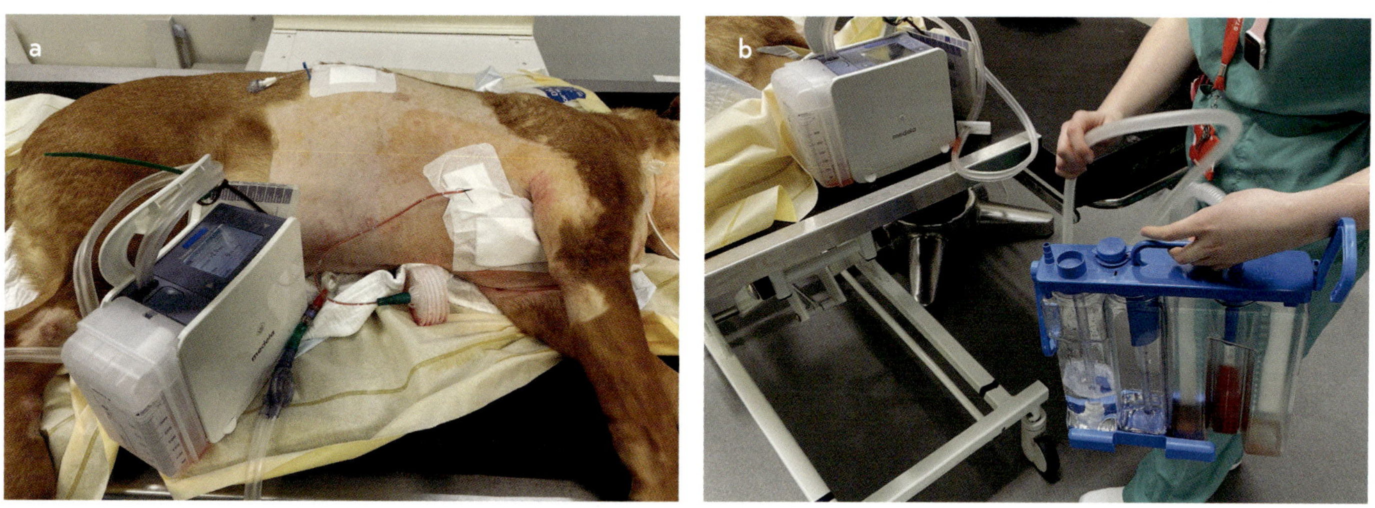

Figure 22.16 (a) Digital chest drainage and monitoring system (Thopaz+) allowing continuous thoracic drainage and monitoring of fluid drainage, air leak, and pressure. (b) Three-chambered chest drainage unit (Thora-Seal) with a water seal chamber and a separate fluid collection chamber.

Large airway lesions may fail to heal spontaneously and require surgical intervention.

The surgical approach is based on the cause of pneumothorax. When the cause has been identified, an intercostal thoracotomy can be performed. However, in cases of primary spontaneous pneumothorax, a median sternotomy is recommended to access both sides of the thorax and has been associated with an improved ability to identify all lesions and low rates of recurrence (13%).[16–18]

In cats, pneumothorax is typically considered a medical condition. Cats tend to develop pneumothorax secondary to extensive or generalized lung pathology, with feline allergic airway disease or asthma often implicated (25% of cases).[15,20,26] Other underlying conditions include pulmonary neoplasia, heartworm infection, pulmonary abscess, or lungworm infection.[26] This condition is managed supportively with oxygen therapy, antibiotics, bronchodilators or steroids, thoracocentesis or thoracostomy tube placement, and/or pleurodesis. High-rise syndrome (falling from height) may also result in development of pneumothorax. This condition is again usually managed supportively unless severe trauma necessitates surgical exploration or fracture stabilization.

Surgical technique: Spontaneous pneumothorax management

1. A median sternotomy is performed (see Chapter 4).
2. Invasive positive-pressure ventilation is essential and can be performed manually or using a mechanical ventilator.
3. The mediastinal attachments to the sternum should be removed to improve exposure.
4. Finochietto retractors are placed to allow visualization of intrathoracic structures.
5. All the surfaces of each lung lobe should be carefully examined.
6. If a primary lesion cannot be identified, the thoracic cavity is filled with warm sterile saline and positive-pressure ventilation (maximum 12 cmH_2O in cats and 16 cm H_2O in dogs) is provided to inflate the lungs, to identify bubbling from the affected lung lobe. Particular attention should be paid to the left and right cranial lung lobes, as 56% of bullae are located in these lobes.[19] Multiple lesions are also a very common finding.[25]
7. Once the lesion has been identified, partial or total lung lobectomy can be performed (Fig. 22.17).
8. Unilateral or bilateral thoracostomy tube placement is performed.
9. The thoracic cavity should be lavaged with warm saline.
10. Sternotomy closure is routine (see Chapter 4).

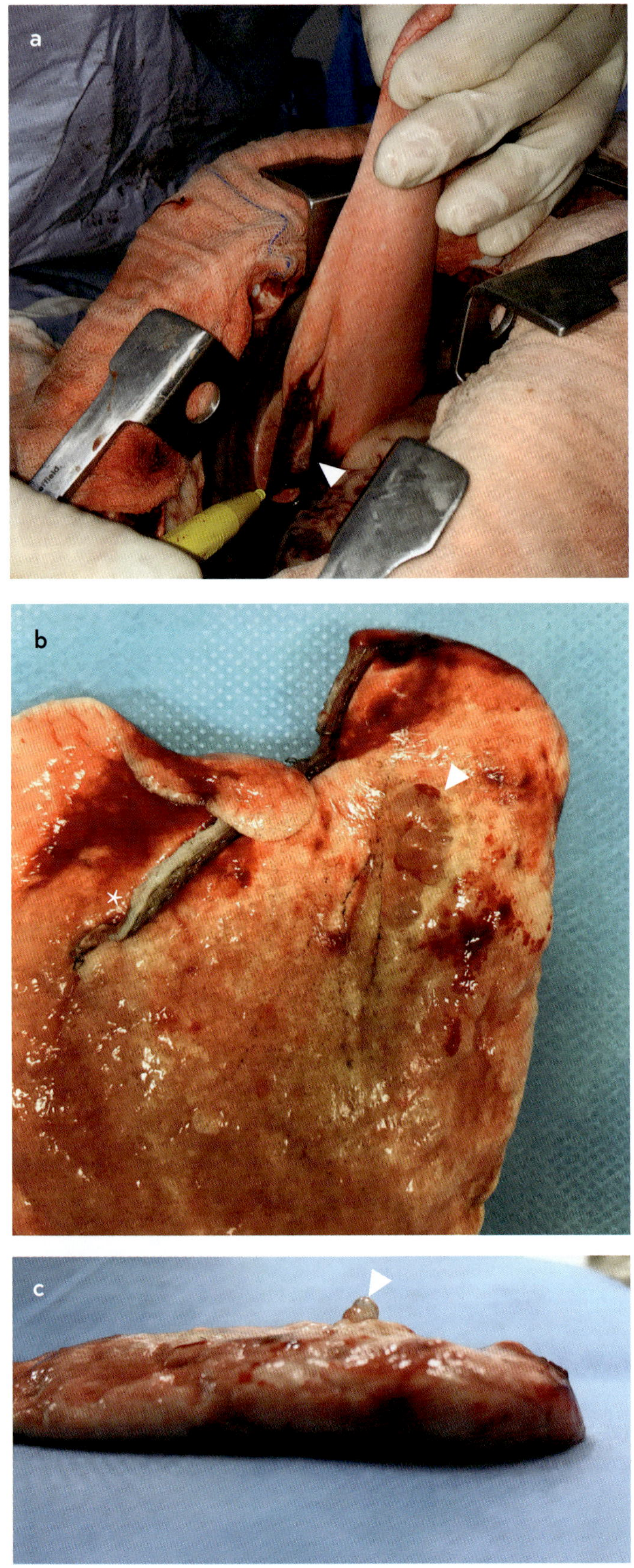

Figure 22.17 Stapled total lung lobectomy in a dog with spontaneous pneumothorax. The cranial lung lobe is partially collapsed and a pulmonary bleb can be seen (arrowhead). The asterisk indicates the staple line.

Surgical technique: Blood patch pleurodesis

In case of diffuse air leakage or if pneumonectomy may be required, pleurodesis can be considered. This procedure obliterates the pleural space by stimulating inflammation and adhesion formation between the parietal and visceral pleural surfaces. This can be achieved by mechanical abrasion of the lung surfaces, chemical sclerosing agents, or autologous blood administration via thoracostomy tube. This has been proven to be effective in human patients, but the use and success in small animals is still controversial. The authors discourage the use of mechanical abrasion and chemical sclerosing agents. Autologous blood pleurodesis, also known as blood patch pleurodesis, works by the mechanical action of coagulated blood adhering to the site of air leakage and the promotion of adhesion formation.

1. The pleural space is evacuated of air.
2. The skin over the jugular vein is clipped and aseptically prepared. Placement of a jugular catheter can be considered.
3. Whole blood (5–10 mL/kg or 5%–10% of body weight) is collected from the jugular vein using a 18- or 20-gauge needle attached to an extension tube, a three-way stopcock, and 20 or 50 mL syringes with no additives.
4. Once collected, the blood is immediately injected into the pleural cavity via the thoracostomy tube. If bilateral tubes are present, half of the blood volume is injected into each tube.
5. The thoracostomy tube is flushed with 10–20 mL of sterile saline to avoid clotting inside the tube. It should not be used for 4 hours following the injection of blood.
6. The patient's position is changed to obtain homogenous distribution of blood within the pleural cavity.

This technique may be an alternative when surgery is not financially feasible. It has been reported as successful in feline[27] and canine[28] cases of persistent pneumothorax, but multiple treatments may be required.[28] In a case series of eight dogs, the reported success rate after a single procedure is 62.5% and increases to 87.5% with multiple treatments.[28]

Postoperative management

Pain management is crucial, especially in patients with traumatic pneumothorax. Intrapleural local anesthesia (bupivacaine 1.5 mg/kg every 6 h) can be used. The use of pulse oximetry and assessment of arterial blood gas in the initial postoperative period is essential for monitoring ventilatory function. If arterial oxygen saturation is lower than 90% with an alveolar–arterial gradient above 20 mmHg, oxygen supplementation is required. Supplemental oxygen therapy is used to support pulmonary function and increase oxygen delivery. If there is severe hypoxemia (arterial partial oxygen pressure <60 mmHg) and hypoventilation (arterial partial carbon dioxide pressure >50 mmHg), ventilation is recommended.

Outcome

Through a combination of stabilization measures, thoracocentesis, thoracostomy tube placement, and appropriate surgical intervention, good outcomes can be achieved. Traumatic pneumothorax generally has a good prognosis in the absence of other complications related to trauma, whereas the prognosis for secondary spontaneous pneumothorax depends on the underlying condition.

Recurrence and mortality rates of surgically treated dogs with primary spontaneous pneumothorax due to pulmonary blebs and bullae are 3%–14% and 12%, respectively.[14–20] In animals that have no recurrence in the first month postoperatively, the risk of recurrence is even lower (3%). The survival rates of patients with spontaneous pneumothorax at 2 and 5 years are 88.4% and 83.5%, respectively.[17] Dogs treated conservatively have a 50% recurrence rate and a 53% mortality rate.

Early surgical intervention is recommended for definitive diagnosis and treatment of dogs with spontaneous pneumothorax and has been associated with a better outcome and lower recurrence rate compared to medically managed dogs.[16–18] If lesions are present in multiple lung lobes and resection cannot be performed, the prognosis is guarded and the risk of recurrence high.

In cats, survival after medical management is greater than that after surgical treatment (54% vs. 20%) and is linked to the degree of underlying lung pathology. Favorable prognostic factors in cats with pneumothorax include absence of dyspnea, no need for thoracocentesis, and normal body temperature at presentation.[15,20,26]

In case of recurrent or persistent air leakage after surgery, blood patch pleurodesis should be considered.

Hemothorax

Hemothorax is characterized by the accumulation of blood within the pleural space. It is commonly defined as a pleural effusion with a packed cell volume of at least 25% that of peripheral blood; however, no standard definition exists in veterinary medicine.[29–33] The source of blood can vary, including the thoracic wall, lung parenchyma, mediastinum, heart, or great vessels. It may result from traumatic or nontraumatic (spontaneous) causes (Table 22.2). In traumatic hemothorax, the most common mechanisms are blunt or penetrating injuries or iatrogenic injury to intra- or extrathoracic structures, resulting in bleeding into the thorax. Nontraumatic causes are less frequent and encompass coagulopathies (defective primary and secondary he-

TABLE 22.2 - COMMON CAUSES OF HEMOTHORAX

Traumatic	Nontraumatic	
	Coagulopathic	Spontaneous (noncoagulopathic)
Road traffic accident Penetrating injury Crush/compression injury (e.g., bite wound) Acceleration/deceleration injury Iatrogenic: • Thoracic surgery • Intrathoracic fine needle aspiration • Jugular puncture or catheter placement	Defective primary hemostasis: • Thrombocytopenia • Thrombocytopathy • Von Willebrand disease Defective secondary hemostasis: • Inherited factor deficiency • Rodenticide intoxication • Hyperfibrinolysis • *Angiostrongylus* infection	Neoplasia: • Thoracic wall neoplasia • Hemangiosarcoma • Mesothelioma • Pulmonary carcinoma • Metastatic neoplasia Lung lobe torsion Infectious disease Thymic hemorrhage

mostasis), neoplasia, lung lobe torsion, or infectious agents (e.g., *Angiostrongylus vasorum*, *Spirocerca lupi*, *Dirofilaria immitis*).

Clinically, traumatic injuries and coagulopathies are the primary causes of hemothorax in dogs, while neoplasia emerges as the most common cause in cases of non-coagulopathic spontaneous hemothorax, with 50% of tumors located on the thoracic wall.[32–34] Reported neoplastic conditions responsible for hemothorax include hemangiosarcoma, mesothelioma, metastatic carcinoma, osteosarcoma, pulmonary carcinoma, and chemodectoma.[32–34] Animals presenting with thoracic wall masses frequently exhibit a significant incidence of hemorrhagic pleural effusion, ranging between 10% and 40%. The development of hemothorax in cases of neoplasia is believed to be multifactorial, with the prevailing theories suggesting that it arises either from tumor invasion into the intercostal vessels or as a consequence of tumor necrosis and rupture.

Hemothorax can also develop postoperatively following any thoracic surgical procedure, but it is more frequently observed after significant cardiac or vascular surgery. It also occurs at a higher rate among patients who are on anticoagulant therapy or those undergoing excision of large masses. Diagnosing postoperative hemothorax and pinpointing its root cause present significant challenges.

Clinical presentation and diagnosis

A thorough clinical history is crucial, as it may offer insights into the potential causes. Hemothorax should be suspected in any animal following blunt or penetrating thoracic trauma, signs of hypovolemia and respiratory distress, or any recent medical procedures including thoracic surgery, thoracocentesis, intrathoracic fine needle aspiration, or jugular catheter placement.[29–31,35,36]

When there is no previous history of trauma or interventions, a spontaneous cause should be considered. Patients with a thoracic mass are typically older, with no breed or sex predilection.

Clinical signs associated with hemothorax can be quite vague and may be similar to those of any pleural effusion. These signs reflect the hemodynamic consequences of the redistribution of a significant blood volume and the respiratory compromise due to lung compression/atelectasis (tachypnea, dyspnea, and collapse). Therefore, rapid loss of 15%–20% of total blood volume may cause signs of hypovolemia without a significant impact on breathing. Breathing difficulties are expected only after accumulation of 20 mL/kg of pleural fluid.[30]

Physical examination may reveal tachycardia, tachypnea, a restricted ventilatory pattern, muffled heart or lung sounds (especially ventrally), and weak pulse quality. Other findings include the presence of external wounds, petechiae, and ecchymoses or external thoracic mass lesions.

Diagnostic investigations should include hematology and serum biochemistry. Hematological findings may quantify the anemia and provide an indication of the regenerative status. Platelet count can indicate thrombocytopenia. Biochemical abnormalities are often nonspecific. A coagulation profile is helpful to evaluate the intrinsic and extrinsic clotting pathways.

Thoracic imaging can confirm the presence of pleural fluid and may detect the cause or origin. In patients in respiratory distress, thoracocentesis can be performed prior to imaging. Thoracic radiographs are a sensitive method to diagnose pleural effusion, even if a small volume of fluid is present. If the animal is dyspneic, a dorsoventral or a standing lateral projection is recommended. Patient stability can represent a limiting factor in obtaining different radiographic projections. The radiographs should be evaluated to detect the origin of the hemothorax, primarily any mass effect of the thoracic wall, cranial and caudal mediastinum, or pulmonary mass.

Thoracic ultrasonography allows detection of pleural fluid without the need of physical or chemical restraint and guides thoracocentesis and aspiration of a mass lesion for cytological evaluation, bacteriology, and tho-

racic drainage. Serial ultrasounds can be used to monitor the progression or resolution of pleural effusion.
Thoracic CT is a more comprehensive method that provides superior resolution of anatomical structures. It allows for evaluation of all the extra- and intrathoracic structures, increasing the chances of detecting the origin of the hemothorax. CT is critical for staging and surgical planning, especially if a neoplasia is diagnosed.
Thoracocentesis and fluid analysis are required to confirm hemothorax. This can be done in a conscious patient with oxygen supplementation in sternal recumbency or a standing position. Thoracocentesis can be diagnostic for hemothorax and therapeutic, alleviating clinical signs. The fluid should not be judged by its gross appearance, as effusion with a packed cell volume of 5% appears hemorrhagic.
Definitive diagnosis of hemothorax is achieved by measuring the packed cell volume of the pleural fluid and comparing it to that of peripheral blood. It is important to note that blood in the pleural space may not clot due to rapid defribrination, hence the fluid may not clot. Iatrogenic, postsurgical, or neoplastic bleeding can be differentiated by the presence of platelets and the lack of erythrophagocytosis.[29,31] In animals with blunt thoracic injury, signs of hypovolemic shock, and free pleural fluid, a presumptive diagnosis of hemothorax can be made.

Treatment

Treatment highly depends on the underlying cause and clinical signs shown by the patient. Rapid evaluation, recognition, and intervention of potential thoracic injuries is essential. Key diagnostic steps include assessment of hemostasis, thoracic imaging, and thoracocentesis for fluid analysis. Animals in respiratory distress or presenting with hypovolemic shock require fluid resuscitation and oxygen supplementation using a face mask, nasal prongs, or flow-by to improve oxygen delivery. Analgesia should be provided to relieve pain and to allow physical examination, vascular access, and therapeutic thoracocentesis. In traumatic cases, unless there is active bleeding or a penetrating injury, conservative and supportive management is usually successful. Fluid resuscitation should be started immediately in the presence of cardiovascular shock. After significant blood loss, a red blood cell transfusion can be considered also to maintain an appropriate level of oxygen delivery. Autotransfusion (from the pleural cavity to the patient's circulation) using an appropriate filter may be considered in some dogs and cats with large-volume hemorrhage and cardiovascular instability, even in case of neoplasia, as it is unlikely that neoplastic cells present in the effusion will significantly worsen the prognosis.[37] Fresh frozen plasma and vitamin K may be indicated if a coagulopathy is present or anticoagulant rodenticide toxicity is suspected. Antifibrinolytics (tranexamic acid or aminocaproic acid) can be considered if the hemorrhage cannot be controlled. If respiratory signs are associated to the volume of hemothorax, enough blood should be removed by thoracocentesis to allow the animal to breathe comfortably. Complete voiding of the thoracic cavity is not necessary, as the remainder of the blood will be reabsorbed over time. Fresh frozen plasma is used for secondary coagulopathies. Oxygen supplementation is instituted if necessary based on the status of the patient.
If the cause of hemothorax is a lung lobe torsion, intercostal thoracotomy and lung lobectomy is the definite treatment, whereas in case of neoplasia (intrathoracic or thoracic wall) staging and surgical excision, if amenable, should be considered. In patients with postsurgical bleeding the choice can be difficult, as it depends on the origin. In case of rapid fluid accumulation, hypotension, and tachycardia, the authors suggest to reexplore the thoracic cavity and reevaluate the surgical site (e.g., staple line or lung hilus). If no bleeding is noted, the authors check the main vessels that could have been damaged during surgery or closure, including the internal thoracic arteries and the intercostal arteries. When an infectious disease is diagnosed, specific treatment is indicated.
Complications, outcome, and prognosis are highly variable based on the underlying cause of hemothorax.

Lung lobe torsion

Lung lobe torsion is a rare and potentially life-threatening condition reported in dogs and cats. It consists of an axial rotation of the bronchovascular pedicle centered close to, or at, the hilus causing airway obstruction and vascular compromise, leading to progressive lobar edema, hemorrhage, necrosis, and consolidation of the affected lung lobe.[38–41] The incidence in small animals is not clear. The pathophysiology is still poorly understood, but it has been linked to factors believed to increase lung lobe mobility such as increased perilobar space, bronchial cartilage dysplasia, lobar pathology, and thoracic conformation. This condition has been documented in dogs and cats of any age and size. The most represented breeds are large with a deep, narrow chest, such as sight hounds, in which the right middle and left cranial lung lobes are most commonly affected, and small breeds such as Pugs, with a tendency to occur in the left cranial lung lobe.[38,42,43] The etiology can be primary (spontaneous or idiopathic), if no predisposing factor is identified, or secondary to an underlying pulmonary or pleural disease. Idiopathic lung lobe torsion appears to be more common in dogs, whereas lung lobe torsion in cats seems to occur more frequently secondary to an underlying thoracic condition.[38–42]

Clinical presentation and diagnosis

Respiratory clinical signs are often present, but vague, nonspecific clinical signs have also been reported. On auscultation, decreased respiratory sounds can be detected over the affected region. Blood cell counts can show neutrophilia with left shift and/or anemia. Serum biochemistry tends to be nonspecific.

Thoracic ultrasound can be used to detect and sample pleural effusion. The affected lung lobe appears as a thoracic soft tissue mass. Absent blood flow within the lobe can be identified on Doppler scanning. Thoracic radiographs show pleural effusion and lung consolidation with an emphysematous pattern and an irregular, blunted or narrow dependent bronchus. It is often necessary to repeat the radiographs after draining the pleural effusion to correctly detect any lung pathology. Thoracic CT findings include pleural effusion, lobar enlargement, collapse/consolidation, vesicular emphysema, and an abrupt termination of the affected lung lobe bronchus (Fig. 22.18).[39] No significant contrast enhancement is noted on the affected lobe. Bronchoscopy shows an obstructed main bronchus.

Treatment

The standard treatment is surgical, with lung lobectomy considered the gold standard in dogs and cats.[38–44] The patient should be stabilized prior to surgery. Initial management includes thoracic drainage, oxygen supplementation, intravenous fluid therapy, and analgesia. Surgery should be performed as soon as the patient is stable enough.

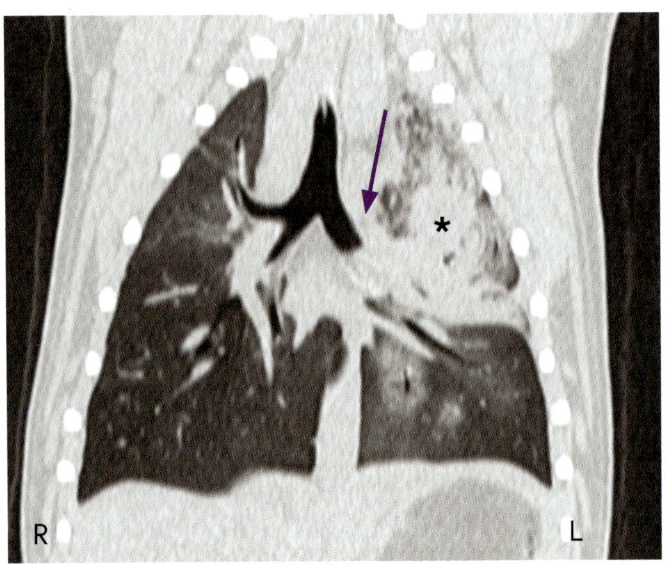

Figure 22.18 Precontrast dorsal computed tomography image of the thorax of a 3-year-old Pug with lung lobe torsion. Note the abrupt termination of the left cranial bronchus (arrow) and the consolidation of the affected lobe (asterisk).

Epidural or local regional blocks (e.g., intercostal nerve blocks) can control pain in the perioperative period without interfering with ventilation. An intercostal thoracotomy ipsilateral to the affected lobe is the preferred open surgical approach. If the exact location cannot be confirmed, a median sternotomy allows complete exploration of the thoracic cavity.

Surgical technique (Fig. 22.19)

1. Mechanical ventilation is required for this procedure.
2. A fifth intercostal thoracotomy ipsilateral to the affected lung lobe is performed (see Chapter 4).
3. Moistened laparotomy swabs are used to isolate the affected lung lobe and to pack the surrounding lung lobes away.
4. To isolate the caudal lung lobes, the pulmonary ligament extending from the caudal edge of the pleura of the hilus to the mediastinal pleura is transected. This can be performed by using Metzenbaum scissors or a diathermy device.
5. The pulmonary vessels and lobar bronchus are identified (this may be difficult in a torsed lung lobe).
6. Total lung lobectomy can be performed using a stapling device or suture ligation as described at the beginning of this chapter. Note that in case of suture ligation the entire pedicle is ligated using one or two encircling sutures (proximally) and a transfixing suture (distally). Derotation of the lung lobe should not be attempted.
7. Before closure, a thoracostomy tube should be placed (see Chapter 5).
8. Closure is routine (see Chapter 4).

Postoperative management

Following thoracotomy, pain, hypoxemia, pleural effusion, and residual pneumothorax should be corrected. Vital parameters, including heart rate, blood pressure, respiratory pattern, and temperature, as well as urine production and electrolytes must be checked for the first 24–48 hours. Blood gas analysis is important in the postoperative period to evaluate ventilation, hypoxemia, and the need for oxygen supplementation. Mechanical ventilation should be continued if necessary. Oxygen supplementation should be given to patients with arterial oxygen saturation below 95% or if the alveolar–arterial oxygen gradient is above 20 mmHg. The patient should recover either in sternal recumbency or in a lateral position laying on the surgical side to allow full expansion of the contralateral side.

The thoracostomy tube should be initially checked with a frequency of 2–4 hours to remove any pleural effusion and/or residual pneumothorax. The amount of air or fluid retrieved should be recorded and the milliliters of fluid/air per kilogram of body weight calculated over a pe-

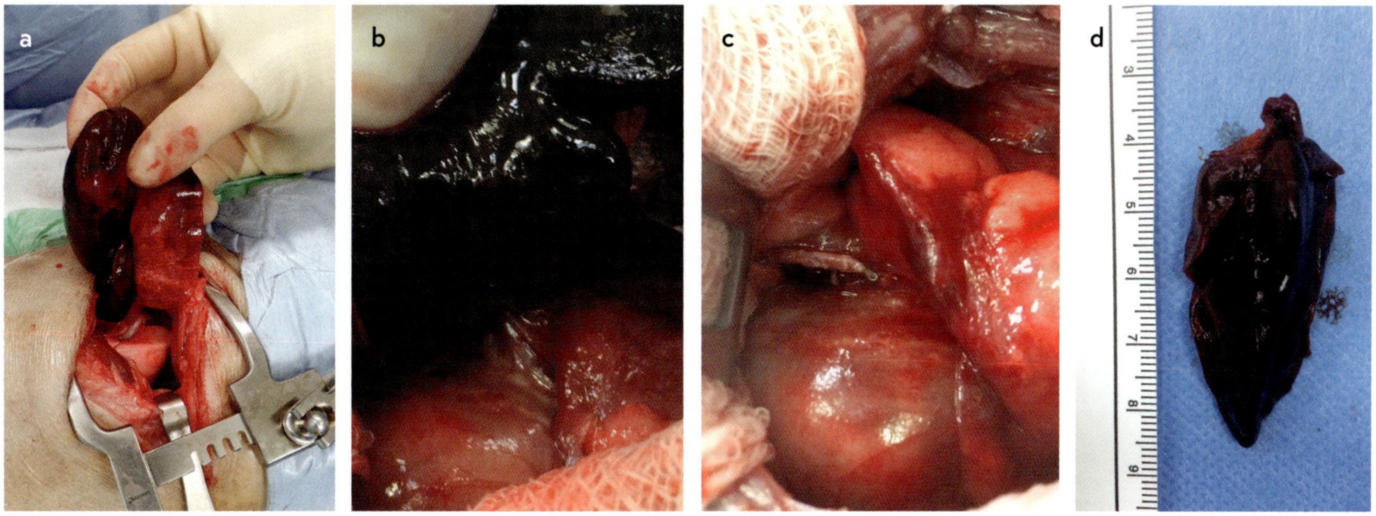

Figure 22.19 Lung lobectomy in a 3-year-old Pug with a left cranial lung lobe torsion. (a) The affected lobe is consolidated and hemorrhagic. (b) The torsed pedicle can be visualized. (c) Lobectomy is performed without derotation. (d) Resected lobe for histopathologic examination.

riod of at least 12 hours. This should guide the surgeon in deciding when to remove the thoracostomy tube.

Pain contributes to reduce pulmonary expansion and ventilation. Opioids (e.g., methadone, fentanyl) and intrapleural bupivacaine or lidocaine can be used for analgesia. If not contraindicated, patients are prescribed nonsteroidal anti-inflammatory drugs for 7–14 days. Paracetamol can also be considered in dogs.

Exercise should be restricted for at least 2 weeks after surgery, with 10–15-minute slow on-leash walks allowed 2–3 times daily. Exercise can be gradually increased after the first 2 weeks. The surgical site should be rechecked 10–14 days postoperatively.

Outcome

The complication rate after lung lobectomy due to lung lobe torsion ranges from 8% to 24%.[38–44] Occurrence of postoperative complications has not been associated with a poorer outcome.[38]

Historically, a fair to guarded prognosis was given to patients presented for this disease; however, recent studies have showed a survival rate ranging from 87% to 95%.[38,40,41,44] Dogs with idiopathic lung lobe torsion have a longer survival after lung lobectomy than dogs with secondary torsion.[38] The largest study in cats with lung lobe torsion revealed high complication (6/10 cats) and mortality (8/10 cats) rates, but animals surviving to follow-up had a good overall outcome.[42]

Diaphragmatic rupture/hernia

The diaphragm is a musculotendinous structure that separates the thoracic and abdominal cavities. It is composed of a strong central tendon surrounded by diaphragmatic muscle, which is divided into pars lumbalis (dorsal), pars sternalis (ventral), and pars costalis (lateral). There are three major openings: aortic hiatus, esophageal hiatus, and caval foramen.

A traumatic diaphragmatic hernia or rupture is a condition that occurs when there is a break or defect in the diaphragm, enabling abdominal organs to move into the thorax. This often occurs due to a sudden increase in intra-abdominal pressure with the glottis open. Trauma caused by motor vehicle injury is the most common (85% of cases) cause of diaphragmatic rupture in cats and dogs. The diaphragmatic costal muscles are more often ruptured. Left-to-right distribution is uniform, with about 15% being bilateral or having multiple tears. The orientation of muscle tears in dogs is circumferential (40%; along the junction of the diaphragm and the rib cage), radial (40%), or a combination (20%), whereas in cats it is mainly circumferential (60%) and rarely radial (20%). The liver is the organ most often herniated (90%), followed by the small intestine, stomach, spleen, omentum, pancreas, colon, cecum, and uterus.[45,46]

Clinical presentation and diagnosis

The clinical signs associated with diaphragmatic hernia can vary considerably, but respiratory signs are the most commonly reported due to lung compression (herniated organs, pleural effusion, hemothorax, pneumothorax) and pain (fractures, contusions) limiting thoracic expansion. After trauma, animals may present with an acute respiratory crisis and require emergency stabilization. Some patients adopt a sitting or standing position, with the elbows abducted and head extended. Vomiting and diarrhea may indicate gastrointestinal involvement, while in chronic cases general signs such

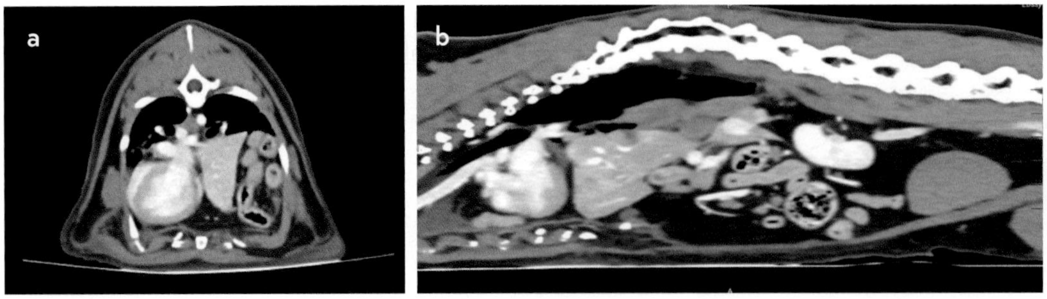

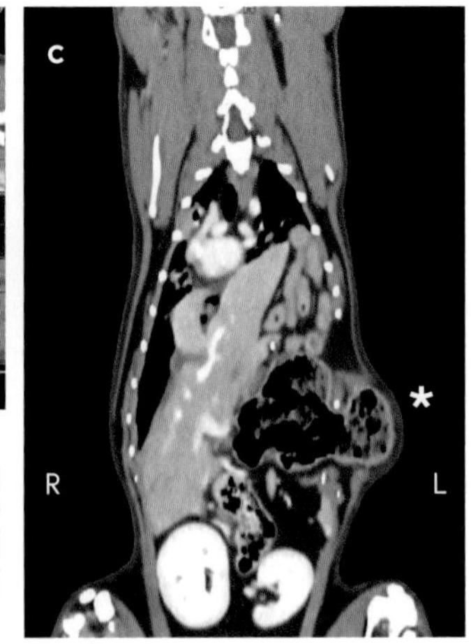

Figure 22.20 Multiplanar reformation/reconstruction (MPR) images in (a) transverse, (b) sagittal, and (c) dorsal planes using maximum intensity projection (MIP) showing diaphragmatic and left lateral body wall rupture in a cat. There is a lack of the outline of the diaphragm. The liver, intestine, and omentum are herniated in the thoracic cavity at the level of the heart. Note the left lateral abdominal wall body rupture (asterisk).

as weight loss or reduced appetite may be more obvious than respiratory changes.

On physical examination, there can be abnormalities on thoracic auscultation such as absence or reduction in normal lung sounds, borborygmi in the thorax, and muffled heart sounds or apical beat in an abnormal position or more apparent on the side contralateral to the hernia. Gastric tympany could indicate herniation of the stomach. Evidence of head trauma, such as cranial fractures and scleral hemorrhage, should be ruled out. It is important to remember that physical examination can be normal in some animals with diaphragmatic hernia.

Diagnosis relies on thoracic imaging, including radiographs, ultrasound, fluoroscopy, or CT (Fig. 22.20).[47,48] Caution is advised during patient restraint due to potential cardiovascular and respiratory compromise. Two orthogonal thoracic radiographs are the most useful test for diagnosis; however, it is important to remember that the appearance of the diaphragm can be influenced by respiration and animal positioning. Standard lateral projections (Fig. 22.21) are optimal and show alteration in the shape of the diaphragm (66%–97%), displacement of abdominal organs into the thorax (intestines in up to 61% of cases; spleen, liver, or stomach in 35%), gas-filled viscera within the thoracic cavity, and loss of thoracic detail/cardiac shadow due to increased soft tissue opacity in the thorax.[48,49] Thoracic radiographs can also be used to assess the presence of pulmonary contusions, pneumothorax, and pleural effusion. Pleural effusion and lung lobe collapse can be readily detected in dorsoventral projections and are found in 20% to 31% of cases. While contrast studies are rarely indicated, the presence of barium-filled organs within the thoracic cavity confirms the diagnosis. Nondiagnostic contrast studies due to gastrointestinal obstruction or delayed transit are possible. Ultrasonography has an accuracy of 93%, particularly in animals with pleural effusion, for detecting the presence of herniated organs such as intestinal loops, liver, or spleen within the thoracic cavity.

Treatment

For effective treatment, monitoring cardiovascular and respiratory parameters, intravenous fluid therapy, and analgesia are necessary. Antibiotic therapy should be considered based on the patient's general status and on the herniated organs (e.g., incarceration of the liver would suggest the use of prophylactic antibiotics). Preoxygenation is recommended in dogs and cats with thoracic disease, aimed at avoiding hypoxemia that may occur at the onset of anesthesia due to respiratory depression and apnea. Oxygen is administered by face mask or oxygen cage for 3–5 minutes prior to anesthetic induction.

Given the direct connection to the thoracic cavity, all the considerations of thoracotomy apply to anesthesia for repair of a ruptured diaphragm even though the surgical approach is a midline laparotomy. Induction should be quick to allow rapid airway control and ventilation. Despite the compression of the lungs by herniated organs, mechanical ventilation is sufficient for adequate lung expansion and oxygenation. Patient positioning is also important; having the head and thorax higher than the rest of the body reduces lung compression caused by the herniated organs. In case of herniation and distention of the stomach

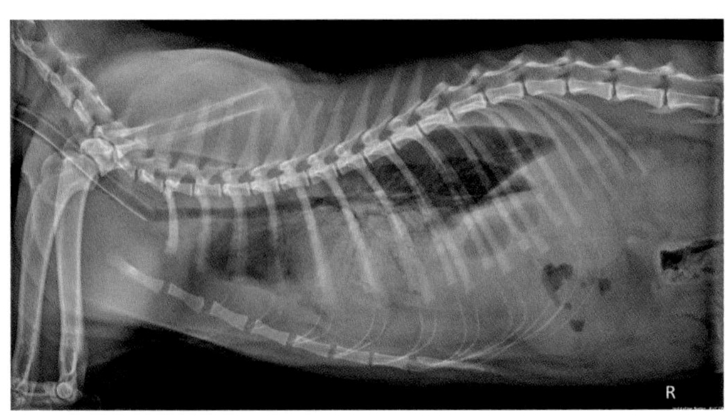

Figure 22.21 Lateral thoracic radiograph of a cat with diaphragmatic rupture. Note the lack of the diaphragmatic silhouette and the presence of abdominal viscera within the thoracic cavity.

(tension gastrothorax), emergency decompression should be immediately done using a wide-bore catheter inserted percutaneously on the left side of the thorax under sedation. Alternatively, an orogastric tube can also be used before surgery.[50]

The timing of surgery should be based on the degree of cardiopulmonary dysfunction, lung parenchyma compression, organ entrapment, and the overall patient condition.[51] However, as a general rule, surgical intervention should be performed as soon as the patient is stable. Indications for immediate surgery include tension gastrothorax, organ incarceration/strangulation, ongoing hemorrhage due to liver or spleen trauma, or unremitting abdominal pain. The patient should be prepared for combined exploratory laparotomy and caudal median sternotomy, with a wide and extended clip. The patient is positioned in dorsal recumbency with the head and thorax slightly elevated to minimize lung compression.

Surgical technique[52–55]

1. A cranial ventral midline celiotomy is performed. The incision can be extended caudally as needed (see Chapter 3).
2. Invasive positive-pressure ventilation is essential at this stage and can be performed manually or using a mechanical ventilator.
3. The falciform fat should be removed to improve exposure.
4. Balfour retractors are placed to allow visualization of cranial abdominal organs.
5. The whole diaphragm should be examined, as multiple tears can be present.
6. Stay sutures can be placed on the edges of the hernia to allow for manipulation of the diaphragm.
7. All the herniated abdominal organs are gently reduced into the abdomen and inspected for damage (Fig. 22.22). Care should be taken at this point, as organs incarcerated by the hernia ring may have become congested and subsequently may be more friable. Also, adhesions may be present in chronic diaphragmatic hernias. Immature serosal adhesions (<14 days) can be gently disrupted because they are primarily composed of fibrin, whereas mature adhesions can be divided with a combination of sharp dissection, electrocautery, and resection of portions of the organ involved (lung, liver, or intestine).
8. If the herniated organs are irreducible due to adhesions, swollen organs, or a small hernia ring, the tear in the diaphragm is enlarged with Metzenbaum scissors in a ventral direction, as this is a safe area (Video 22.8). Care should be taken dorsally, toward the major blood vessels that cross the diaphragm (i.e., caudal vena cava, aorta, and azygous vein). A caudal median sternotomy may be necessary in case of intrathoracic adhesions (see Chapter 4).

Video 22.8. Diaphragmatic rupture in a cat. An attempt is first made to gently reduce the herniated organs into the abdomen. The diaphragmatic tear is then enlarged with Metzenbaum scissors to allow the hernia contents (omentum and spleen) to be repositioned into the abdomen. Note the ventrolateral diaphragmatic defect.

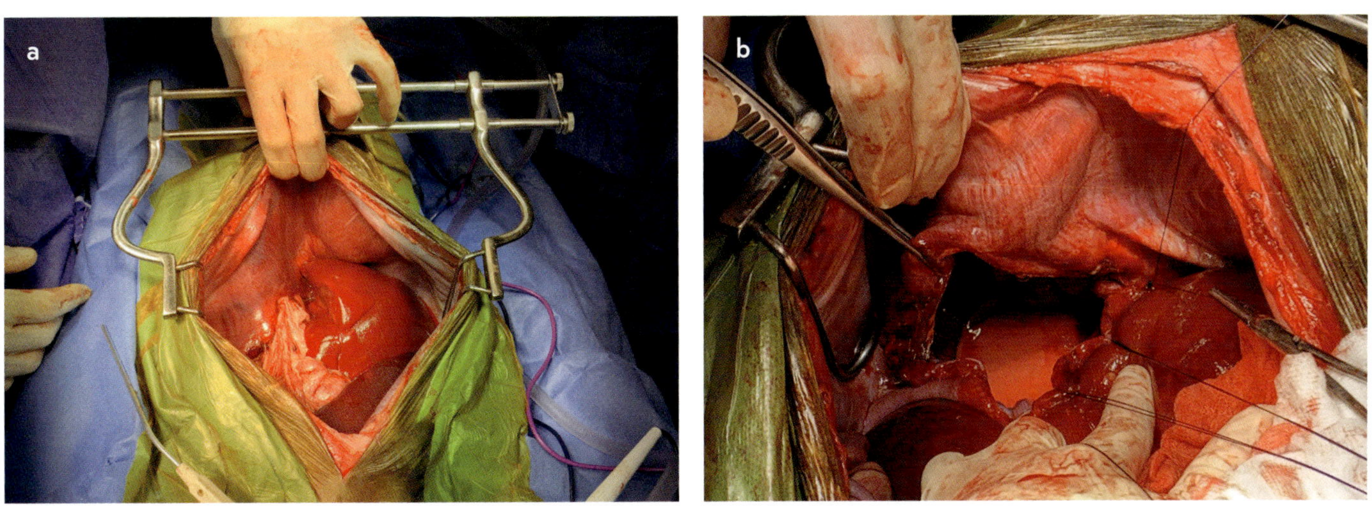

Figure 22.22 Diaphragmatic rupture in a dog. (a) Exploratory laparotomy revealing a tear in the lateral aspect of the diaphragm and herniated liver lobes, omentum, and small intestine. (b) Diaphragmatic defect after reduction of abdominal contents. Note the stay sutures on the edge of the diaphragm to aid in manipulation.

9. Once all the hernia contents have been repositioned, large moistened laparotomy swabs are used to retract the abdominal organs caudally in order to examine the thoracic cavity through the tear and inspect the diaphragm for further damage.
10. The thoracic cavity can be lavaged if needed and all the fluid aspirated.
11. Debridement of the edges of the defect to stimulate healing is controversial. Current opinion is that it is not essential, even in chronic hernias, as it increases the size of the defect and may reduce the holding power of sutures.
12. The diaphragm is repaired using either simple continuous (preferably), simple interrupted, or cruciate mattress sutures with 4-0 (in cats and small dogs) to 2-0 absorbable monofilament (e.g., polydioxanone, polyglyconate). The first suture is placed on the most dorsal aspect of the hernia. The ends of this suture can be left long, acting as a stay suture for manipulation.
    - For circumcostal diaphragmatic tears with not enough muscle available, the diaphragm can be anchored to the ribs (circumcostal suture) or along the body wall.
    - For tears that extend toward the caudal vena cava, suture knots should be positioned far enough from the vessel to avoid constriction of the vessel and subsequent venous return obstruction. The same principle applies to the aortic and esophageal hiatus.
13. Closure should continue in a ventral direction. No tension across the defect should be present, and enough bite (3–5 mm) should be taken from the hernia edges. In chronic diaphragmatic ruptures, or when primary repair is complicated by tension and contraction of native diaphragm muscles, alternative closure methods may be required, including omental flaps, pericardium, muscle flaps (transversus abdominis, rectus abdominis, latissimus dorsi), fascia, or synthetic mesh.
14. Prior to herniorrhaphy completion, the thoracic cavity should be evacuated using:
    - A thoracostomy tube (see Chapter 5). This allows gradual drainage as well as instillation of local anesthetics postoperatively.
    - An 18-gauge catheter or a butterfly needle with a three-way tap placed through the diaphragm.[56] This allows emptying of residual air from the thoracic cavity only once before closure. Care should be taken to prevent trauma to the lung tissue during this process.
    - A pediatric feeding tube with a three-way tap placed through the diaphragmatic closure and exiting the celiotomy incision.
15. A swab count should be performed before closure.
16. Closure is routine.

Postoperative management

Postoperative cardiovascular and respiratory monitoring is essential. Oxygen supplementation using an oxygen cage or nasal tube is recommended for several hours after anesthesia. Pain can lead to significant hypoventilation; management options include opioids, nonsteroidal anti-inflammatory drugs, and/or local anesthetics tailored to the patient's individual needs. Intravenous fluid therapy should continue until the animal is eating consistently.

Reestablishing negative pressure is not necessary and can even be detrimental. Residual pneumothorax should only be addressed if it compromises respiration and removal of residual pleural fluid or air should occur gradually as the patient demonstrates the ability to ventilate without support. Small volumes of residual air will slowly be reabsorbed without clinical significance. Chronically collapsed lungs should be allowed to gradually expand over several hours postoperatively; rapid expansion of these lungs should be avoided, as this can cause reperfusion injury and development of pulmonary edema. Cardiovascular support, oxygen, diuretics, and bronchodilators can be used if rapid lung expansion leads to complications. Preventing this scenario is advisable due to the guarded prognosis associated with reperfusion injury.

In the event of ongoing pneumothorax, thoracocentesis or thoracostomy tube placement should be considered. However, identifying and treating (e.g., lung lobectomy) the underlying cause is paramount. If a thoracostomy tube is already in place, regular assessment every 4 hours is recommended, with removal if insignificant quantities of air or fluid (<2–3 mL/kg/day) are produced.

Outcome

Approximately 15% of animals die to complications before presentation and surgery, due to hypoventilation, lung compression, shock, organ failure, and cardiac dysrhythmias. Medical stabilization prior to anesthesia and surgical intervention is strongly recommended to improve survival. Surgery should be performed promptly once the patient is stable enough. Intraoperative mortality is believed to be associated with poor anesthetic management and inadequate ventilation. If the animal survives the early postoperative period (12–24 hours), the prognosis is excellent, with recent studies reporting survival rates of 79%–100% for traumatic herniation, acute or chronic, in dogs and cats.[46,57–60] Recurrence is uncommon with proper surgical technique.[45,46] In recent studies, increased anesthetic duration, increased surgical duration, perioperative oxygen dependence, concurrent soft tissue or orthopedic injuries, and occurrence of intra- and postoperative complications were all associated with an increased risk of death both in cats and dogs.[58–60]

KEEP IN MIND

Pyothorax

- Surgical management is typically used in dogs or in case of identification of a primary cause, failed medical management, persistence of pleural effusion beyond 3–7 days, or presence of filamentous bacteria or migrating plant material on cytology.
- Current evidence suggests parapneumonic spread may be the most common route of infection in cats.
- Prognosis in dogs and cats can be good, with overall survival rates of 83% in dogs and 62% in cats.

Pneumothorax

- Rupture of pulmonary blebs or bullae is the most common cause of spontaneous pneumothorax in dogs but has not been reported in cats.
- Conservative management of spontaneous pneumothorax is often unsuccessful. Surgical exploration is indicated if air accumulation continues for more than 2–5 days or if an underlying cause is identified.
- In dogs with spontaneous pneumothorax, early surgical intervention has been associated with better outcomes and lower recurrence rates than medical management.

Hemothorax

- Hemothorax is defined as a pleural effusion with a packed cell volume approximately equivalent to that of peripheral blood; however, no standard definition exists in veterinary medicine.
- Treatment (conservative vs. surgical), outcome, and prognosis are highly variable based on the underlying cause.

Lung lobe torsion

- Vesicular emphysema and an abrupt termination of the affected lung lobe bronchus on diagnostic imaging are diagnostic.
- Lung lobectomy should be performed without attempting to derotate the lobe.
- Prognosis in dogs is good, whereas cats have high rates of complications and mortality.

Diaphragmatic hernia/rupture

- Immediate surgery is indicated in case of tension gastrothorax, organ incarceration/strangulation, ongoing hemorrhage, or unremitting abdominal pain.
- Exploratory surgery, replacement of abdominal organs in the correct position, and herniorrhaphy should be performed as soon as the patient is stable enough.
- The prognosis for animals surviving the early postoperative period is excellent, and recurrence is uncommon with proper surgical technique.

References

1. Stillion JR, Letendre JA. A clinical review of the pathophysiology, diagnosis, and treatment of pyothorax in dogs and cats. *J Vet Emerg Crit Care (San Antonio)*. 2015; 25(1):113–129.
2. Krämer F, Rainer J, Bali MS. Short- and long-term outcome in cats diagnosed with pyothorax: 47 cases (2009–2018). *J Small Anim Pract*. 2021; 62(8):669–676.
3. Tobias KM, Darrow BG, Radlinsky MG. Thoracic cavity. In: Johnston SA, Tobias KM (eds.). *Veterinary Surgery: Small Animal Expert Consult*, 2nd ed. St. Louis, MO: Elsevier; 2017. pp. 2019–2048.
4. Lee KCL. Surgical or medical management of pyothorax in dogs? *Vet Rec*. 2014; 174(24):605–606.
5. Bach JF, Balakrishnan A. Retrospective comparison of costs between medical and surgical treatment of canine pyothorax. *Can Vet J*. 2015; 56(11):1140–1143.
6. Demetriou JL et al. Canine and feline pyothorax: A retrospective study of 50 cases in the UK and Ireland. *J Small Anim Pract*. 2002; 43(9):388–394.
7. MacPhail CM. Medical and surgical management of pyothorax. *Vet Clin North Am Small Anim Pract*. 2007; 37(5):975–988.
8. Meakin LB et al. Prevalence, outcome and risk factors for postoperative pyothorax in 232 dogs undergoing thoracic surgery. *J Small Anim Pract*. 2013; 54(6):313–317.
9. Mellanby RJ, Villiers E, Herrtage ME. Canine pleural and mediastinal effusions: A retrospective study of 81 cases. *J Small Anim Pract*. 2002; 43(10):447–451.
10. Robertson SA et al. Thoracic empyema in the dog: A report of twenty-two cases. *J Small Anim Pract*. 1983; 24(2):103–119.
11. Rooney MB, Monnet E. Medical and surgical treatment of pyothorax in dogs: 26 cases (1991–2001). *J Am Vet Med Assoc*. 2002; 221(1):86–92.
12. Johnson MS, Martin MW. Successful medical treatment of 15 dogs with pyothorax. *J Small Anim Pract*. 2007; 48(1):12–16.
13. Boothe HW et al. Evaluation of outcomes in dogs treated for pyothorax: 46 cases (1983–2001). *J Am Vet Med Assoc*. 2010; 236(6):657–663.

14. Holtsinger RH, Beale BS, Bellah JR, King RR. Spontaneous pneumothorax in the dog: A retrospective analysis of 21 cases. *J Am Anim Hosp Assoc.* 1993; 29:195–210.
15. Cooper ES, Syring RS, King LG. Pneumothorax in cats with a clinical diagnosis of feline asthma: 5 cases (1990–2000). *J Vet Emerg Crit Care.* 2003; 13(2):95–101.
16. Dickson R et al. Surgical management and outcome of dogs with primary spontaneous pneumothorax: 110 cases (2009–2019). *J Am Vet Med Assoc.* 2021; 258(11):1229–1235.
17. Howes CL et al. Long-term clinical outcomes following surgery for spontaneous pneumothorax caused by pulmonary blebs and bullae in dogs—a multicentre (AVSTS Research Cooperative) retrospective study. *J Small Anim Pract.* 2020; 61(7):436–441.
18. Puerto DA, Brockman DJ, Lindquist C, Drobatz K. Surgical and nonsurgical management of and selected risk factors for spontaneous pneumothorax in dogs: 64 cases (1986–1999). *J Am Vet Med Assoc.* 2002; 220(11):1670–1674.
19. Lipscomb VJ, Hardie RJ, Dubielzig RR. Spontaneous pneumothorax caused by pulmonary blebs and bullae in 12 dogs. *J Am Anim Hosp Assoc.* 2003; 39(5):435–445.
20. Mooney ET, Rozanski EA, King RG, Sharp CR. Spontaneous pneumothorax in 35 cats (2001–2010). *J Feline Med Surg.* 2012; 14(6):384–391.
21. Lisciandro GR et al. Evaluation of a thoracic focused assessment with sonography for trauma (TFAST) protocol to detect pneumothorax and concurrent thoracic injury in 145 traumatized dogs. *J Vet Emerg Crit Care.* 2008; 18(3):258–269.
22. Boysen S, McMurray J, Gommeren K. Abnormal curtain signs identified with a novel lung ultrasound protocol in six dogs with pneumothorax. *Front Vet Sci.* 2019; 6:291.
23. Dickson R et al. Computed tomography in two recumbencies aides in the identification of pulmonary bullae in dogs with spontaneous pneumothorax. *Vet Radiol Ultrasound.* 2020; 61(6):641–648.
24. Reetz JA et al. Sensitivity, positive predictive value, and interobserver variability of computed tomography in the diagnosis of bullae associated with spontaneous pneumothorax in dogs: 19 cases (2003–2012). *J Am Vet Med Assoc.* 2013; 243(2):244–251.
25. Baudin Tréhiou C et al. CT is helpful for the detection and presurgical planning of lung perforation in dogs with spontaneous pneumothorax induced by grass awn migration: 22 cases. *Vet Radiol Ultrasound.* 2020; 61(2):157–166.
26. Liu DT, Silverstein DC. Feline secondary spontaneous pneumothorax: A retrospective study of 16 cases (2000–2012). *J Vet Emerg Crit Care (San Antonio).* 2014; 24(3):316–325.
27. Bersenas AM, Hoddinott KL. Allogenic blood patch pleurodesis for continuous pneumothorax in three cats. *JFMS Open Rep.* 2020; 6(2):2055116920945595.
28. Oppenheimer N et al. Retrospective evaluation of the use of autologous blood-patch treatment for persistent pneumothorax in 8 dogs (2009–2012). *J Vet Emerg Crit Care (San Antonio).* 2014; 24(2):215–220.
29. Prittie J, Barton L. Hemothorax and sanguineous effusions. In: King LG (ed.). *Textbook of Respiratory Diseases in Dogs and Cats.* St. Louis, MO: Saunders; 2004; pp. 610–616.
30. Allerton F. Diagnosing and treating haemothorax in dogs and cats. *In Pract.* 2019; 41(8):349–360.
31. Epstein SE, Balsa IM. Canine and feline exudative pleural diseases. *Vet Clin North Am Small Anim Pract.* 2020; 50(2):467–487.
32. Nakamura RK, Rozanski EA, Rush JE. Non-coagulopathic spontaneous hemothorax in dogs. *J Vet Emerg Crit Care.* 2008; 18(3):292–297.
33. Azfar Ali H, Lippmann M, Mundathaje U, Khaleeq G. Spontaneous hemothorax: A comprehensive review. *Chest.* 2008; 134(5):1056–1065.
34. Rutherford L, Stell A, Smith K, Kulendra N. Hemothorax in three dogs with intrathoracic extracardiac hemangiosarcoma. *J Am Anim Hosp Assoc.* 2016; 52(5):325–329.
35. Simpson SA, Syring R, Otto CM. Severe blunt trauma in dogs: 235 cases (1997–2003). *J Vet Emerg Crit Care (San Antonio).* 2009; 19(6):588–602.
36. Vnuk D et al. Feline high-rise syndrome: 119 cases (1998–2001). *J Feline Med Surg.* 2004; 6(5):305–312.
37. Higgs VA, Rudloff E, Kirby R, Linklater AK. Autologous blood transfusion in dogs with thoracic or abdominal hemorrhage: 25 cases (2007–2012). *J Vet Emerg Crit Care (San Antonio).* 2015; 25(6):731–738.
38. Rossanese M et al. Long-term survival after treatment of idiopathic lung lobe torsion in 80 cases. *Vet Surg.* 2020; 49(4):659–667.
39. Tobias KM, Johnston SA. Lung lobe torsion. In: *Veterinary Surgery: Small Animal.* St. Louis, MO: Elsevier; 2017. pp. 1993–1994.
40. Park KM et al. Lung lobe torsion in dogs: 52 cases (2005–2017). *Vet Surg.* 2018; 47(8):1002–1008.
41. Benavides KL, Rozanski EA, Oura TJ. Lung lobe torsion in 35 dogs and 4 cats. *Can Vet J.* 2019; 60(1):60–66.
42. Tindale C et al. Clinical characteristics and long-term outcome of lung lobe torsions in cats: A review of 10 cases (2000–2021). *J Feline Med Surg.* 2022; 24(10):1072–1080.
43. Neath PJ, Brockman DJ, King LG. Lung lobe torsion in dogs: 22 cases (1981–1999). *J Am Vet Med Assoc.* 2000; 217(7):1041–1044.
44. Wainberg SH et al. Evaluation of risk factors for mortality in dogs with lung lobe torsion: A retrospective study of 66 dogs (2000–2015). *Can Vet J.* 2019; 60(2):167–173.
45. Banz AC, Gottfried SD. Peritoneopericardial diaphragmatic hernia: A retrospective study of 31 cats and eight dogs. *J Am Anim Hosp Assoc.* 2010; 46(6):398–404.
46. Besalti O, Pekcan Z, Caliskan M, Aykut ZG. A retrospective study on traumatic diaphragmatic hernias in cats. *Ankara Üniv Vet Fak Derg.* 2011; 58(3):175–179.
47. Das J, Jena B, Behera SS. Surgical management of feline traumatic diaphragmatic hernia—a case report. *J Livestock Sci.* 2016; 7:107–110.
48. Hyun C. Radiographic diagnosis of diaphragmatic hernia: Review of 60 cases in dogs and cats. *J Vet Sci.* 2004; 5(2):157–162.
49. Stokhof AA. Diagnosis and treatment of acquired diaphragmatic hernia by thoracotomy in 49 dogs and 72 cats. *Vet Q.* 1986; 8(3):177–183.
50. Rossanese M, Pivetta M, Pereira N, Burrow R. Congenital pleuroperitoneal hernia presenting as gastrothorax in five cavalier King Charles spaniel dogs. *J Small Anim Pract.* 2019; 60(11):701–704.
51. Boudrieau RJ, Muir WW. Pathophysiology of traumatic diaphragmatic hernia in dogs. *Compend Contin Educ Pract Vet.* 1987; 9(4):379–385.
52. Fossum TW. Surgery of the lower respiratory system: Pleural cavity and diaphragm. In: Fossum TW (ed.). *Small Animal Surgery*, 5th ed. Philadelphia, PA: Elsevier; 2019. pp. 916–956.

53. Garson HL, Dodman NH, Baker GJ. Diaphragmatic hernia. Analysis of fifty-six cases in dogs and cats. *J Small Anim Pract*. 1980; 21(9):469–481.
54. Minihan AC, Berg J, Evans KL. Chronic diaphragmatic hernia in 34 dogs and 16 cats. *J Am Anim Hosp Assoc*. 2004; 40(1):51–63.
55. Schmiedt CW, Tobias KM, Stevenson MA. Traumatic diaphragmatic hernia in cats: 34 cases (1991–2001). *J Am Vet Med Assoc*. 2003; 222(9):1237–1240.
56. De Bastiani D et al. Complications and outcome of traumatic diaphragmatic hernia repair without post-operative chest drain: Retrospective study in 90 cats. *Open Vet J*. 2023; 13(6):677–683.
57. Hunt GB, Johnson KA. Diaphragmatic hernias. In: Tobias KM, Johnston SA (eds.). *Veterinary Surgery: Small Animal*, 1st ed. St. Louis, MO: Elsevier; 2013. pp. 1380–1390.
58. Sullivan M, Reid J. Management of 60 cases of diaphragmatic rupture. *J Small Anim Pract*. 1990; 31(9):425–430.
59. Gibson TW, Brisson BA, Sears W. Perioperative survival rates after surgery for diaphragmatic hernia in dogs and cats: 92 cases (1990–2002). *J Am Vet Med Assoc*. 2005; 227(1):105–109.
60. Legallet C, Thieman Mankin K, Selmic LE. Prognostic indicators for perioperative survival after diaphragmatic herniorrhaphy in cats and dogs: 96 cases (2001–2013). *BMC Vet Res*. 2017; 13(1):16.

Chapter 23

Chest wall emergencies

Ben Kaye

Thoracic trauma

Injury involving the thoracic chest wall can affect the skin, musculature, neurovascular structures, ribs, and sternum, but also the intrathoracic structures and pleural space. Damage to the critical cardiopulmonary structures encased in the thorax, which are essential for life, can have major associated morbidity or mortality.[1]

Thoracic injury is a frequent presentation in dogs and cats. The most common causes are penetrating injury (e.g., animal bite wounds and lacerations, gunshot wounds, impalement with sharp objects), high-rise syndrome, road traffic or motor vehicle accidents, and major blunt or crushing trauma.[2–5]

Penetrating thoracic injuries can severely affect the chest wall and lung tissue, resulting in impaired oxygenation, pneumothorax, and hemothorax. Damage to the heart and/or great vessels can result in rapid cardiovascular decompensation and death. Animal bite wounds can be challenging to treat due to the often innocuous appearance of the injury. Deep laceration and compression injury to the chest wall is common, with concomitant rib fractures and intrathoracic involvement.[5,6] Furthermore, inoculation of bacteria poses a risk of infection and sepsis, warranting early decontamination and empirical antimicrobial therapy. Gunshot wounds are often treated conservatively with appropriate wound management. If gunshot-related hemothorax and pneumothorax are not amenable to thoracostomy drainage, then exploratory thoracotomy is indicated.[3] Generally, penetrating injuries are associated with very favorable survival outcomes if early treatment is implemented. See Chapter 9 for further information on penetrating injuries.

High-rise syndrome in cats and dogs is defined as a fall from a height of two or more stories that results in polytrauma. Cats tend to suffer less severe global injury due to their righting reflex and smaller body mass. The most frequent thoracic conditions associated with high-rise syndrome are pneumothorax and pleural effusion.[7]

The most common sequelae of blunt trauma to the thorax include pulmonary contusions, pneumothorax, pneumomediastinum, hemothorax, rib fractures, (pseudo)flail chest, and diaphragmatic rupture and hernia. Blunt trauma to the thoracic cavity can result in injury via direct force, deceleration injury, and/or compression injury. Lung contusion is an entity involving injury to the alveolar capillaries without any tear or cut in lung tissue. This results in accumulation of blood and other fluids within the lung tissue. The pathophysiology of lung contusion includes ventilation–perfusion mismatch, increased intrapulmonary shunting, pulmonary edema, segmental lung damage, and a loss of compliance.[8–10]

Clinical presentation and diagnosis

Animals that present following thoracic trauma can have varied clinical signs of different severity. The clinical absence of thoracic wall injury does not preclude intrathoracic trauma. Animals that do have damage to the thoracic wall are more likely to have injury to intrathoracic structures. This is particularly important if there are rib fractures or (pseudo)flail chest present. Patients with pleural space disease (e.g., hemothorax, pneumothorax) or marked pain from chest wall injury or rib fractures will often have short, shallow breathing patterns. Conversely, animals with primary pulmonary disease (e.g., pulmonary contusion) will have larger, deeper breaths with a more notable abdominal component. In case of marked respiratory distress, fatigue, or flail chest, paradoxical breathing may be present (Video 23.1).[11]

Depending on the injury type, animals may present with extensive wounds to the thoracic wall or have visible impaled foreign bodies. In case of bite wounds, there may be only small puncture wounds or severe disruption of the chest wall. If the integrity of the pleural space is

Video 23.1. Marked paradoxical breathing pattern due to disruption of the sternum in an anesthetized German Short-haired Pointing Dog with severe thoracic trauma. Note the inward motion of the ventral thoracic wall overlying the sternum during inspiration and marked breathing effort.

Video 23.2. Computed tomographic reconstruction of the same dog as in Video 23.1, highlighting the 3rd–4th and 5th–6th sternal fracture–luxations.

compromised, patients will be unable to ventilate due to pneumothorax.

Diagnostic imaging can greatly assist clinicians in qualifying thoracic injury and can help direct treatment. The most common imaging modalities used when evaluating an animal with thoracic trauma are point-of-care ultrasonography, plain thoracic radiography, and computed tomography (CT) (Video 23.2). In the emergency setting, CT imaging increases the sensitivity of detecting pleural effusion, pneumothorax, and pulmonary contusions. It is important for clinicians to note that pulmonary contusions usually take 4–6 hours (or even up to 48 hours in some instances) before being radiographically detectable. Thoracocentesis can be used as a diagnostic and therapeutic procedure, particularly with trauma-induced pneumo- and hemothorax.[12]

Treatment

Animals presenting with thoracic trauma must be triaged and treated with a systemic, global approach to maximize a successful outcome. Life-threatening injury should be prioritized. Patients with thoracic trauma will often have clinically significant cardiopulmonary injury, and these body systems should be stabilized first, in addition to appropriate analgesia.

Analgesia should always be administered to trauma animals either intravenously or via parenteral injection, to avoid the ongoing deleterious physiological effects of pain. Multimodal analgesia and sedation protocols including combinations of opioids, alpha-2 adrenoreceptor agonists, N-methyl-D-aspartate (NMDA) receptor antagonists, dissociative anesthetics, or local anesthetics (e.g., nerve blocks, constant-rate infusions) are often indicated.

Oxygen supplementation should be given to animals with dyspnea following thoracic trauma and is very helpful in case of shock due to hypoxemia. It can be administered via flow-by, nasal prongs or cannulas, oxygen masks, or oxygen cages. Parameters indicating poor respiratory function include oxygen saturation below 95% (measured via pulse oximetry), partial pressure of arterial oxygen below 80 mmHg or less than around 4–5 times that of fraction of inspired oxygen (generally 21% at room air), partial pressure of carbon dioxide above 60 mmHg, or marked respiratory effort, despite supplemental oxygenation.[13]

All soft tissue lacerations should be inspected under general anesthesia for the selection of appropriate treatment (superficial vs. deep/open wound).

- Simple, superficial soft tissue lacerations, without communication into the pleural space, should be treated with the basic principles of wound management. Wounds are decontaminated with isotonic crystalloid flushing and mechanical debridement of devitalized tissue as appropriate. Depending on the degree of trauma and contamination, simple wounds can be primarily closed, providing adequate drainage as needed, or left to heal via secondary intention with appropriate dressings and bandaging. Bacteriology of wounds can help guide empirical antibiotic therapy as needed and should be performed following debridement and flushing.
- Open wounds communicating with the pleural space can lead to pneumothorax and should be addressed as an emergency. Prior to stabilization and definitive treatment, plastic or nonair permeable wraps can be circumferentially applied to a patient in an acute emergency setting, creating an "airtight" seal. Clinically, significant pleural effusion or pneumothorax can be rapidly alleviated via thoracocentesis.
- More significant injury to the thoracic wall, especially if there is major soft tissue crushing injury, pleural cavity involvement, unstable sternal or rib fractures, devitalized tissue, or a concern over contamination and sepsis, warrants more intensive treatment. Specific management of rib fractures and flail chest is described below. See Chapters 7, 9, and 22 for further information on bite wounds, penetrating injury, and pleural effusion and pneumothorax, respectively.
- Traumatized but healthy viable musculature can be repaired primarily, and doing so will often restore the pleural space. Intercostal muscle lacerations can be repaired via circumcostal sutures of adjacent ribs, similar to that of a standard intercostal thoracotomy (see Chapter 4). Multiple intercostal lacerations can be repaired using a basket-weave pattern (Fig. 23.1).
- Depending on the type of trauma and extent of soft tissue injury, primary repair can be augmented by axial pattern flaps, subdermal plexus flaps, local muscular rotation flaps (e.g., latissimus dorsi, external abdominal oblique, or internal abdominal oblique muscle flaps), or mobilization of omental pedicle grafts from the abdomen.[9]
- Sternal fractures or luxations can be stabilized with interfragmentary wiring or plate fixation (Fig. 23.2). Reconstruction of the thoracic wall and sternum may be required to restore structural rigidity of the thoracic cavity and reestablish the pleural space.

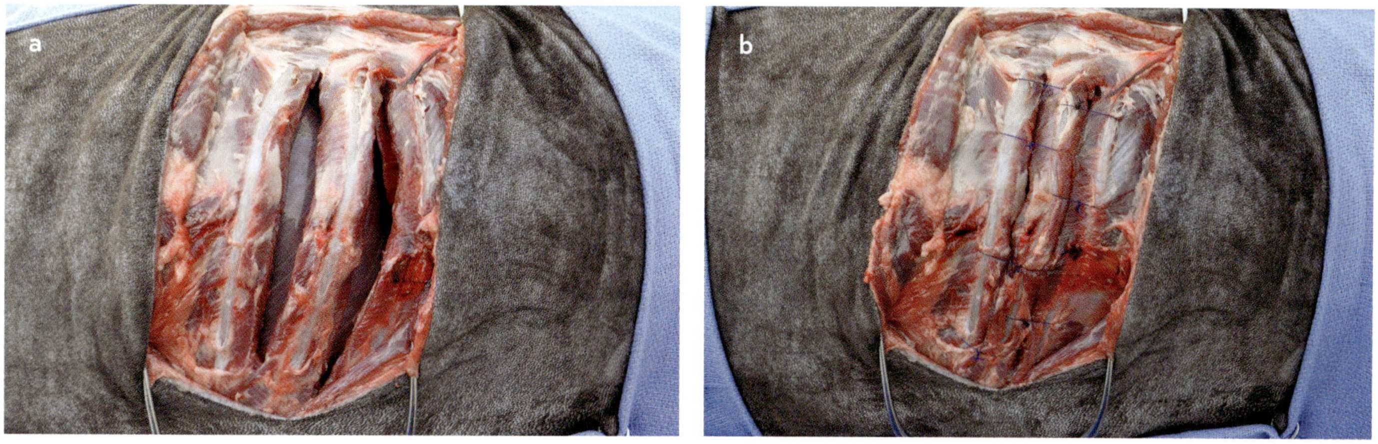

Figure 23.1 Basket-weave pattern for repair of multiple intercostal lacerations. (a) Lacerations between the 8th, 9th, and 10th ribs have been created in a 35 kg Rottweiler cadaver to mimic severe penetrating trauma to the chest wall. The animal is in left lateral recumbency, with the head to the right of the image. The diaphragm and caudal edge of the right caudal lung lobe can be seen. Note that the latissimus dorsi and external abdominal oblique muscles have been reflected to improve visualization. (b) Multiple basket-weave or staggered circumcostal sutures have been used to appose the lacerated intercostal musculature, using size 0 or 3-0 polydioxanone. Note that the goal is to appose the musculature together and not the ribs themselves. An airtight seal is subsequently created via reconstruction and repair of the overlying soft tissues.

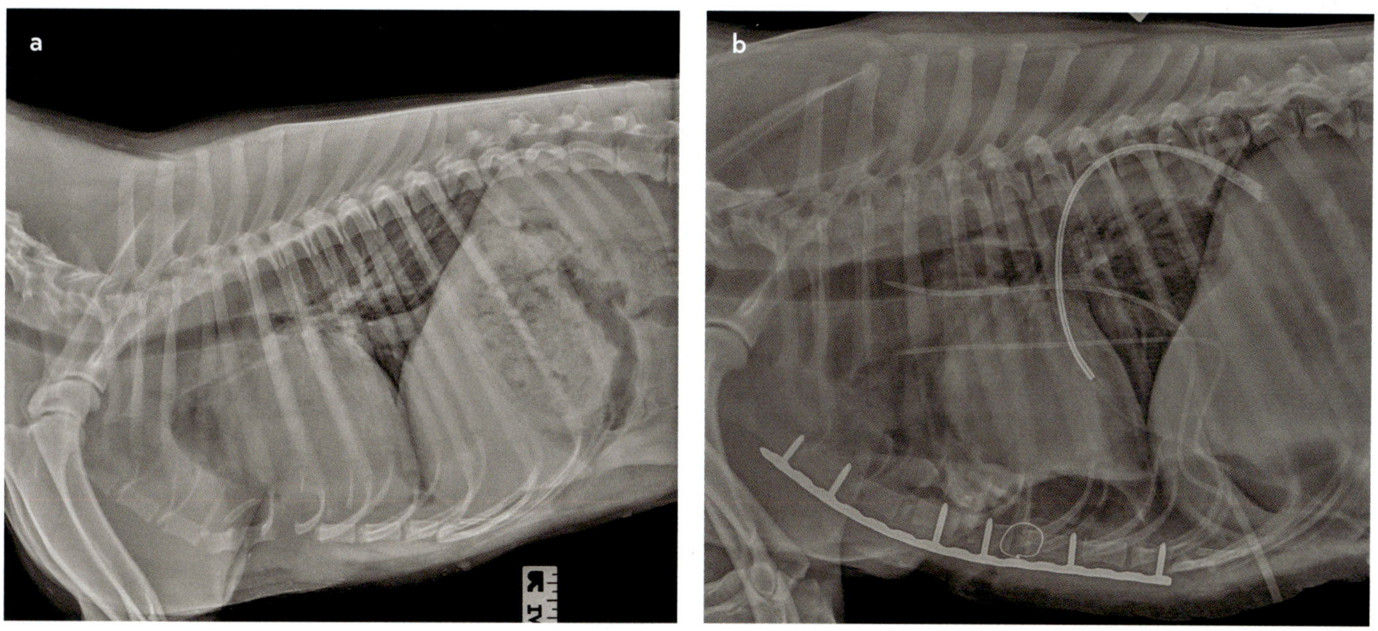

Figure 23.2 Lateral radiographs of the same dog as in Video 23.1 (a) before and (b) after stabilization of the 3rd–4th and 5th–6th sternal fracture–luxations with a combination of interfragmentary orthopedic wiring and internal plate fixation (3.5 mm Synthes locking compression plate).

Outcome

Animals that have sustained thoracic trauma generally have very good outcomes provided early stabilization is performed. Feline high-rise syndrome has an excellent prognosis, with survival rates exceeding 90%. Patients with penetrating injury have improved overall survival rates compared to those suffering from blunt trauma; however, both carry favorable prognoses with early, appropriate treatment.[3,4,7]

Rib fractures

Rib fractures are frequently encountered in veterinary practice, due to high-velocity blunt or low-velocity crushing trauma to the thorax.[14] The main causes are road traffic accidents (>50%), other blunt force trauma, or animal bite wounds.[5,15] Iatrogenic rib fractures can occur during thoracic surgery, particularly if incorrect techniques are used. These fractures can be associated with significant morbidity and mortality and are indicative of the severity and force of the inciting trauma.[16] They can cause considerable pain, hemothorax, and pneumothorax, and sharp fractured ends can lacerate intrathoracic structures, worsening clinical signs. Marked pain can reduce thoracic wall excursion, reducing the ability to ventilate and resulting in hypoxemia or hypercarbia. This can subsequently worsen any primary insult to the lungs, such as pulmonary contusions. Hemothorax can result in acute hypovolemic shock, reducing global delivery of oxygen. As pneumothorax progresses, the ability of the lungs to expand, and thus ventilation, is reduced.

Clinical presentation and diagnosis

Patients with rib fractures will have clinical signs consistent with pain and any underlying comorbidities associated with the trauma. The respiratory signs are more often due to pulmonary injury (e.g., contusions) rather than to the fractures themselves. However, pain may decrease thoracic wall excursion, further impairing ventilation. Animals may exhibit shallow rapid breathing, tachypnea, cyanosis, and paradoxical movement of the chest wall. Labored breathing with paradoxical abdominal movement may indicate imminent respiratory failure.

Rib fractures can be palpated or diagnosed with conventional radiography or CT (Fig. 23.3). Dogs that sustain rib fractures from motor vehicle accidents tend to have a dorsal fracture location (39%) and an even spread across the thorax. Conversely, those that sustain injury through dog bites tend to have multiple (>1) fractured ribs (35%), occurring midthorax (71%). Rib fracture characteristics are not associated with outcome.[14]

Treatment

It is of critical importance that patients be completely evaluated to determine whether surgical stabilization of rib fractures or nonoperative management is warranted. Rib fractures, and the associated trauma, can result in self-limiting, mildly clinical hemothorax, pneumothorax and hypoventilation from pain.

Initial management should include supplemental oxygen, analgesia, intravenous fluid therapy (volume resuscitation or blood products, as indicated), and treatment of any life-threatening injury focusing on the cardiovascular and respiratory systems. Point-of-care ultrasonography, thoracic radiography, or CT can assist with diagnosing intrapleural disease and guiding thoracocentesis or chest drain placement. Following initial management, continuous critical monitoring is recommended. Patients may rapidly deteriorate, needing intubation and mechanical ventilation if oxygenation is inadequate.

Ongoing nonsurgical management of rib fractures should include exercise restriction for 6–8 weeks, oral analgesia, and monitoring for worsening cardiovascular or respiratory disease. Soft padded thoracic bandaging may be used to reduce pain and immobilize fractures; however, care must be taken to avoid impairment to thoracic wall excursion (thus causing hypoventilation) or further displacement of the fracture.

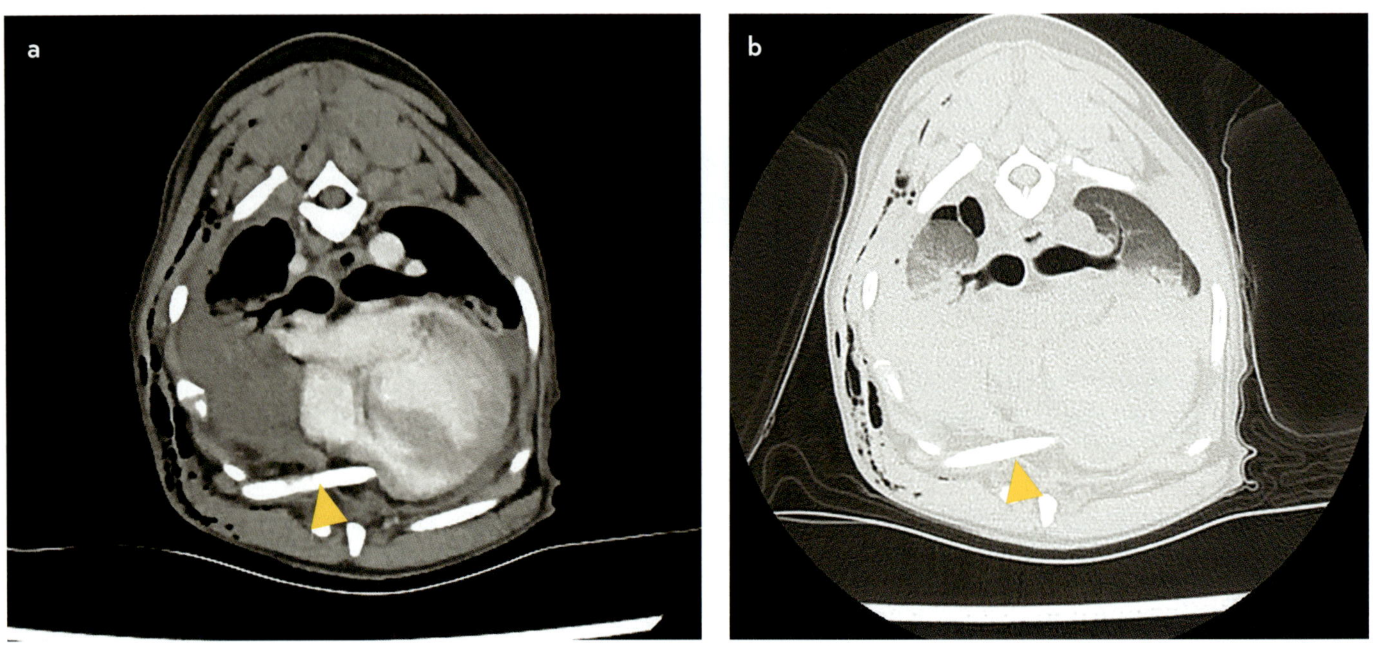

Figure 23.3 Postcontrast (a) soft tissue window and (b) lung window computed tomography images in a transverse plane showing a displaced rib fracture (arrowhead) compressing the heart in a 2-year-old Dachshund that sustained a road traffic accident. Images courtesy of Matteo Rossanese.

It is the author's experience that internal fixation of rib fractures is rarely required. Conservative management of up to three consecutive rib fractures can be employed successfully via external bandaging, multimodal analgesia, exercise restriction, and ongoing symptomatic treatment for the initial trauma. Internal fixation should be considered if more than three consecutive ribs are fractured; the fractured ends are displaced, unstable, and there is ongoing risk of internal laceration of vital structures; or there is extensive soft tissue injury associated with the rib fractures, which may reduce healing capabilities. Rib resection should also be considered if fixation is not achievable, the viability of the region is questionable, or there is comminution.

Reported techniques for internal fixation of rib fractures generally include interfragmentary wiring with small-gauge orthopedic pins and wire, or an intramedullary pin. The exact pin and wire configuration depends on the fracture configuration and location. These techniques provide nonrigid interfragmentary fixation permitting rapid secondary bone healing. The use of pins and wires is a quick method of repair, which is advantageous in the compromised patient; surgery and general anesthesia time should be kept to a minimum. Should the fracture configuration warrant rigid fixation, or not be appropriate for pin and wire stabilization, then internal fixation with locking plates can be utilized. The objective of any internal fixation of a rib fracture is to restore semirigid competency of the thoracic wall. This enables adequate thoracic excursion, improving ventilation.[16–20]

There is very limited data providing optimal timings for surgical repair of fractured ribs. Ultimately, surgical fixation should be performed as soon as the patient is stable enough for general anesthesia. For acute rib fractures, it has been suggested that fixation should occur within the first 7 days, ideally within the first 3 days after trauma. This timeframe minimizes any callus formation, therefore making fracture reduction easier and stabilization less technically challenging.[17] It is important to note that many pulmonary contusions can progress over the first 48 hours, but thereafter respiratory signs tend to improve.

Surgical technique

1. Following identification of which ribs require surgical stabilization, the procedure is performed under general anesthesia with full aseptic preparation. Patients will likely require positive-pressure mechanical ventilation because the noninjured lung is dependent during lateral recumbency, a pneumothorax is created when entering the thoracic cavity, and primary lung trauma such as contusions may be present.
2. Patient positioning is determined by the location of the fractured ribs; generally, lateral recumbency with the affected ribs upwards is used. The thoracic limbs may need to be secured in an extended position if access to the cranial ribs is required.
3. An incision is made over the affected rib fractures; this can be guided by previous imaging or palpation. Surgeons should be familiar with the approach to and the anatomy of the thoracic wall, especially the overlying musculature and neurovascular structures. Muscle-sparing techniques should be used to minimize further trauma and pain. This involves longitudinal muscle splitting, parallel to muscle fiber orientation. Where possible, muscles should be gently retracted, rather than transected (e.g., dorsal retraction of latissimus dorsi muscle).
4. Reduction of rib fractures can be assisted by Freer or periosteal elevators, bone reduction grasping forceps, right-angled forceps, or manually. The overlying periosteum should be preserved to reduce the risk of devitalization. Fracture stabilization can be achieved with pins and wires, intramedullary pins, and/or plates (Fig. 23.4).
   - Orthopedic pins or wires can be placed for temporary or permanent stabilization depending on fracture stability. Small drill holes can help facilitate placement of interfragmentary wiring. Care must be taken to avoid damage to intrathoracic structures.
   - An intramedullary pin can be placed retrogradely into the more mobile distal fragment first, and then into the proximal fragment. The natural rib curvature will vary significantly between breeds, thus intramedullary pin contouring may be required.

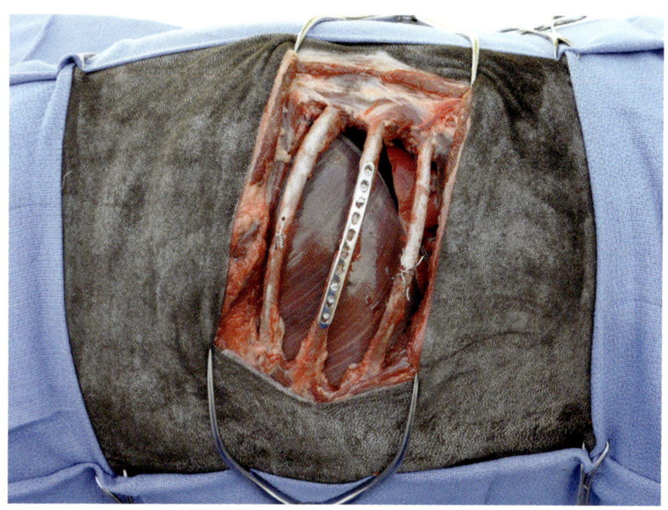

Figure 23.4 The same rib fractures as in Figure 23.1 have been repaired via internal fixation. Crossed 1.2 mm wires with 21-gauge orthopedic wiring, a contoured 10-hole 2.4 mm locking compression plate, and interfragmentary wiring through two bone tunnels have been used to stabilize ribs 8, 9, and 10, respectively.

- Low-profile contoured locking plate implants can be placed on the outer surface of the rib. From basic orthopedic principles, a target of 4–6 cortices in each fragment are recommended; however, conventional osteosynthesis plates far exceed bending stiffness of ribs.[17]

5. Rib resection must be considered in case of irreducible, complicated, or displaced rib fractures.
6. Routine wound closure is performed with an attempt to provide adequate coverage of implants with musculature.
7. Thoracic drains should be placed to monitor for ongoing pneumo- or hemothorax and can also be used to provide analgesia with local anesthetics.

Postoperative management

The level of care will depend on patient stability. A focus on cardiovascular and respiratory systems is important. Adequate hydration and intravascular volume are ensured with intravenous fluid therapy. Should there be persistent hypotension or anemia, vasopressor/inotropic support or blood products can be considered, respectively. Respiratory function may be compromised for many reasons related to the index trauma, progression of pulmonary contusions, anesthesia, or surgery itself, and animals may require ongoing supplemental oxygen to avoid hypoxemia. Sufficient multimodal analgesia is required to ensure patients are comfortable and able to ventilate adequately. If there are severely contaminated or infected wounds, appropriate antibiotic therapy is warranted. Patients should be exercise restricted and rested for 6–8 weeks, and, if needed, plain radiography can be performed to ensure adequate bone healing.

Outcome

Patients with cardiovascular and respiratory stability and less than three simple rib fractures, treated conservatively, are expected to have excellent clinical outcomes. However, the presence of rib fractures should raise suspicion of serious intrathoracic injury. Dogs presenting with rib fractures are 11.2 times more likely to require an exploratory thoracotomy procedure.[5] The animal trauma triage score can provide prognostic information, although it is not specific to rib fractures.[14]

It is not known whether surgical stabilization or conservative management of rib fractures provides the best outcomes. Clinical judgement should be used on a case-by-case basis.

Flail chest

Flail chest is defined as two or more fractures per rib in at least two or more adjacent ribs. The resultant flail segment is partly detached from the thoracic wall and moves in a paradoxical manner to the rest of the chest cavity.[21] That is, during inspiration and thoracic wall excursion, the flail segment is drawn inward, whereas during expiration the flail segment moves outwards. A pseudoflail chest is defined as multiple sequential rib fractures; depending on fracture stability, there may also be paradoxical movement (Video 23.1).[5]

The majority of rib fracture considerations apply to flail chest. A flail segment can significantly contribute to poor ventilation. When the segment is in an internal position (i.e., during inspiration), there is reduced intrapleural space, restricting lung expansion. The movement of the flail segment is associated with pain, which can reduce thoracic wall excursion. Furthermore, pulmonary contusions are highly likely to be present subsequent to the inciting trauma. These can all reduce efficient ventilation, causing hypoxemia via perfusion-induced low ventilation–perfusion mismatch.[16]

An experimental (nontrauma) flail chest study showed that internalization of the flail segment resulted in reduced tidal volume, increased respiratory rate, and reduced minute volume. Whilst there were significant changes to ventilatory parameters, hypoxemia and hypercarbia were not observed.[22] This suggests that the primary pulmonary pathology sustained during initial trauma (e.g., pulmonary contusion), in addition to the deleterious changes in ventilatory parameters, results in severe respiratory compromise in clinical patients with flail chest.

Clinical presentation and diagnosis

Animals with a flail chest are often in marked respiratory distress, with paradoxical movement during respiration. Clinical findings reported include tachypnea, dyspnea, pain, paradoxical movement of the flail segment, subcutaneous emphysema, hemoptysis, pulmonary contusions, reduced respiratory function causing hypoxemia or hypoventilation, pneumothorax, hemothorax, and pneumomediastinum.

Flail segments can be diagnosed on physical examination or via radiography or CT, which have the added advantage of providing information on intrathoracic pathology (Fig. 23.5). In dogs suffering from thoracic bite wounds, pulmonary contusions and pneumothorax are concurrently diagnosed with flail chest via plain radiography in more than 50% of cases.[14] Whilst providing precise and more sensitive detail compared to plain radiography, thoracic CT requires deep sedation or general anesthesia, both potentially deleterious to acute trauma patients in marked respiratory distress.[23]

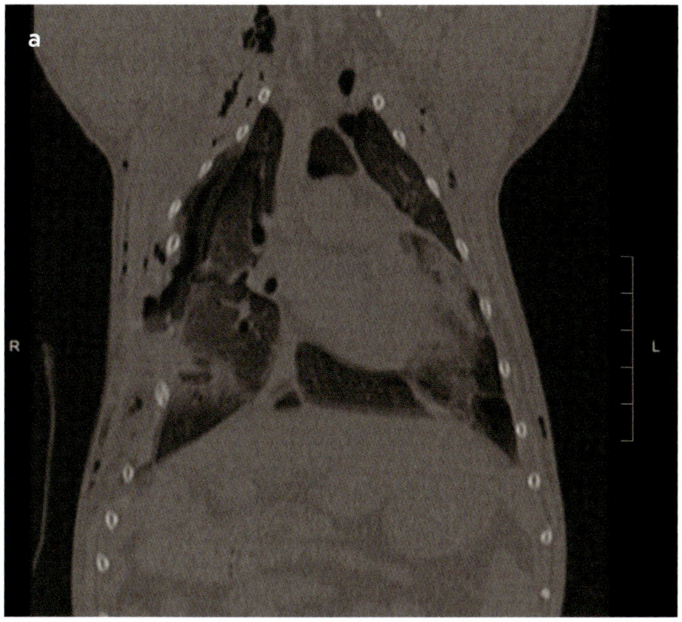

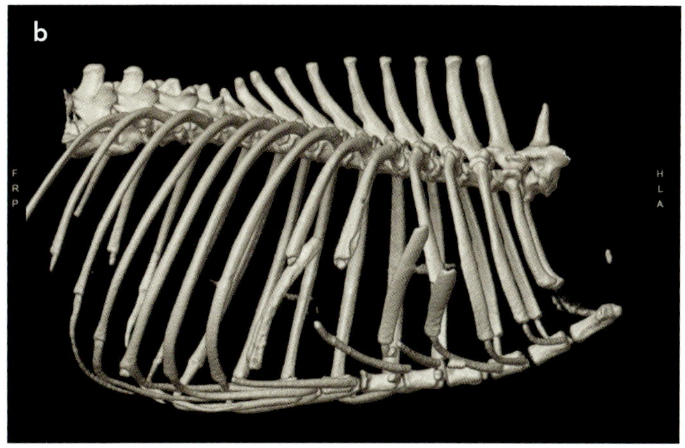

Figure 23.5 Computed tomography images (a) in a dorsal plane and (b) 3D reconstruction showing a large defect in the right thoracic wall associated with rib fractures (4th–7th) consistent with a flail chest in an 8-year-old Miniature Pinscher attacked by a dog. Images courtesy of Matteo Rossanese.

Treatment

Initial management is based upon initial triage and physical examination and is similar to that outlined in the "Thoracic trauma" section above. More specifically to flail chest, patients should be placed in lateral recumbency with the flail segment down. This reduces outward segment movement, particularly during expiration, and thus diminishes pain.[16] The segment, however, is still free to move inwards during inspiration.

Point-of-care ultrasonography can be utilized to diagnose pneumothorax or pleural effusion or to evidence pulmonary contusion or consolidation. Furthermore, ultrasonography can guide thoracocentesis to evacuate the pleural space of clinically significant air or fluid. If this imaging modality is not available, thoracocentesis can be performed blindly (see Chapter 22).

Supplemental oxygen should always be administered to patients in respiratory distress. Increasing the percentage of fraction of inspired oxygen in trauma patients will often improve hypoxemia due to hypoventilation or impaired gaseous exchange.

Due to the severity of trauma to intrathoracic structures and the flail chest, animals nearing respiratory failure may require emergency intubation and positive-pressure mechanical ventilation; despite ongoing flail segment movement, the paradoxical nature will be abolished.

Once the patient has been stabilized, the flail segment can either be externally splinted or surgically stabilized via internal fixation. External splinting can be a definitive stabilization technique until complete rib healing, or temporary prior to internal fixation. To date, there is very limited research and evidence to promote one treatment method over another. Clinicians must judge on a case-by-case basis. Given the traumatic nature of a flail chest and variation of intrathoracic injury, an approach that restores adequate cardiorespiratory function, whilst reducing pain from flail movement, should be considered. In one clinical study, there was a 16.7% overall mortality rate; 33% for surgical stabilization compared to 6.3% for external splinting.[21]

Bandaging and external splinting

Following stabilization of the patient, bandaging of a flail segment can markedly improve fracture stability, reducing pain and decreasing the risk of lung and intercostal or internal thoracic vascular injury. Although bandaging will minimize paradoxical motion, the external compressive nature of the bandage will likely internalize the flail segment, reducing ventilatory parameters.[22]
External splinting can be a definitive stabilization technique until bone union or provide temporary fixation prior to internal fracture repair. The decision may be influenced by soft tissue trauma, cardiorespiratory compromise of the patient, degree of instability of the flail segment, and flail stability afforded by the external splint alone.[16]

Technique: Bandaging[24]

The purpose of the dressing and bandage is to address the primary wounds, often caused by animal bite injury, and to reduce the associated morbidity of paradoxical abduction of the flail segment.

1. Bandaging is often performed under general anesthesia or heavy sedation and should only be performed once the patient's major body systems are stable.
2. The affected injury site is widely clipped and cleaned, via flushing or mechanical removal of debris.

3. The wounds should be appropriately managed with sterile dressings, which can be secured with skin tape.
4. Soft padding (e.g., swabs, cotton wool, or conforming bandage) can be placed gently within the defect of the flail segment to the level of the adjacent skin. This ensures reduced flail segment abduction during paradoxical movement. Again, this can be secured with tape.
5. A circumferential bandage can then be placed, ensuring there is no respiratory restriction.

Surgical technique: External splinting (Figs. 23.6 and 23.7)

1. The procedure is performed under general anesthesia, once the patient's major body systems are stable.
2. The affected injury site is widely clipped and aseptically prepared.
3. External frames can be fashioned from many materials, but they should be lightweight, malleable or adjustable to fit the flail segment, and provide adequate rigidity.
4. Percutaneous, heavy-gauge circumcostal sutures (2-0 to 1 monofilament based on patient size) are

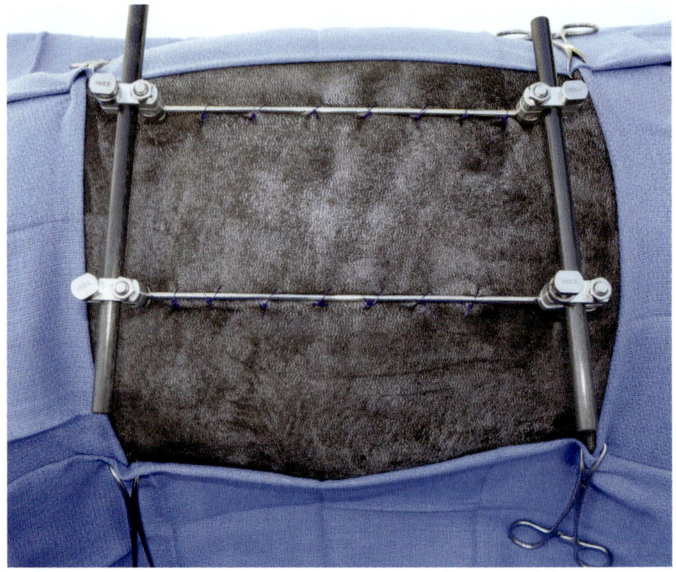

Figure 23.6 External splinting in a 35 kg Rottweiler cadaver. The animal is in left lateral recumbency, with the head to the right of the image. An external skeletal frame has been fashioned to stabilize a 3-rib flail segment. Fourteen (7 dorsal, 7 ventral) percutaneous circumcostal sutures (size 1 or 4-0 polydioxanone) have been placed across 7 ribs. The middle sutures (3 dorsal, 3 ventral) are placed to support the flail segment. The most cranial and caudal sutures (2 dorsal, 2 ventral) are placed around nonfractured ribs to provide more rigid support.

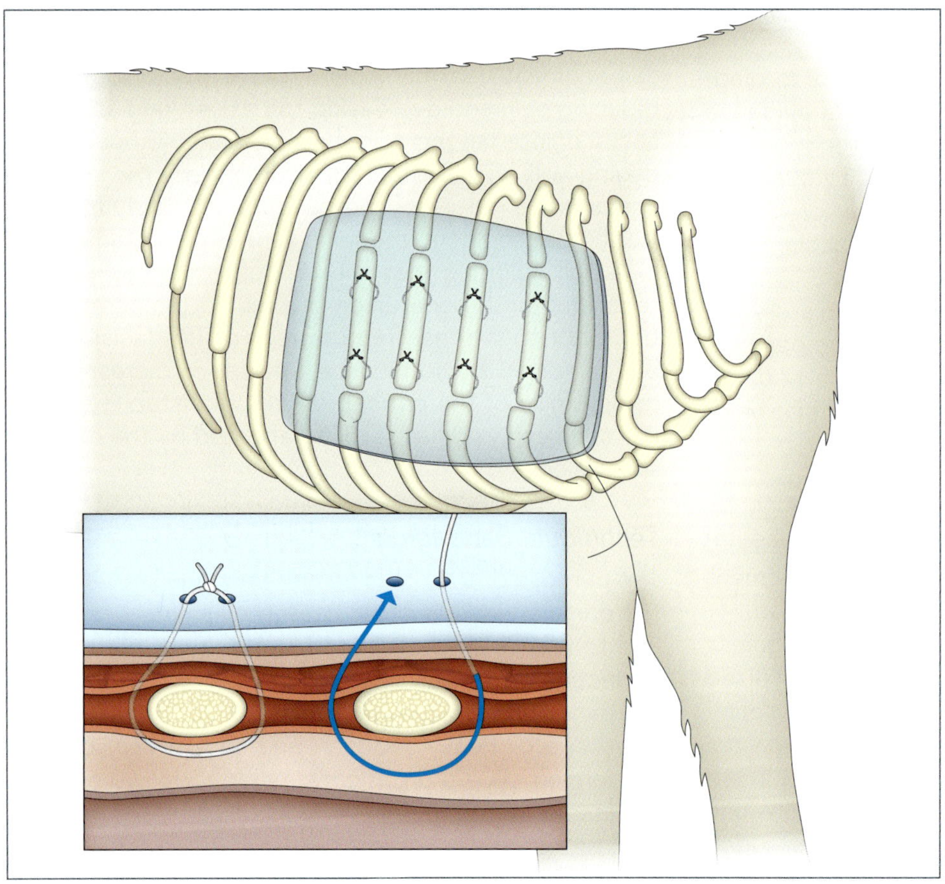

Figure 23.7 Schematic representation illustrating the repair of a flail chest by securing the affected ribs to a sheet of plastic splinting material. The sutures are placed circumferentially around the affected ribs and through holes in the splinting material.

placed around the ribs and external splint and tied securely. Ideally, two circumcostal sutures are placed per rib segment of the flail segment. If possible, the two ribs cranial and caudal to the flail segment should also be incorporated. When placing these sutures, care should be taken to avoid iatrogenic trauma to the underlying lung lobes and the intercostal arteries and veins running along the caudal edge of the ribs. Larger perforating vessels (e.g., thoracodorsal artery and vein) are located caudal to the shoulder region.
5. Depending on the degree of trauma and external splint placement, an indwelling thoracostomy tube can be placed to monitor for pneumo- or hemothorax.
6. A circumferential bandage can then be placed for protection, ensuring there is no respiratory restriction.

Surgical stabilization of a flail segment

Surgical repair is indicated if clinical signs associated with the flail segment do not resolve. The techniques for flail fixation are similar to those for rib fixation (see above). Again, the goal of surgical stabilization of a flail segment is to improve ventilatory parameters (tidal volume, respiratory rate, minute volume) by reducing the internalization of the flail segment during paradoxical motion.[22] Fracture stability will also reduce associated pain.

Postoperative management

Peri- and postoperative care is similar to that described in the "Rib fractures" section above; however, the external bandage or splint should be regularly assessed to monitor for complications. Regardless of the stabilization technique used, fibrocartilaginous callus formed during secondary bone healing will develop and mature over 2–6 weeks, whilst complete bone union occurs in 8–12 weeks. External splints can be removed 2–4 weeks after placement, depending on patient recovery and flail segment stability.[18] Healing may be dependent on vascularity and soft tissue trauma to the affected area.

Outcome

No adverse effects or complications were noted in external splinting in a report of two dogs and one cat with traumatically induced flail chest.[25] Furthermore, there was no significant difference in mortality between patients undergoing conservative management or flail segment stabilization. Similarly, the use of silk fiber-reinforced polycaprolactone plates in multiple rib fractures has showed good biocompatibility and mechanical strength leading to healing in an experimental model.[26] Cats with flail chest, pleural effusion, or diaphragmatic hernia are significantly more likely to die than cats without each injury.[8]

Currently, it is not possible to provide specific recommendations regarding patients with flail chest. Irrespective of the stabilization method utilized, a good outcome is expected with appropriate cardiopulmonary treatment, supportive care, and ongoing monitoring. A flail chest is more indicative of the degree of trauma the patient has sustained.

Penetrating thoracic injury

Penetrating injury to the thorax is frequently encountered in dogs and cats, with animal bite wounds being the most common form.[2] Other types of penetrating trauma include lacerations, gunshot injury, or impalement with sharp objects. The most common sharp objects causing penetrating chest injuries are wooden foreign bodies, typically sticks that have been chased; however, other reports include migrating grass seeds or awns and porcupine quills.[3,27]
Each type of penetrating injury is associated with slightly different pathology and morbidity. Animal bite injury causes initial soft tissue penetration by teeth and crushing injury. This can be followed by laceration (tension and compression forces) of the deeper tissues, as animals will often shake their head during the bite. Bite injury will often contaminate the thoracic wall or intrathoracic structures with bacteria, posing a risk for sepsis. Bite wounds can vary in visual presentation depending on the bite force and size and the degree of shaking causing lacerating injury.[28]
Impalement injury with wooden sticks can be visually impressive, with large foreign material visible within the soft tissues of the thoracic wall. There may be large amounts of organic contamination. Conversely, gunshot wounds may have minimal external evidence of trauma. These wounds tend to cause trauma deeper within the chest cavity and are often associated with hemothorax, pneumothorax, or massive hemorrhage.[4]

Clinical presentation and diagnosis

If there is significant injury to the thoracic wall or penetration into the thoracic cavity, animals can present with a wide range of clinical signs, varying in their clinical severity. Patients can exhibit dyspnea, tachypnea, hypoxemia, altered breathing patterns, or be close to respiratory fatigue and arrest.
Diagnosis of penetrating thoracic injury can be challenging depending on the type of inciting trauma. Pneumothorax or pneumomediastinum, pleural effusion (e.g., hemothorax), rib fractures, flail chest, lung contusions, subcutaneous gas, and radiodense or radiolucent foreign bodies can be visualized on plain orthogonal radiographs. CT with systemic contrast provides a higher degree of sensitivity and detail when evaluating tho-

racic trauma. If available, and if the patient is stable for sedation or anesthesia, it is the author's preference to perform a whole-body CT scan.[12]

Treatment

Initial major body system assessment followed by stabilization of the cardiopulmonary system are of critical importance. Supplemental oxygen, adequate multimodal analgesia, and judicious use of intravenous fluid therapy are commonly required and implemented during initial stabilization. Serial secondary and tertiary assessments determine further injury to other body systems (e.g., musculoskeletal). If large impalement foreign bodies (e.g., sticks) are in situ on presentation, they should not be removed initially. The foreign body may assist with hemostasis via tamponade of blood vessels, and removal may cause further trauma and massive bleeding. The foreign body should be removed in a controlled setting, usually during surgical exploration under anesthesia, when potential severe hemorrhage can be addressed in a controlled and safe manner.

Due to the nature of penetrating injuries, initial respiratory distress may result from loss of integrity of the pleural space causing pneumothorax, bleeding causing hemothorax, direct trauma to the lung (contusion or laceration), or pain from chest wall and rib fractures.

Surgical intervention of dogs suffering from gunshot wounds is based on the degree of intrathoracic trauma to vital structures, and whether pneumothorax or hemothorax can be managed adequately via thoracostomy tube alone. Stabilization of the patient and appropriate wound management is generally adequate for most gunshot wounds. Exploratory thoracotomy with the purpose of bullet removal is not indicated, even in stable patients.

Following stabilization, treatment can vary depending on the cause of penetration. Penetrating injury to the thorax should be assessed for intrathoracic disorders via radiography, CT, thoracocentesis, or focused ultrasonography. Clinically significant hemothorax or pneumothorax should be therapeutically drained until the animal's respiratory function improves. Concerns for impaired respiration and ventilation capabilities include oxygen saturation below 95% (measured via pulse oximetry), partial pressure of arterial oxygen below 80 mmHg or less than around 4–5 times that of fraction of inspired oxygen (generally 21% at room air), partial pressure of carbon dioxide above 60 mmHg, or marked respiratory effort, despite supplemental oxygenation.[13]

Indications for thoracic bite wound exploration include suspected severe injury to the soft tissues of the chest wall, rib fractures, presence of flail segment, and presence of hemothorax or pneumothorax. Decontamination should be performed as soon as possible; however, the animal should ideally be stabilized over a period of at least 2–4 hours prior to anesthesia and surgery.[28]

Early porcupine quill removal is recommended to prevent secondary migration. Removal is substantially easier if performed early, as quills may weaken.[3]

Penetrating injuries generally warrant antimicrobial therapy. Empirical broad-spectrum antibiotics should be initiated on presentation and then be dictated further by bacterial culture and sensitivity results, particularly if the animal is immunocompromised or the wounds are from bite injury. It is recommended that the wound is cultured at the time of surgery, following debridement and flushing. For deep wounds, tissue samples can also be submitted for culture and sensitivity testing.

Surgical technique (Fig. 23.8)

1. Once the patient has been anesthetized, sterile water-soluble gel is placed within the wound to minimize further contamination. The region should be clipped from the wound edges to well beyond any visible bruising or trauma. Wide clipping is of great importance when dealing with wound management, as it reduces ongoing contamination, allows a wide region to be draped in the surgical field so the true extent of penetrating injury can be explored, and permits ongoing assessment of soft tissue viability. Due to the nature of the tension, compression, and crushing injury in bite wounds, nonviable skin and underlying soft tissues can take weeks to completely declare themselves. The surrounding skin should be aseptically prepared using standard protocols (e.g., 0.05% chlorhexidine diacetate solution). At therapeutic concentrations, most antiseptics are cytotoxic to fibroblasts and keratinocytes, impairing wound healing.[29] It is acceptable for open wounds to be directly cleaned until gross debris is removed.
2. Further decontamination of the wound with large volumes of sterile crystalloid fluids at around 8–15 psi can be utilized to overcome adhesive forces of bacteria to the wound. This is also strong enough to flush away unwanted debris without causing further trauma to healthy tissue. Low to moderate manual force using a 35 mL syringe coupled to an 18–20-gauge syringe generates adequate pressure for wound irrigation.[30]
3. Penetrating wounds should be explored to their complete extent, even if this involves exploration of the thoracic cavity. All questionable or nonviable soft tissue should be excised.
4. Primary closure or reconstruction of the traumatic defect should only be performed if there is tension-free closure and the soft tissues are healthy. It is recommended to use absorbable suture and to utilize the least amount of suture required to minimize bacterial

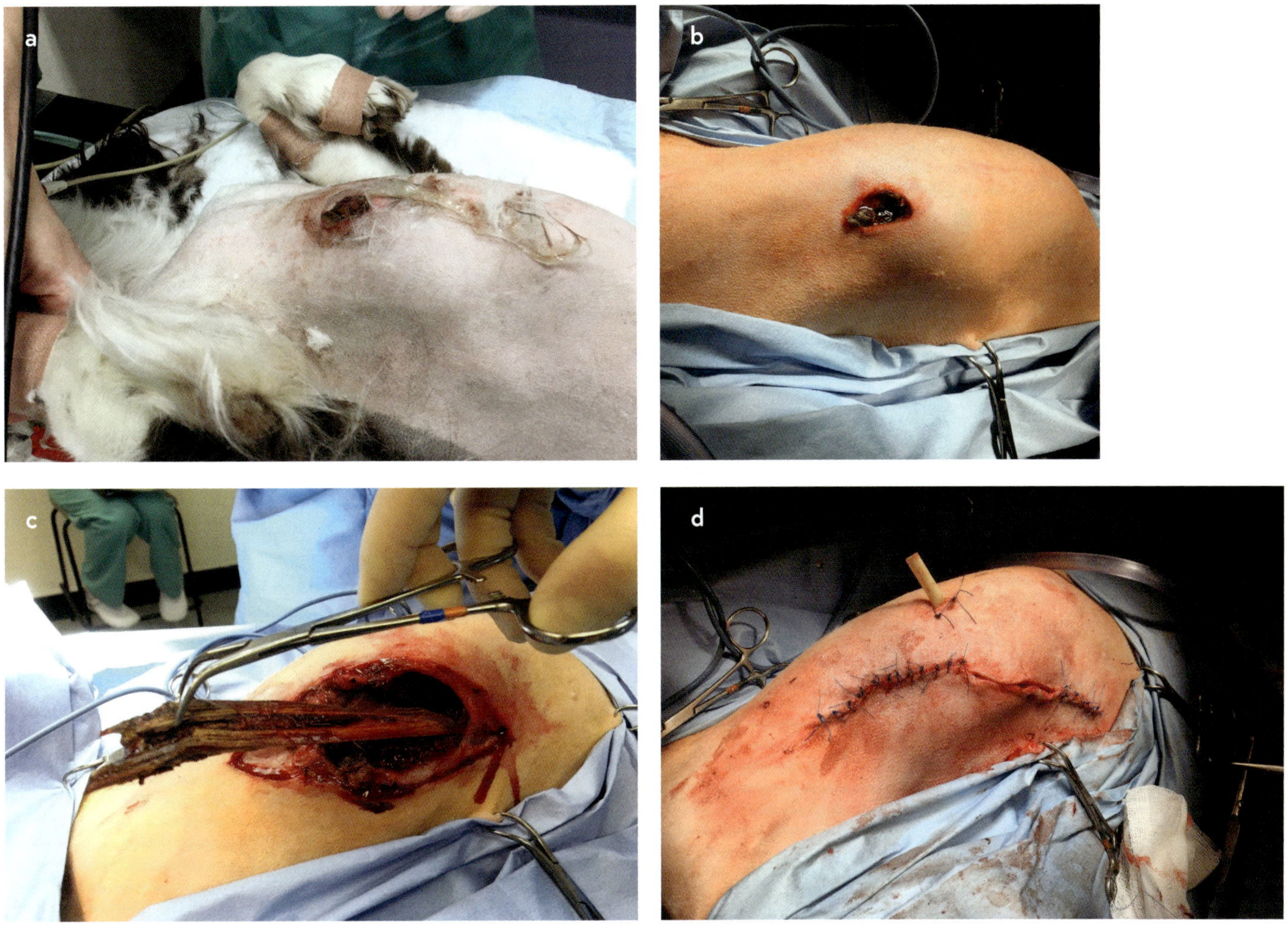

Figure 23.8 Surgical treatment of a penetrating thoracic wall injury over the mid to right lateral thorax of an English Springer Spaniel dog. Cranial is to the left of the images. (a) Placement of sterile water-soluble gel within the wound to minimize further contamination. (b) Patient aseptically prepared for exploratory surgery. Note that wide clipping has been performed (as the foreign material and true extent of the wound are not known), the area has been cleaned, and the surgical site has been draped widely. The foreign material is left in situ for safe surgical removal and wound evaluation. (c) Removal of the sharp wooden foreign body. (d) Primary wound closure after mechanical debridement and flushing with isotonic crystalloids. The midsection has not been closed to facilitate drainage and will heal via secondary intention. Note that one end of a Penrose drain has been exited ventrally to further facilitate drainage.

contamination. Thoracic wall reconstruction to maintain integrity of the pleural space as best as possible should be prioritized. This can involve circumcostal rib sutures in a basket-weave pattern (see above) if there is intercostal muscle laceration. Ipsilateral diaphragmatic advancement can be useful for reconstructing thoracic defects from caudal ribs 8 to 13.[9] Larger thoracic wall defects can be reconstructed using latissimus dorsi, rectus abdominis, or external abdominal oblique muscle flaps. Myofascial flaps permit more robust autologous closure that does not rely upon potentially already compromised soft tissues. Fractured ribs can be internally stabilized (see above) or small fragments removed if comminution is present. Commercial products (e.g., polypropylene or polytetrafluoroethylene mesh) and an overlying abdominal omental pedicle flap can be utilized; however, the risk of implant infection, particularly following a bite wound, needs to be carefully considered.[9]

5. Penetrating injury and subsequent debridement can leave significant dead space. Drains can be placed to reduce potential fluid accumulation, which can reduce wound healing and increase infection risk. Both active and passive drains can be successfully used for management of penetrating injuries. If there is likely to be significant ongoing fluid production, the trauma involves the ventral or most gravity-dependent region of the thorax, or there is intrathoracic cavity involvement, it is the author's preference to use closed active drains. For open wounds, negative-pressure wound therapy can also be considered.[31]

Postoperative management

Animals may often require intensive monitoring and ongoing critical care. Kirby's rule of 20 is a useful and comprehensive checklist for practitioners to follow when supporting animals postoperatively.[32] Specifically to penetrating injury to the thorax, the cardiorespiratory function, adequate pain control, wound healing and bandages, drains, appropriate antibiotics, and nutrition status are prioritized.

If there is massive trauma, animals must be monitored for systemic inflammatory response syndrome and sepsis. Postoperative deterioration could be caused by a "second-hit" phenomenon; that is, animals are subjected to systemic inflammation from the inciting trauma, contamination, or infection (first hit), while the subsequent debriding and reconstructive surgery generate further inflammation (second hit).[33]

Outcome

With appropriate stabilization and treatment, penetrating injuries to the thorax are associated with a good outcome, and survival is reported in up to 92% of cases. In dogs suffering from thoracic bite wounds, the presence of pleural effusion on initial presentation and positive bacterial cultures were associated with a 12.1 and 23.4 times higher odds of mortality, respectively. Reported survival rates are around 85%, with sepsis or systemic inflammatory response syndrome being the most common cause of mortality (80%). In cats suffering from thoracic dog bite wounds, specific wound management type did not influence mortality; survival rates are reported to be 73%–79%. Animals suffering from gunshot wounds had an overall survival rate of 86%; however, this was not exclusive to thoracic injury.[4–6,34]

KEEP IN MIND

- Common presentations of animals with thoracic trauma are related to impaired respiratory function, due to pain, chest wall disease, or pulmonary contusion, or thoracic wall injury, including devitalized, contaminated, or septic open wounds.
- Thoracic trauma severe enough to cause rib fractures or flail chest in dogs and cats is likely associated with clinically significant intrathoracic injury.
- Most rib fractures can be managed with nonsurgical, conservative management, prioritizing analgesia and cardiopulmonary support.
- A flail segment is detached from the thoracic wall and moves in a paradoxical manner to the rest of the chest cavity, reducing respiratory parameters.
- External bandaging or splinting of a flail segment and chest can improve clinical signs.
- Flail segments can be surgically fixated or stabilized concurrently, via plate fixation or interfragmentary wiring, but the best technique has not yet been established.
- Bite wounds may have severe soft tissue and intrathoracic involvement even if externally they only appear as cutaneous puncture wounds.
- Wooden sticks and other impalement foreign bodies should be removed in a controlled setting, usually during surgical exploration under general anesthesia.
- Indications for surgical exploration of penetrating wounds include significant injury to the chest wall and presence of rib fractures, flail segment, hemothorax, or pneumothorax.
- Irrespective of etiology, penetrating injury to the thorax can have very good outcomes with appropriate management. Reported survival for cats and dogs is around 73%–92%.

References

1. Piegari G et al. Cardiac laceration following non-penetrating chest trauma in dog and cat. *Forensic Sci Int*. 2018; 290:e5–e8.
2. Risselada M, de Rooster H, Taeymans O, van Bree H. Penetrating injuries in dogs and cats. A study of 16 cases. *Vet Comp Orthop Traumatol*. 2008; 21(5):434–439.
3. Mehler SJ. Penetrating injury in the dog and cat. In: Aronson LR (ed.). *Small Animal Surgical Emergencies*, 2nd ed. Wiley Blackwell; 2022. pp. 600–612.
4. Olsen LE, Streeter EM, DeCook RR. Review of gunshot injuries in cats and dogs and utility of a triage scoring system to predict short-term outcome: 37 cases (2003–2008). *J Am Vet Med Assoc*. 2014; 245(8):923–929.
5. Frykfors von Hekkel AK, Pegram C, Halfacree ZJ. Thoracic dog bite wounds in dogs: A retrospective study of 123 cases (2003–2016). *Vet Surg*. 2020; 49(4):694–703.
6. Frykfors von Hekkel AK, Halfacree ZJ. Thoracic dog bite wounds in cats: A retrospective study of 22 cases (2005–2015). *J Feline Med Surg*. 2020; 22(2):146–152.
7. Lefman S, Prittie JE. High-rise syndrome in cats and dogs. *J Vet Emerg Crit Care (San Antonio)*. 2022; 32(5):571–581.
8. Kraje BJ et al. Intrathoracic and concurrent orthopedic injury associated with traumatic rib fracture in cats: 75 cases (1980–1998). *J Am Vet Med Assoc*. 2000; 216(1):51–54.

9. Hunt G. Thoracic wall. In: Johnston SA, Tobias KM (eds.). *Veterinary Surgery: Small Animal*, 2nd ed. St. Louis, MO: Elsevier; 2018. pp. 2001–2018.
10. Ganie FA et al. Lung contusion: A clinico-pathological entity with unpredictable clinical course. *Bull Emerg Trauma*. 2013; 1(1):7–16.
11. Sigrist NE, Adamik KN, Doherr MG, Spreng DE. Evaluation of respiratory parameters at presentation as clinical indicators of the respiratory localization in dogs and cats with respiratory distress. *J Vet Emerg Crit Care (San Antonio)*. 2011; 21(1):13–23.
12. Dozeman ET, Prittie JE, Fischetti AJ. Utilization of whole body computed tomography in polytrauma patients. *J Vet Emerg Crit Care (San Antonio)*. 2020; 30(1):28–33.
13. Grubb T et al. 2020 AAHA anesthesia and monitoring guidelines for dogs and cats. *J Am Anim Hosp Assoc*. 2020; 56(2):59–82.
14. McCarthy D et al. Use of the animal trauma triage score, RibScore, modified RibScore and other clinical factors for prognostication in canine rib fractures. *Vet Comp Orthop Traumatol*. 2018; 31(4):239–245.
15. Shahar R, Shamir M, Johnston DE. A technique for management of bite wounds of the thoracic wall in small dogs. *Vet Surg*. 1997; 26(1):45–50.
16. Orton EC. *Small Animal Thoracic Surgery*. Philadelphia, PA: Williams & Wilkins; 1995.
17. Fokin AA et al. Surgical stabilization of rib fractures: Indications, techniques, and pitfalls. *JBJS Essent Surg Tech*. 2020; 10(2):e0032.
18. Hunt GB. Thoracic wall anatomy and surgical approaches. In: Brockman DJ, Holt DE (eds.). *BSAVA Manual of Canine and Feline Head, Neck and Thoracic Surgery*. Gloucester, United Kingdom: British Small Animal Veterinary Association; 2005. pp. 135–143.
19. Slatter DH. *Textbook of Small Animal Surgery*, 3rd ed. Philadelphia, PA: WB Saunders; 2003.
20. Tobias KM et al. Thoracic cavity. In: Johnston SA, Tobias KM (eds.). *Veterinary Surgery: Small Animal*, 2nd ed. St. Louis, MO: Elsevier; 2018. pp. 2019–2047.
21. Olsen D et al. Clinical management of flail chest in dogs and cats: A retrospective study of 24 cases (1989–1999). *J Am Anim Hosp Assoc*. 2002; 38(4):315–320.
22. Gyhra A et al. Experimental flail chest: Ventilatory function with fixation of flail segment in internal and external position. *J Trauma*. 1996; 40(6):977–979.
23. Dancer SC, Le Roux C, Fosgate GT, Kirberger RM. Radiography is less sensitive relative to CT for detecting thoracic radiographic changes in dogs affected by blunt trauma secondary to a motor vehicle accident. *Vet Radiol Ultrasound*. 2019; 60(6):648–658.
24. McCarthy D et al. Flail chest: Diagnosis & bandaging. Clinician's Brief, last updated November 2016. Available at https://www.cliniciansbrief.com/article/flail-chest-diagnosis-bandaging.
25. McAnulty JF. A simplified method for stabilization of flail chest injuries in small animals. *J Am Anim Hosp Assoc*. 1995; 31(2):137–141.
26. Huang KN et al. Stabilization of multiple rib fractures in a canine model. *J Surg Res*. 2014; 192(2):621–627.
27. Bufalari A et al. Intracardiac porcupine quill migration in a dog: Multimodality imaging findings and surgical management. *Vet Sci*. 2022; 9(12):700.
28. Holt D, Thawley V. Bite wounds. In: Aronson LR (ed.). *Small Animal Surgical Emergencies*, 2nd ed. Wiley Blackwell; 2022. pp. 575–685.
29. Damour O et al. Cytotoxicity evaluation of antiseptics and antibiotics on cultured human fibroblasts and keratinocytes. *Burns*. 1992; 18(6):479–485.
30. Chatterjee JS. A critical review of irrigation techniques in acute wounds. *Int Wound J*. 2005; 2(3):258–265.
31. Nolff MC, Pieper K, Meyer-Lindenberg A. Treatment of a perforating thoracic bite wound in a dog with negative pressure wound therapy. *J Am Vet Med Assoc*. 2016; 249(7):794–800.
32. Kirby R, Linklater A (eds.). *Monitoring and Intervention for the Critically Ill Small Animal: The Rule of 20*. John Wiley & Sons; 2016.
33. Tschoeke SK et al. The early second hit in trauma management augments the proinflammatory immune response to multiple injuries. *J Trauma*. 2007; 62(6):1396–1403.
34. Cabon Q et al. Thoracic bite trauma in dogs and cats: A retrospective study of 65 cases. *Vet Comp Orthop Traumatol*. 2015; 28(6):448–454.

Chapter 24

Pericardial disease

Matteo Rossanese, Daniel J. Brockman

The pericardium is a double-layered sac that encloses the heart and the major blood vessels at the base of the heart. The pericardial space found between the two layers normally contains a small amount of serous fluid, which serves as a lubricant to facilitate heart motion. The pericardium plays an important role in maintaining the heart's normal position within the thorax, helping to balance the output of the right and left ventricles, and preventing acute distension of the heart.[1–4]

Diseases of the pericardium are typically caused by an abnormal accumulation of fluid within the pericardial space: a pericardial effusion. The pericardium is relatively inelastic and noncompliant, although it can become distended over time. Thus, acute small-volume pericardial effusion and chronic large-volume pericardial effusion can both disrupt normal cardiac function by causing cardiac tamponade and impairing cardiac filling. Although myocardial contractility is not directly affected, reduced coronary perfusion can occur during tamponade, which reduces myocardial perfusion directly and impairs systolic and diastolic function, ultimately reducing cardiac output and perfusion of distant organs and leading to cardiogenic shock and death.[5] Pericardial effusion in small animals is most commonly associated with either cardiac or pericardial neoplasia or is idiopathic hemorrhagic effusion. Trauma, rupture of the left atrium secondary to degenerative mitral valve disease, anticoagulant intoxication, and pericarditis are among other possible causes. In the absence of an identifiable underlying cause, the effusion is considered idiopathic.

Clinical presentation and diagnosis

Pericardial effusion is more common in older and larger breeds of dogs, with the Golden Retriever and St. Bernard breeds overrepresented. Clinical signs may vary depending on the rate of accumulation of the fluid and its overall volume. Dogs with cardiac tamponade may present with collapse due to hypotension or progressive right-sided congestive heart failure, reflecting poor cardiac output and venous congestion that frequently results in ascites. Other clinical signs are exercise intolerance, weakness, lethargy, anorexia, coughing, dyspnea, abdominal distension, and vomiting.

On physical examination, classic features of cardiac tamponade include the (Beck's) triad of muffled heart sounds, jugular vein distension, and pulsus paradoxus (variation in peripheral pulse quality associated with the respiration phase). Other findings include weak femoral pulses, tachycardia, hepatomegaly, free peritoneal fluid, and pleural effusion associated with respiratory signs. Animals presenting with cardiogenic shock have increased capillary refill time, pale mucous membranes, weak pulses, and tachycardia.

On thoracic radiographs, acute pericardial effusion may not result in any appreciable changes, whereas chronic pericardial effusion results in an enlargement of the cardiac silhouette, with sharp borders and the classic globoid shape seen on lateral and ventrodorsal projections. Other findings associated with cardiac tamponade include pleural effusion, caudal vena cava distension, hepatomegaly, and ascites.

ECG may reveal sinus rhythm along with rhythmic changes in the size of the QRS complex (electrical alternans) as the heart changes position within the fluid-filled pericardium. Supraventricular arrhythmias can occur as can ST segment elevation, indicating myocardial hypoxia.

Hematology and serum biochemistry may reveal nonregenerative (or poorly regenerative) anemia in animals with hemorrhagic effusion and prerenal azotemia, secondary to low cardiac output.

Ultrasound examination is the diagnostic test of choice, as it is highly sensitive for detecting small volumes of pericardial effusion, identifying an underlying mass or cardiac condition, and documenting tamponade. A thoracic point-of-care ultrasound (tPOCUS) exam should be initially performed to identify any pericardial effusion, described as an anechoic space between the epicardium and pericardial sac (Fig. 24.1; Video 24.1). Collapse of the right atrium, and sometimes the right ventricle, during diastole suggests increased intrapericardial pressure and cardiac tamponade.

Video 24.1. Right parasternal long axis and right parasternal short axis echocardiographic views in a dog with pericardial effusion. Note the anechoic fluid between the heart and the pericardial sac. Video courtesy of Brogan Atkinson.

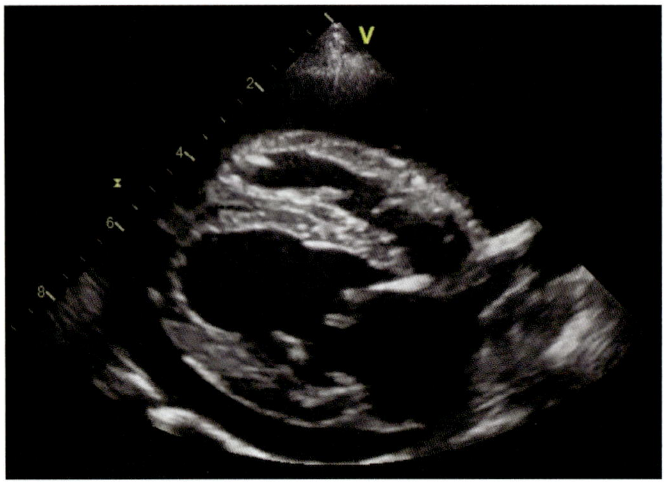

Figure 24.1 Right parasternal long axis view in a dog with pericardial effusion. Note the anechoic fluid between the heart and the pericardial sac. Image courtesy of Brogan Atkinson.

Treatment

In the case of cardiac tamponade that is not caused by an atrial rupture secondary to myxomatous mitral valve disease, initial stabilization requires immediate pericardiocentesis with a needle or catheter via a right lateral thoracic approach (5th intercostal space) under ultrasound guidance (Fig. 24.2).[5] Full aseptic technique, sedation, and local anesthetic infiltration should be used. Continuous ECG monitoring is recommended to rapidly identify ventricular arrhythmias in case of contact of the needle or catheter with the heart. In hypotensive animals without underlying heart disease, an initial intravenous crystalloid fluid bolus of 10–20 mL/kg along with continuous monitoring should be considered to support cardiac output and blood pressure. Once the needle or catheter is in position, the fluid in the pericardial sac should be drained and submitted for cytology, biochemical analysis, and bacteriology (Video 24.2). Resolution of cardiac tamponade should lead to decreased heart rate, increased amplitude of QRS complexes on ECG, decreased central venous pressure, and improved pulse quality (Video 24.3). Pericardiectomy should be considered if pericardial effusion recurs and repeated pericardiocentesis is required. Pericardiectomy can be curative for idiopathic pericardial effusion and palliative for neoplastic pericardial effusion, as it increases the surface area for fluid absorption (pleural cavity) and prevents cardiac tamponade.[1,4,6] Different techniques and

Video 24.2. Pericardiocentesis using a centesis catheter in the same patient as in Figure 24.2. An over-the-needle catheter is advanced into the pericardial space. The needle/stylet is removed and the centesis catheter advanced and connected to a closed system with a one-way valve. This prevents fluid from flowing back into the pericardium and allows accurate fluid measurement and rapid draining maintaining sterility. Video courtesy of Hannah Brodie Leigh and Simon Cook.

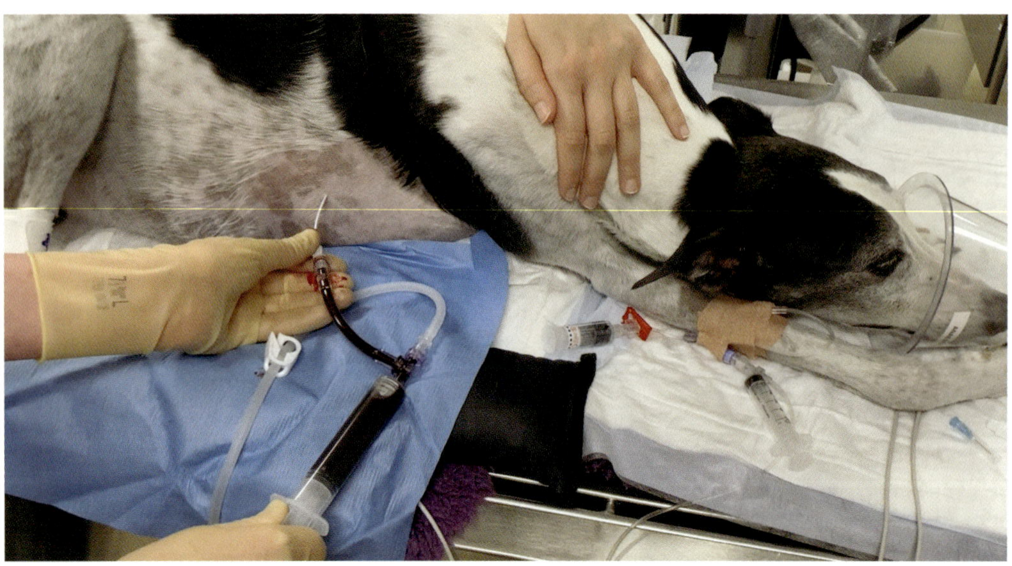

Figure 24.2 Pericardiocentesis using a centesis catheter connected to a closed collection system. Note that the procedure is being performed with the patient sedated; oxygen is provided via an oxygen mask. Image courtesy of Hannah Brodie Leigh and Simon Cook.

Video 24.3. Intraoperative video of a dog with pericardial effusion. Note the improvement in blood pressure and heart rate after the opening of the pericardium.

Video 24.4. Subphrenic (subtotal) pericardiectomy using a vessel-sealing device.

approaches are available for pericardiectomy in dogs and cats;[6,7] this chapter describes subphrenic pericardiectomy through a right intercostal thoracotomy.

Surgical technique

1. Intermittent positive-pressure ventilation (IPPV) is required for this procedure.
2. A right 5th intercostal thoracotomy is performed (see Chapter 4). A left 5th intercostal thoracotomy or a median sternotomy can also be used.
3. Moist swabs are used to retract the right lung lobes and expose the heart.
4. The right phrenic nerve should be identified and retracted dorsally (Fig. 24.3).
5. Pericardiectomy should be performed using electrosurgery, a harmonic instrument, or a vessel-sealing device to reduce bleeding. Curved Metzenbaum scissors can also be used. Care should be taken to avoid phrenic nerve injury.
6. An initial window in the pericardium is made by grasping the pericardium with a pair of forceps and retracting it away from the heart (Fig. 24.3; Video 24.4).
7. The fluid in the pericardial sac should be aspirated and submitted for cytology, biochemical analysis, and bacteriology.
8. A T-shaped incision is made in the pericardium (Video 24.5):
   - The first incision is made ventral and parallel to the right phrenic nerve and heart base. The two incisions can be interchanged (Fig. 24.4).
   - The second incision is made from the base to the apex of the heart (Fig. 24.5).
9. Stay sutures (2-0 or 3-0 absorbable or nonabsorbable monofilament) can be placed in the pericardial incision edges to help with manipulation and orientation (Fig. 24.6).
10. The incision should continue around the base of the heart ventral to the right phrenic nerve (Fig. 24.7).
11. The heart can be retracted and elevated by an assistant to improve visualization of the contralateral side of the pericardium. Communication with the anesthetist is critical to manage any hemodynamic changes (reduction in venous return and systemic blood pressure).

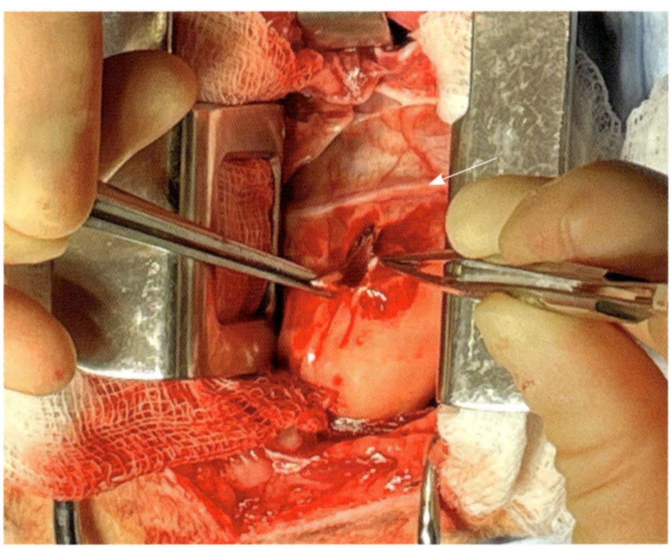

Figure 24.3 The pericardium has been opened (between the forceps) to alleviate the pression caused by the pericardial effusion. The right phrenic nerve is identified (arrow); this represents the dorsal landmark for performing a subphrenic pericardiectomy. The approach was through a right 5th intercostal thoracotomy.

Video 24.5. Subphrenic pericardiectomy in a 6-year-old Maine Coon. Note the initial pericardial window made to release the pericardial fluid. Pericardiectomy was performed with a vertical incision followed by a horizontal incision ventral and parallel to the phrenic nerve.

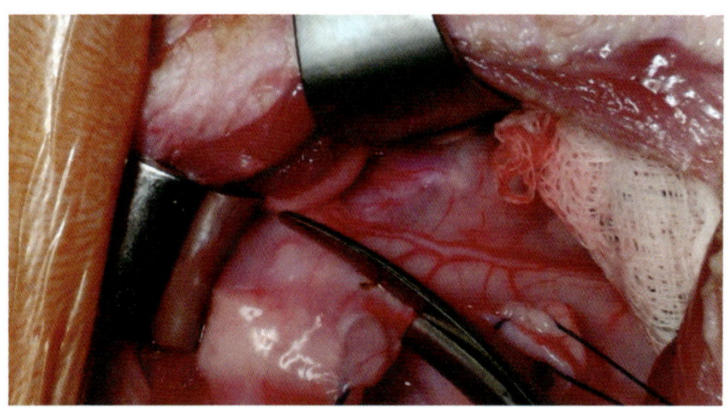

Figure 24.4 Horizontal incision of the pericardium ventral and parallel to the right phrenic nerve using a pair of Metzenbaum scissors.

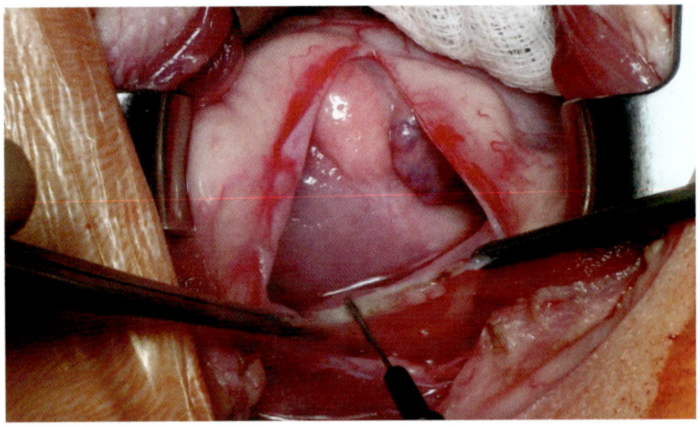

Figure 24.5 Vertical incision of the pericardium toward the apex of the heart using electrocautery. Care should be taken to protect the epicardium.

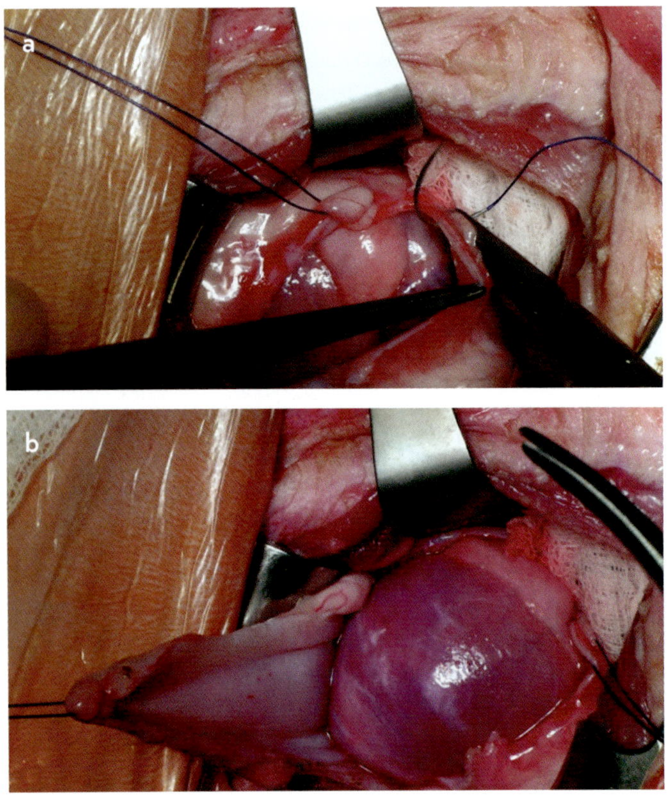

Figure 24.6 (a) Placement of two stay sutures on the edges of the incision. (b) This helps manipulate the pericardium during excision.

12. The pericardiophrenic ligament is transected using electrosurgery, a harmonic instrument, or a vessel-sealing device.
13. The cut edges of the pericardium should be inspected for bleeding.
14. Before closure, a thoracostomy tube should be placed (see Chapter 5).
15. The swabs retracting the lungs are removed from the thorax, and a swab count must be performed.

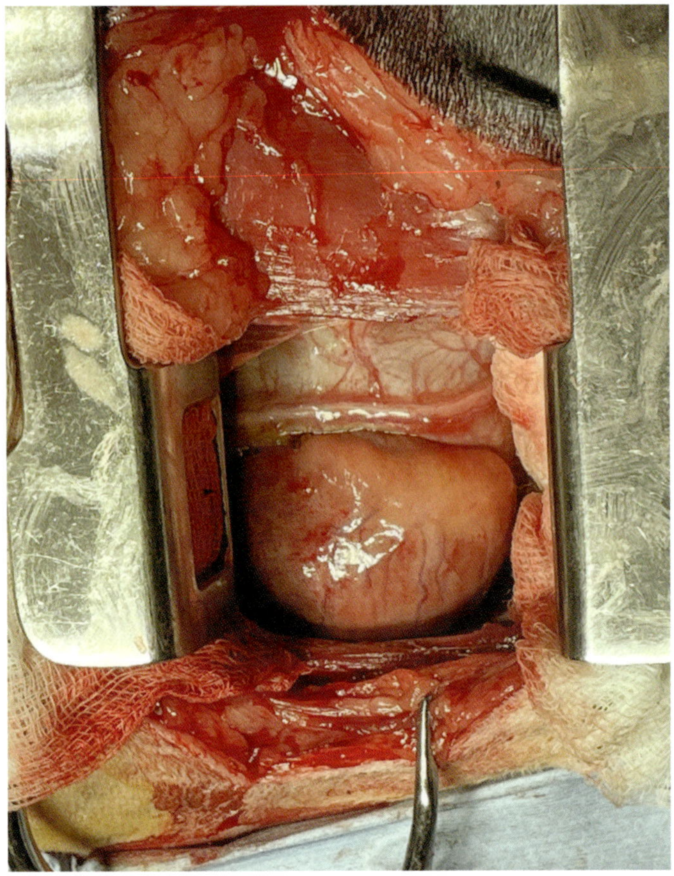

Figure 24.7 Intraoperative appearance following subphrenic pericardiectomy. Note the horizontal incision running parallel to the right phrenic nerve.

16. Routine postoperative thoracotomy care is recommended (see Chapter 5).
17. Closure is performed as described in Chapter 4.

Postoperative management

After pericardiectomy, postoperative monitoring for the first 24–48 hours is essential. Pain, hypoxemia, pleural effusion, and residual pneumothorax should be corrected. Vital signs including heart rate, blood pressure, respiratory pattern, and temperature must be checked for the first 24–48 hours. Oxygen supplementation should be given to patients with arterial oxygen saturation lower than 95% or if the $P(A–a)O_2$ gradient is higher than 20 mmHg.

The thoracostomy tube should be checked every 2–4 hours initially to remove any pleural effusion and/or residual pneumothorax. The amount of air or fluid retrieved should be recorded and the milliliters of fluid and air per kilogram of body weight should be calculated over a period of at least 8–12 hours; this guides the surgeon on when to remove the thoracostomy tube. Pain management options may include opioids, nonsteroidal anti-inflammatory drugs, or interpleural local anesthetics, depending on the patient's individual needs. The surgical incision should be monitored closely for any signs of infection or dehiscence, and appropriate patient activity restrictions should be implemented postoperatively.

Outcome

Complications associated with subphrenic pericardiectomy include hemorrhage, phrenic nerve injury, and recurrence of either pericardial or pleural effusion. Specifically, pleural effusion is the most common complication, with a poor prognosis reported for dogs developing pleural effusion more than 30 days after pericardiectomy.[1,4,6,9] The prognosis for animals undergoing pericardiectomy for pericardial effusion depends on the underlying disease process.[3,9] The procedure is considered curative for idiopathic pericardial effusion, with an excellent long-term (>3 years) outcome reported in 70%–100% of animals. Surgery is considered successful at palliating clinical signs in dogs with aortic body tumors, with a reported median survival time of 730 days, whereas it is not recommended as sole treatment for pericardial effusion secondary to hemangiosarcoma due to the grave prognosis; serial pericardiocentesis without pericardiectomy is more appropriate if the primary tumor is left in situ.[3,9]

KEEP IN MIND

- In case of cardiac tamponade, immediate pericardiocentesis through the right 5th intercostal space under ultrasound guidance is crucial.
- The phrenic nerve is the main landmark for a subphrenic (subtotal) pericardiectomy.
- Prognosis for patients undergoing pericardiectomy for pericardial effusion depends on the underlying disease process: curative for idiopathic pericardial effusion, palliative for neoplastic pericardial effusion.

References

1. Brockman DJ. Surgery of the heart, pericardium and great vessels. In: Brockman DJ, Holt DE, Haar GT (eds.). *BSAVA Manual of Canine and Feline Head, Neck and Thoracic Surgery*, 2nd ed. BSAVA; 2018.
2. Ware WA, Bonagura JD, Scansen BA. Pericardial diseases and cardiac tumors. In: Ware WA, Bonagura JD (eds.). *Cardiovascular Disease in Companion Animals: Dog, Cat, and Horse*, 2nd ed. CRC Press; 2022.
3. Dunning D, Monnet E, Orton EC, Salman MD. Analysis of prognostic indicators for dogs with pericardial effusion: 46 cases (1985–1996). *J Am Vet Med Assoc*. 1998; 212(8): 1276–1280.
4. Tobias AH, McNiel EA. Pericardial disorders and cardiac tumors. In: Tilley LP, Smith FWK, Oyama MA, Sleeper MM (eds.). *Manual of Canine and Feline Cardiology*, 4th ed. St. Louis, MO: Saunders/Elsevier; 2005.
5. Humm KR, Keenaghan-Clark EA, Boag AK. Adverse events associated with pericardiocentesis in dogs: 85 cases (1999–2006). *J Vet Emerg Crit Care (San Antonio)*. 2009; 19(4):352–356.
6. Aronsohn MG, Carpenter JL. Surgical treatment of idiopathic pericardial effusion in the dog: 25 cases (1978–1993). *J Am Anim Hosp Assoc*. 1999; 35(6):521–525.
7. De Ridder M et al. Transdiaphragmatic pericardiectomy in dogs. *Vet Rec*. 2017; 180(4):95.
8. Case JB, Maxwell M, Aman A, Monnet EL. Outcome evaluation of a thoracoscopic pericardial window procedure or subtotal pericardectomy via thoracotomy for the treatment of pericardial effusion in dogs. *J Am Vet Med Assoc*. 2013; 242(4):493–498.
9. Ehrhart N et al. Analysis of factors affecting survival in dogs with aortic body tumors. *Vet Surg*. 2002; 31(1):44–48.

Chapter 25

Patent ductus arteriosus

Matteo Rossanese, Daniel J. Brockman

Patent ductus arteriosus (PDA) is a congenital heart defect that results from the persistence of the ductus arteriosus, a fetal blood vessel that connects the descending aorta with the main pulmonary artery (Fig. 25.1). During normal development, this vessel closes shortly after birth. In animals with PDA, however, the ductus arteriosus remains open, allowing blood to flow from the aorta to the pulmonary artery (left-to-right shunting), resulting in increased blood flow to the lungs and overloading of the left heart. This causes left atrial and ventricular dilatation and progressive left-sided congestive heart failure (Fig. 25.2).[1–4]

The exact cause of PDA is not fully understood, but it is believed to be multifactorial, with both genetic and environmental factors playing an important role. A morphometric analysis of PDAs in dogs determined that hypoplasia of the duct muscle mass and an eccentric distribution of muscular and elastic fibers were the main abnormalities causing the failure of the normal closure mechanism.[1–4] Some pure dog breeds, such as Maltese, Poodle, Keeshond, Cocker Spaniel, and Welsh Corgi, among others, are overrepresented. Female dogs also have a higher prevalence of PDA than male dogs, although the reason for this is unclear. In cats, PDA is rare and occurs most frequently in purebred cats, particularly in Siamese cats. Over the years, there have been several advances in the diagnosis and management of PDA in small animals, and numerous studies have been conducted to evaluate the effectiveness of various treatment options.[5–10]

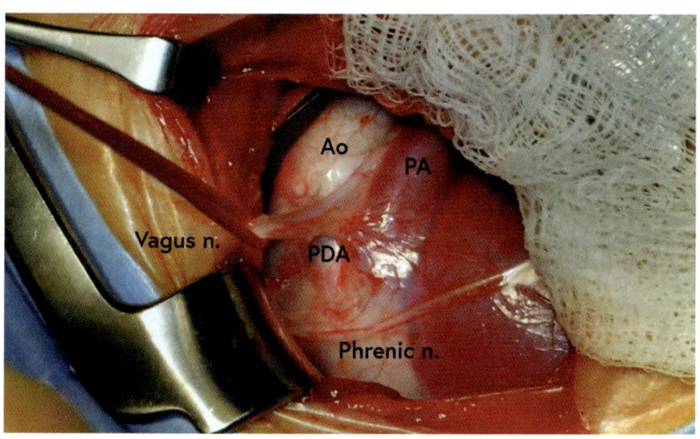

Figure 25.1 Intraoperative image of a patent ductus arteriosus (PDA) in a dog. Note the vagus nerve running over the PDA. Ao, aorta; PA, pulmonary artery.

Clinical presentation and diagnosis

Recognizing the clinical presentation and achieving a prompt diagnosis of PDA in dogs and cats can be critical for effective management. The clinical features vary in severity depending on the PDA's size and on the volume of blood passing through the vessel. Some animals may remain asymptomatic, while others can present with heart failure. Frequently, the characteristic murmur created by continuous left-to-right flow of blood is detected on routine physical examination at the time of vaccination. Common clinical features of left-to-right PDA include exercise intolerance, lethargy, coughing, tachypnea, and/or dyspnea. Typically, affected animals develop left-sided congestive heart failure within the first 12 months of life.

Definitive diagnosis of PDA requires a combination of physical examination and imaging. On auscultation, a characteristic machinery heart murmur is present in the left fourth intercostal space, and a palpable thrill can be felt. Pulmonary crackles may be present in dogs with left heart failure. Other abnormal findings include hyperkinetic (bounding/tall and narrow) arterial pulses and pale mucous membranes. Imaging techniques, such as thoracic radiographs and echocardiography, are critical in the diagnosis and characterization of PDA. Thoracic radiographs may reveal left heart dilatation, left atrial and auricular enlargement, and a bulge in the descending aorta caused by the ductus aneurysm/diverticulum, best seen in a high-quality dorsoventral radiograph. Signs of pulmonary overcirculation, such as pulmonary artery enlargement or pulmonary edema, may also be present. Echocardiography is the best non-invasive way to confirm PDA, as it allows visualization of the shunt and assessment of any associated cardiac abnormalities such as mitral valve regurgitation or persistent left cranial vena cava (Fig. 25.3; Video 25.1). Findings supporting the diagnosis include left heart, aorta and pulmonary trunk dilatation, mitral valve regurgitation, increased aortic ejection velocity, and di-

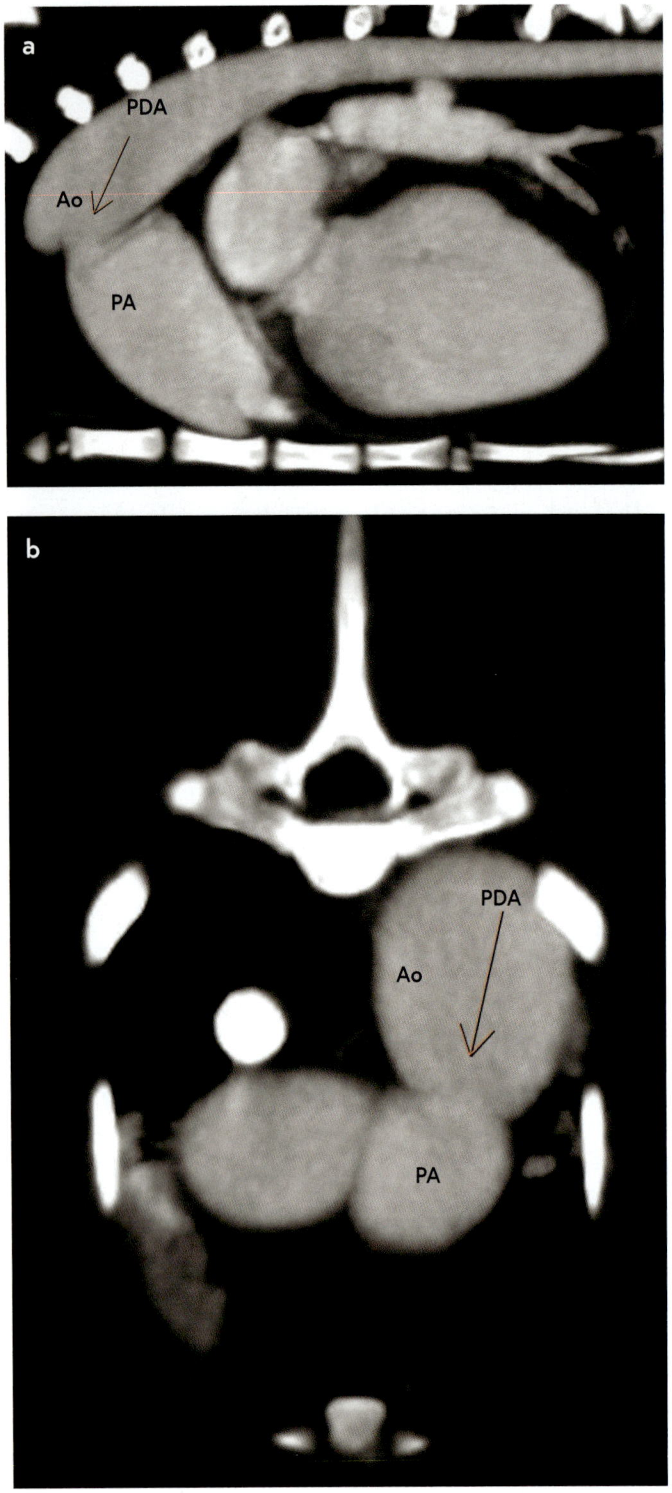

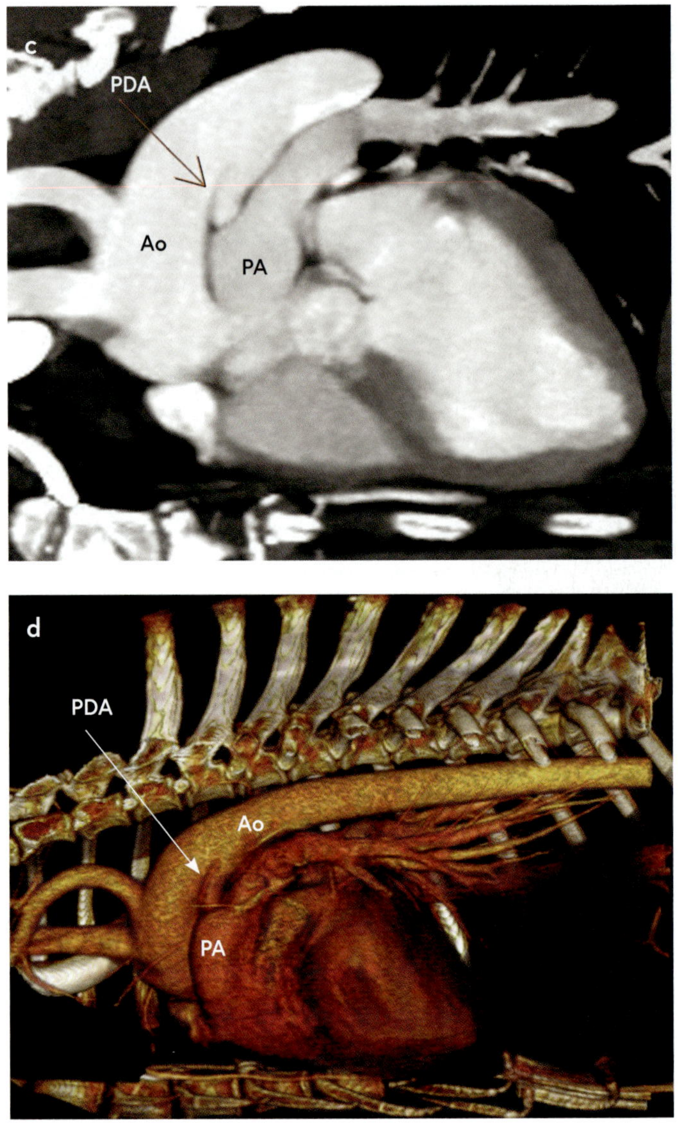

Figure 25.2 Multiplanar reformation/reconstruction (MPR) images in (a) sagittal and (b) transverse planes using maximum intensity projection (MIP), acquired by ECG-gated 320 MDCT angiography, showing a left-to-right patent ductus arteriosus (PDA) connecting the descending aorta (Ao) with the main pulmonary artery (PA) in a 1.5-year-old domestic shorthair cat. The main PA and left ventricle are markedly dilated. (c) MPR image in a sagittal plane using MIP and (d) 3D volume rendering, acquired by non-ECG-gated 320 MDCT angiography, showing an incidentally found left-to-right type IIA PDA connecting the descending Ao with the main PA in a 7-year-old German Shepherd Dog. Images courtesy of Cesar Llanos.

Video 25.1. Left cranial echocardiographic view optimized to visualize the pulmonary artery, with and without color-flow Doppler, demonstrating left-to-right shunting through a patent ductus arteriosus. See Figure 25.3 for identification of the anatomical structures. Video courtesy of Brogan Atkinson.

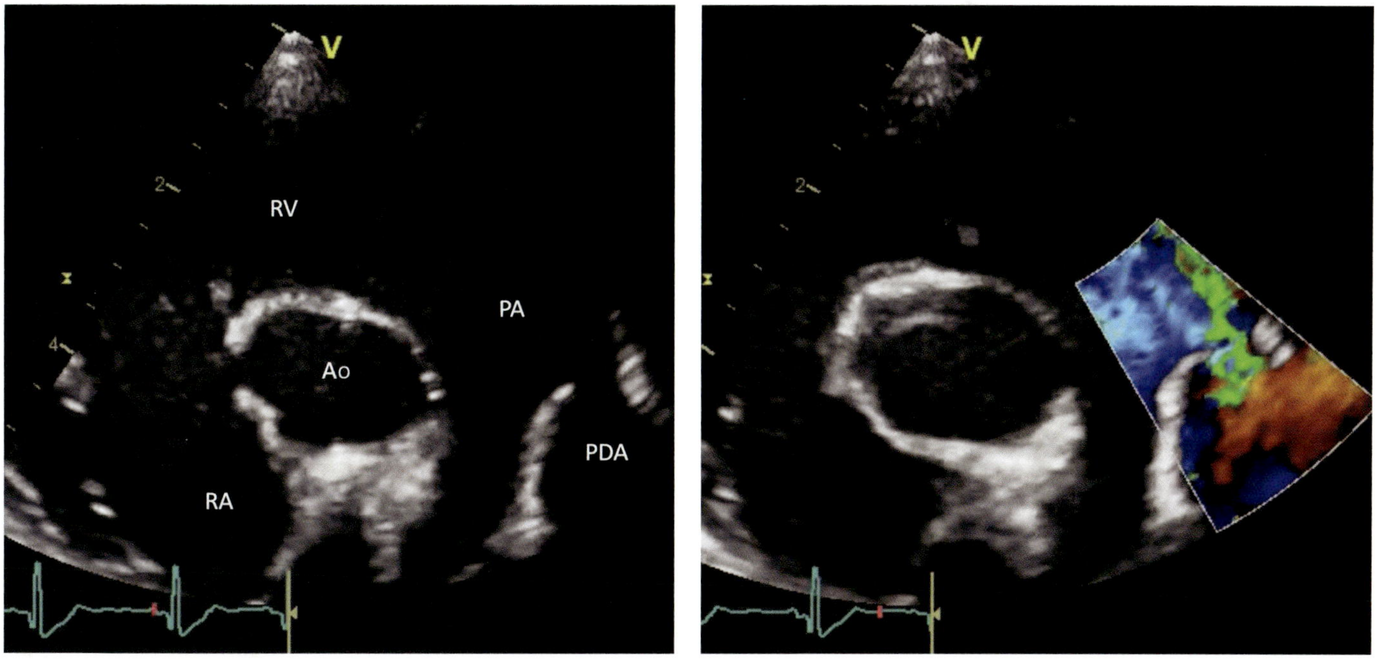

Figure 25.3 Left cranial echocardiographic view optimized for visualization of the main pulmonary artery (PA), with and without color-flow Doppler, demonstrating left-to-right shunting (green flow) through a patent ductus arteriosus (PDA). Ao, aorta; RA, right atrium; RV, right ventricle. Images courtesy of Brogan Atkinson.

rect visualization of the PDA between the pulmonary artery and the descending aorta. Doppler analysis may reveal a characteristic pattern of continuous turbulent flow in the pulmonary artery. Electrocardiography may show tall R waves and wide P waves in lead II, but these findings are not always present (approximately 60%).

Treatment

The treatment of PDA depends on several factors, including the size and severity of the shunt, the overall health of the animal, and the presence of any concurrent cardiac abnormalities. PDA closure is the treatment of choice for dogs and cats with a left-to-right shunt, but it is contraindicated in animals with pulmonary hypertension or a permanent right-to-left shunt. The procedure involves either PDA ligation through a thoracotomy or PDA occlusion using interventional radiology techniques. Although PDA closure can be performed at any age, preferably it should be carried out before 16 weeks of age. Older animals should undergo surgery as soon as possible after the diagnosis is confirmed. Animals that present with congestive heart failure should initially be treated with loop diuretics (e.g., furosemide) and then undergo PDA closure as soon as they are stable, usually within 24–48 hours. Animals with pulmonary hypertension can undergo surgery if the pulmonary artery pressure is not suprasystemic (right-to-left shunting is not present). Pulmonary vasodilators (e.g., sildenafil) can be used in these patients in an attempt to balance or reverse the flow (from right-to-left to left-to-right).

Surgical technique (Video 25.2)

1. Invasive positive-pressure ventilation is essential for this procedure and can be performed manually or using a mechanical ventilator.
2. A left fourth intercostal thoracotomy is typically performed in dogs. In cats, a left fourth or fifth intercostal thoracotomy is employed (see Chapter 4). The decision should be based on the evaluation of the position of the PDA relative to the chest wall on the preoperative radiographs.
3. Moist swabs are used to retract the left cranial lung lobe caudally and expose the heart.
4. The left vagus nerve should be identified coursing over the PDA. It represents the first landmark for the procedure.
5. The vagus nerve should be dissected free at the level of the PDA and retracted ventrally using a silicone vessel loop, or similar, around it.

Video 25.2. Patent ductus arteriosus ligation through a left fourth intercostal thoracotomy. Note the use of two 2-0 silk sutures and one 5-0 polypropylene suture for ligation.

6. The mediastinum should be gently dissected over the PDA using cotton buds.
7. The most cranial and most caudal aspect of the PDA between the main pulmonary artery and the descending aorta should be identified (these are critical landmarks).
8. To improve PDA visualization, a moist umbilical tape or a silicone vessel loop is placed loosely around the aorta just caudal to the PDA. Retraction of the aorta will aid visualization and dissection of the caudal aspect of the PDA (Fig. 25.4).
9. The space caudal to the PDA, between the pulmonary artery and the aorta, is gently dissected and opened with a pair of right-angle forceps or curved mosquito forceps. A direction parallel to the PDA toward the contralateral mediastinum should be maintained.
10. The space cranial to the PDA is then dissected and opened in the same manner, remaining parallel to the PDA toward the contralateral mediastinum.
11. The aorta can be retracted with the umbilical tape to allow better visualization during the dissection of the caudomedial aspect of the PDA.
12. Dissection of the medial aspect of the PDA is the most critical step (extreme care should be taken during this part of the procedure). When completed, a pair of right-angle forceps should be gently placed under and around the PDA from cranial to caudal or from caudal to cranial (Fig. 25.5).
13. Two 3-0 or 2-0 silk sutures should be passed around the PDA using a pair of right-angle forceps. A 5-0 nonabsorbable suture (e.g., polypropylene) can also be added to minimize the risk of return of flow associated with the degradation of silk over time.
14. The PDA is closed by slowly tying these sutures: the suture on the aortic side is tied first, followed by the suture on the pulmonary artery side (Fig. 25.6). Closure of the PDA can result in the Branham reflex (a reflex decrease in heart rate following an increase in blood pressure) (Video 25.3).

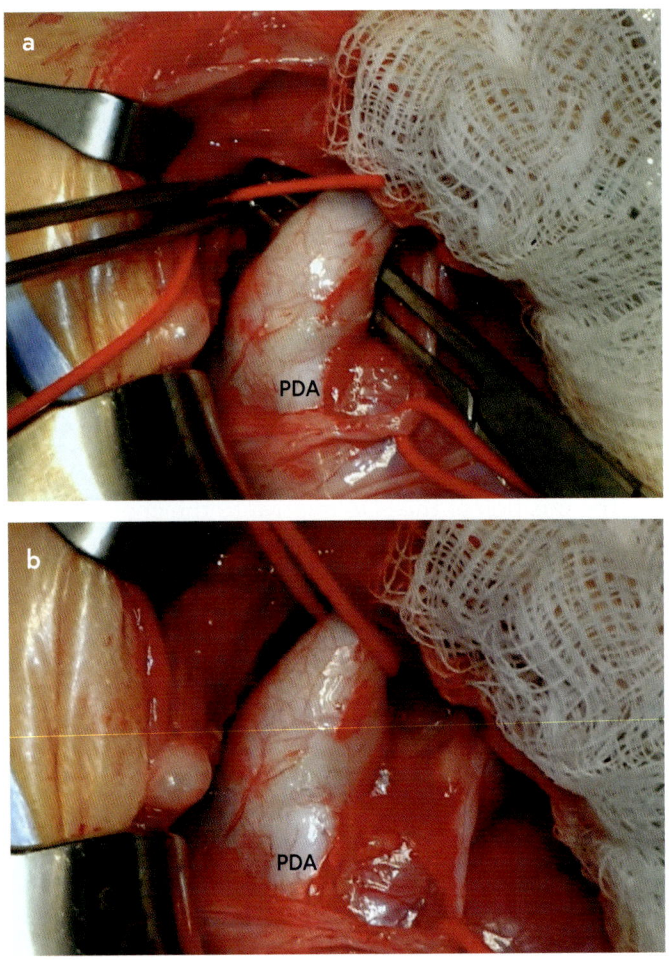

Figure 25.4 (a) Dissection of the aorta caudal to the patent ductus arteriosus (PDA) for the placement of a silicone vessel loop. (b) Retraction of the aorta aids visualization and dissection of the caudal aspect of the PDA.

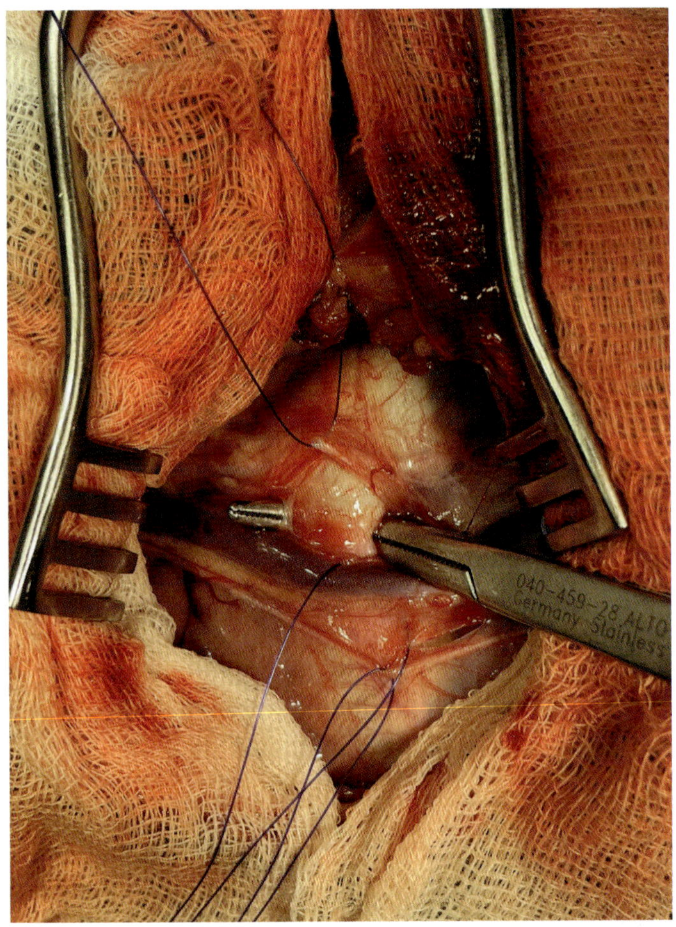

Figure 25.5 A pair of right-angle forceps are gently placed under and around the patent ductus arteriosus (PDA) from caudal to cranial. Note a persistent left cranial vena cava, ventral to the PDA. This should not be ligated or divided. Image courtesy of Filippo Cinti.

Video 25.3. Branham reflex after ligation of a patent ductus arteriosus. Note the increase in blood pressure (mainly mean and diastolic) and the decrease in heart rate. Video courtesy of Cristina Parra Martínez.

15. Before chest closure, a thoracostomy tube should be placed (see Chapter 5).
16. The swabs retracting the lungs should be removed from the thorax and a swab count performed.
17. Chest closure is performed as described in Chapter 4.

Postoperative management

After surgical correction of PDA, postoperative monitoring for the first 24–48 hours is essential. Oxygen supplementation should be considered in patients with arterial oxygen saturation below 95% or if the alveolar–arterial oxygen gradient (PA–aO_2) is higher than 20 mmHg. The patient's vital signs, including heart rate, respiratory rate, blood pressure, and temperature, should be monitored closely to detect any signs of complications, such as hemorrhage, arrhythmias, or hypothermia. Pain management options may include opioids, nonsteroidal anti-inflammatory drugs, or local anesthetics, depending on the patient's individual needs. Typically, the thoracostomy tube is removed once the chest has been completely evacuated. The surgical incision should be monitored closely for any signs of infection or dehiscence. Appropriate activity restrictions should be implemented postoperatively to prevent excessive activity or stress on the cardiovascular system, which could compromise healing or lead to complications. Cardiac function should be assessed postoperatively using echocardiography to evaluate the adequacy of PDA closure, detect any residual shunt, and assess overall cardiac function. Follow-up evaluations are essential to monitor for long-term complications, such as pulmonary hypertension or recurrence of the PDA.

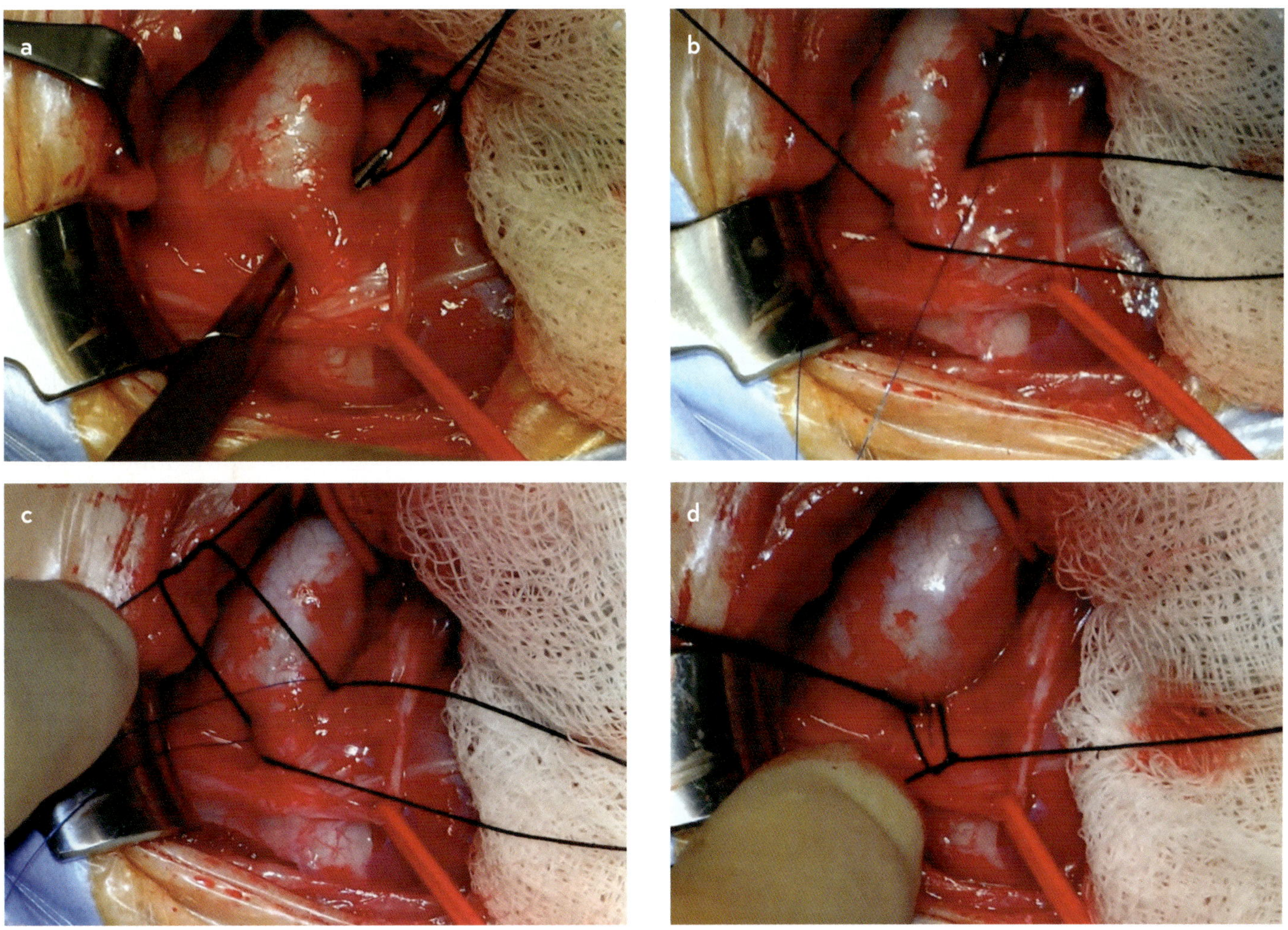

Figure 25.6 Sequential photographs of patent ductus arteriosus (PDA) ligation. (a) Two silk sutures are passed around the PDA using a pair of right-angle forceps. (b) One suture is placed on the aortic side and the other on the pulmonary artery side (note the polypropylene suture in between). (c) The suture on the aortic side is tied first, (d) followed by the suture on the pulmonary artery side.

Outcome

The success rate of surgical correction of PDA in dogs and cats exceeds 92%, with the mortality rate approaching 0% when performed by experienced surgeons. However, major complications can occur in approximately 10% of cases.[7,9,11–15] Rupture of the PDA resulting in severe hemorrhage is the most common cause of perioperative mortality and typically occurs during dissection of the craniomedial aspect of the PDA.[15,16] Cardiac arrhythmias may also occur postoperatively due to changes in cardiac function and physiology, requiring medical management or additional interventions. Residual ductal flow has been reported and could contribute to persistent volume overload and predispose to PDA recanalization or endocarditis.[5] However, in the vast majority of animals, this flow is insignificant, and additional procedures are not necessary. The use of an additional nonabsorbable encircling suture between the silk ligatures can be beneficial in case the silk fails over time.

In general, the prognosis for dogs and cats undergoing surgical correction of PDA is excellent, with a high success rate independent of the type of intervention.[11–15] The outcome of the procedure depends on many factors, including the severity of the shunt, the patient's overall health, and the surgeon's expertise and experience. Regular follow-up appointments and ongoing monitoring may be necessary to ensure the long-term success of the procedure.

Ligation of the PDA is considered curative in dogs and cats when performed at an early age (<6 months), and a normal lifespan is expected. Mitral valve regurgitation and apparent myocardial dysfunction may reverse postoperatively in response to the new loading conditions, whereas secondary changes in older dogs may not reverse remodel so effectively. Nonetheless, surgery is still indicated in these older dogs due to its beneficial palliative effect.

KEEP IN MIND

- Echocardiography is the best noninvasive way to confirm a patent ductus arteriosus (PDA), as it allows visualization of the shunt and assessment of any associated cardiac abnormalities.
- PDA closure is the treatment of choice for animals with a left-to-right shunt but is contraindicated in patients with pulmonary hypertension or a permanent right-to-left shunt.
- The left vagus nerve is the first landmark to identify for the procedure. It courses over the PDA.
- Extreme care should be taken during dissection of the medial aspect of the PDA.

References

1. Brockman DJ. Surgery of the heart, pericardium and great vessels. In: Brockman DJ, Holt DE, Haar GT (eds.). *BSAVA Manual of Canine and Feline Head, Neck and Thoracic Surgery*, 2nd ed. BSAVA; 2018.
2. Buchanan JW, Patterson DF. Etiology of patent ductus arteriosus in dogs. *J Vet Intern Med.* 2003; 17(2):167–171.
3. Buchanan JW. Patent ductus arteriosus morphology, pathogenesis, types and treatment. *J Vet Cardiol.* 2001; 3(1):7–16.
4. Fox PR. Pathophysiology and management of patent ductus arteriosus in dogs. *J Vet Cardiol.* 2010; 12(2):85–91.
5. Stanley BJ, Luis-Fuentes V, Darke PG. Comparison of the incidence of residual shunting between two surgical techniques used for ligation of patent ductus arteriosus in the dog. *Vet Surg.* 2003; 32(3):231–237.
6. Goodrich KR, Kyles AE, Kass PH, Campbell F. Retrospective comparison of surgical ligation and transarterial catheter occlusion for treatment of patent ductus arteriosus in two hundred and four dogs (1993–2003). *Vet Surg.* 2007; 36(1):43–49.
7. Hutton JE et al. Surgical and nonsurgical management of patent ductus arteriosus in cats: 28 cases (1991–2012). *J Am Vet Med Assoc.* 2015; 247(3):278–285.
8. Grimes JA, Thieman Mankin KM. Surgical ligation of patent ductus arteriosus in dogs: Incidence and risk factors for rupture. *Vet Surg.* 2022; 51(4):592–599.
9. Wustefeld-Janssens BG et al. Clinical findings and treatment outcomes for cats diagnosed with patent ductus arteriosus in the UK: A retrospective study of 19 cases (2004–2012). *Vet Rec.* 2016; 179(1):17.
10. Bascuñán A et al. Patent ductus arteriosus in cats (Felis catus): 50 cases (2000–2015). *J Vet Cardiol.* 2017; 19(1):35–43.
11. Bureau S, Monnet E, Orton EC. Evaluation of survival rate and prognostic indicators for surgical treatment of left-to-right patent ductus arteriosus in dogs: 52 cases (1995–2003). *J Am Vet Med Assoc.* 2005; 227(11):1794–1799.
12. Van Israël N, French AT, Dukes-McEwan J, Corcoran BM. Review of left-to-right shunting patent ductus arteriosus and short term outcome in 98 dogs. *J Small Anim Pract.* 2002; 43(9):395–400.
13. Van Israël N, Dukes-McEwan J, French AT. Long-term follow-up of dogs with patent ductus arteriosus. *J Small Anim Pract.* 2003; 44(11):480–490.
14. Saunders AB, Gordon SG, Boggess MM, Miller MW. Long-term outcome in dogs with patent ductus arteriosus: 520 cases (1994–2009). *J Vet Intern Med.* 2014; 28(2):401–410.
15. McNamara KL et al. Risk factors for intraoperative hemorrhage and perioperative complications and short- and long-term outcomes during surgical patent ductus arteriosus ligation in 417 dogs. *J Am Vet Med Assoc.* 2023; 261 (8):1–7.
16. Hunt GB et al. Intraoperative hemorrhage during patent ductus arteriosus ligation in dogs. *Vet Surg.* 2001; 30(1):58–63.

Chapter 26

Dentoalveolar emergencies

Ingrid Tundo, Boaz Arzi

Dental trauma

Dental traumatic injuries include lesions affecting dental tissues: enamel, dentin, pulp, and cementum.[1] Complicated crown fractures refer to dental fractures exposing the dental pulp and are the most common type of traumatic dental injury.[2] Immature permanent teeth, characterized by an open apex and very thin dentinal walls, are a real dental emergency if conservative treatment (tooth preservation) is considered.[3] In fact, pulp survival is essential for normal root development, closing of the apex, and initial thickening of the tooth walls.[4–6]

In dogs and cats, the prevalence of dental and periodontal trauma is approximately 26%, notably higher in dogs than in cats.[2,3] Maxillofacial trauma increases the likelihood of concurrent dental/periodontal injury, which can be seen in up to 72% of patients with maxillofacial trauma.[7,8]

Common causes of dentoalveolar trauma include fights, vehicular trauma, falls from height (especially in cats), collisions with moving objects (e.g., frisbee, balls, stones), and mastication of hard objects (e.g., stones, bones, wood, hard plastic objects, ice cubes, cage bars).[2] The canine and incisor teeth are the most frequently affected by trauma in dogs and cats due to their exposed position.[2]

Following a trauma causing pulp exposure, immediate invasion of the pulp by oral bacteria occurs, leading to inflammation, infection, and, with time, necrosis of the internal tissues of the tooth.[9] If not promptly treated, pulpitis can progress to involve periapical periodontal structures, resulting in the invasion of the periodontal space by bacteria, toxins, and inflammatory mediators after crossing the apical delta.[9,10] It has been experimentally demonstrated in dogs that a periapical lesion may develop within 20 days of pulpal exposure.[11]

Hematogenous infection of the necrotic pulp tissue is also possible without pulp exposure following concussion, with a similar evolution.[9] Inflammation and periapical infection induce bone resorption and inflammatory root resorption in the affected area.[9,12,13] Bacterial presence in the periapical area is essential for the development of periapical lesions such as an abscess of dental origin.[9]

Clinical presentation and diagnosis

Although acute complicated crown fractures cause pain, clinical signs are often nonspecific and/or hardly noticeable.[2,3] Diagnosis is frequently underestimated, as clinically recognizable complications may develop long after the traumatic event. Dental trauma is diagnosed mainly through clinical examination and diagnostic imaging, particularly radiographic examination or cone-beam computed tomography (CT).[14,15] Upon oral examination, a fractured tooth's surface appears rough with a pink-red spot in the center (pulp tissue) (Fig. 26.1).[2]

The diagnosis of a complicated crown fracture is confirmed under general anesthesia using a sharp dental explorer on the fractured surface to assess exposure of the pulp cavity.[1] Radiographic examination is necessary to evaluate the structures that are not clinically visible (roots, alveolar bone, endodontic system, and periodontal space). Trauma causing crown lesions can also induce radicular and periodontal lesions, detectable only through radiographic assessment.[1] Periapical lesions can only be detected radiographically several weeks after trauma.[2]

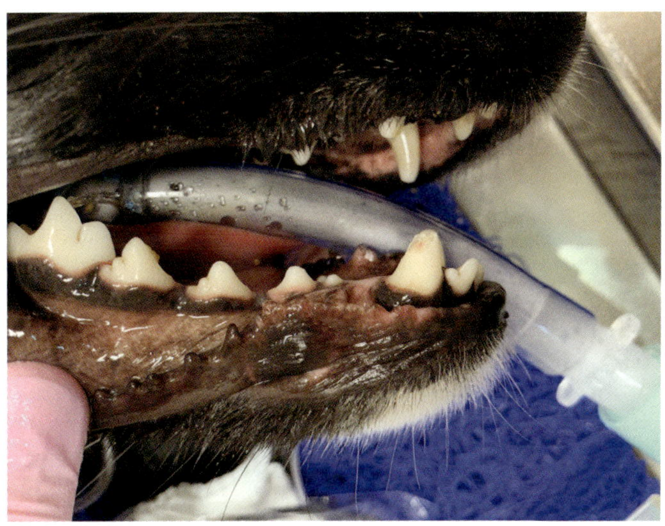

Figure 26.1 2-year-old dog presented with a complicated crown fracture of the right mandibular canine tooth. The fractured tooth's surface appears rough and has a pink-red spot in the center (pulp tissue).

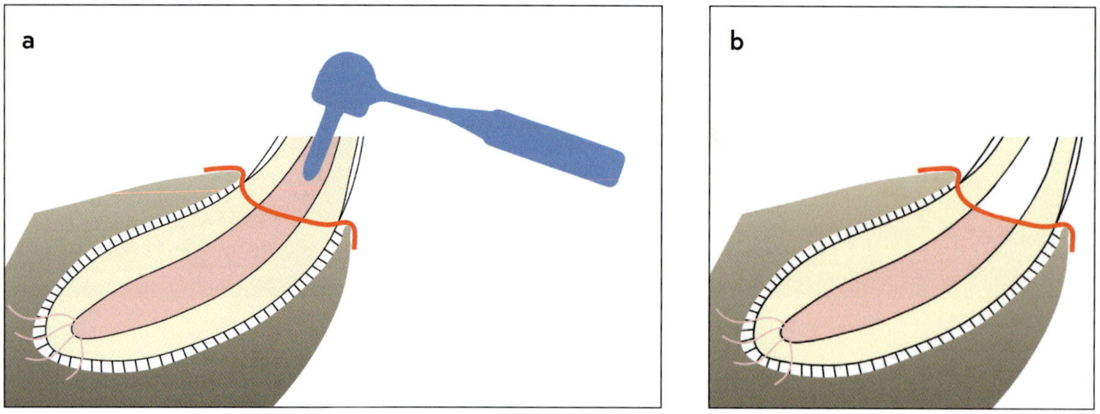

Figure 26.2 Approximately 6–7 mm of the coronal pulp tissue is removed using a round diamond bur on a high-speed handpiece with distilled water cooling.

Treatment

Dental trauma involving pulp tissue always requires treatment.[2] Treatment options may differ depending on the tooth and the type and extent of trauma, among other factors.[16] In particular, extraction may be the treatment of choice depending on the patient's circumstances (e.g., concurrent diseases, compliance), owner's financial restrictions, clinician's professional capabilities, and equipment limitations.[17]

The treatment plan (e.g., exodontic or endodontic treatment and type of endodontic treatment) also depends on the patient's general health and age.[2] Extraction is the treatment of choice when trauma affects primary dentition.[18]

Pulp exposure in patients younger than 12–18 months of age is considered a dental emergency.[1,3] Vital pulpectomy is an emergency procedure, as the success rate of the treatment declines rapidly after pulp exposure.[3] This procedure aims to treat reversible pulpal injuries and maintain pulp vitality and function.[3] Immature permanent teeth, which still have an open apex and very thin dentinal walls, are the primary candidates to be treated with vital pulp therapy if conservative treatment (tooth preservation) is considered.[3]

Surgical technique: Vital pulp therapy

Vital pulp therapy consists of removing only the superficial and infected part of the pulp (pulpectomy) in a delicate and sterile manner and applying specific materials to the remaining pulp, followed by a sealing restoration.[3,17,19] Pain management includes preoperative regional nerve block with either lidocaine, mepivacaine, or bupivacaine and postoperative nonsteroidal anti-inflammatory drugs (if appropriate).[3]

1. The acutely fractured tooth is radiographically assessed with at least two intraoral radiographs: occlusal (ventrodorsal) and lateral/orthogonal projections.[3]
2. The tooth is ultrasonically scaled and polished with fluoride-free pumice. A rubber dam and draping with sterile towels, sterile instruments, and burs are used to maintain an aseptic endodontic field throughout the procedure.[3]
3. Approximately 6–7 mm of the coronal pulp tissue is removed using a round diamond bur on a high-speed handpiece with distilled water cooling (Fig. 26.2). The blunt end of a sterile paper point is moistened with saline (0.9% NaCl) solution, inserted into the canal, and pressed gently against the pulp tissue.[3]
4. After achieving hemostasis, a 2–3 mm thick layer of mineral trioxide aggregate (MTA) is placed over the exposed pulp tissue, followed by a 1 mm intermediate layer of glass ionomer restorative to cover the pulp dressing material.[3]
5. The remainder of the cavity is then acid etched, bonded, and restored with a 2–4 mm layer of hybrid composite restoration material (Fig. 26.3).[3]

Postoperative management

Teeth should be radiographically checked at 3–6 months postoperatively and ideally annually to evaluate progress and absence of complications.[3]

Outcome

Outcome is determined according to the guidelines for radiographic assessment of vital pulp therapy established by the European Society of Endodontology.[20] The three possible outcomes are as follows:

- Successful: Radiographic evidence of continued root formation (secondary dentin production and apical closure when applicable), absence of clinical and radiographic signs of apical periodontitis, and absence of internal or external root resorption (Fig. 26.4).
- No evidence of failure: Fulfilling success criteria, except for the width of the apical periodontal ligament, which could be wider but not greater than double the width of the periodontal ligament in other areas.

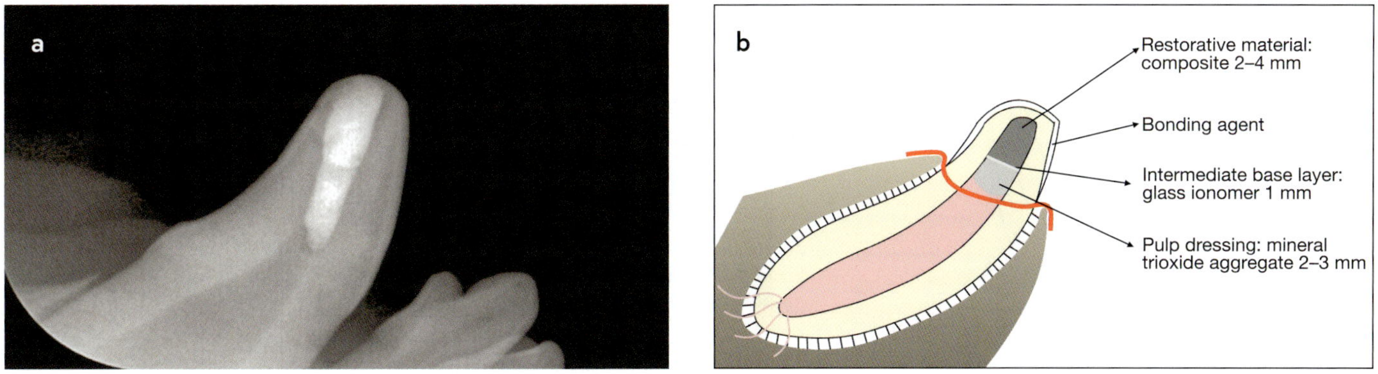

Figure 26.3 (a) Lateral radiographic view of the crown of a right mandibular canine tooth obtained immediately after vital pulp therapy. (b) Four different layers are applied: pulp dressing, an intermediate base layer, a bonding agent, and restorative material.

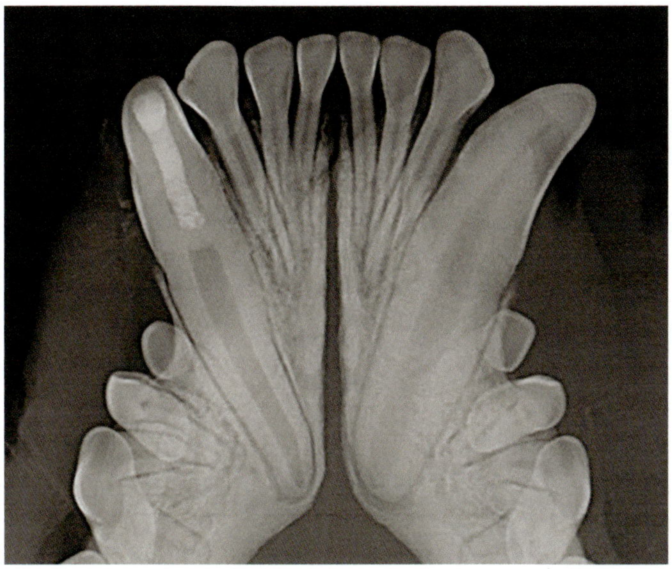

Figure 26.4 Occlusal radiographic view of a right mandibular canine tooth treated with vital pulp therapy obtained at 12-month follow-up. Tertiary dentin bridge formation is evident.

- Failed: Secondary dentin production ceased, root formation in immature teeth discontinued, or periapical lesion or root resorption developed by the time of follow-up.

A study reported a vital pulp therapy success rate of around 92% when teeth are treated with MTA within the first 24–48 hours.[3] In another study involving a 36-month follow-up period of 97 mature canine teeth with complicated crown fractures, based on the results of radiographic examination, 88.2% of teeth were vital when treated within 48 hours, 41.4% when treated within 1 week, and 23.5% when treated within 3 weeks after pulp exposure.[17]

Periodontal trauma

Traumatic injuries affecting the periodontal tissues involve the supporting structures of the teeth, including the gingiva, periodontal ligament, alveolar bone, and cementum.[1] Common causes include fights, car accidents, falls from a height, blunt trauma, and chewing on hard materials.[2] Periodontal injuries may be associated with tooth trauma, but not exclusively (teeth may not be damaged but rather displaced), and are classified as concussion, subluxation, luxation (lateral, intrusive, or extrusive), and avulsion.[21] Concussion and subluxation are not considered emergencies, while luxation and avulsion (see below) are considered an emergency if conservative treatment (tooth preservation) is elected.[21] Luxation and avulsion are time-sensitive situations, as the periodontal ligament begins to necrotize after 60 minutes of extraoral time.[22]

Clinical presentation and diagnosis

Diagnosis is mainly based on clinical examination and diagnostic imaging, such as intraoral radiographs, CT, or cone-beam CT.[1–2,14] The most common clinical signs are soft tissue laceration, gingival bleeding, and tooth displacement. Concomitant injuries, such as crown or root fractures, are commonly reported.[21]

Luxation is the partial displacement of a tooth. There are three types of tooth luxation (Fig. 26.5):

- Lateral luxation: Displacement of a tooth in a horizontal direction, usually accompanied by comminution or fracture of the alveolus and laceration of mucogingival tissues.[1] It is the most diagnosed type of periodontal injury in dogs.[21] Radiographic signs include widening of the periodontal space and displacement of the lamina dura. These changes may not be visible depending on the angle of the X-ray beam.[24,32] Hence, advanced diagnostic imaging, such as CT or cone-beam CT, is likely to have higher diagnostic yield.
- Intrusive luxation or intrusion: Apical displacement of a tooth into the alveolus.[1] Intrusive trauma is uncommon in dogs and cats.[2] This type of injury is usually accompanied by fracture of the alveolus and

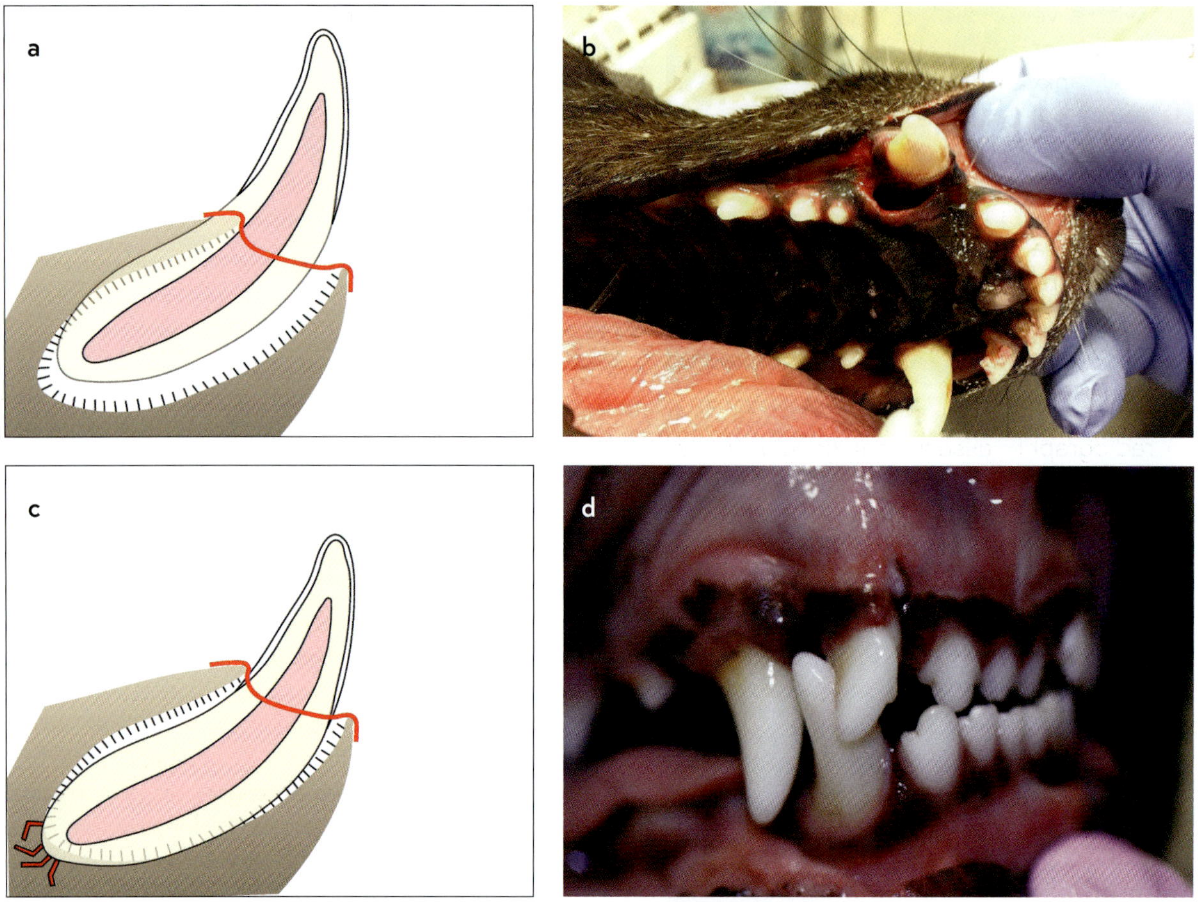

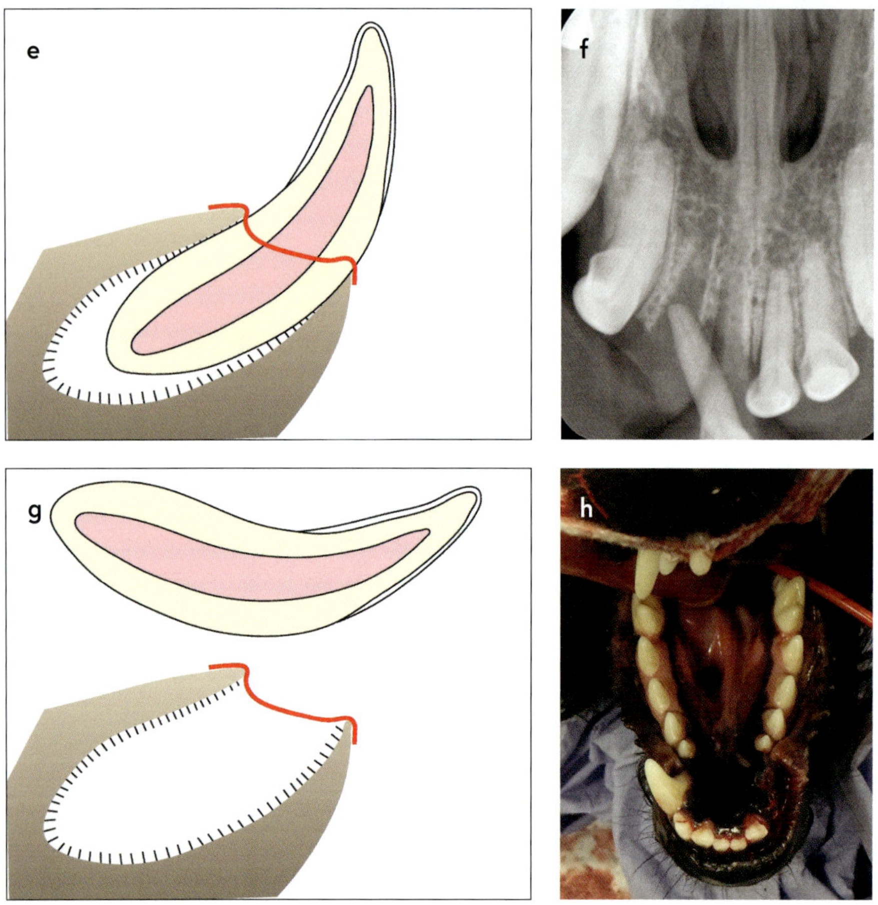

Figure 26.5 (a,b) Lateral luxation; right maxillary canine tooth. (c,d) Intrusion; right maxillary first and second incisor teeth and left maxillary first incisor tooth. (e,f) Extrusion; right maxillary second incisor tooth. (g,h) Avulsion; left mandibular canine and third incisor teeth.

associated with a very high incidence of complications such as pulp canal obliteration, pulp necrosis, root resorption, ankylosis, and marginal bone loss. Intrusive luxation bears a poor prognosis.[25–27]

- Extrusive luxation or extrusion: Partial displacement of a tooth out of its alveolus.[1] The tooth may appear clinically "elongated" and there may be bleeding from the periodontal tissues. Radiographic examination reveals an increased width of the periodontal ligament space, particularly in the periapical area.[26,32]

Avulsion, or exarticulation, is the complete displacement of the tooth from the alveolus (Fig. 26.5).[1] Following trauma, a radiographic assessment should always be performed to differentiate avulsion from severe intrusion or root retention. Radiographically, the tooth is absent, and the alveolus appears empty.[32] Bony fractures may be present. The incidence of dental avulsion in veterinary patients is unknown.[21]

Following facial trauma, all teeth should be assessed for abnormal mobility suggesting displacement or jaw fracture. Diagnostic imaging is necessary to evaluate the degree of dental displacement, presence of preexisting periodontal disease, extent of root development, size of the pulp cavity, presence of root or bony fractures, and presence of tooth fragments and foreign bodies lodged in the soft tissues.[1,28,29] Multiple radiographic projections at different angles may be necessary to fully evaluate tooth displacement.[23] Given that maxillofacial trauma does not typically result in isolated or obvious injuries, advanced diagnostic imaging in the form of CT or cone-beam CT is recommended.

Treatment

Treatment choice depends on several factors, including patient age, oral and general health, extent of dental damage, timing between trauma and treatment, type of affected tooth, periodontal health of affected and adjacent teeth, veterinarian's experience, and availability of materials and equipment for advanced treatments.[2]

The guidelines of the American Association of Endodontists and of the International Association of Dental Traumatology are applicable with some modification for the treatment of displaced teeth in veterinary patients.[30,31] Differences are mainly due to the need for general anesthesia for veterinary dental procedures. Treatment includes repositioning (for luxation) or reimplantation (for avulsion) of the tooth in its alveolus, management of bony and soft tissue injuries, and endodontic treatment, given the disrupted blood supply to the pulp as a consequence of the trauma.[2,32] These procedures should be performed promptly and with great care.[21,30] The tooth should be minimally manipulated, handled by the crown, and reinserted into the alveolus without effort, minimizing further damage to the periodontal ligament fibers and cementum.[21] Curettage of either the root or the alveolus should be avoided to prevent the healthy periodontal ligament from being removed.[33,34]

Surgical technique (Fig. 26.6)[21]

1. To arrest any hemorrhage and avoid contamination of the surgical field with dental materials, lacerated soft tissues should be sutured, and bony fractures should be stabilized during repositioning (luxation) or reimplantation (avulsion) before splinting the displaced teeth.
2. Scaling and polishing of the teeth to be included in the splint should be performed. Nonfluoride pumice is used for polishing, as fluoride interferes with the setting of the composite and resin materials.
3. After radiographic confirmation that the displaced tooth has been correctly repositioned, it should be attached to adjacent teeth, ideally using a nonrigid splint.
4. Splinting of the displaced tooth to the adjacent teeth using orthodontic or stainless steel wire is performed. The splint should extend one to three teeth mesially and distally from the displaced tooth. The size of the wire depends on the size of the dog and teeth. The wire is shaped with orthodontic pliers to passively conform to the dental surface. It is positioned a few millimeters coronal to the gingival margin to avoid contact with the soft tissue. Occlusal interference should be avoided. If the wire and the bulk of the resin interfere with occlusion, it should be placed on the buccal side of the maxillary teeth or the lingual side of the mandibular teeth. If no interference is expected, the wire may be placed on either side of the teeth. In brachycephalic breeds, positioning may be different given their skull configuration.
5. Acid etching of the surface of the teeth to be included in the device should be performed with phosphoric acid etching gel or liquid for 15 seconds. Acid etching can be avoided if the shape of the teeth included in the splint assures good mechanical retention for the splinting material.
6. A bonding material is applied to the teeth and the wires. Application of bonding material can be avoided if the shape of the teeth included in the splint assures good mechanical retention for the splinting material.
7. Composite material or acrylic resin is applied to secure the wire. Polymerization of light-cured composite is started from the noninjured teeth and finished at the displaced tooth, which can be held in position by digital pressure. After polymerization,

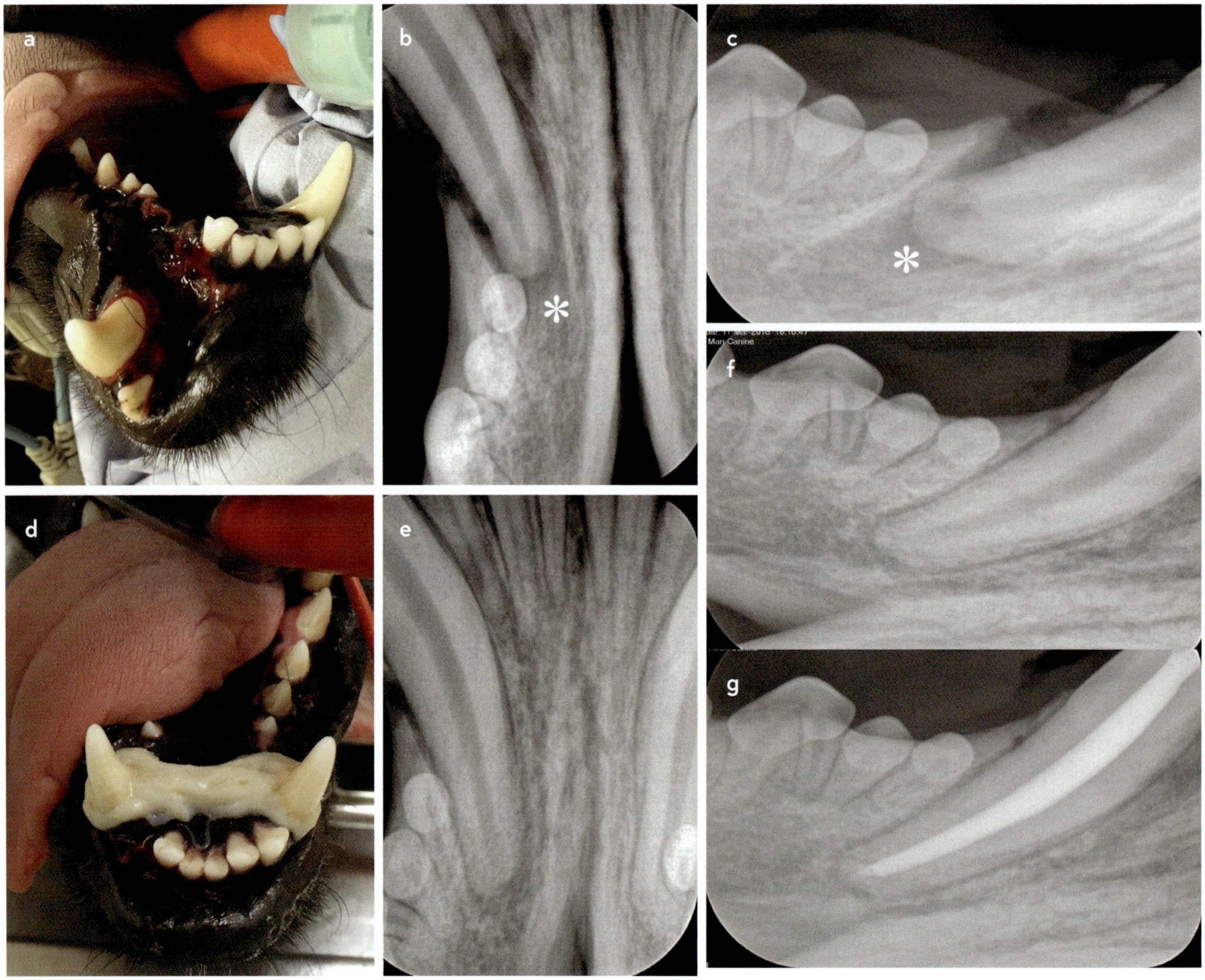

Figure 26.6 (a) Lateral luxation of the right mandibular canine tooth (404) and third incisor tooth (403) in a 2-year-old Labrador Retriever. Preoperative radiographic examination in (b) occlusal and (c) lateral (c) projections. Note the increased distance between the tooth root and the alveolar walls (asterisk). (d) The incisor tooth (403) was extracted, and a wire and composite resin were applied between the canines. Postoperative radiographic evaluation in (e) occlusal and (f) lateral projections. (g) Root canal treatment (tooth 404) was performed 2 weeks following splint placement.

the distal ends of the wire may be smoothed with a burr. The acrylic or composite material should not contact the soft tissues to avoid inflammation.

8. Final radiographs are taken to assess the repositioning.
9. The splint is trimmed and smoothed.
10. The patient's occlusion should be assessed before allowing them to recover.

Postoperative management

In the postoperative period, systemic antibiotics (to minimize the occurrence of inflammatory resorption and pulp infection) and analgesics should be prescribed. Biting should be minimized, chew toys withdrawn, and a soft diet offered. Oral home care (e.g., tooth brushing and rinsing with a 0.12% diluted chlorhexidine gluconate solution) should be recommended. As luxation and avulsion injuries frequently result in pulp necrosis, root canal therapy of injured teeth is necessary. It is recommended to perform it during splint removal (avulsion) or at least 10–14 days after repositioning (luxation). In the latter case, it may be accomplished through the splint.[21] Splinting duration should be as short as possible, as minimizing splinting time improves the treatment outcome and reduces complications such as dentoalveolar ankylosis and periodontitis. Recommendations in human patients entail a splinting time of 4–6 weeks for luxated teeth and 7–10 days for avulsed teeth. However, splinting time for large avulsed teeth, such as canine teeth in dogs, may be longer to allow for complete periodontal healing.[21]

Outcome

Potential long-term complications following treatment of displaced teeth include inflammatory root resorption, dentoalveolar ankylosis, and root replacement resorption. Repositioned and replanted teeth should therefore be followed-up radiographically for an extended period. Because of the possible development of late complications, radiographic follow-up examinations are recommended in humans for 2–5 years after replantation.[21] Further studies are needed to evaluate the incidence and rate of development of late complications in veterinary patients.[21] Deciduous teeth should not be repositioned or replanted due to the potential damage to the underlying developing permanent teeth and the innate short longevity of the tooth.[21]

KEEP IN MIND

- Pulp exposure in patients younger than 12–18 months of age requires treatment within 24–48 hours.
- Up to 72% of patients presenting for maxillofacial trauma have concurrent dental and periodontal trauma.
- Complicated crown fractures in mature patients (with closed apex) must always be treated with either endodontic or exodontic treatment.
- Dental radiography or computed tomography is an essential tool for the diagnosis of dental and periodontal trauma.

References

1. Andersson L, Andreasen JO. Traumatic dental injuries. In: Andersson L, Kahnberg KE, Pogrel MA (eds.). *Oral and Maxillofacial Surgery*. Oxford: Wiley-Blackwell; 2010. pp. 799–816.
2. Soukup JW, Hetzel S, Paul A. Classification and epidemiology of traumatic dentoalveolar injuries in dogs and cats: 959 injuries in 660 patient visits (2004–2012). *J Vet Dent*. 2015; 32(1):6–14.
3. Luotonen N et al. Vital pulp therapy in dogs: 190 cases (2001–2011). *J Am Vet Med Assoc*. 2014; 244(4):449–459.
4. Hennet PR, Harvey CE. Craniofacial development and growth in the dog. *J Vet Dent*. 1992; 9(2):11–18.
5. Wilson G. Timing of apical closure of the maxillary canine and mandibular first molar teeth of cats. *J Vet Dent*. 1999; 16(1):19–21.
6. Watanabe K et al. The formation of apical delta of the permanent teeth in dogs. *J Vet Med Sci*. 2001; 63(7):789–795.
7. Soukup JW, Mulherin BL, Snyder CJ. Prevalence and nature of dentoalveolar injuries among patients with maxillofacial fractures. *J Small Anim Pract*. 2013; 54(1):9–14.
8. Bonner SE, Reiter AM, Lewis JR. Orofacial manifestations of high-rise syndrome in cats: A retrospective study of 84 cases. *J Vet Dent*. 2012; 29(1):10–18.
9. Lin LM, Huang GTJ. Pathobiology of the periapex. In: Hargreaves M, Cohen S (eds.). *Cohen's Pathways of the Pulp*. St. Louis, MO: Mosby Elsevier; 2011. pp. 529–558.
10. Kortegaard HE et al. Consequences of crown shortening canine teeth in Greenland sled dogs. *J Small Anim Pract*. 2015; 56(4):264–269.
11. Kovacević M et al. The transition from pulpitis to periapical periodontitis in dogs' teeth. *Aust Endod J*. 2008; 34(1):12–18.
12. Constantaras ME, Charlier CJ. Diagnostic imaging in veterinary dental practice. Dental disease in a cat. *J Am Vet Med Assoc*. 2013; 243(12):1691–1694.
13. DeForge DH. Images in veterinary dental practice. Osteolysis of the apices of the distal and mesiobuccal roots of the tooth. *J Am Vet Med Assoc*. 2004; 224(6):841–842.
14. Gracis M. Management of periodontal trauma. In: Verstraete F, Lommer M (eds.). *Oral and Maxillofacial Surgery in Dogs and Cats*, 1st ed. Edinburgh: Saunders Elsevier; 2012. pp. 201–215.
15. White SC, Pharoah MJ. Trauma to teeth and facial structures. In: White SC, Pharoah MJ (eds.). *Oral Radiology: Principles and Interpretation*, 5th ed. St. Louis, MO: Mosby; 2004. pp. 615–638.
16. Luskin IR, Kressin DJ. Endodontic decisions based on radiographic appearance. *Clin Tech Small Anim Pract*. 2001; 16(3):173–181.
17. Clarke DE. Vital pulp therapy for complicated crown fracture of permanent canine teeth in dogs: A three-year retrospective study. *J Vet Dent*. 2001; 18(3):117–121.
18. Flores MT et al. Guidelines for the evaluation and management of traumatic dental injuries. *Dent Traumatol*. 2001; 17(3):97–102.
19. Niemiec BA. Assessment of vital pulp therapy for nine complicated crown fractures and fifty-four crown reductions in dogs and cats. *J Vet Dent*. 2001; 18(3):122–125.
20. European Society of Endodontology. Quality guidelines for endodontic treatment: consensus report of the European Society of Endodontology. *Int Endod J*. 2006; 39(12):921–930.
21. Gracis M. Management of periodontal trauma. In: Verstraete F, Lommer M (eds.). *Oral and Maxillofacial Surgery in Dogs and Cats, 2nd ed*. Edinburgh: Saunders Elsevier; 2020. pp. 218–231.
22. Pettiette M, Hupp J, Mesaros S, Trope M. Periodontal healing of extracted dogs' teeth air-dried for extended periods and soaked in various media. *Endod Dent Traumatol*. 1997; 13(3):113–118.
23. Mulligan TW, Aller MS, Williams CA. *Atlas of Canine and Feline Dental Radiography*. Trenton, NJ: Veterinary Learning System; 1998.
24. Gracis M, Orsini P. Treatment of traumatic dental displacement in dogs: Six cases of lateral luxation. *J Vet Dent*. 1998; 15(2):65–72.

25. Ebeleseder KA et al. An analysis of 58 traumatically intruded and surgically extruded permanent teeth. *Endod Dent Traumatol.* 2000; 16(1):34–39.
26. Turley PK, Joiner MW, Hellstrom S. The effect of orthodontic extrusion on traumatically intruded teeth. *Am J Orthod.* 1984; 85(1):47–56.
27. Turley PK, Crawford LB, Carrington KW. Traumatically intruded teeth. *Angle Orthod.* 1987; 57(3):234–244.
28. Trope M, Blanco L, Chivian N, Sigurdsson A. The role of endodontics after traumatic injuries. In: Cohen S, Hargreaves KM (eds.). *Pathways of the Pulp*, 9th ed. St. Louis, MO: Elsevier Mosby; 2006. pp. 610–649.
29. Nakane S, Kameyama Y. Root resorption caused by mechanical injury of the periodontal soft tissues in rats. *J Periodontal Res.* 1987; 22(5):390–395.
30. The Recommended Guidelines of the American Association of Endodontists for the Treatment of Traumatic Dental Injuries. American Association of Endodontists, revised September 13, 2013. Available at https://www.aae.org/specialty/wp-content/uploads/sites/2/2019/02/19_TraumaGuidelines.pdf.
31. International Association of Dental Traumatology. Dental Trauma Guidelines. https://www.iadt-dentaltrauma.org/for-professionals.html
32. Grossman LI, Oliet S, del Rio CE. Replantation, transplantation, and endodontic implants. In: Grossman LI, Oliet S, del Rio CE (eds.). *Endodontic Practice*, 11th ed. Philadelphia, PA: Lea & Febiger; 1988. pp. 329–348.
33. Trope M. Clinical management of the avulsed tooth. *Dent Clin North Am.* 1995; 39(1):93–112.
34. Löe H, Waerhaug J. Experimental replantation of teeth in dogs and monkeys. *Arch Oral Biol.* 1961; 3:176–184.

Chapter 27

Maxillofacial trauma and temporomandibular joint emergencies

Ingrid Tundo, Boaz Arzi

Maxillofacial trauma

Maxillofacial fractures in dogs and cats commonly result from motor vehicle trauma or dog bites. Addressing jaw fractures requires initial systemic stabilization, followed by a comprehensive assessment of all injuries before proceeding to general anesthesia. Analgesics and temporary bone support (e.g., a muzzle) should be provided on an emergency basis to all patients.[1–5] Nutritional support, including feeding tube placement, along with other supportive therapies like antibiotic therapy and fluid therapy should be considered.

Jaw fractures should be carefully evaluated via oral and dental examination and diagnostic imaging, preferably conventional computed tomography (CT) or cone-beam CT, with the patient under general anesthesia if/once the patient is stable.[6] The animal should then receive definitive fracture fixation as soon as possible, as this provides the opportunity for the optimal outcome. Some fractures, especially those in juvenile animals, are frequently best treated conservatively to avoid interference with the ongoing growth of the jaws and teeth.

Soft tissue injuries of the oral cavity and face, such as lip avulsion or midline palatal fracture/separation with tearing of palatal soft tissues, should be treated as soon as possible by wound debridement and lavage, soft tissue repair as indicated, and, usually, systemic antibiotic support. The full extent of the soft tissue necrosis resulting from chemical and electrical burns may only be visible within days of the traumatic event. A conservative approach is therefore warranted in these cases, but supportive care should be established on an emergency basis.[1–5]

Clinical presentation and diagnosis

Following stabilization of the patient, jaw fractures and soft tissue trauma are evaluated by inspection and palpation of the mandibular and maxillary bones, temporomandibular joints (TMJs), lips, cheeks, tongue, palate, and oral and pharyngeal mucosal linings. The head is examined for asymmetry and discontinuity, exophthalmos or enophthalmos, lip avulsions, and facial wounds, whilst the oral cavity is inspected for mucosal lacerations, hematomas and hemorrhage, fractured/displaced teeth, and malocclusion.[1] Lip avulsion injuries are common consequences of orofacial trauma, with bilateral rostral upper lip avulsion being more common in dogs and bilateral rostral lower lip avulsion being more frequent in cats (Fig. 27.1).[2] Diagnostic imaging, by means of CT or cone-beam CT, in trauma patients should be performed under general anesthesia or heavy sedation after stabilization of the animal. CT is superior to conventional head radiography for identifying maxillofacial traumatic injuries in dogs and cats,[6] providing 3D rendering of images for better spatial understanding of the fractures and surgical planning. The CT DICOM files can be converted to stereolithography files for 3D printers to create models that can be used in treatment planning or fabrication of fixation devices or jigs (Fig. 27.2).[7]

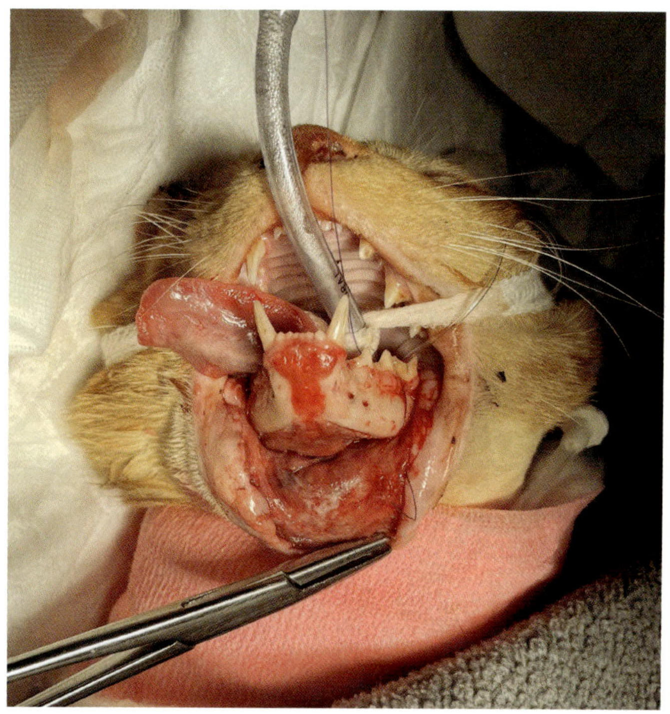

Figure 27.1 Bilateral avulsion of the mandibular lip and associated labial mucosa from the adjacent gingiva in a 6-year-old cat. Image courtesy of Filippo Cinti.

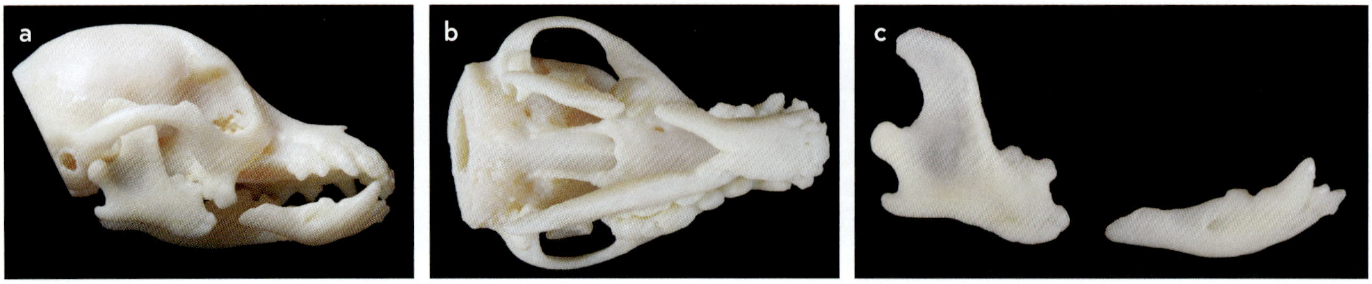

Figure 27.2 3D printed models of a dog that had a fracture nonunion of the right mandible. (a) Lateral and (b) ventrodorsal views of the skull model. (c) Lateral view of the right mandible model.

Treatment

The primary goals in managing maxillofacial fractures are restoring functional, nonpainful occlusion and preventing dental, vascular, and nerve damage during repair. Ideally, the fracture fixation method should result in quick return to normal function and prevent recurrence.[5]

Maxillofacial trauma is most successfully managed by early definitive fracture fixation. Oral and maxillofacial trauma should be considered an urgent rather than an emergency indication for surgery. Trauma to the head may also involve traumatic brain and/or cervical spine injury. In the face of any neurological deficits or uncertainty about the patient's neurological status, surgery should be delayed to enable diagnosis of other life-threatening issues that could place the animal at risk with early anesthesia and surgery. This short delay allows for a more thorough evaluation and coordination of a multidisciplinary approach to patient care. In human maxillofacial trauma, "early" and "late" repairs are defined as less and more than 48 hours from admission to surgery, respectively. In both cases, the hospitalization length and complication rate (e.g., infection) are similar, which further supports a judicious approach.[8] Managing jaw fractures involves the consideration of many variables, including patient's age, fracture type and location, presence and condition of the teeth for device anchorage, jawbone quality, available stabilization methods, and surgeon's skill and preference.[3–5]

Surgical technique: Lip avulsion repair (Fig. 27.3)

Soft tissue injuries, including lacerations and lip avulsions, can be treated under general anesthesia once the patient is stable.

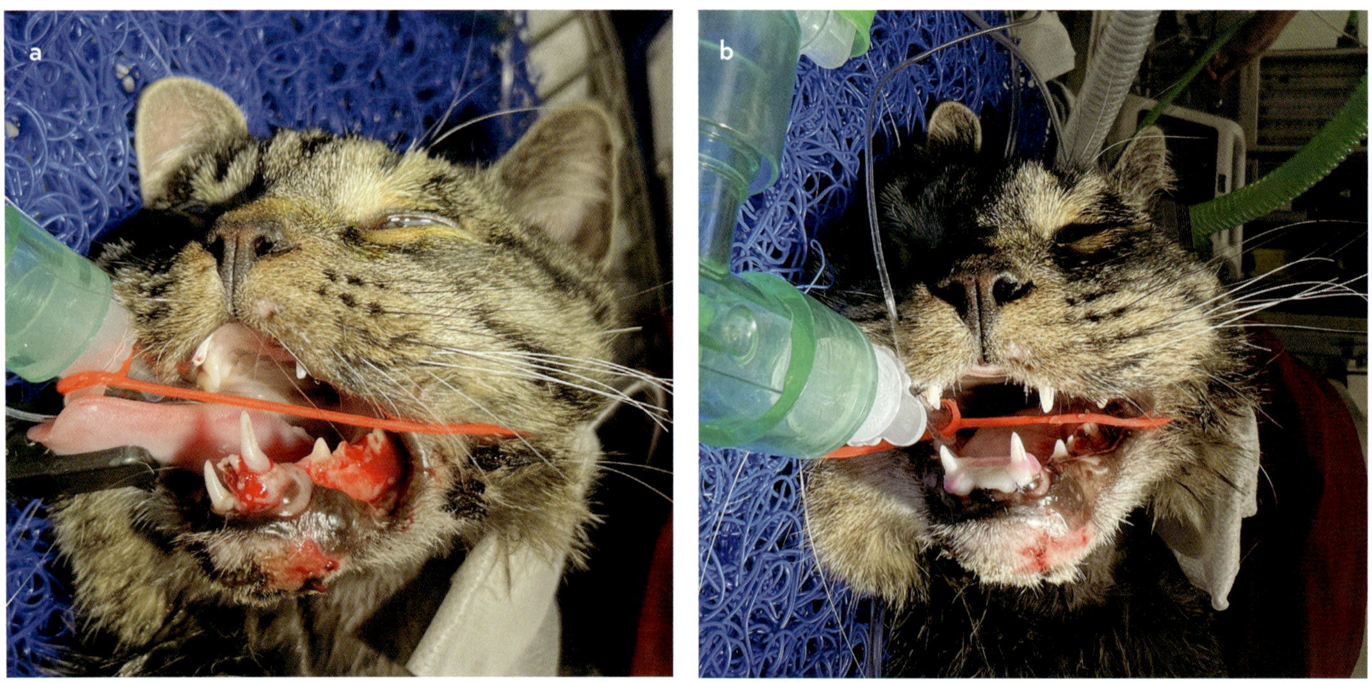

Figure 27.3 Symphyseal separation and unilateral rostral and caudal lower lip avulsion in a 4-year-old cat that was hit by a car. Appearance (a) before surgery and (b) after debridement of oral tissues, interproximal simple interrupted suturing, and placement of a wire and acrylic splint between the mandibular canine teeth.

1. The avulsed lip is debrided and lavaged with sterile saline.
2. Appositional repair of the lip and the mandibular/maxillary mucosa is performed with simple interrupted and/or horizontal mattress sutures (occasionally around the teeth for additional anchorage) using rapidly absorbable material such as 3-0 to 4-0 poliglecaprone 25.[2]
3. Small holes may be drilled through the mandible to provide anchor points for the suture if the incisors are absent or if a large defect is present.
4. The submucosal tissue on the avulsed lip is secured to the mandible via the bone tunnels using absorbable suture material (3-0 to 2-0 poliglecaprone 25) in a simple interrupted pattern or interrupted mattress pattern.
5. Apposition of the mucosal and gingival tissue is maintained with a smaller-gauge suture in a simple continuous pattern (3-0 to 4-0 poliglecaprone 25).
6. A passive or active drain can be placed for 3–5 days, but this is usually not necessary.
7. Nutritional support, including feeding tube placement (nasogastric or esophagostomy tube), is recommended.

Surgical technique: Stabilization of jaw fractures

Noninvasive and minimally invasive maxillofacial fracture repair

The maxilla and mandible have features that allow for different repair techniques compared with other areas of the body. The teeth can be used as anchors for attaching various materials or devices to aid in fracture stabilization.[5] When addressing mandibular fractures, tension forces primarily occur along the dorsal (alveolar) aspect of the bone due to the pulling of the masticatory muscles, the influence of gravity, and the mechanical force exerted by food boluses. Simultaneously, these forces create compression on the ventral aspect of the mandible. Consequently, mandibular fractures may be treated with fixation techniques, focusing on neutralizing tension forces at the dorsal aspect of the bone. The ventral aspect will naturally compress, requiring less direct effort for stabilization.[9]

Techniques falling under the categories of noninvasive and minimally invasive interventions involve minimal manipulation of the fractured bones to achieve alignment, resulting in immobility that allows tissue healing. Among these procedures are maxillomandibular apposition (via muzzle or labial button), maxillomandibular fixation (interarch splinting/bonding), and interdental wiring and composite splinting. The advantages of these techniques include preservation of the periosteum and any callus or hematoma that has started to form, less surgical pain, and prioritization of occlusion. The limitation of noninvasive techniques is the creation of a less rigid fixation compared with more invasive methods, thereby resulting in the potential formation of a larger callus. Also, the less invasive the technique, the greater the probability of prolonged healing times and variation in final teeth occlusion, which may result in traumatic malocclusion.

Maxillomandibular apposition via custom-fitted tape muzzle (Fig. 27.4)

1. An appropriate length of adhesive tape (2 in or 5 cm in large dogs, 1 in or 2.5 cm in small dogs) is folded

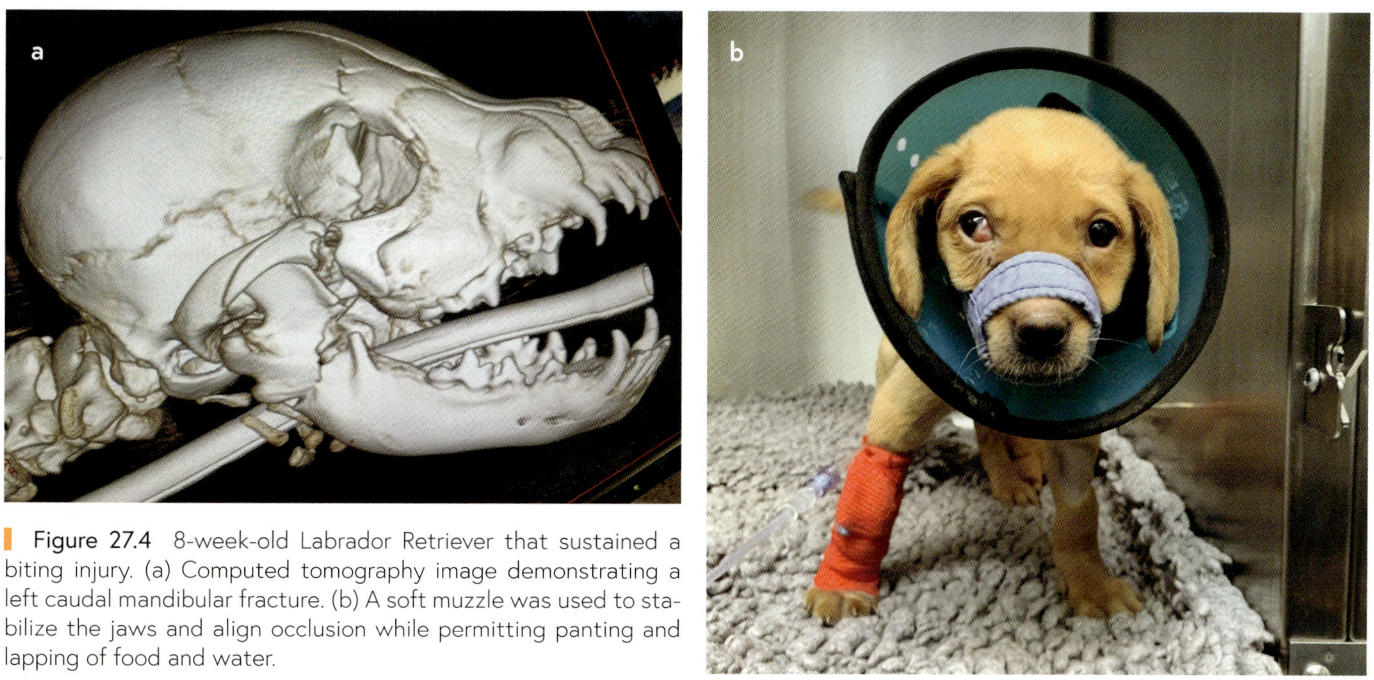

Figure 27.4 8-week-old Labrador Retriever that sustained a biting injury. (a) Computed tomography image demonstrating a left caudal mandibular fracture. (b) A soft muzzle was used to stabilize the jaws and align occlusion while permitting panting and lapping of food and water.

on itself so that the nonstick surface interfaces with the skin of the muzzle. The tape should limit the patient's ability to open their mouth while allowing the tongue to protrude between the incisor teeth (drink water and eat gruel-consistency food).
2. Side tapes are adhered to the muzzle tape and then tied behind the occipital region. The side tapes should be tied to a tightness level that barely allows the veterinarian's index finger between the tapes and the patient's skin.
3. A third tape (optional) can be applied around the muzzle tape, coursing between the patient's eyes, and attached to the tapes at the occipital region.
4. Placement of a feeding tube (nasogastric or esophagostomy) should be considered (see Chapter 5).
5. The tape muzzle is removed after 14–20 days.

Maxillomandibular apposition via labial button technique (Fig. 27.5)

1. The dislocated canine teeth are reduced to their normal position.
2. Nonabsorbable suture material is used to close the lips in a mattress pattern.
   a. First, the suture material is placed through the buttons to distribute the pressure and tied loosely.
   b. It is then passed through the lips, at their base at the mucogingival junction.
   c. Finally, it is placed rostral to the canine teeth on both sides of the upper lip and through the midline of the lower lip.

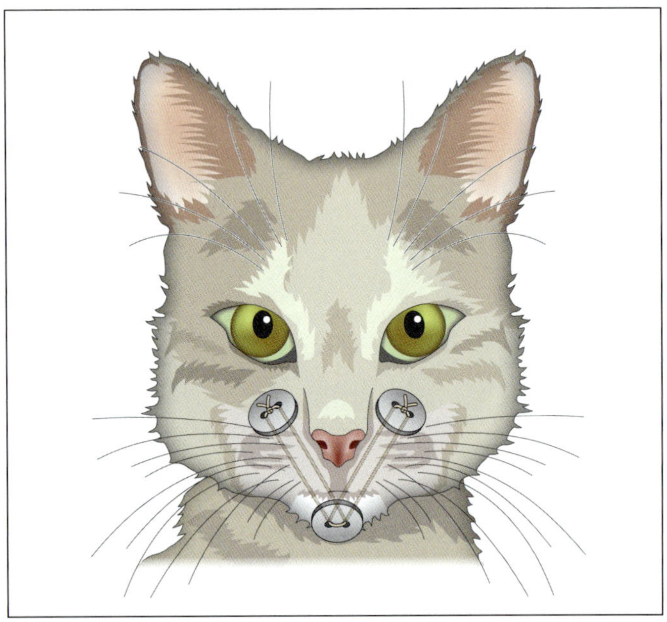

Figure 27.5 Labial button technique in a cat. The jaws are closed using a labial reverse suture through buttons, ensuring dental occlusion.

3. The suture is tied loosely enough to allow the patient to lap up fluid with their tongue.
4. Placement of a feeding tube (nasogastric or esophagostomy) should be considered (see Chapter 5).
5. The buttons are removed after 8–10 days.

Maxillomandibular fixation (interarch splinting/bonding) (Fig. 27.6)

Occlusal alignment and stabilization of caudal mandibular fractures or chronic TMJ displacement may be achieved with bis-acryl composite bridges placed between the maxillary and mandibular canines.

1. The canine teeth are cleaned and acid etched.
2. After placing the canine teeth in occlusion, the mouth is opened and the canine teeth are positioned to overlap by approximately one-third to one-half of the length of the crowns, allowing enough space for drinking and eating gruel-consistency food.
3. A self-curing acrylic resin or composite is applied circumferentially around the teeth forming two posts or pillars of splinting material engaging the canine teeth.

Alternatively, an elastic chain anchored to orthodontic buttons on the mandibular and maxillary canines can be used for maxillomandibular fixation (see Fig. 27.6b).

Interdental wiring (modified Stout loop pattern) and composite splinting (Figs. 27.7 and 27.8)

1. A length of wire is placed and twisted between the teeth with a resultant loop at the interdental space. Repetitive loops are placed around a minimum of two teeth on either side of the fracture.
2. The loops are twisted tight as the wire is held tight in place along the teeth.
3. The loops are twisted in a dorsal direction to lie flat against the coronal surface, with the wire twists located on the lingual/palatal aspect.
4. Acrylic resin is applied on the teeth and wire. Occlusal interference should be avoided.

Invasive maxillofacial fracture repair

Invasive methods of fracture fixation require exposure of the fracture site and/or involve applying internal fixation to the bones. The two primary techniques employed are interfragmentary (intraosseous) wiring and bone plate fixation. External skeletal fixation is rarely indicated but may be used in infected or highly comminuted fractures.[10,11]

Interfragmentary (intraosseous) wiring

Depending on the patient's size, interfragmentary wiring is performed using 18- to 20-gauge and 20- to 24-gauge orthopedic wire in dogs and cats, respectively, with flexibility in pilot hole placement to avoid tooth

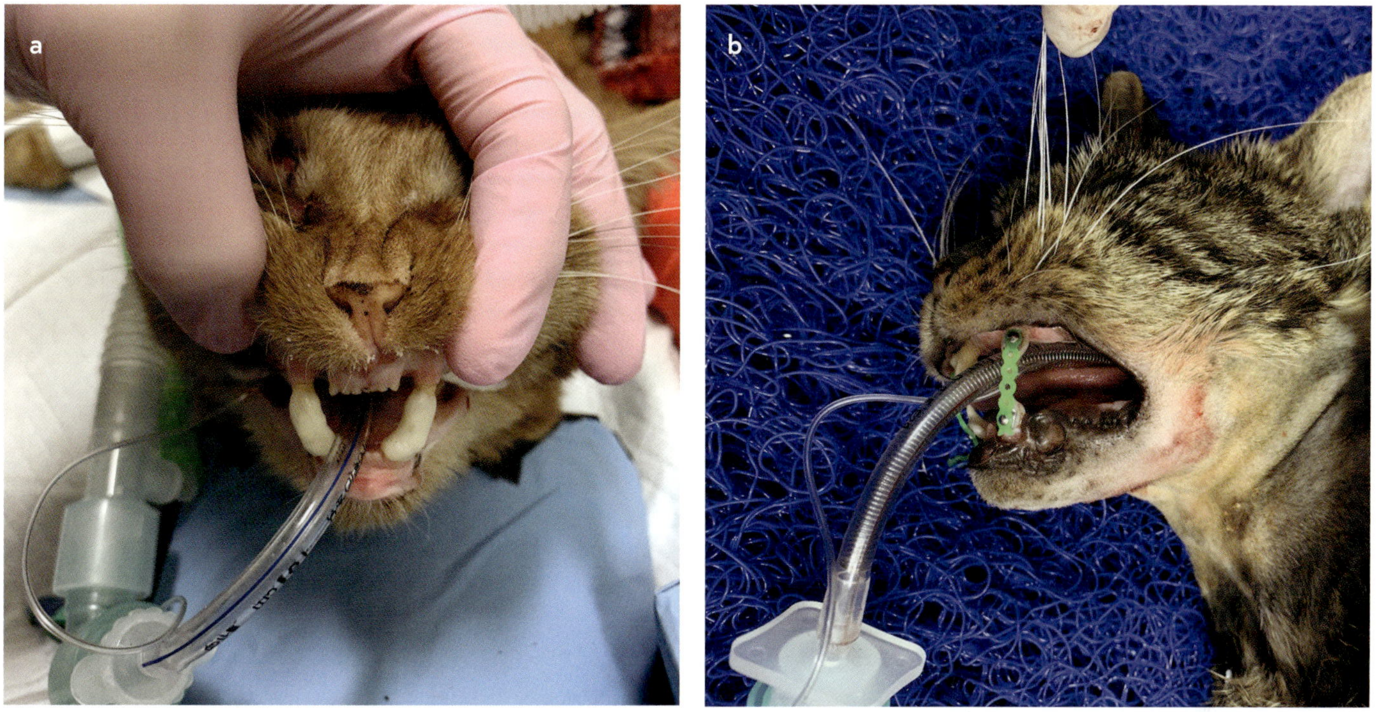

Figure 27.6 Maxillomandibular splinting for treatment of caudal mandibular fractures in two cats. (a) Rigid fixation with dental composite. (b) Elastic fixation with orthodontic buttons and an elastic chain.

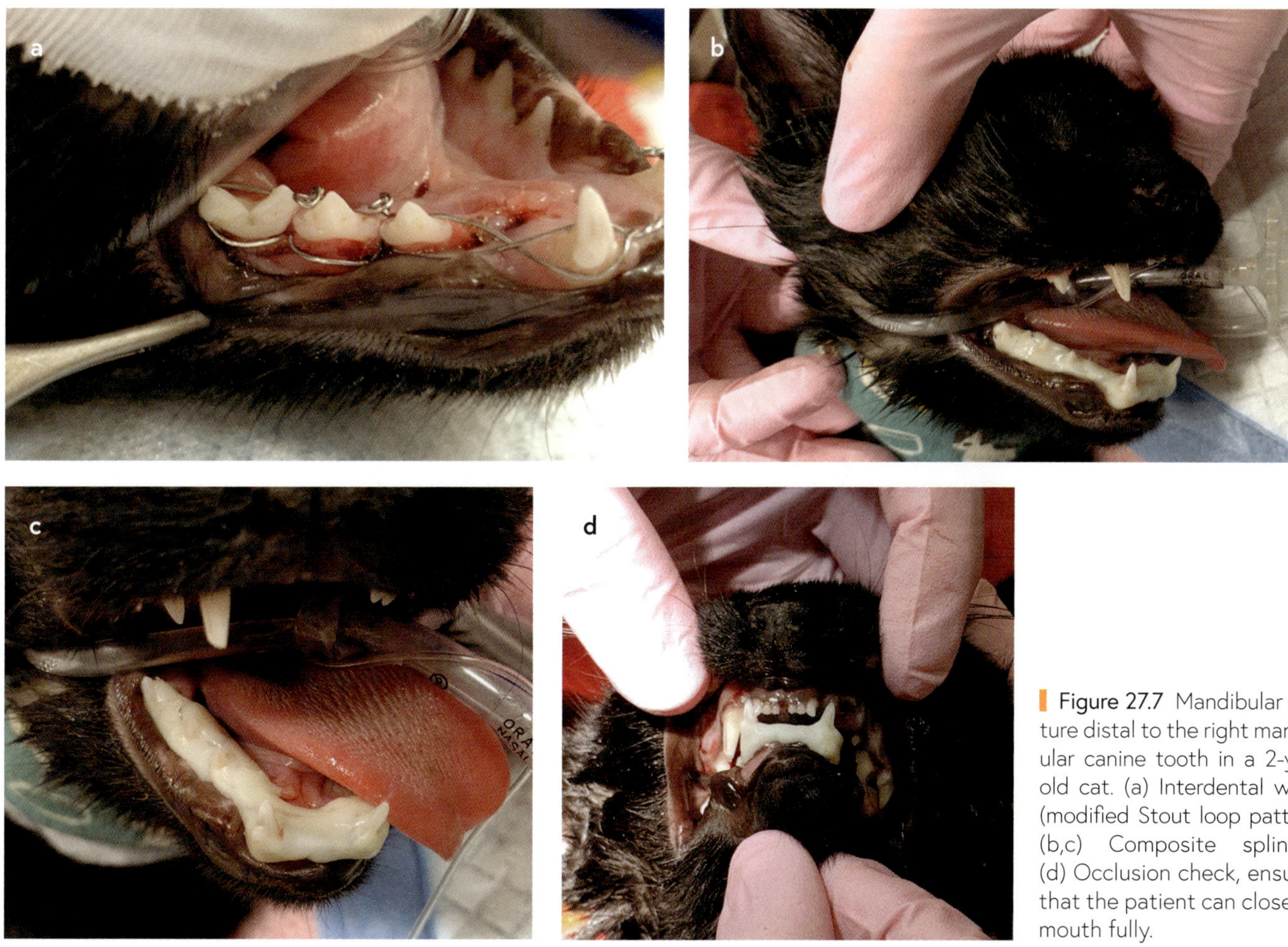

Figure 27.7 Mandibular fracture distal to the right mandibular canine tooth in a 2-year-old cat. (a) Interdental wiring (modified Stout loop pattern). (b,c) Composite splinting. (d) Occlusion check, ensuring that the patient can close the mouth fully.

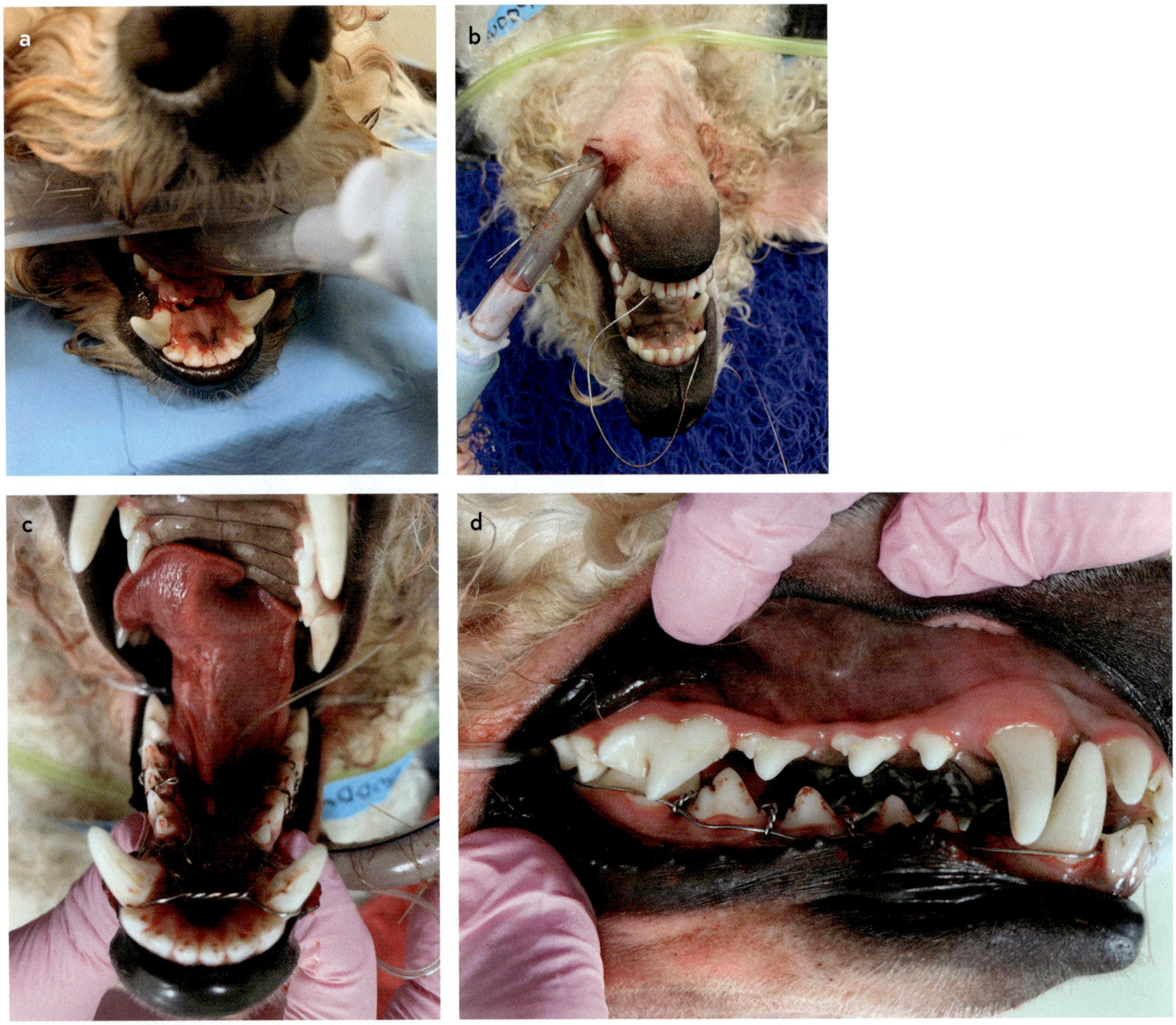

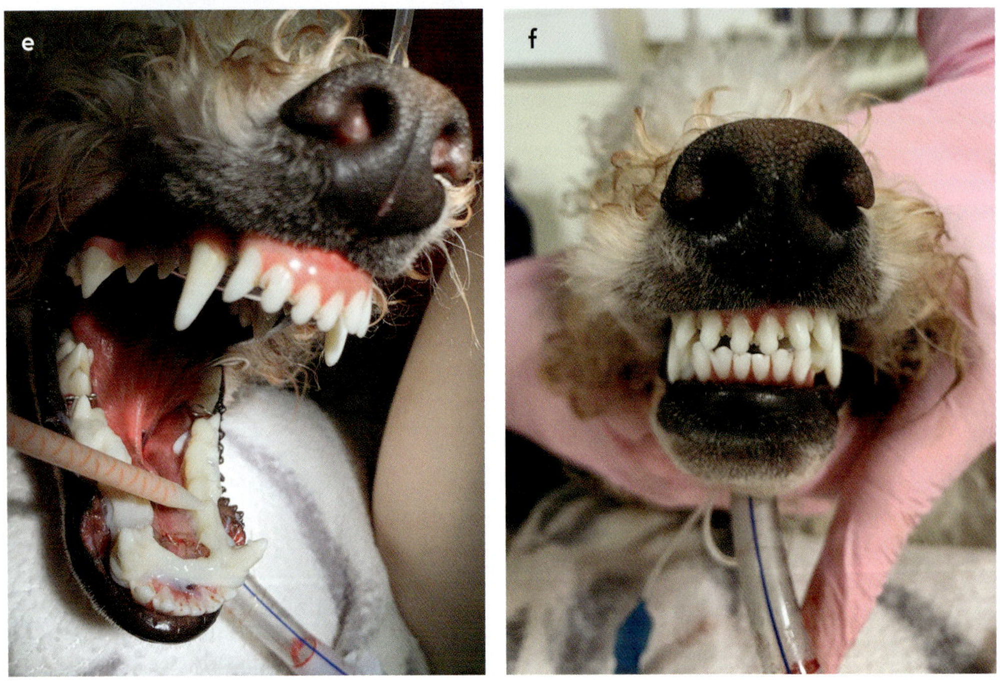

Figure 27.8 Rostral mandibular fracture in a 2-year-old dog. (a) Preoperative appearance. (b) Extraoral (transmylohyoid) intubation. (c,d) Interdental wiring technique (modified Stout loop pattern). (e) Composite splinting. (f) Intraoperative occlusion check.

roots and neurovascular structures. However, this is considered a semirigid form of fixation with poor compression. This technique may be used for repair of a single, interdigitating, and unilateral mandibular fracture. Two sets of pilot holes with wires are typically used at an angle, placed perpendicular to the fracture plane to prevent telescoping.[12,13]

Bone plate fixation (Figs. 27.9 and 27.10)

Titanium miniplates or locking reconstruction plates are frequently used in maxillofacial trauma and reconstruction in human patients and are becoming increasingly common in veterinary medicine. Veterinary-specific applications for craniomaxillofacial repair have been reported clinically in patients and experimentally (biomechanically) in the literature.[14–17] Titanium locking reconstruction plates accept 2.4 mm and 3 mm locking screws, while 2 mm locking miniplates accept 2 mm locking screws. Miniplate constructs are categorized based on the type of plate and the screw–plate relationship. Adaptation plates, locking plates, and reconstruction plates vary in their biomechanical properties and warrant specific surgeon training and familiarity to select optimal constructs. In human medicine, research regarding root repair after damage due to screw insertion for orthodontic miniplate placement has shown that limited root damage has the potential to heal, while extensive root damage may not.[18] Therefore, the precise position of insertion of the miniplates is of utmost importance for achieving successful outcomes.[18]

1. The patient is intubated via pharyngostomy or transmylohyoid intubation, and temporary maxillomandibular fixation is applied to keep the animal in occlusion throughout the surgery (Fig. 27.11).

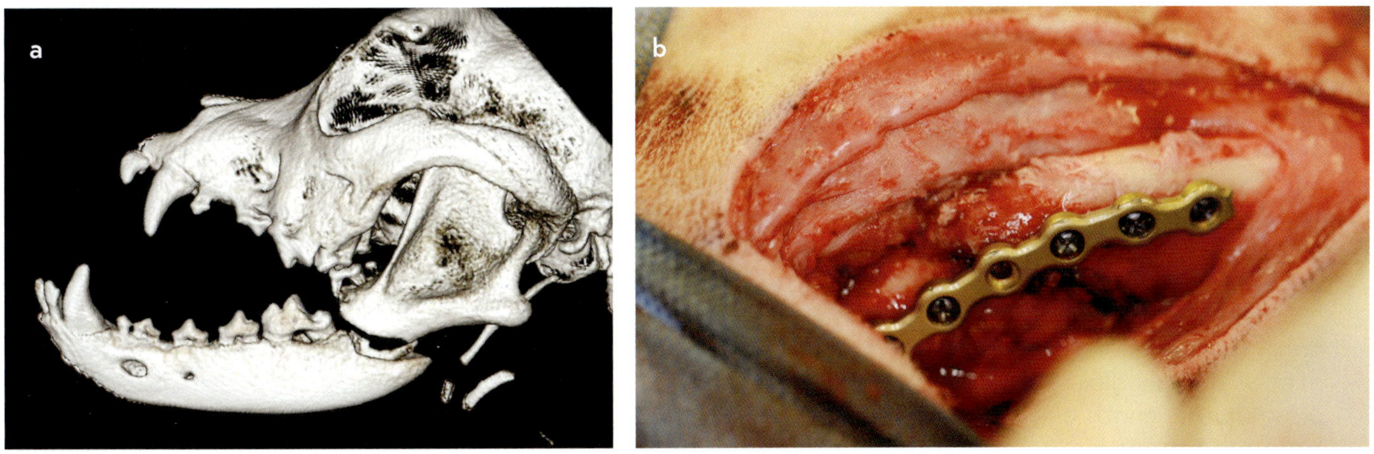

Figure 27.9 Caudal mandibular fracture in a 10-month-old dog. (a) Preoperative computed tomography image. (b) Open reduction of the fracture and internal fixation with a 2.0 mm locking miniplate.

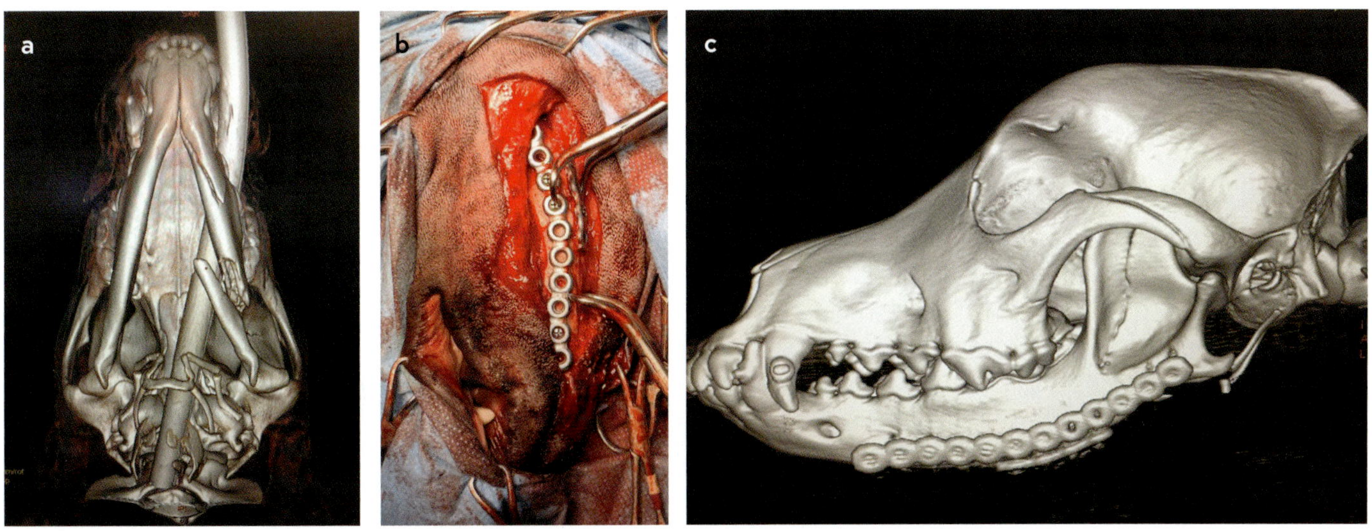

Figure 27.10 Mandibular fracture in a 9-year-old dog. (a) Preoperative computed tomography image. (b) Open reduction of the fracture and internal fixation with two locking plates. (c) Postoperative computed tomography image.

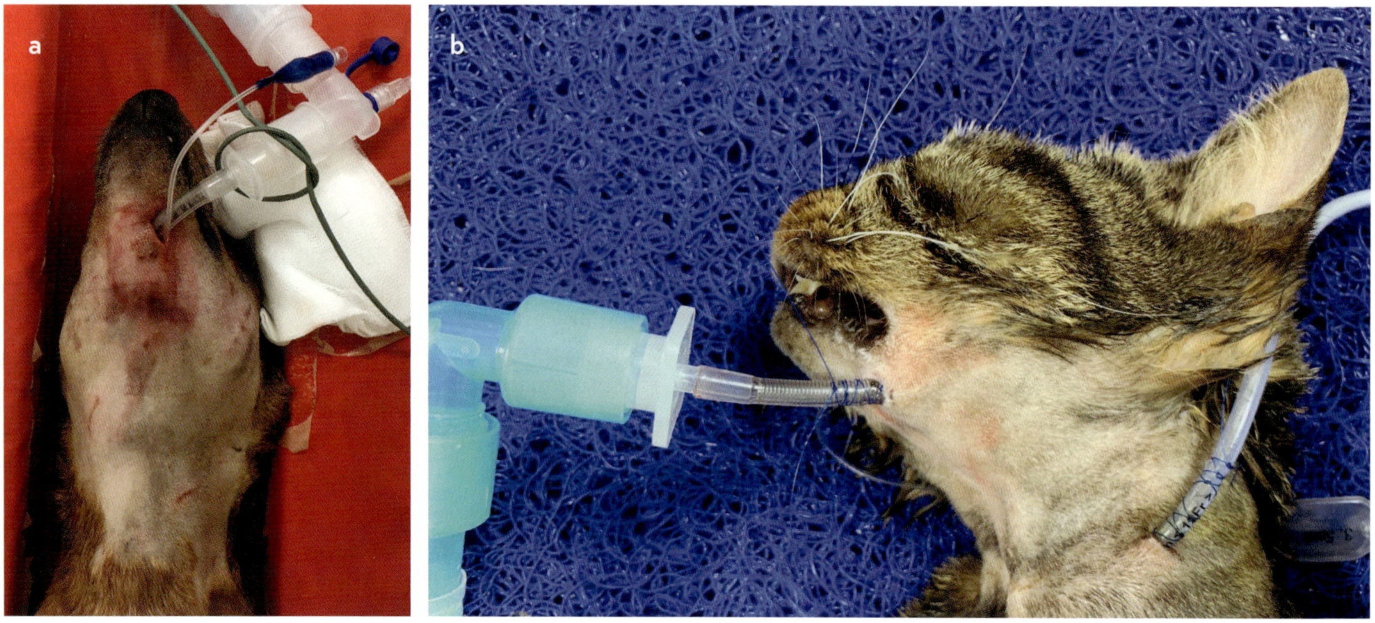

Figure 27.11 Extraoral transmylohyoid intubation for mandibular surgery in (a) a dog and (b) a cat. Images courtesy of Filippo Cinti.

2. A ventral extraoral approach to the mandible is performed. In bilateral fractures, it is recommended to approach each mandible separately (i.e., not through a single midline incision).
3. A single 2.0 mm locking miniplate (cats and small dogs) or a single 2.4 mm/3.0 mm titanium locking reconstruction plate (medium- and large-breed dogs) is fitted and secured on the ventrobuccal aspect of the mandible with titanium locking screws of adequate length and size. The use of "alveolar plates" is not needed, as it is likely to cause dental damage and plate exposure. The use of stainless steel plates and screws in the maxillofacial region is discouraged.
4. Closure of the surgical approach is routine in three layers (3-0 to 4-0 poliglecaprone 25).
5. Nutritional support, including feeding tube placement (nasogastric or esophagostomy tube), should be considered (see Chapter 5).

Postoperative management

Noninvasive maxillofacial fracture repair

The type of fixation device influences postoperative care recommendations for patients undergoing noninvasive repair methods. Patients with intraoral splints should be restricted from chewing or playing with hard objects. To minimize oral soft tissue inflammation due to the accumulation of food debris, intraoral splints should be flushed with tap water or 0.12% chlorhexidine gluconate oral rinse after each meal. Some patients may benefit from an Elizabethan collar to prevent them from chewing or self-traumatizing in an attempt to remove an intraoral splint or maxillomandibular fixation from their mouth. Owners of patients treated with muzzle coaptation must be instructed to change and clean the muzzles daily to reduce the risk of dermatitis (the median time for tape muzzle removal is 2–3 weeks).[5]

Invasive maxillofacial fracture repair

Patients treated with internal rigid fixation typically resume eating and drinking within 24 hours after surgery, limited only by the degree of pain and/or postoperative swelling. Soft food or kibble presoaked with water should be offered during this period. Chewing on hard objects or playing with chew toys is not permitted for the first 4–6 weeks postoperatively.[5] Titanium plates and screws are typically not removed unless infection is noted.

Outcome

The prognosis of lip avulsion injuries treated surgically is excellent.[2] The most common short-term complication is wound dehiscence. Most lip avulsions heal uneventfully if the tissues are properly handled, debrided, and lavaged prior to wound closure. Otherwise, complications such as infection, abscess formation, necrosis, and dehiscence may occur. Failure to achieve tension-free closure will undoubtedly result in partial dehiscence, especially in the lower lip area, where gravity and the bilateral lateral labial frenula create a more ventral pull on the tissues.[2]

The outcome and prognosis after maxillofacial trauma depend on several factors. Regardless of the technique used, achieving good fracture stabilization and functional occlusion contribute to a favorable outcome. The most common complication of noninvasive techniques is delayed union or nonunion. Delayed healing, exuberant callus formation, and fracture nonhealing are also possible. The most frequent complications of invasive techniques are dehiscence, plate exposure, and infection.[5]

Evaluation of the teeth in the fracture line at the time of repair is essential to assess periodontal and endodontic health. The goal of fracture treatment does not end with confirmation of bone healing. Endodontic health of the teeth in the fracture line or teeth affected by disruption to the alveolar neurovascular structures should be evaluated with serial radiographs 3–12 months apart and monitored for continued tooth maturation and development.[5]

Temporomandibular joint emergencies

The inability to close or open the mouth in animals should be addressed on an emergency basis owing to the potential for severe disability and pain. The causes of this inability can vary widely, and an accurate diagnosis based on clinical examination and diagnostic imaging (CT or cone-beam CT) must first be established. A patient may not be able to close their mouth due to maxillofacial trauma with TMJ dislocation or due to TMJ dysplasia or instability resulting in open-mouth jaw locking. Various factors, including foreign bodies, tumors, dislocated teeth, large dental calculus on the teeth's crowns, sublingual sialocele (ranula), and trigeminal neuropathy, may also prevent closing of the mouth. Similarly, reasons for the inability to open the mouth may be related to TMJ lesions (ankylosis), masticatory myositis, severe middle ear disease, foreign bodies, tumors, retrobulbar diseases, or tetanus.[19]

Clinical presentation and diagnosis

Fractures and luxations

TMJ fractures and luxations typically occur as a result of trauma.[20–22] Luxations may be unilateral or bilateral, often with rostrodorsal displacement. Caudal displacement is rare and typically, but not always, involves a fracture of the retroarticular process. This condition may be seen in combination with other maxillofacial injuries, especially in the cat.[19] A complete physical examination, including assessment of cranial nerves, should be performed to search for other injuries secondary to trauma. The most common findings in patients with TMJ subluxation, luxation, or fracture are the inability to close the mouth completely and various degrees of mandibular drift.[19] Oral examination of an animal unable to close their mouth will be challenging without sedation or general anesthesia due to the pain and discomfort.[19] After anesthetic induction, oral examination is performed, focusing on oral wounds and open fractures. The mandibles and maxilla should be gently palpated and the mandible manipulated. Palpable crepitus suggests fracture, and gentle pressure will usually allow mouth closure. Malocclusion and inability to close the mouth by manipulation may suggest TMJ luxation.[19] Commonly, unilateral rostrodorsal TMJ luxation, with the condylar process moving rostrally and dorsally, results in the mandible shifting laterorostrally toward the contralateral side, manifesting in the patient as an acute inability to close their mouth fully due to the abnormal contact between the maxillary and mandibular teeth on the opposite side (Video 27.1).[23]

CT is essential for a comprehensive assessment of the TMJs, which is important for formulating a precise treatment plan (Fig. 27.12). With luxation, the condylar process of the mandible is displaced from the mandibular fossa of the temporal bone, most commonly in a rostrodorsal direction.[19]

Video 27.1. 1-year-4-month-old domestic short-haired cat presented with left TMJ luxation (rostrodorsal displacement). Note the inability to close the mouth, hematoma on the left caudal mucosa and the mandibular drift.

Open-mouth jaw locking

True dysplasia of the hard and/or soft tissue structures forming the TMJ can be congenital or acquired and has primarily been reported in Basset Hounds and Persian cats but may also occur in other dog and cat breeds.[24] Often, TMJ instability, resulting in open-mouth jaw locking, may be seen without radiological evidence of dysplasia. Instability of the TMJ results in abnormal movement of the mandible where the coronoid process engages the zygomatic arch, resulting in a "lock" that can be ventral or lateral to the zygomatic arch (Fig. 27.13).

Clinical signs typically manifest in young adults (6 months to 5 years of age),[25] with locking episodes happening multiple times a day or over several weeks or months. When these episodes occur, most dogs will vocalize, shake the head, paw at the muzzle, and rub the muzzle on the ground until the locking is spontaneously reduced, whereas cats may seek seclusion. Initially, locking episodes are of short duration and self-correcting by opening the mouth wider, allowing the coronoid process to disengage the zygomatic arch and return to its physiological position. As the insta-

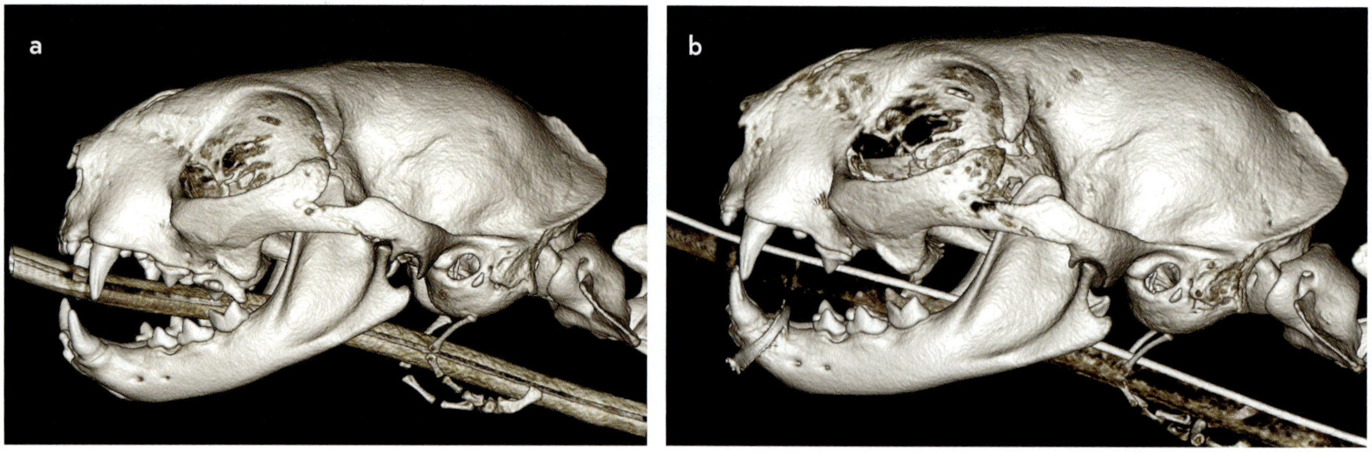

Figure 27.12 Cone-beam computed tomography images of a 7-year-old domestic shorthair cat that sustained maxillofacial trauma resulting in left-sided rostrodorsal temporomandibular joint (TMJ) luxation and symphysis separation. (a) Preoperative appearance. (b) Follow-up 2 weeks after manual reduction of the TMJ luxation and rigid maxillomandibular fixation, confirming that the TMJ was in place. The maxillomandibular fixation device was subsequently removed.

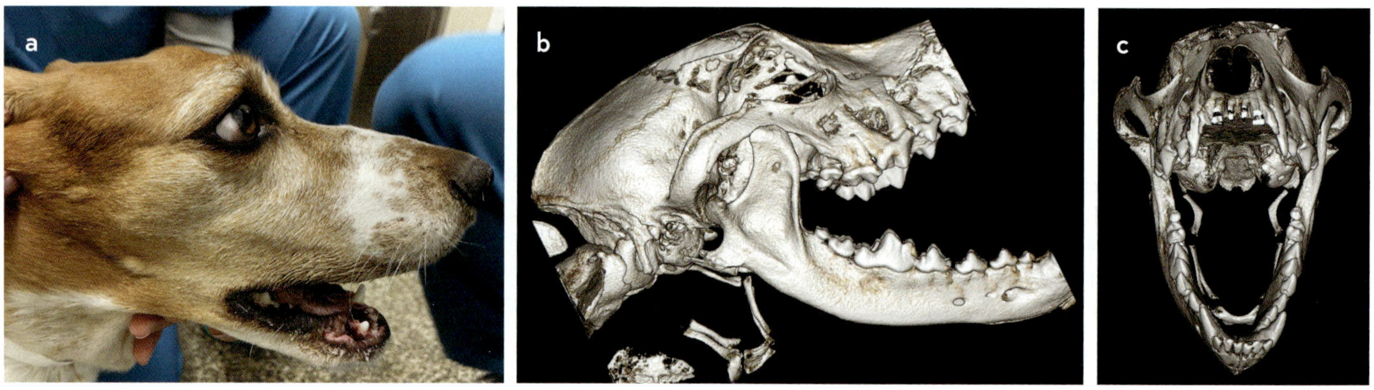

Figure 27.13 Open-mouth jaw locking due to temporomandibular joint dysplasia in a 3-year-old Basset Hound dog. (a) Clinical appearance. Note the bulge on the right side due to the coronoid process locking lateral to the zygomatic arch. (b) Right lateral and (c) rostral 3D cone-beam computed tomography images demonstrating the locking of the coronoid process lateral to the zygomatic arch.

bility progresses and the episodes of coronoid process engagement with the zygomatic arch become more frequent, periosteal reaction on both bones increases, resulting in larger surface area for engagement. Consequently, this leads to a failure of spontaneous reduction and/or more frequent locking episodes. When a history of head trauma is reported, the locking may be attributed to a healed depressed fracture of the zygomatic arch. This healed fracture interferes with the movement of the coronoid process, giving rise to locking episodes that closely resemble those caused by TMJ dysplasia/instability.[25,26]

The diagnosis of TMJ dysplasia/instability and the resultant open-mouth jaw locking heavily relies on a thorough physical examination and manipulation of the mandibles (i.e., creating the lock, on both sides) under general anesthesia. Attempting to manipulate the mandibles to induce a lock under heavy sedation may fail if complete muscle relaxation is not achieved and is not recommended. During an episode of open-mouth jaw locking, examination shows a patient with an open mouth very resistant to manipulation of the lower jaw. A palpable and visible bulge on the side of the face becomes evident when the coronoid process is displaced ventrally or laterally to the zygomatic arch. The lower jaw is shifted toward the side where the lock has occurred, and there is a noticeable tilt, resulting in the mandibular body being slightly displaced ventrally to the locked side.[25]

CT is currently considered the gold standard imaging modality for diagnosing TMJ disorders.[21,22,25–28] Magnetic resonance imaging may be used if soft tissue pathology is suspected (e.g., TMJ disc abnormality). Advanced imaging may allow the detection of subtle anatomic abnormalities and a comparison between both joints of the patient. The use of CT is of crucial value in the evaluation

In recurrent cases, treatment consists of surgical correction.[20,29] The goal of surgical treatment is to prevent further locking episodes rather than to stabilize the TMJ. Both sides may be affected.

1. Locking of the apparently unaffected side should be attempted under general anesthesia during the diagnostic phases and confirmed via CT prior to surgery. Both sides require surgery if locking can be elicited on either side.
2. An incision is made along the zygomatic arch.
3. The masseter muscle origin and temporal muscle insertions are elevated from the bone, and the coronoid process is identified.
4. A rim excision or segment of the zygomatic arch is removed, ideally with a piezoelectric surgical unit.
5. The same instrument is then used to remove a portion of the coronoid process large enough to stop future locking.
6. The surgical site is closed routinely.

If surgery is performed in patients with the mouth locked open, it is helpful to release any muscle attachments from the coronoid process and grasp the process with bone holding forceps, so that it can be readily found after partial zygomectomy.[24,25,29]

Postoperative management

After condylectomy, coronoidectomy, and zygomectomy, soft food is recommended and oral activity should be limited to eating and drinking for the first 2 weeks postoperatively. Normal oral activity may resume thereafter.[25] Nutritional support, including feeding tube placement (nasogastric or esophagostomy tube), should be considered.

Outcome

A small seroma may develop at the surgery site secondary to jaw movement. This usually does not require treatment. If the entire height of the zygomatic arch is excised, some facial asymmetry may result, with the operated side appearing flatter compared to the normal side. Recurrence of locking episodes after unilateral surgery may indicate inadequate removal or regrowth of the zygomatic arch, inadequate reduction of coronoid process height, undetected bilateral disease, need for surgery on the opposite side, or initial misdiagnosis of the involved side.[25]

The prognosis is generally good after unilateral or bilateral surgery, assuming that enough bone was removed to prevent recurrence. Owners should be informed about the possibility of undetected bilateral disease and the need for additional surgery should locking episodes recur. Long-term results do not indicate further clinical complications associated with the dysplastic or unstable TMJs.[25,26]

KEEP IN MIND

- The goals of maxillofacial fracture management are restoring functional, nonpainful occlusion and avoiding dental, vascular, and nerve damage during repair.
- Maxillofacial fractures in immature patients are best treated with noninvasive techniques to avoid disturbance of dental development and growth.
- Extraoral intubation is helpful to avoid interference with intraoperative occlusion assessment.
- In adult patients, internal rigid fixation is associated with less postoperative complications and faster return to normal function compared with noninvasive techniques.

References

1. Reiter AM. Dental and oral diseases. In: Little SE. *The Cat: Clinical Medicine and Management*, 1st ed. St. Louis, MO: Saunders; 2012. pp. 329–370.
2. Saverino KM, Reiter AM. Clinical presentation, causes, treatment, and outcome of lip avulsion injuries in dogs and cats: 24 cases (2001–2017). *Front Vet Sci.* 2018; 5:144.
3. Umphlet RC, Johnson AL. Mandibular fractures in the dog. A retrospective study of 157 cases. *Vet Surg.* 1990; 19(4): 272–275.
4. Kitshoff AM, de Rooster H, Ferreira SM, Steenkamp G. A retrospective study of 109 dogs with mandibular fractures. *Vet Comp Orthop Traumatol.* 2013; 26(1):1–5.
5. Boudrieau R, Arzi B, Verstraete F. Principles of maxillofacial trauma repair. In: Verstraete F, Lommer M, Arzi B (eds.). *Oral and Maxillofacial Surgery in Dogs and Cats*, 2nd ed. St. Louis, MO: Saunders (Elsevier); 2020. pp. 252–261.
6. Bar-Am Y, Pollard RE, Kass PH, Verstraete FJ. The diagnostic yield of conventional radiographs and computed tomography in dogs and cats with maxillofacial trauma. *Vet Surg.* 2008; 37(3):294–299.
7. Winer JN et al. The application of 3-dimensional printing for preoperative planning in oral and maxillofacial surgery in dogs and cats. *Vet Surg.* 2017; 46(7):942–951.
8. Weider L, Hughes K, Ciarochi J, Dunn E. Early versus delayed repair of facial fractures in the multiply injured patient. *Am Surg.* 1999; 65(8):790–793.
9. Howard PE. Tape muzzle for mandibular fractures. *Vet Med Small Anim Clin.* 1981; 76(4):517–519.
10. Owen MR et al. Mandibular fracture repair in dogs and cats using epoxy resin and acrylic external skeletal fixation. *Vet Comp Orthop Traumatol.* 2004; 17(4):189–197.
11. Woodbridge N, Owen M. Feline mandibular fractures: A significant surgical challenge. *J Feline Med Surg.* 2013; 15(3):211–218.

Chapter

Septic

A positive synovial culture or the identification of intracellular bacteria in synovial fluid cytology is currently the gold standard for diagnosis of bacterial septic arthritis. However, the reported sensitivities of synovial tissue/fluid bacterial culture are relatively low, with false-negative results ranging from 20% to 50% in dogs.[1–3,7,8,11] Intracellular bacteria are only observed in about 50%–60% of samples that culture positively for bacterial growth; no association between identification of bacteria on a synovial fluid smear and a positive culture result has been reported.[1,2,7] Skin commensals are the most common type of bacteria cultured in cases of septic arthritis. In dogs, *Staphylococcus* spp. is the most frequently cultured species, followed by *Streptococcus* spp.; in cats, organisms like *Pasteurella multocida* and *Bacteroides* spp. are more common, reflecting the oral flora and the suspicion of bite wounds being a route of infection.[1–3,8,9]

Despite the challenges in diagnosing septic arthritis, arthrocentesis should be performed in a sterile manner, and synovial fluid analysis and cytology should be performed, with the remaining sample submitted for bacterial culture. If only a small amount of fluid is obtained, preparing slides for microscopic examination should be prioritized.[12,13] Cytological examination shows an increase in total nucleated cell counts, with a shift in the cell population to polymorphonuclear leukocytes. Intracellular bacteria are observed.[1–3,12] Typically, septic joints have a total nucleated cell count above 5000 cells/μL, whereas normal joints should have less than 3000 cells/μL.[4] Neutrophils often comprise more than 90% of the total nucleated cell count (Table 28.1).[1,2,5,7]

A diagnosis of septic arthritis can still be considered even if bacteriology results are negative, as long as the clinical signs and cytology findings strongly support the presence of infective arthritis.

There is controversy regarding the impact of antibiotic administration prior to sample collection on culture results. Some studies suggest an association between antibiotic therapy and false-negative culture results,[3,8,9] while others have found no such association.[1,2,7] Synovial fluid lactate concentration has been evaluated as a marker for septic arthritis in dogs. In one study, a lactate concentration below 6.5 mmol/L was exclusionary for a diagnosis of septic arthritis, suggesting that a low synovial fluid lactate level is inconsistent with a diagnosis of septic arthritis.[14]

Radiographs of the affected joint are rarely helpful to establish a diagnosis of septic arthritis. By the time significant radiographic changes appear, there is usually already loss of bone, cartilage erosion, and cartilage matrix breakdown present. Early radiographic findings include joint effusion and soft tissue swelling. Late radiographic changes are characterized by joint surface irregularities, subchondral bone sclerosis and lysis, and periosteal new bone formation (Fig. 28.2).[15]

Treatment

Early diagnosis and treatment are crucial to prevent irreversible damage to the articular cartilage caused by the release of proteolytic enzymes and decreased nutrient exchange/tissue oxygenation due to accumulation of intra-articular exudate.[4,6] Systemic sepsis secondary to an articular infection has been rarely reported in dogs, further supporting the recommendation for early treatment of septic arthritis.[2]

Treatment options for septic arthritis include medical management alone or with joint flushing/surgical intervention. Medical management involves at least 4 weeks of parenteral antimicrobial therapy, ideally based on culture and sensitivity results. In more advanced cases, treatment may need to be continued for 6–8 weeks.[4] A broad-spectrum antimicrobial that is effective against *Staphylococcus* and *Streptococcus* (e.g., ampicillin–sulbactam) is a good initial choice while culture results are pending. Many studies have reported successful treatment with antibiotics as the sole therapy in patients with septic arthritis.[1–3,5,8,9,16] Interestingly, in a rabbit model of septic arthritis, adding a nonsteroidal anti-inflammatory medication decreased cartilage glycosaminoglycan and collagen loss when compared to

TABLE 28.1 - SYNOVIAL FLUID COMPOSITION IN INFECTIVE ARTHRITIS

Parameter	Normal	Bacterial arthritis
Consistency	Clear, ropy, long strand	Cloudy, tan, pink-tinged, less viscous
Total protein	<3 g/dL	>3 g/dL
Glucose (compared to serum)	Same	Lower
Lactate (compared to serum)	Same	Higher
Cell count (cells/μL)	<3000	>5000
Cell type	Mononuclear	>75% neutrophils

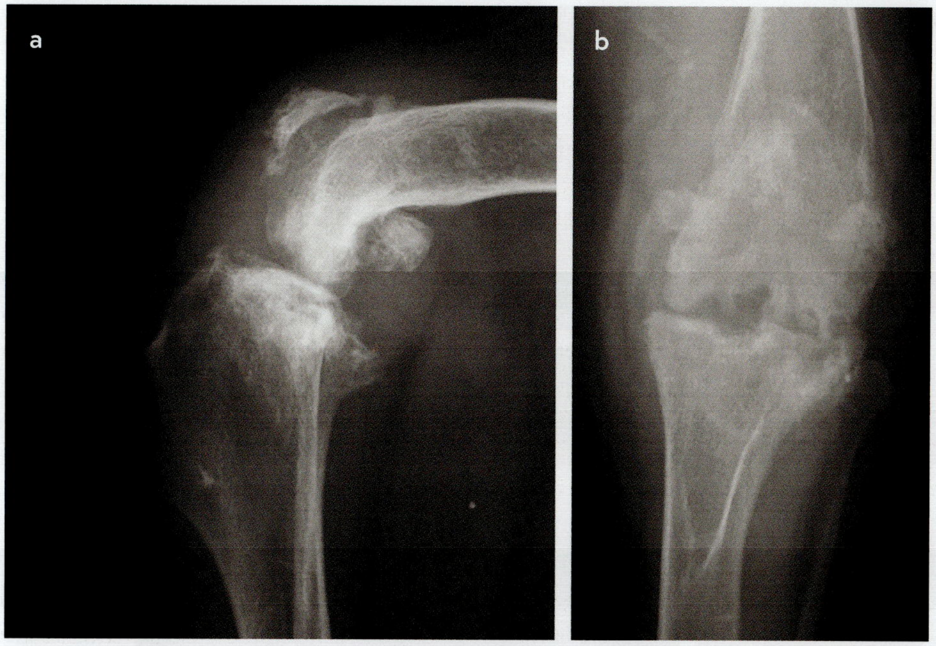

Figure 28.2 (a) Mediolateral and (b) craniocaudal radiographs of the right stifle joint of a 4-year-old 35 kg Cane Corso with septic arthritis after extracapsular suture stabilization to treat cranial cruciate ligament rupture. Images courtesy of Luca Vezzoni.

antibiotic therapy alone.[17] Therefore, it may be prudent to consider the coadministration of a nonsteroidal anti-inflammatory drug if patient factors allow.

The recommendation for joint flushing is clinician dependent and likely based on the severity of the clinical signs. The rationale for joint flushing and/or debridement includes the removal of suppurative material to improve tissue oxygenation and decrease inflammation, debridement of necrotic tissue, and removal of implants that may serve as a nidus of infection (Figs. 28.3 and 28.4).[4] In human medicine, it is recommended that all septic joints are flushed and debrided via arthroscopy or arthrotomy, although no prospective studies have been published comparing drainage to nondrainage procedures.[18–20]

Outcome

Initial successful management is frequently reported, but multiple studies have found that many dogs have residual long-term lameness. This is especially common in dogs with underlying osteoarthritis.[1,2,9,16] Treatment success parameters vary, but, generally, successful treatment is reported in 78%–100% of cases documented in the literature. Successful treatment is more likely with early intervention compared to chronic septic arthritis and delayed treatment.[1,8] Increasing body weight has been associated with poorer outcomes following either medical or surgical treatment of septic arthritis.[1,8]

Recurrence of septic arthritis in the same joint or a different joint has been reported, although this appears

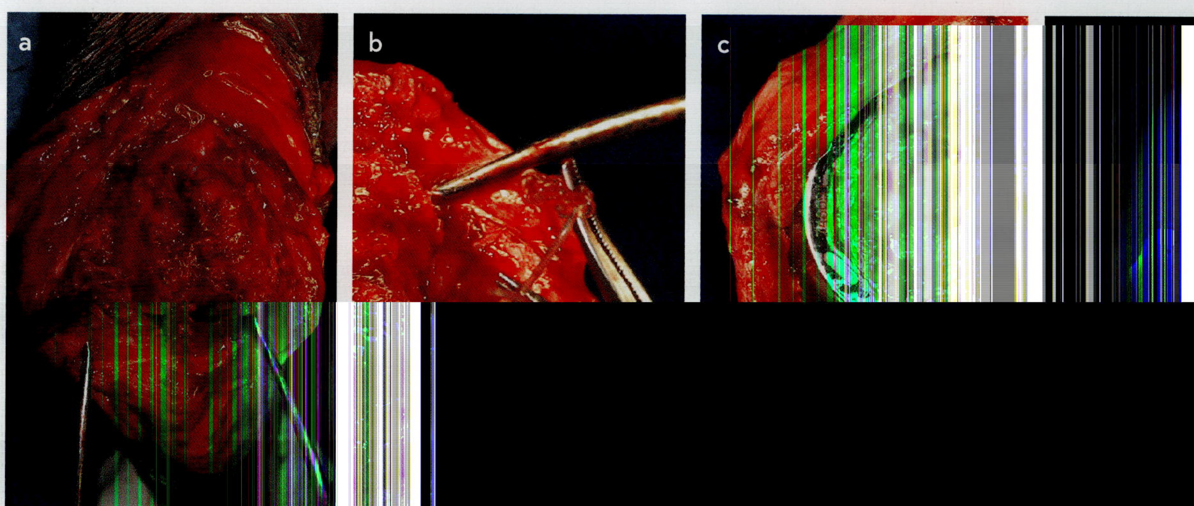

Figure 28.3 Same patient as in Fig...

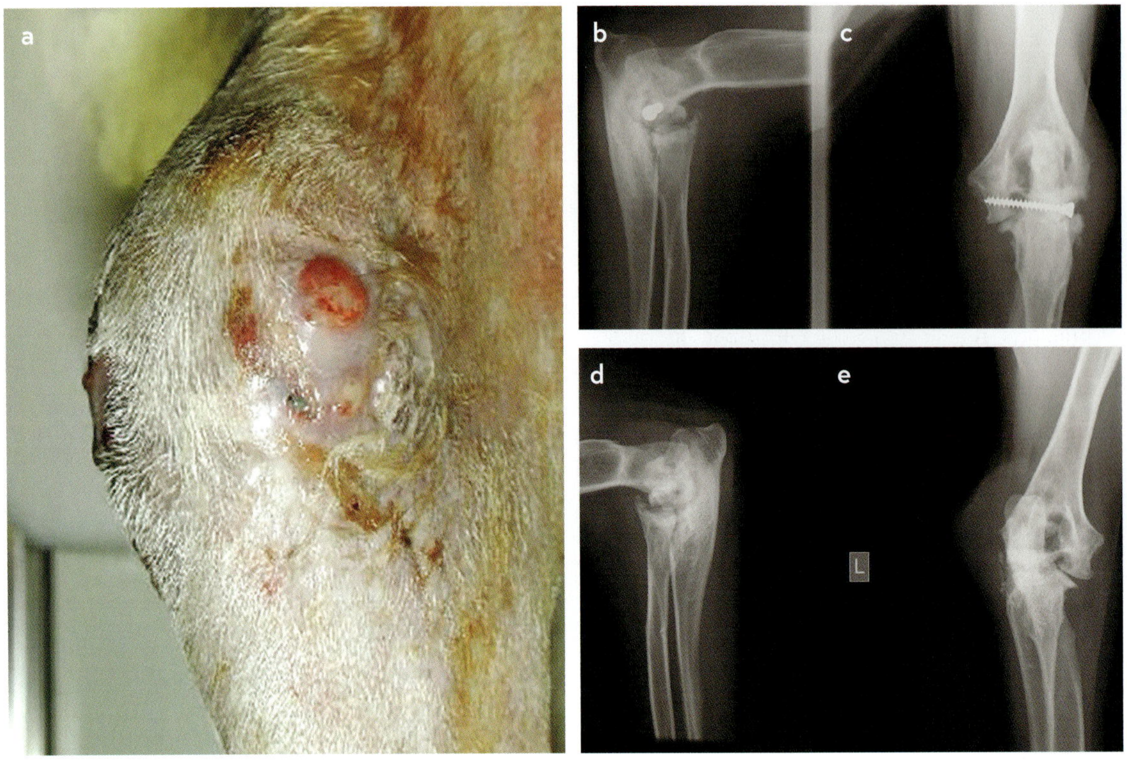

Figure 28.4 Septic arthritis of the elbow in a dog. The patient was treated for an intercondylar humeral fracture by a referral veterinarian, but septic arthritis developed a few months later. (a) A draining tract is present, and the implant is visible. (b,c) Mediolateral and craniocaudal radiographs are consistent with septic arthritis. (d,e) Revision surgery was performed in a different hospital and the implant (screw) was removed. Images courtesy of Luca Vezzoni and Aldo Vezzoni.

to be relatively uncommon (0%–11%).[1,2] Spontaneous septic arthritis with concurrent elbow osteoarthritis was associated with a higher recurrence rate (25%) in one study, with preexisting osteoarthritis proposed to be a recrudescence mechanism of infection.[2] Another study supported this mechanism and found a significant association between recurrent septic arthritis and preexisting osteoarthritis.[8] Additionally, recurrence may be associated with other comorbidities, such as lupus erythematosus, diabetes mellitus, urinary tract infection, or skin infection.[2] It is suggested that a lack of surgical intervention significantly increases the risk of recurrence of septic arthritis in human retrospective studies,[20] but no such association has been reported in veterinary medicine.

In conclusion, septic arthritis should be recognized and treated quickly to achieve the best patient outcome. In veterinary medicine there is no clear advantage of surgical treatment over antibiotic therapy alone, and the choice of treatment is likely clinician dependent. Many clinicians, at the author's institution, use medical therapy initially and consider joint flushing or arthroscopy if the patient does not improve. While dogs with septic arthritis generally have a good prognosis, owners should be informed that many patients may experience long-term lameness, especially if underlying joint disease is present.

KEEP IN MIND

- Most animals with septic arthritis present with a monoarthropathy and mild to severe lameness.
- Septic joints are usually associated with previous articular surgery, underlying osteoarthritis, or trauma to the joint.
- Diagnosis is supported by synovial fluid cytology and bacterial culture of synovium or synovial fluid.
- Treatment includes at least 4 weeks of parenteral broad-spectrum antibiotic administration based on bacterial culture results. It is unknown if joint flushing or debridement results in a more favorable outcome than antibiotic therapy alone.
- Early diagnosis and treatment is important to prevent irreversible changes to the articular cartilage.

References

1. Clements DN et al. Retrospective study of bacterial infective arthritis in 31 dogs. *J Small Anim Pract.* 2005; 46(4):171–176.
2. Mielke B, Comerford E, English K, Meeson R. Spontaneous septic arthritis of canine elbows: Twenty-one cases. *Vet Comp Orthop Traumatol.* 2018; 31(6):488–493.
3. Marchevsky AM, Read RA. Bacterial septic arthritis in 19 dogs. *Aust Vet J.* 1999; 77(4):233–237.
4. Greene CE, Bennett D. Joint infections In: Sykes JE, Greene CE (eds.). *Infectious Diseases of the Dog and Cat*, 4th ed. Elsevier; 2011. pp. 908–911.
5. Benzioni H, Shahar R, Yudelevitch S, Milgram J. Bacterial infective arthritis of the coxofemoral joint in dogs with hip dysplasia. *Vet Comp Orthop Traumatol.* 2008; 21(3):262–266.
6. Goldstein R. Swollen joints and lameness. In: Ettinger S, Feldmman E (eds.). *Textbook of Veterinary Internal Medicine*, 7th ed. Elsevier; 2010. pp. 130–133.
7. Scharf VF et al. Retrospective evaluation of the efficacy of isolating bacteria from synovial fluid in dogs with suspected septic arthritis. *Aust Vet J.* 2015; 93(6):200–203.
8. Phillips TF, Bleyaert HF. Retrospective evaluation of 103 cases of septic arthritis in dogs. *Vet Rec.* 2022; 190(5):e938.
9. Bennett D, Taylor DJ. Bacterial infective arthritis in the dog. *J Small Anim Pract.* 1988; 29(4):207–230.
10. Bennett D, Taylor DJ. Bacterial endocarditis and inflammatory joint disease in the dog. *J Small Anim Pract.* 1988; 29(6):347–365.
11. Montgomery RD et al. Comparison of aerobic culturette, synovial membrane biopsy, and blood culture medium in detection of canine bacterial arthritis. *Vet Surg.* 1989; 18(4):300–303.
12. MacWilliams PS, Friedrichs KR. Laboratory evaluation and interpretation of synovial fluid. *Vet Clin North Am Small Anim Pract.* 2003; 33(1):153–178.
13. Gibson NR et al. Value of direct smears of synovial fluid in the diagnosis of canine joint disease. *Vet Rec.* 1999; 144(17):463–465.
14. Proot JL, de Vicente F, Sheahan DE. Analysis of lactate concentrations in canine synovial fluid. *Vet Comp Orthop Traumatol.* 2015; 28(5):301–305.
15. Lemetayer J, Taylor S. Inflammatory joint disease in cats: Diagnostic approach and treatment. *J Feline Med Surg.* 2014; 16(7):547–562.
16. Fitch RB, Hogan TC, Kudnig ST. Hematogenous septic arthritis in the dog: Results of five patients treated nonsurgically with antibiotics. *J Am Anim Hosp Assoc.* 2003; 39(6):563–566.
17. Smith RL, Kajiyama G, Schurman DJ. Staphylococcal septic arthritis: Antibiotic and nonsteroidal anti-inflammatory drug treatment in a rabbit model. *J Orthop Res.* 1997; 15(6):919–926.
18. Sammer DM, Shin AY. Comparison of arthroscopic and open treatment of septic arthritis of the wrist. Surgical technique. *J Bone Joint Surg Am.* 2010; 92 Suppl 1 Pt 1:107–113.
19. Lauper N et al. Native septic arthritis is not an immediate surgical emergency. *J Infect.* 2018; 77(1):47–53.
20. Uçkay I et al. Short parenteral antibiotic treatment for adult septic arthritis after successful drainage. *Int J Infect Dis.* 2013; 17(3):e199–e205.

Chapter 29

Open fracture management

Anna M. Massie

Open fractures involve disruption of soft tissue integrity and subsequent exposure of a fractured bone to environmental contamination.[1] They are frequently seen in veterinary medicine, representing 14% and 29% of traumatic fractures in dogs and cats, respectively.[2] Although not established in cats, open fractures are most commonly a sequela to high-impact trauma in dogs.[2]
Open fractures present a unique challenge, as disruption of both bone and soft tissues must be addressed, and the degree of damage to each has a substantial effect on the local tissue vascularity and healing potential.[3] The introduction of microorganisms and potential foreign bodies into the wound increases the risks involved, including, but not limited to, infection, delayed healing, and nonunion fracture formation.[3,4]
The incidence of open fractures is reported to be higher in sexually intact dogs and cats, suspectedly due to the propensity for these animals to roam and thus be at risk for a traumatic event. Although younger dogs are more likely to sustain a traumatic fracture, in older dogs such fractures are more likely to be open. The risk of open fractures is also higher in larger dogs than in those with a lower body weight. Even though this could be sampling bias, it may be due to the greater traumatic forces required to break the bones of large dogs. Bones particularly at risk for open fractures include the scapula, radius, ulna, tibia, fibula, and tarsus in dogs, and the tarsus and bones distal to the tarsus in cats.[2] Tarsal degloving injuries are particularly common in small animals and are frequently associated with fractures of the associated bones.[5] As open fractures are generally secondary to high-energy, high-velocity trauma, they are frequently comminuted.[2]
It is imperative to individually assess and classify open fractures due to the high variability in tissue damage and contamination, including skin, muscles, bone, tendons, vasculature, nerves, and articular cartilage. Prevention of infection is paramount, as is wound management and fracture stabilization.[3,4] Owners as well as veterinarians should be prepared for prolonged management and the potential for multiple surgical procedures.

Clinical presentation and diagnosis

Open fractures in dogs and cats are frequently due to high-impact trauma, including vehicular trauma or falls from significant heights. Because of this, a full systemic evaluation and assessment for comorbidities is critical and should be prioritized. Open fractures should be covered with sterile dressing to prevent nosocomial infection as patient stabilization is pursued. The diagnosis of an open fracture is made on physical examination by noting disruption of the skin and soft tissues in association with a fractured bone. Alternatively, if emphysema is noted subcutaneously or in the deep tissues on radiographic evaluation, the skin should be more carefully examined for disruption and appropriate diagnosis.
Multiple open fracture classification schemes have been established to both document the degree of associated damage and help to establish treatment and prognosis more objectively. The most commonly used classification system in veterinary medicine was established by Gustilo and Anderson, dividing open fractures into three categories (Table 29.1).[1,6]

- Type I have a wound smaller than or equal to 1 cm in diameter, with mild or moderate contusion to the surrounding soft tissues. This wound is frequently caused by a sharp bone fragment penetrating the tissues and skin (i.e., from the inside out).
- Type II involve a wound larger than 1 cm in diameter, without extensive soft tissue damage, flaps, or avulsions. In these cases, the skin is generally penetrated by the high-energy external force (i.e., from the outside in).
- Type III include three subcategories and are defined as having extensive soft tissue damage including tissue avulsion and degloving injuries.
    - Type IIIA indicate the soft tissue envelope can be closed over the bone.
    - Type IIIB lack adequate soft tissues to cover the bone and encompasses many shearing injuries (Figs. 29.1 and 29.2).
    - Type IIIC have extensive soft tissue damage, with arterial injury that requires repair (Fig. 29.3). Due to the need for vascular reconstruction/anastomosis, these fractures frequently result in amputation in veterinary patients.

However, the Gustilo and Anderson classification system lacks strong intraobserver variability, making treatment assumptions and prognosis difficult to elucidate.[7]

TABLE 29.1 - THE GUSTILO AND ANDERSON OPEN FRACTURE CLASSIFICATION SCHEME[1]	
Classification	**Description**
Type I	Puncture wound ≤1 cm diameter Minimal soft tissue injury Minimal wound contamination and muscle crushing
Type II	Wound >1 cm diameter Moderate soft tissue injury Adequate soft tissue coverage of the bone
Type IIIA	Extensive soft tissue damage Adequate soft tissue coverage of the bone
Type IIIB	Extensive soft tissue damage Periosteal stripping and bone exposure Inability to close soft tissue envelope
Type IIIC	Extensive soft tissue damage Inability to close soft tissue envelope Arterial injury requiring repair

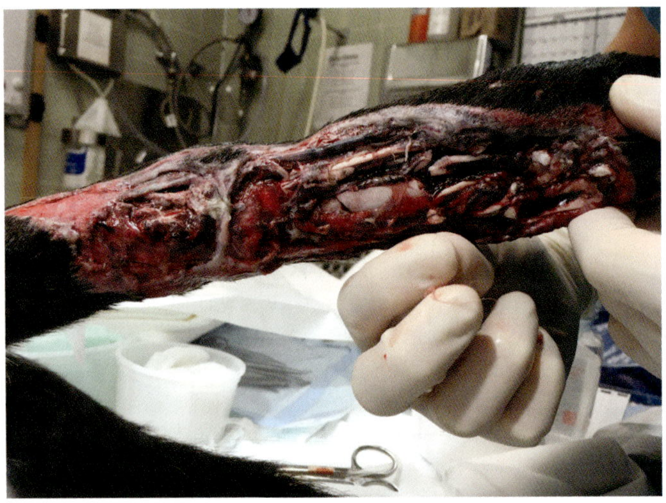

Figure 29.1 Type IIIB open fracture (Gustilo–Anderson classification) due to a shearing injury to the tarsus of a dog. Significant soft tissue damage has occurred, with the inability to close the soft tissue envelope over the fractured bones.

This has led to the development of other classification schemes, most notably the one proposed by the Orthopedic Trauma Association in 2010.[8–10] This system documents five factors: skin defect, muscle injury, arterial injury, bone loss, and contamination. Each of these has three subcategories: mild, moderate, and severe. While not yet commonly adopted in veterinary medicine, this scheme allows for a more specific assessment of fractures and their numerous qualities. While peer-reviewed data assessing this system remains lacking in veterinary medicine, this option may allow more objec-

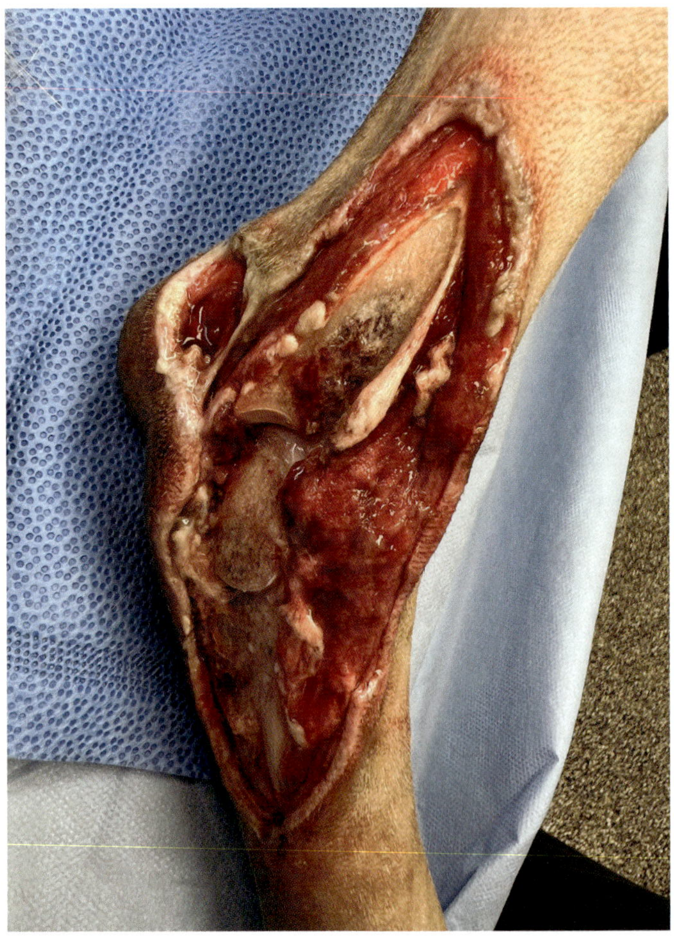

Figure 29.2 Another example of type IIIB open fracture (Gustilo–Anderson classification) due to a shearing injury to the medial tarsus in a dog. Extensive soft tissue and bone loss is visible, and there is not enough soft tissue to close the wound.

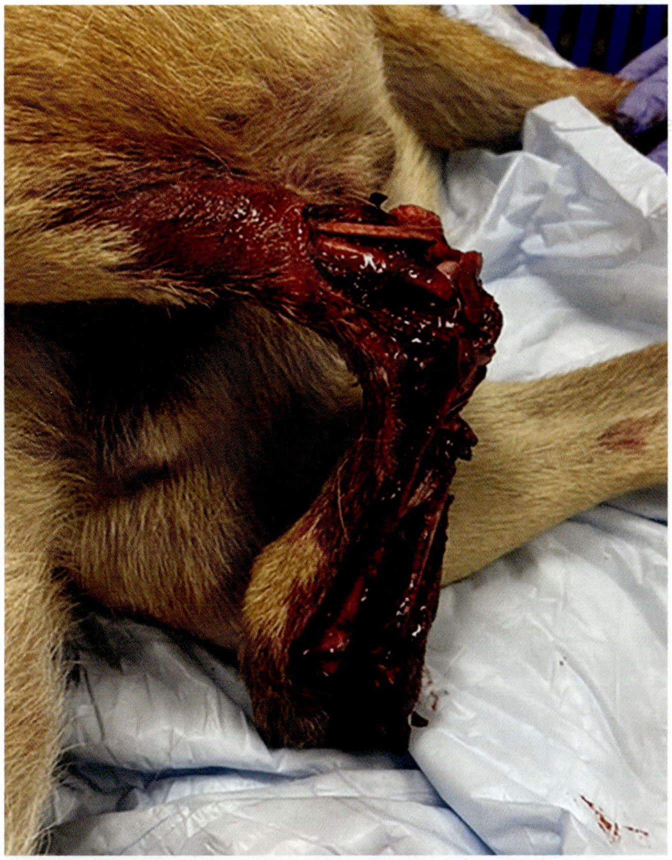

Figure 29.3 Type IIIC open fracture (Gustilo–Anderson classification), defined by significant soft tissue disruption as well as arterial injury requiring repair. In this case, arterial disruption was visible, and there was absence of pulse or active bleeding in the digits. While the digits were palpably cold, this parameter alone is not adequate to assess vascular integrity.

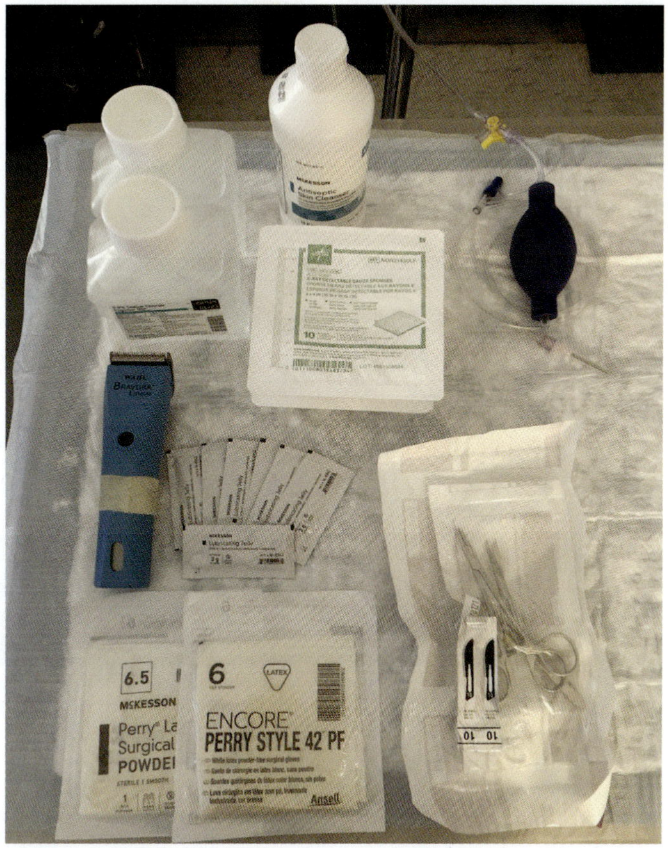

Figure 29.4 Example of the procedural setup for open fracture wound management, including lubrication, surgical clippers, lavage fluid, and sterile surgical equipment for debridement. Following debridement, a deep tissue culture should be obtained.

tive recommendations regarding treatment, prognosis, and owner expectations.

Treatment

Once an open fracture is identified, early decontamination of the wound should be performed (Fig. 29.4). This consists of wide clipping of the fur and copious lavage of the wound. The optimal amount of lavage, delivery method/pressure, and ideal irrigation solution have not been well established.[3] Following lavage, surgical debridement is critical to remove nonviable tissue and any foreign material, as these would enhance bacterial growth and interfere with the defense mechanisms of the host. Any cortical bone fragments without soft tissue attachments should also be removed to avoid future sequestra. Frequently, a second debridement is required 24–48 hours after presentation, as it make take time for tissues to declare their viability (Fig. 29.5).

Wound closure of open fractures is generally not recommended for 3–7 days after the initial trauma to avoid creation of an anaerobic environment, facilitate drainage, and allow repeated debridement procedures.[3] A sterile dressing and bandage should be maintained during this time, with regular dressing changes and reassessment. While some wounds, particularly type I and II open fractures, may heal by second intention, others may require surgical closure or soft tissue reconstructive techniques. Early empirical broad-spectrum antibiotic therapy should be promptly started, as delayed administration of systemic antibiotics in humans has been demonstrated to significantly increase the risk of infection.[11] A deep tissue culture should be obtained after wound irrigation and debridement to help guide early antimicrobial therapy.[12] It is important to note, however, that this often fails to isolate the causative agent of subsequent infection; a culture taken before debridement is particularly insensitive and not recommended.[12]

Orthogonal radiographs under sedation are warranted to assess the fracture and guide definitive stabilization. Additional projections including oblique images and/or stress radiographs of the joints should be considered

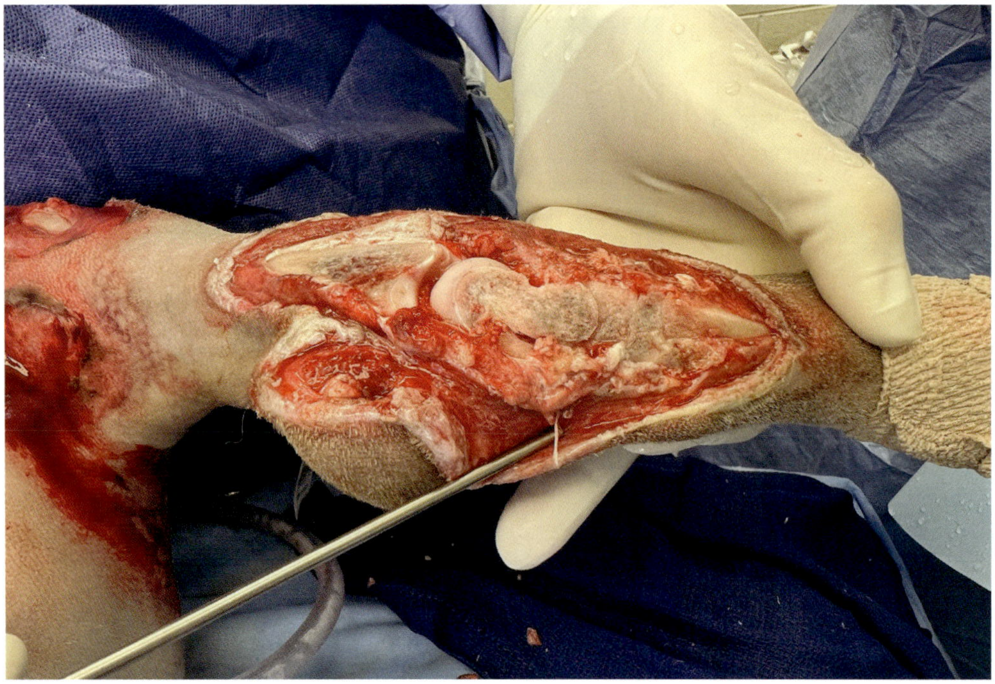

Figure 29.5 Same wound from Figure 29.2 following aggressive surgical debridement and lavage. There is loss of the medial malleolus and medial talar ridge. This dog had an external splint placed while the wound was managed with serial tissue debridement and bandage changes. Once the wound was free of gross infection and there was no ongoing tissue loss, a pantarsal arthrodesis was performed.

to further assess fracture configuration and stability associated with periarticular ligamentous disruption. Temporary stabilization is recommended (e.g., external coaptation/splinting) to decrease further soft tissue damage in the time leading up to surgical stabilization. Definitive fracture stabilization is critical to allow bone healing while protecting the soft tissues from further injury. The most appropriate method for stabilization of open fractures is controversial in both human and veterinary medicine and depends largely on the fractured bone, fracture location (e.g., articular vs. diaphyseal), and extent and location of the soft tissue injury. While originally thought that external fixation was ideal in these cases, this theory has largely been disproven. Studies have found no difference in fracture site infection or bone healing rates between internal and external fixation for treatment of open diaphyseal fractures in humans.[13,14] External fixation may in fact increase the risk of major complications.[15] The surgeon must therefore carefully select the method for temporary or definitive fracture stabilization based on multiple mechanical, biological, and client factors. Priority should be given to providing appropriate stability to the fracture site, allowing access to wounds for soft tissue care, and preserving all remaining viable soft tissues (Fig. 29.6).[1,16] Continued soft tissue wound management should be pursued medically or surgically as indicated.

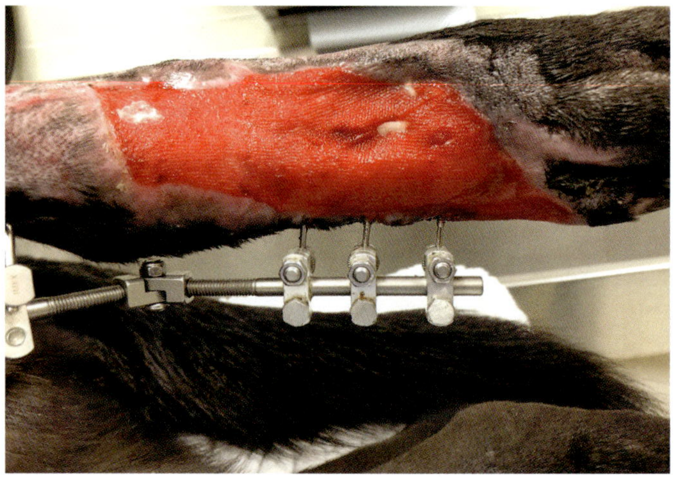

Figure 29.6 Same type IIIB open fracture from Figure 29.1 after surgical stabilization with external fixation and extensive wound care including multiple debridement procedures and negative-pressure wound therapy. A healthy bed of granulation tissue is present, allowing further surgical reconstruction or healing by second intention.

Surgical technique

1. The wound is protected with sterile water-based lubricant while the fur surrounding the open wound is clipped with wide margins. These skin margins are cleaned with dilute chlorhexidine and saline solutions.
2. Copious lavage of the wound should be performed, ideally with sterile irrigation solution.
3. Surgical debridement is performed, removing nonviable tissue and any foreign material. Any cortical bone fragments without soft tissue attachments should also be removed. A second debridement procedure is usually required 24–48 hours after presentation.

4. A deep tissue culture is obtained after irrigation and debridement.
5. Wound closure is generally not recommended for 3–7 days after the initial trauma, during which a sterile dressing and bandage should be applied and changed frequently.
6. Empirical broad-spectrum antibiotics should be promptly administered and later adjusted based on culture and sensitivity results.
7. Radiographs under sedation (orthogonal ± oblique or stress projections) are obtained to assess fracture configuration and guide further treatment plans.

Postoperative management

Reducing postoperative infection is a major focus when managing open fractures. Systemic antibiotic administration is recommended, although the timeline has not been well established. Despite the controversy regarding antibiotic selection and duration, it is recommended to start empirical systemic antibiotics immediately, adjust them as needed based on subsequent culture and sensitivity results, and maintain the treatment at least through the time of soft tissue closure.[11,17] Total antibiotic therapy duration should be based on the degree of soft tissue damage and culture and sensitivity testing results of surgically obtained deep tissue.

Regular radiographic monitoring is recommended to ensure the bone is active and healing is progressing appropriately. In the case of delayed healing, early bone grafting may be recommended, with ideal timing ranging from 2 to 6 weeks after soft tissue coverage.[18,19]

Outcome

The outcome following treatment of open fractures is variable and not well established in the veterinary literature. The variability in both bone and soft tissue damage, largely associated with the grade of the open fracture, plays a significant role in the outcome and prognosis, and much of this veterinary data has been extrapolated from the human literature.

Owners should be prepared for the potential of implant removal after fracture healing. In one retrospective study evaluating the use of internal fixation for open fracture management, implant removal occurred in 18% of dogs and 50% of cats with open fractures (21.25% of total cases).[16] Approximately 65% of the explants (accounting for 13.8% of total cases) were due to recurrent draining tracts, osteomyelitis, implant-associated infection, or implant exposure, whereas 30% of implants were removed secondary to implant failure, breakage, or migration.[16] The overall complication rate was 42.5%, with a major complication rate of 28.75%.[16]

Complications can be minimized by ensuring adequate fracture stabilization, early debridement with maintenance of viable soft tissues, appropriate antimicrobial therapy, and continuous monitoring with adjustment of the treatment plan as needed.

KEEP IN MIND

- Early diagnosis and appropriate decontamination of open fractures are imperative for treatment success.
- Empirical broad-spectrum antibiotics should be started as early as possible.
- A deep tissue culture should be obtained after cleaning and debridement of the wound to improve sensitivity and guide long-term antibiotic treatment.
- Orthogonal radiographs under sedation should be taken to assess fracture configuration and joint stability and to guide stabilization recommendations. Oblique and/or stress projections should be considered when appropriate.
- Complications of open fractures can be minimized by ensuring adequate fracture stabilization, early debridement with maintenance of viable soft tissues, appropriate antimicrobial therapy, and continuous monitoring with adjustment of the treatment plan as needed.

References

1. Gustilo RB, Anderson JT. Prevention of infection in the treatment of one thousand and twenty-five open fractures of long bones: Retrospective and prospective analyses. *J Bone Joint Surg Am.* 1976; 58(4):453–458.
2. Millard RP, Weng HY. Proportion of and risk factors for open fractures of the appendicular skeleton in dogs and cats. *J Am Vet Med Assoc.* 2014; 245(6):663–668.
3. Zalavras CG, Patzakis MJ. Open fractures: Evaluation and management. *J Am Acad Orthop Surg.* 2003; 11(3):212–219.
4. Zalavras CG. Prevention of infection in open fractures. *Infect Dis Clin North Am.* 2017; 31(2):339–352.
5. Beardsley SL, Schrader SC. Treatment of dogs with wounds of the limbs caused by shearing forces: 98 cases (1975–1993). *J Am Vet Med Assoc.* 1995; 207(8):1071–1075.
6. Kim PH, Leopold SS. Gustilo–Anderson classification. *Clin Orthop Relat Res.* 2012; 470(11):3270–3274.
7. Horn BD, Rettig ME. Interobserver reliability in the Gustilo and Anderson classification of open fractures. *J Orthop Trauma.* 1993; 7(4):357–360.
8. OTA Open Fracture Classification (OTA-OFC). *J Orthop Trauma.* 2018; 32 Suppl 1:S106.

9. Agel J et al. The OTA open fracture classification: A study of reliability and agreement. *J Orthop Trauma*. 2013; 27(7):379–384.
10. Orthopaedic Trauma Association: Open Fracture Study Group. A new classification scheme for open fractures. *J Orthop Trauma*. 2010; 24(8):457–464.
11. Wilkins J, Patzakis M. Choice and duration of antibiotics in open fractures. *Orthop Clin North Am*. 1991; 22(3):433–437.
12. Lee J. Efficacy of cultures in the management of open fractures. *Clin Orthop Relat Res*. 1997; (339):71–75.
13. Tornetta P 3rd et al. Treatment of grade-IIIb open tibial fractures. A prospective randomised comparison of external fixation and non-reamed locked nailing. *J Bone Joint Surg Br*. 1994; 76(1):13–19.
14. Henley MB et al. Treatment of type II, IIIA, and IIIB open fractures of the tibial shaft: A prospective comparison of unreamed interlocking intramedullary nails and half-pin external fixators. *J Orthop Trauma*. 1998; 12(1):1–7.
15. Major Extremity Trauma Research Consortium (METRC). Modern external ring fixation versus internal fixation for treatment of severe open tibial fractures: A randomized clinical trial (FIX-IT study). *J Bone Joint Surg Am*. 2022; 104(12):1061–1067.
16. Sandness BM, Perry KL, Bruce M. Single institution retrospective study evaluating the frequency of implant removal and associated risk factors following open fracture fixation in 80 cases (2010–2020). *BMC Vet Res*. 2023; 19(1):119.
17. Patzakis MJ, Wilkins J. Factors influencing infection rate in open fracture wounds. *Clin Orthop Relat Res*. 1989; (243):36–40.
18. Edwards CC, Simmons SC, Browner BD, Weigel MC. Severe open tibial fractures. Results treating 202 injuries with external fixation. *Clin Orthop Relat Res*. 1988; (230):98–115.
19. Blick SS et al. Early prophylactic bone grafting of high-energy tibial fractures. *Clin Orthop Relat Res*. 1989; (240):21–41.

Chapter 30

Elbow and hip luxation

Anna M. Massie

Luxation is defined as the separation of articular surfaces, with traumatic luxation occurring in conjunction with tearing of the joint capsule and collateral or other supporting ligament(s). This requires a significant amount of energy, most commonly secondary to high-force trauma (e.g., vehicular trauma, fall from a height). Prompt and complete diagnosis of the joint luxation and associated soft tissue disruption is critical to the success of reduction and return to function. Without timely reduction and stabilization, permanent injury to the cartilage, periarticular fibrosis, and loss of range of motion with chronic osteoarthritis results. Chronic luxations greater than 1–2 weeks' duration require open reduction or salvage procedures depending on the degree of cartilage damage and soft tissue fibrosis.[1]

A full systemic evaluation is paramount, as traumatic luxations are generally secondary to high-force trauma. Once the patient has been stabilized, a full orthopedic examination should be performed to carefully assess all joints and long bones. Luxations may be masked by local soft tissue swelling and/or regional damage. Luxation is then confirmed by obtaining sedated orthogonal radiographs of the joint of interest. If an obvious luxation is not present, oblique and stressed projections should be obtained to more thoroughly evaluate joint integrity. These images should also be carefully evaluated for osteochondral and ligamentous avulsion fractures, as this may change management recommendations. Preexisting disorders including dysplastic disease, previous fracture/malunion, or congenital (sub) luxation should be diagnosed, particularly in cases of more low-impact trauma or chronic history of lameness. The patient's problem list should be carefully prioritized, as comorbidities may supersede the ability to immediately address the luxation. In this case, temporary immobilization of the joint is recommended to decrease motion and further damage to the cartilage and soft tissue structures while more pressing issues are treated. For elbow luxation, this entails a soft tissue bandage or Spica splint extending above the shoulder joint (incorporating a chest bandage). As the hip joint cannot be immobilized in such a fashion, an Ehmer sling is recommended for craniodorsal luxations to decrease motion.

Elbow luxation

Clinical presentation and diagnosis

The elbow joint possesses significant intrinsic stability due to the interlocking "puzzle piece" nature of the anconeus, olecranon fossa, and humeral epicondyles. This stability makes fractures more common than luxation.[1] The medial and lateral collateral ligaments connect the humerus, radius, and ulna, with secondary support from the olecranon ligament, oblique ligament, and annular ligament.[2] A more rounded lateral epicondyle, a larger more cuboidal medial epicondyle, and a more robust lateral collateral ligament lead to traumatic luxations almost always occurring in the lateral direction (Fig. 30.1).[2,3]

Animals with luxated elbows generally present non-weight-bearing, with abduction, supination, and mild flexion of the limb. An irregular angulation/contour of the elbow is generally observed.[4,5]

Treatment

Small avulsion fractures of the lateral collateral ligament are frequently seen on radiographic evaluation of the luxated elbow (see Fig. 30.1). When present, these are rarely large enough to allow surgical fixation. With the lack of any significant fractures, closed reduction is recommended while the patient is under sedation for the radiographs.

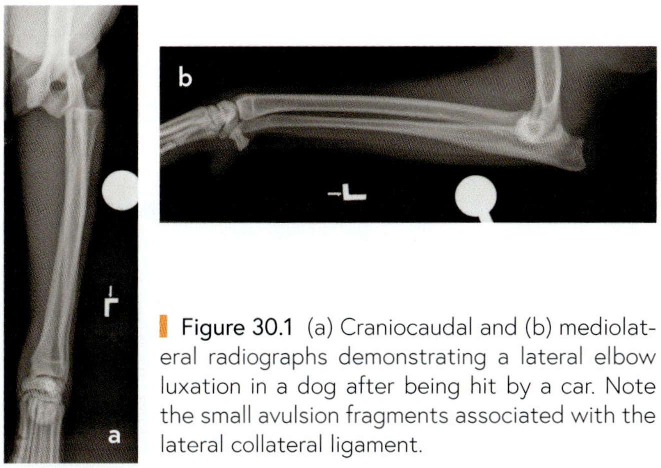

Figure 30.1 (a) Craniocaudal and (b) mediolateral radiographs demonstrating a lateral elbow luxation in a dog after being hit by a car. Note the small avulsion fragments associated with the lateral collateral ligament.

Technique: Closed reduction

1. The animal is placed under heavy sedation or general anesthesia.
2. The next step varies depending on the degree of dislocation:
   - If the anconeal process is lateral to the lateral epicondylar crest, the elbow is flexed beyond 90 degrees and the distal limb inwardly rotated and adducted to allow the anconeal process to engage the lateral epicondyle. Digital pressure is then applied laterally with continued pronation and slow extension, resulting in reduction of the anconeal process into the olecranon fossa.[4,5] Radial head reduction can be assisted with direct medial pressure on the radial head while the elbow is pronated and abducted.
   - If the anconeal process is still within the anconeal fossa, the elbow is slowly flexed to approximately 100 degrees while applying medial pressure to the olecranon. The elbow is then pronated and abducted with medial pressure to the radial head.
3. The elbow is gently assessed for stability.
   - If gross instability is noted, open reduction should be performed.
   - If stable, the limb may be placed in a Spica splint (see below).

Postreduction management

A Spica splint with the elbow extended to approximately 140 degrees is recommended following closed reduction to allow fibrosis and healing of periarticular support structures.[6] Maintaining the limb in extension keeps the anconeal process within the olecranon fossa, preventing lateral translation of the joint. The duration of Spica splint wear is not well established, but a general guideline is 5–7 days followed by passive range-of-motion exercises and controlled weight-bearing activities for 2–4 weeks.[3,5,7] It should be borne in mind that prolonged immobilization of a joint has detrimental effects on the articular cartilage and may be associated with muscular contracture and pain.[8,9]

Outcome

Prognosis after closed elbow reduction is good to excellent in 47%–88.5% of dogs, with reluxation being more common in case of multiple orthopedic injuries.[10–12] Generally, the prognosis following closed reduction is considered better than if open reduction is required.[10,13] If closed reduction cannot be achieved or gross instability is noted after reduction, open reduction and stabilization is recommended.[4,5,7] If the elbow is stable following closed reduction, there is no benefit of open over closed reduction.[10,11] Concurrent additional orthopedic injury to the limb may be a risk factor for reluxation in the canine elbow.[12]

In cats, reluxation has been reported in 61% of cases following closed reduction, and this rate increases as the duration from injury to reduction increases.[14] As with dogs, outcome is considered good to excellent in most cases regardless of the reduction technique employed.[14]

Coxofemoral luxation

Clinical presentation and diagnosis

Hip (coxofemoral) joints are the most common joint to luxate in dogs and cats.[15] Primary stabilizers of the coxofemoral joint include the ligament of the head of the femur, the joint capsule, and the dorsal acetabular rim; secondary stabilizers are the labrum, the ventral acetabular ligament, and the surrounding musculature.[15] The hip most frequently (approximately 90% of cases) luxates in a craniodorsal direction (Fig. 30.2), with caudoventral luxations being much less frequent (Fig. 30.3).[15] Luxation in other directions is very uncommon and usually associated with significant instability and periarticular soft tissue disruption.[3] Animals with a craniodorsal luxation stand with the limb externally rotated and abducted, whereas caudoventral luxations result in internal rotation and an elongated limb.[16] On examination, normal hip anatomy can be identified by creating a shallow triangle or V between three landmarks: the craniodorsal wing of the ilium, the greater trochanter, and the ischial tuberosity (Fig. 30.4).[17] The dorsal displacement of the greater trochanter in a craniodorsal luxation will create a straight line between these landmarks, whereas the greater trochanter may not be palpable in case of caudoventral luxation due to medialization of the femoral head. Pain, decreased range of motion, and crepitus are noted on manipulation of the joint.

Treatment

Radiographs should be thoroughly assessed for any concurrent pathology of the hip, including fracture of the greater trochanter, femoral neck, capital physis, or acetabulum. Avulsion fractures of the ligament of the head of the femur may be present and preclude closed reduction. Additionally, degenerative conditions such as hip dysplasia and Legg–Calves–Perthes disease may preclude closed reduction or change the prognosis.[15–17] In the absence of concurrent pathologies, closed reduction is recommended.

Technique: Closed reduction

1. The patient is placed under general anesthesia and positioned in lateral recumbency. A narrow sling is

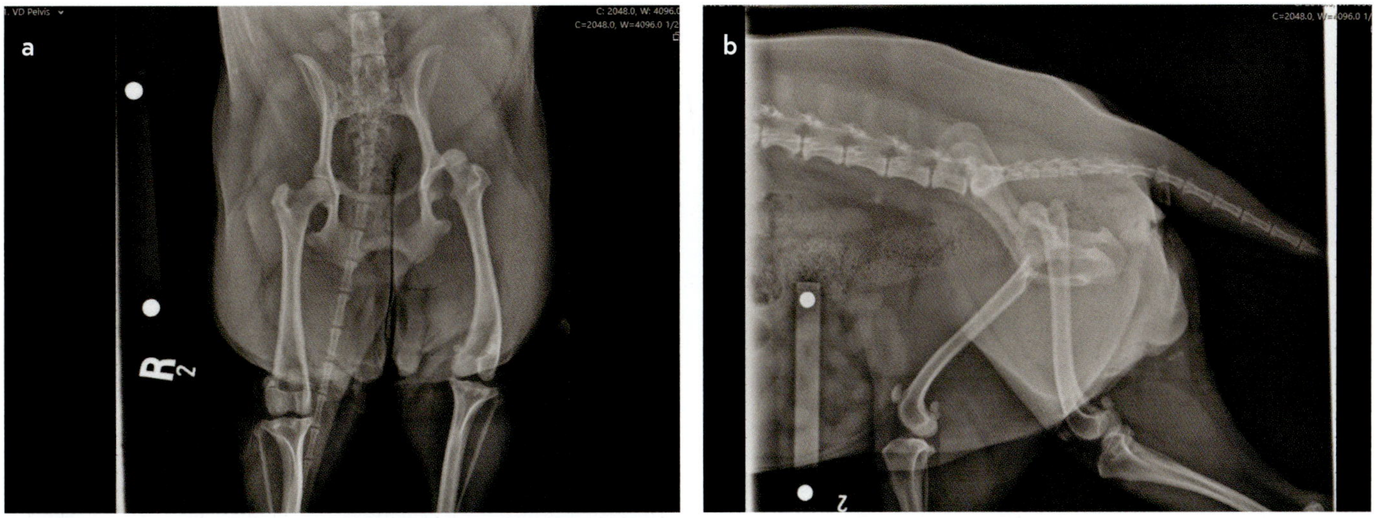

Figure 30.2 (a) Ventrodorsal and (b) lateral radiographs of the pelvis of a dog with a craniodorsal hip luxation after unknown trauma.

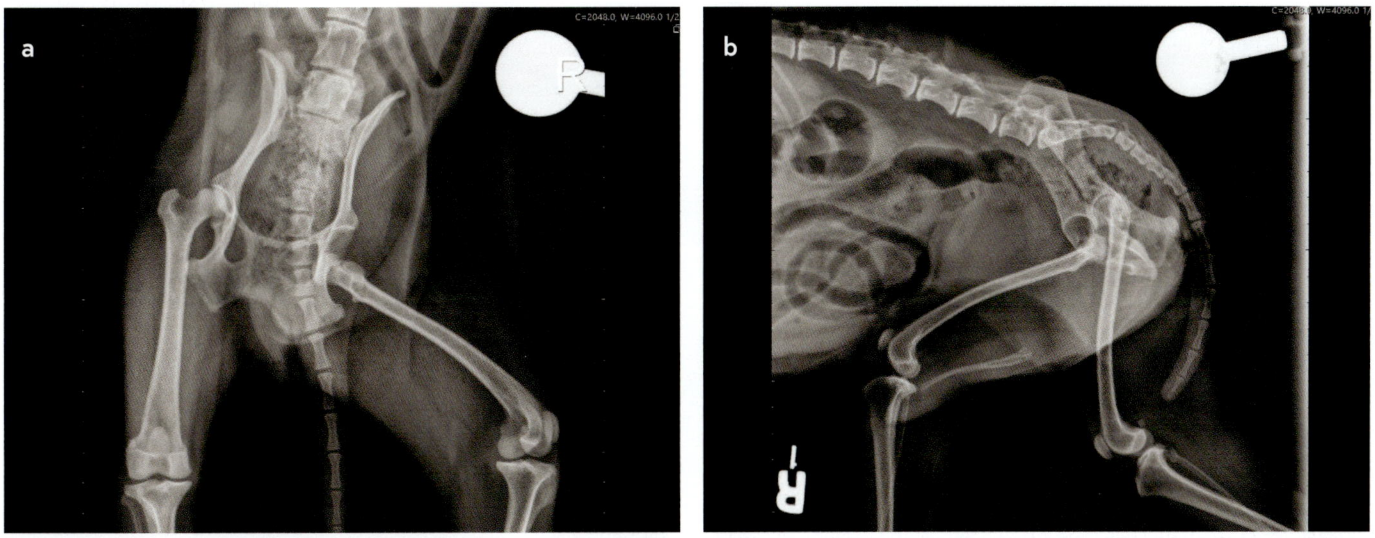

Figure 30.3 (a) Ventrodorsal and (b) lateral radiographs of the pelvis of a small-breed dog with a caudoventral hip luxation after falling off a bed. While this is the second most common direction of coxofemoral luxation, it is relatively rare. Prognosis is not well established but is anecdotally superior to that of craniodorsal luxations.

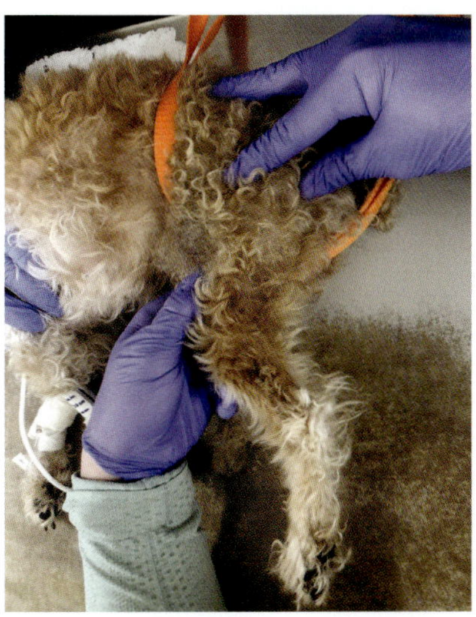

Figure 30.4 The craniodorsal wing of the ilium, greater trochanter, and ischial tuberosity are used as landmarks to help determine whether a hip luxation has occurred. In a normal or reduced hip, these three points, marked by the gloved fingers, should create a shallow triangle or V as demonstrated in this photograph. The points aligning in a straight line suggests craniodorsal luxation of the hip joint. In caudoventral luxations, the greater trochanter is often difficult or impossible to palpate on examination due to medial displacement.

placed around the inguinal region and held by an assistant at the animal's back.
2. The next step varies depending on the direction of dislocation:
   - For craniodorsal luxations, the distal limb is pulled distally and externally rotated while lateral pressure is applied to the greater trochanter. As the femoral head is pulled over the rim of the acetabulum, the limb is internally rotated to allow reduction. This may be associated with an audible or palpable "clunk."
   - For caudoventral luxations, distal and lateral traction is applied to the femur to move the femoral head out of the obturator foramen. Continued lateral traction lifts the femoral head over the ventral acetabular wall into the acetabulum.
3. After hip reduction, pressure is maintained on the greater trochanter while the limb is placed through a range of motion and circumduction for approximately 5 minutes, encouraging displacement of the fracture hematoma, joint capsule, and fibrous tissues from the intra-articular space.
4. Reduction is confirmed by repeat radiographs.

Postreduction management

For craniodorsal luxations, an Ehmer sling or modified Ehmer sling is recommended following reduction (Fig. 30.5). This creates internal rotation and abduction while the joint capsule fibroses. Due to the risk of wounds and serious complications, it is critical that the sling is assessed by a veterinarian every 3–4 days after application. Bandage-associated injuries are reported in approximately 50% of cases, with 40% of these being severe.[18] The sling can be made from elastic tape and cotton, or, alternatively, commercial products are available. It is generally maintained for 7–10 days followed by limited weight-bearing or use of a Robinson sling for 2 weeks. Ehmer slings prove difficult to maintain on cats and have not been associated with reluxation rates; strict cage rest is generally considered adequate in this species.[19,20]

Caudoventral luxation reduction can be followed by hobbles for 2–3 weeks to prevent abduction of the joint (Fig. 30.6). Alternatively, strict cage confinement may be adequate in the recovery period.

Outcome

Closed reduction of craniodorsal hip luxation carries a 35%–50% success rate in both dogs and cats.[15,16,21] The prognosis following closed reduction of caudoventral luxations is not known but may be more successful than that of craniodorsal luxations.[1,3] Open reduction and stabilization is warranted when gross instability is noted after reduction, in the presence of concurrent fracture or degenerative changes to the hip, or if closed reduction fails.[15–17] In case of significant damage to the articular surface, salvage procedures including femoral head and neck excision or total hip arthroplasty are recommended. The selection and specifics of these procedures are beyond the scope of this book, but they generally carry a good to excellent prognosis.

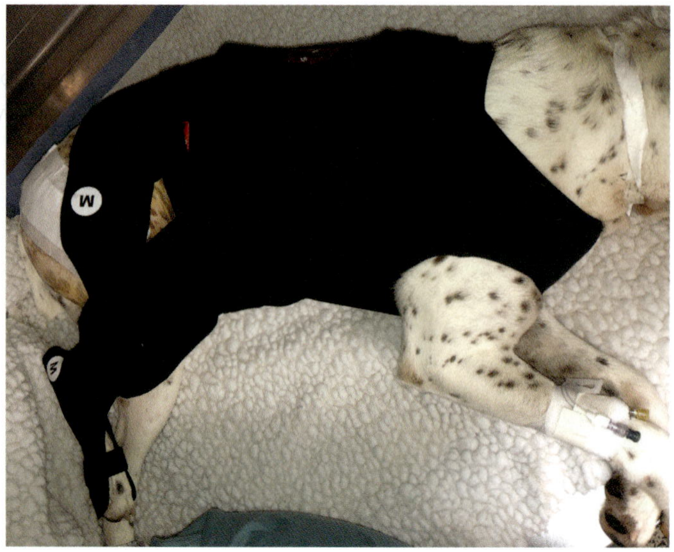

Figure 30.5 Ehmer slings are generally recommended after closed reduction of a craniodorsal hip luxation in the dog. They can be created with elastic tape and cotton, or a commercially available sling, as the one shown in the photograph, can be applied.

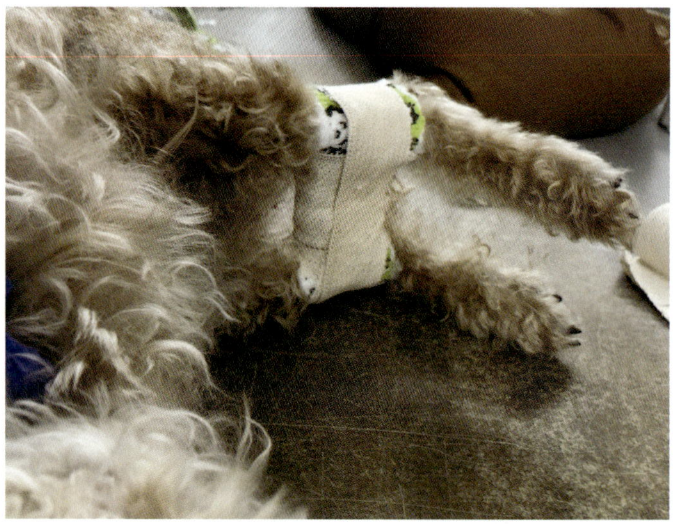

Figure 30.6 Hobbles should be considered after closed reduction of a caudoventral hip luxation. They can be created with tape and cotton, as shown here, or commercially available hobbles can be employed.

KEEP IN MIND

- Without timely reduction and stabilization, luxation may result in permanent injury to the cartilage, periarticular fibrosis, and loss of range of motion with chronic osteoarthritis.
- Luxation is generally secondary to high-energy trauma. A thorough systemic evaluation and full orthopedic examination to assess for comorbidities is paramount.
- Elbow luxations are relatively uncommon due to the inherent instability of the joint. Prompt closed reduction carries a good to excellent prognosis.
- Hip luxations most frequently occur in a craniodorsal direction. Closed reduction has a success rate of approximately 50% and should be selected carefully in the absence of concurrent fracture or significant degenerative changes to the joint.
- If instability is palpated following closed reduction, concurrent fracture is noted on radiographic evaluation, the joint has been chronically luxated, or a patient fails closed reduction, open reduction or salvage procedures should be considered.

References

1. Hulse D. Biomechanics of luxation. In: Bojrab M, Monnet E (eds.). *Mechanisms of Disease in Small Animal Surgery*, 3rd ed. Teton NewMedia; 2010. pp. 693–702.
2. Vogelsang RL et al. Structural, material, and anatomic characteristics of the collateral ligaments of the canine cubital joint. *Am J Vet Res*. 1997; 58(5):461–466.
3. Bordelon JT, Reaugh HF, Rochat MC. Traumatic luxations of the appendicular skeleton. *Vet Clin North Am Small Anim Pract*. 2005; 35(5):1169–1194.
4. Dassler C, Vasseur P. Elbow luxation. In: Slatter D (ed.). *Textbook of Small Animal Surgery*, 3rd ed. WB Saunders; 2003. pp. 1919–1927.
5. Piermattei D, Flo G. The elbow joint. In: *Handbook of Small Animal Orthopedics and Fracture Repair*. WB Saunders; 1997. pp. 288–320.
6. Griffon D. Surgical diseases of the elbow. In: Tobias K, Johnston S (eds.). *Veterinary Surgery: Small Animal*, 1st ed. Elsevier Saunders; 2010. pp. 724–735.
7. Johnson A, Hulse D. Traumatic elbow luxation. In: Fossum T (ed.). *Small Animal Surgery*, 2nd ed. Mosby; 2002. pp. 1079–1084.
8. Josefsson PO, Gentz CF, Johnell O, Wendeberg B. Surgical versus non-surgical treatment of ligamentous injuries following dislocation of the elbow joint. A prospective randomized study. *J Bone Joint Surg Am*. 1987; 69(4):605–608.
9. Bruce WJ et al. A comparison of the effects of joint immobilisation, twice-daily passive motion, and voluntary motion on articular cartilage healing in sheep. *Vet Comp Orthop Traumatol*. 2002; 15(1):23–29.
10. Schaeffer IGF et al. Traumatic luxation of the elbow in 31 dogs. *Vet Comp Orthop Traumatol*. 1999; 12(1):33–39.
11. O'Brien MG, Boudrieau RJ, Clark GN. Traumatic luxation of the cubital joint (elbow) in dogs: 44 cases (1978–1988). *J Am Vet Med Assoc*. 1992; 201(11):1760–1765.
12. Sajik D et al. Multi-centre retrospective study of long-term outcomes following traumatic elbow luxation in 37 dogs. *J Small Anim Pract*. 2016; 57(8):422–428.
13. Campbell JR. Luxation and ligamentous injuries of the elbow of the dog. *Vet Clin North Am*. 1971; 1(3):429–440.
14. Williams H et al. Multi-centre retrospective study of the long-term outcome following suspected traumatic elbow luxation in 32 cats. *J Small Anim Pract*. 2020; 61(6):354–362.
15. Holsworth I, DeCamp C. Coxofemoral luxation. In: Slatter D (ed.). *Textbook of Small Animal Surgery*, 3rd ed. WB Saunders; 2003. pp. 2002–2008.
16. Piermattei DL, Flo GL, DeCamp CE. The hip joint. In: *Brinker, Piermattei and Flo's Handbook of Small Animal Orthopedics and Fracture Repair*, 4th ed. Saunders Elsevier; 2006. pp. 461–511.
17. Johnson A, Hulse D. Coxofemoral luxation. In: Fossum T (ed.). *Small Animal Surgery*, 2nd ed. Mosby; 2002. pp. 1102–1109.
18. Schlag AN et al. Analysis of outcomes following treatment of craniodorsal hip luxation with closed reduction and Ehmer sling application in dogs. *J Am Vet Med Assoc*. 2019; 254(12):1436–1440.
19. Duff SR, Bennett D. Hip luxation in small animals: An evaluation of some methods of treatment. *Vet Rec*. 1982; 111(7):140–143.
20. Meeson RL, Strickland R. Traumatic joint luxations in cats: Reduce, repair, replace, remove. *J Feline Med Surg*. 2021; 23(1):17–32.
21. LeFloch MD, Coronado GS. Outcome of coxofemoral luxation treated with closed reduction in 51 cats. *J Feline Med Surg*. 2022; 24(8):709–714.

Chapter 31

Eyelid lacerations

Maria-Christine Fischer

Eyelid lacerations are characterized by a partial- or full-thickness defect in the eyelid and occur due to two main mechanisms. The first mechanism involves sharp penetration, for example, due to bite wounds, cat claw injuries, and foreign bodies. The second mechanism involves avulsion injuries resulting from blunt trauma, such as that caused by balls or motor vehicle accidents.

Clinical presentation and diagnosis

Irrespective of the etiology, injuries to lid structures should prompt comprehensive investigations to determine if the eyelid laceration is simple or complicated. Complicated eyelid lacerations are extensive, involve the nasolacrimal drainage system, and are accompanied by head trauma or other ocular injuries. Other ocular injuries that may not be apparent at the initial presentation are corneal ulceration, disruption of the lacrimal drainage unit, globe rupture, and orbital fractures. In cases suspected of globe injury, significant subconjunctival or intraocular hemorrhage, swelling around the eye, or intracranial injury, CT or MRI scans are recommended prior to commencing surgery. Bacterial culture and sensitivity testing should be considered, especially for contaminated and bite wounds.

Treatment

Once complicated ocular or cranial injuries have been ruled out, and the patient's general condition is stable, eyelid lacerations should be repaired promptly.[1,2]

Simple eyelid lacerations

If the eyelid margin is not involved, the wound can be treated as a simple skin laceration. Simple interrupted sutures are placed 2–3 mm apart using 6-0 monofilament or coated polyglactin 910 on a reverse cutting needle.

Careful reconstruction of the eyelid anatomy is required if the eyelid margin is involved. The surgical technique is described below.

Surgical technique: Reconstruction of simple eyelid lacerations involving the eyelid margin

1. The surgical field is gently clipped, taking care to avoid causing any further tissue trauma.
2. The patient is positioned in ventral or lateral recumbency, and the patient's head is stabilized in a deflated vacuum cushion. Alternatively, towels, sandbags, and adhesive tape can be used to maintain the patient's head in the desired position.
3. The eyelids and ocular surface are aseptically prepared and any foreign material removed. The ocular surface and the conjunctival sac are copiously flushed with 1:50 diluted povidone iodine for 3 minutes. The eyelid is gently wiped with a swab soaked with 1:10 diluted povidone iodine; the swab should not contact the ocular surface to avoid damage to the corneal epithelium. Finally, the conjunctival sac is flushed with 0.9% saline, and the eyelids are dried with sterile swabs. It is important to remember that iodine solutions must not be used in cases suspected of corneal perforation and globe rupture.
4. Thick lubrication should be placed only on the ocular surface of the contralateral eye. The affected eye can be flushed with 0.9% saline intraoperatively to prevent desiccation.
5. The surgical field is draped avoiding distortion of the eyelid configuration.
6. Local anesthetic (e.g., proparacaine hydrochloride) eye drops are applied to the ocular surface.
7. Minimal tissue debridement should be performed, only by flushing, avoiding mechanical debridement or tissue excision.[1–3] The aim of this is to maintain as much eyelid margin and tissue as possible. Reapposition of lid tissue, even if it is severely traumatized, usually results in a better postoperative outcome than excision of tissue and subsequent reconstructive surgery.[3] The extensive vascular supply of the eyelids protects them against necrosis.
8. Wound closure should start at the eyelid margin and then focus on approximating key areas.
   a. The eyelid margin is closed in a figure-of-eight pattern using 6-0 monofilament or coated polyglactin 910 on a reverse cutting needle (Fig. 31.1).

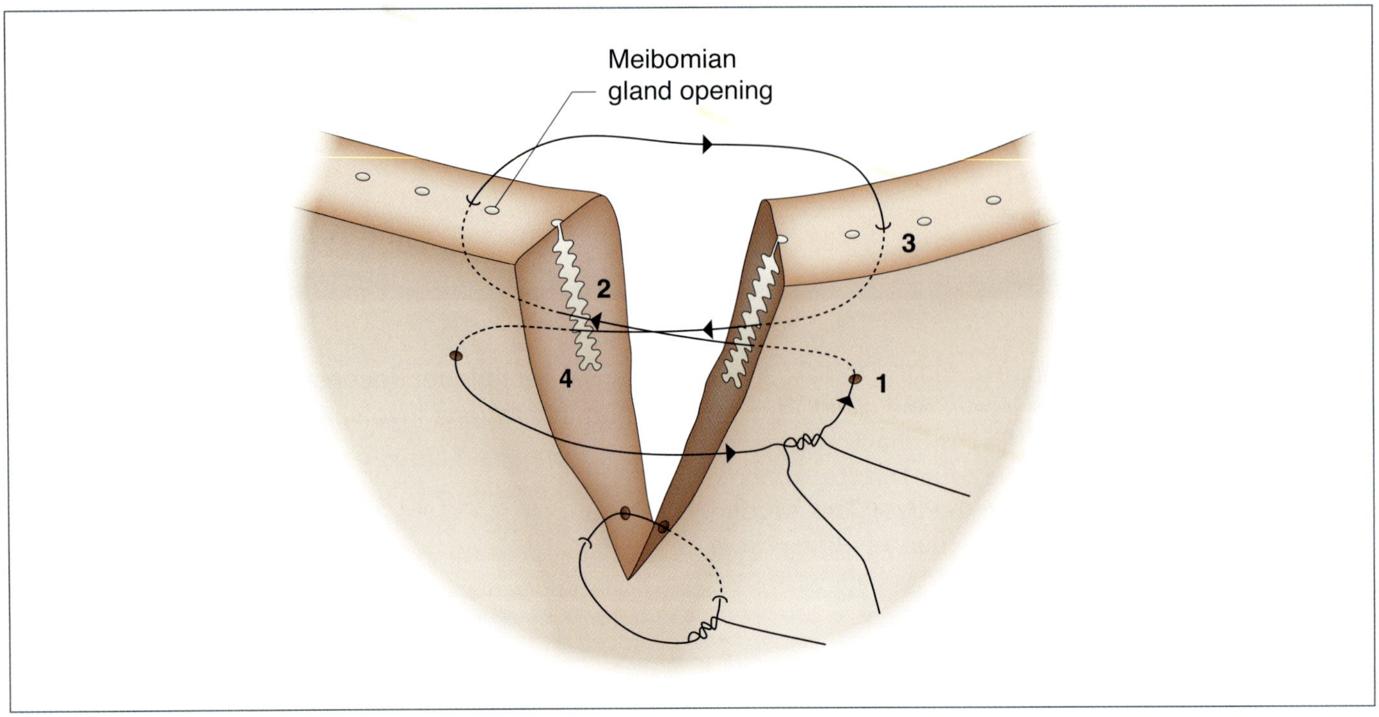

Figure 31.1 Figure-of-eight suture of an eyelid margin wound. The first suture bite is directed into the skin 4 mm below the eyelid margin and 2 mm away from the wound edge, and it exits the interstitial tissue of the wound. The second bite enters the interstitial tissue on the opposite side 2 mm below the eyelid margin and exits the eyelid margin in line with the meibomian glands 1 mm away from the wound edge. For the third bite, the needle enters the eyelid margin in line with the meibomian glands on the opposite side of the wound 1 mm away from the wound edge. This bite exits the interstitial tissue of the wound 2 mm away from the eyelid margin. The last, fourth bite enters the interstitial tissue on the opposite side and is directed to exit the skin 4 mm away from the eyelid margin and 2 mm away from the wound edge. The aim is that the suture entry and exit points are mirror images of each other. Before the knot is tied, vertical and horizontal apposition should be evaluated; even with minimal imperfections, the suture has to be replaced.

Care should be taken that the eyelid margin is perfectly aligned.[1,2] Horizontal or vertical misalignment of the eyelid margin is not acceptable, as it can cause chronic corneal and conjunctival irritation and ulceration.[3]

b. The remaining wound is closed in a two-layered fashion using the same suture material.[1,2] The deep layer can be closed with mattress sutures or in a simple continuous pattern, taking care not to perforate the conjunctival sac. The skin is closed with simple interrupted sutures.
c. The suture ends of the figure of eight and the simple interrupted skin sutures can be tied into the knots of the sutures further away from the eyelid, making sure that they are kept away from the globe to prevent corneal injury (Fig. 31.2).

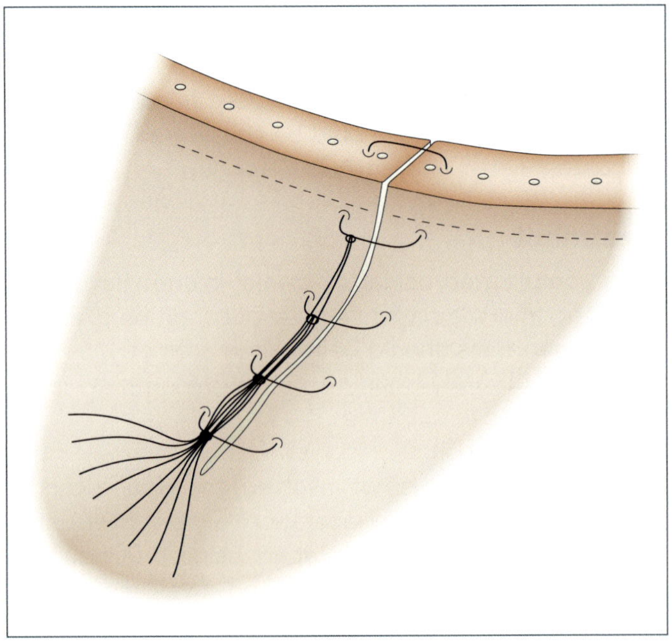

Figure 31.2 The suture ends of the figure of eight and the simple interrupted sutures are tied into the knots of the sutures further away from the eyelid. This keeps them away from the globe and prevents irritation and injury to the cornea.

Complicated eyelid lacerations

If the defect is more extensive than one-third of the eyelid margin, plastic surgical repair using different grafting techniques may be required. If the medial canthal region is involved, the lacrimal puncta should be

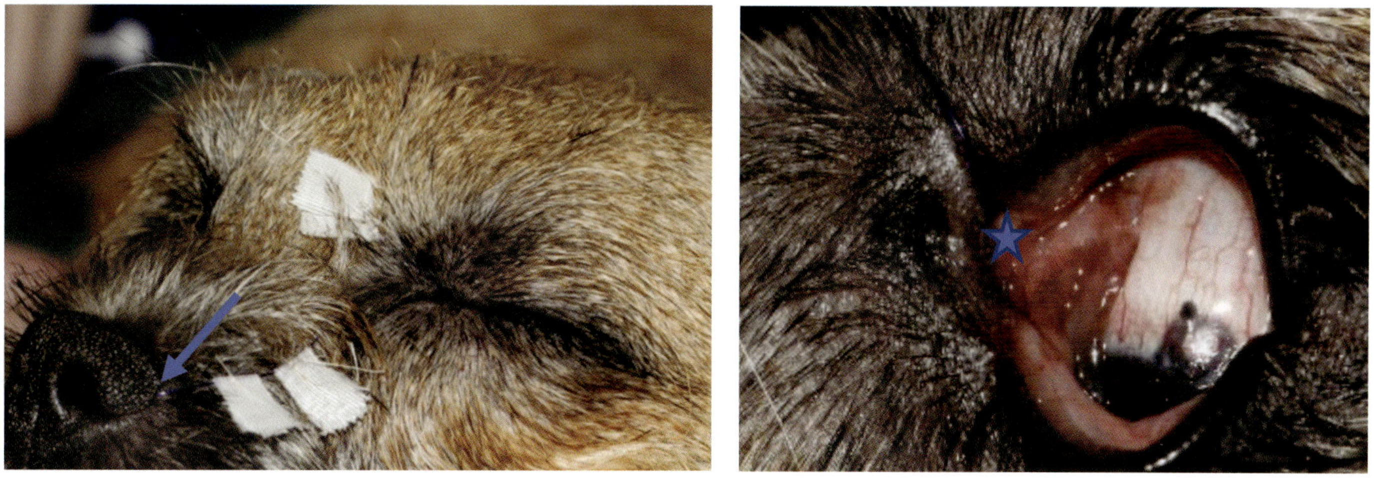

Figure 31.3 Stent in the nasolacrimal duct. Note the 2-0 nylon suture placed in the nasolacrimal duct exiting the left nostril (arrow) and the upper lacrimal punctum (star).

identified, cannulated, and flushed.[2] Lacerations of the nasolacrimal system should be repaired, if possible, by placing a stent (e.g., 0.7–1.3 mm diameter circular silicone tubing or a 2-0 or 3-0 nylon suture) in the nasolacrimal duct (Fig. 31.3).[2,3] The stent is left in place for 2–6 weeks. This allows continuous drainage of tears over the nasolacrimal duct and prevents periocular dermatitis secondary to scarification and nasolacrimal duct obstruction.

Referral to a veterinary ophthalmologist should be considered if the eyelid laceration has been classified as complicated (e.g., an extensive wound that requires advancement flaps, reconstruction of the nasolacrimal drainage system, and globe repair), as magnification and experience are usually required for reconstruction.[1–3]

Postoperative management

As eyelid laceration wounds are often irritating during the healing phase,[1] it is important to prevent self-mutilation by placing an Elizabethan collar and provide systemic anti-inflammatory and broad-spectrum antibiotic treatment. After 10–14 days, the skin sutures can be removed in case of suture reaction.

Outcome

The outcome of an eyelid laceration in dogs can vary depending on its severity, location, and duration. Prompt intervention is essential once the patient has been stabilized, aiming for a perfectly aligned eyelid margin to minimize ongoing irritation and corneal ulceration, and performing minimal tissue debridement to preserve eyelid function. Even severely traumatized eyelid tissue can heal favorably due to the extensive vascular supply of the eyelids.[3]

KEEP IN MIND

- Meticulous anatomical reapposition is mandatory to enhance cosmesis and ensure postoperative eyelid function and corneal health.
- Even in severely traumatized cases, reapposition rather than excision of lid tissue results in a better postoperative outcome.
- Eyelid reapposition is started at the eyelid margin using a figure-of-eight pattern. The orifices of the meibomian glands can be used as landmarks for the suture bites.

References

1. Bettenay SV, Müller RS, Maggs DJ. Diseases of the eyelids. In: Maggs DJ, Miller PE, Ofri R (eds.). *Slatter's Fundamentals of Veterinary Ophthalmology*, 6th ed. Saunders; 2017. pp. 127–157.
2. Gelatt KN, Gelatt JP, Plummer CE. Surgery of the eyelids. In: *Veterinary Ophthalmic Surgery*, 2nd ed. Saunders; 2021. pp. 102–147.
3. Stades FC, van der Woerdt A. Diseases and surgery of the canine eyelid. In: Gelatt KN (ed.). *Veterinary Ophthalmology*, 6th ed. Wiley-Blackwell; 2021. pp. 923–987.

Chapter 32
Globe proptosis

Maria-Christine Fischer

Proptosis is the forward displacement of the eye, with entrapment of the eyelids behind the equator of the globe, as a result of sudden trauma (Fig. 32.1).

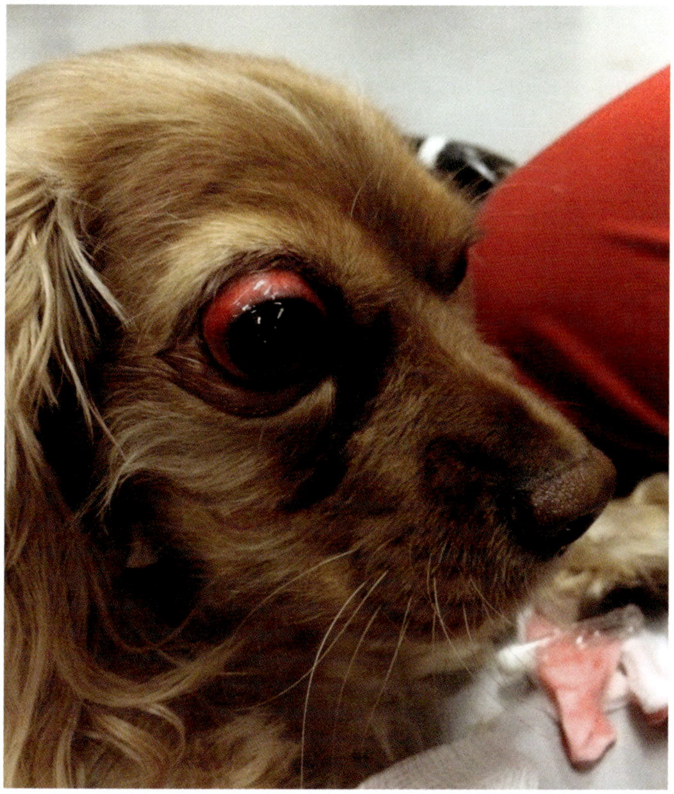

Figure 32.1 Proptosis in a dog. Note the marked anterior displacement of the right globe and the eyelids that are rolled inwards and entrapped behind the equator of the globe. The eyelid margin is not visible. The globe was repositioned promptly. A lateral canthotomy was required. The eye remained visual.

Clinical presentation and diagnosis

The most apparent sign of globe proptosis is the visible anterior displacement of the eye from the socket. The patient is unable to close the eyelids over the protruded eye, and the eyelid margins are not visible because they are entrapped. The periocular area may exhibit swelling and bruising depending on the underlying cause. It is important to consider the patient's skull conformation for prognosis and triage of the case. Relatively little force is required to cause globe proptosis in brachycephalic dog breeds. In meso- and dolichocephalic dogs and cats, extreme forces are required.[1] In these cases, concurrent head trauma with facial fractures and potential systemic injuries may result in life-threatening conditions that require attention and investigation prior to addressing the protruded globe. A detailed ophthalmic examination will help to determine further prognostic indicators (Box 32.1).[1–5] When in doubt about whether a globe can be salvaged, if the owners are willing to provide long-term care if required, an attempt to preserve the eye should be made.[1]

Treatment

Globe proptosis is an ophthalmic emergency that requires prompt surgical management.[1] Until surgical repositioning, the owner and the veterinarian should keep the affected eye moist with saline, water, petroleum jelly, ointments, or viscous gels to prevent corneal desiccation.[1]

Surgical technique

Replacement of the globe should be performed under general anesthesia.[2] The surgical site is aseptically prepared as described for eyelid lacerations (see Chapter 31).

BOX 32.1 - PROGNOSTIC INDICATORS IN PATIENTS WITH PROPTOSIS

Positive prognostic indicators	Negative prognostic indicators that warrant enucleation
• Brachycephalic skull conformation (controversial) • Presence of vision at presentation • Pupillary light reflexes at presentation • Minimal damage to the extraocular muscles (medial rectus muscle avulsion most common), with voluntary eye movement • Absent or minimal intraocular hemorrhage	• Ruptured or blood-filled eye, loss of shape and turgor of the globe • Avulsion of the optic nerve • Owners cannot provide potential long-term postoperative care • Extensive damage to the extraocular muscles (rupture of more than two or three muscles) causing irreversible compromise of the vascular and nervous supply to the anterior segment of the eye

1. Globe replacement without canthotomy should be attempted first (Fig. 32.2).[1,2]
   a. The central eyelid margin is grasped with atraumatic tissue forceps (e.g., Allis tissue or von Graefe forceps).
   b. Thick lubrication should be applied on the ocular surface.
   c. A Jaeger lid plate or the smooth, flat end of a scalpel handle is placed onto the ocular surface.
   d. While applying gentle pressure to the ocular surface and pushing the globe back into the orbit, the eyelid margins are pulled up and away from the globe. If excessive tension is required, a lateral canthotomy should be performed.
2. A lateral canthotomy can be performed if simple replacement was not successful (Fig. 32.3).[1,2]
   a. Using Metzenbaum scissors, a 1–2 cm horizontal incision is started at the outer corner of the eye and extended laterally.
   b. The lid margins are rolled out and repositioned over the globe.
   c. The conjunctival sac is flushed with sterile 0.9% saline and the cornea lubricated.
   d. For canthotomy closure, a 6-0 monofilament or coated polyglactin 910 on a reverse cutting needle is used in a figure-of-eight pattern (see Fig. 31.1). Care should be taken that the eyelid margin is perfectly aligned. The remaining wound is apposed in a simple interrupted pattern using the same suture material. The suture ends of the figure of eight can be tied into the knots of the simple interrupted sutures (see Fig. 31.2).
3. Temporary tarsorrhaphy sutures are placed to close the palpebral fissure (Fig. 32.4).[1,2]
   a. The eyelid is grasped with atraumatic tissue forceps.
   b. Two or three mattress sutures are placed using 4-0 to 6-0 nylon (depending on the size of the patient), passing the needle through the outer half thickness of the eyelid. It should be ensured that the needle exits and enters the eyelid margin at the level of the openings of the meibomian glands and not the palpebral conjunctiva. This prevents the suture material from rubbing on the cornea.
   c. A small opening can be left in the medial aspect for postoperative topical medication.
   d. After placing all the sutures, these should be tightened so that no gap remains between the eyelids. This avoids irritation of the ocular surface by the suture material. If periocular swelling is pronounced and results in excessive tension on the sutures, stents (e.g., intravenous tubing or buttons) can be placed to help prevent pressure necrosis of the skin from the suture material.

Postoperative management

Aftercare consists of systemic antibiotics and nonsteroidal anti-inflammatories.[1,2] If a corneal ulcer is present, topical antibiotics and topical cycloplegic medication (e.g., cyclopentolate 1% or atropine 1% eye drops) should be applied to reduce pain. The patient's activity should be restricted, and an Elizabethan collar is required until suture removal.

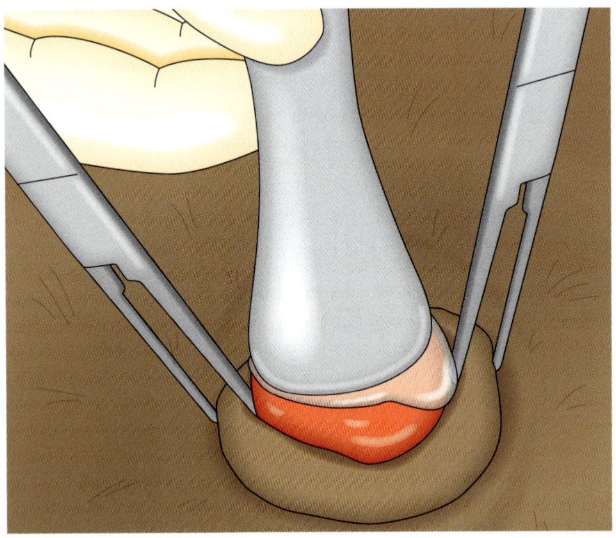

Figure 32.2 Replacement of a proptosed globe. The eyelids are grasped at the midpoint using forceps, and a Jaeger lid plate is placed on the heavily lubricated cornea. The eyelids are then gently pulled outwards and upwards while the Jaeger lid plate provides gentle counterpressure.

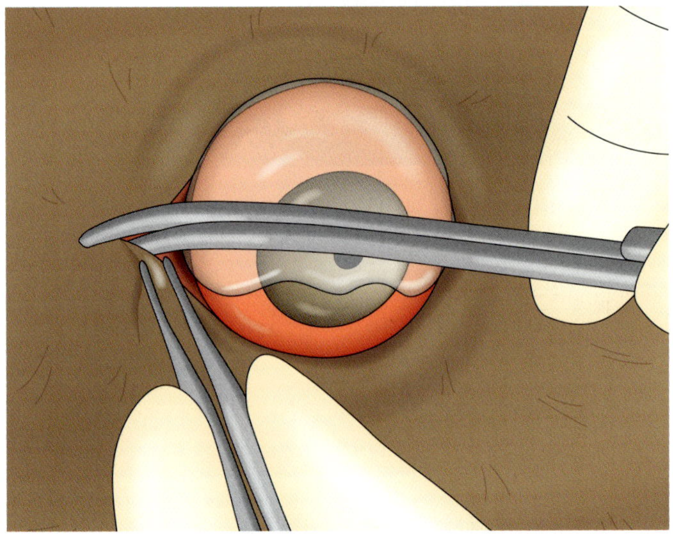

Figure 32.3 Lateral canthotomy. Metzenbaum scissors are inserted into the lateral canthus and an approximately 1 cm horizontal cut is made. This widening of the palpebral fissure after canthotomy reduces tension and enables globe repositioning.

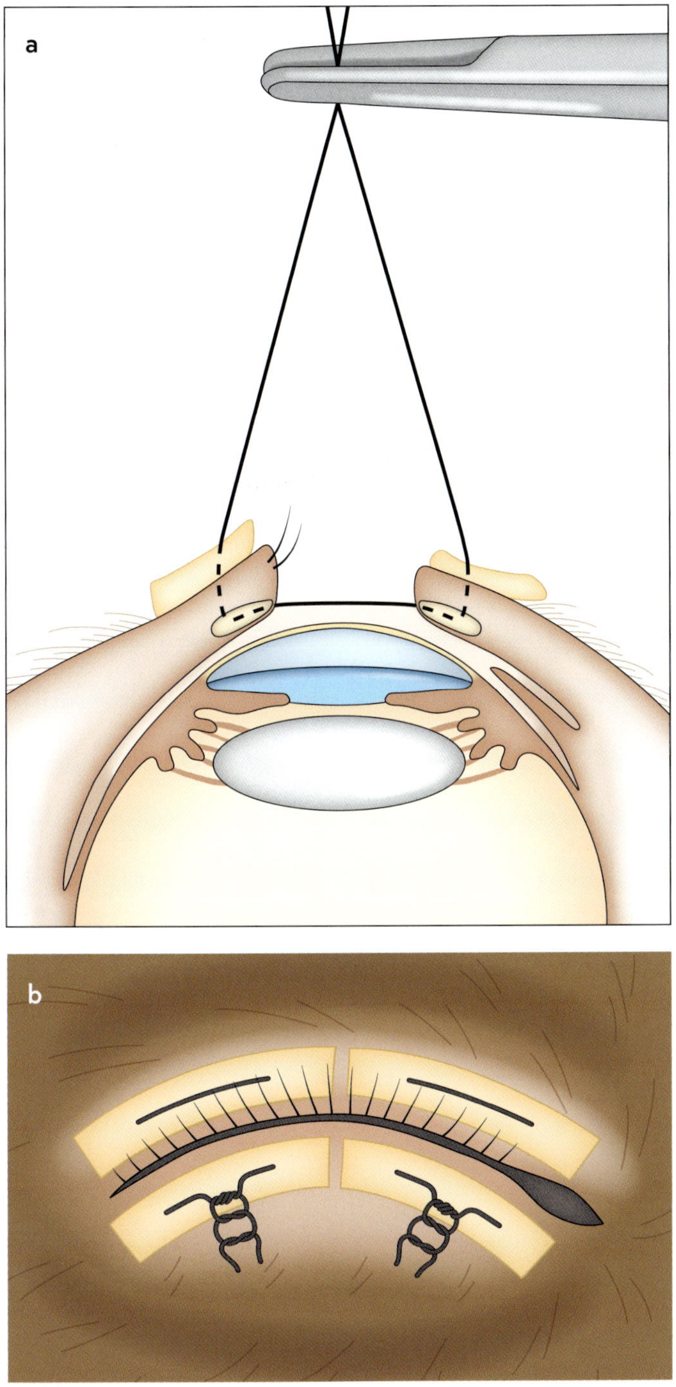

Figure 32.4 Temporary tarsorrhaphy. (a) Partial-thickness sutures are applied in the eyelids, entering and exiting the eyelid margin in the line of the openings of the meibomian glands. (b) Two or three horizontal mattress sutures and stents (intravenous fluid lines for example) are placed. Note that the medial canthus remains open for topical medication administration.

The temporary tarsorrhaphy sutures are left for 2–3 weeks until orbital swelling has resolved and palpebral function recovered.[1] The owners should monitor closely for any gaps between the upper and lower eyelid, as rubbing of the suture material on the cornea can result in corneal ulceration. If gapping occurs, the sutures require immediate removal and should be replaced if orbital swelling and lagophthalmos (inability to fully close the eyelid) persist. Removal of the absorbable canthotomy sutures is not required unless suture reaction is noted. Schirmer tear tests and fluorescein staining should be performed at suture removal and a month later, as keratoconjunctivitis sicca and corneal ulceration are common complications.

A bilateral medial canthoplasty and, if required, a permanent lateral tarsorrhaphy should be considered in patients with a macropalpebral fissure.[1,2] These surgical procedures not only reduce exposure of the ocular surface in lagophthalmic eyes but also act as a preventative measure to lower the risk of recurrent globe prolapse as well as occurrence in the contralateral eye.

Outcome

Proptosed globes can often be salvaged for cosmetic purposes; however, due to damage to the optic nerve the majority of the repositioned globes are blind.[3] No cat and less than a third of dogs has been reported to be visual after repositioning.[3–5] Maintaining vision has been correlated with the presence of direct and indirect pupillary light reflexes at admission,[4,5] with vision at presentation,[4] and with the involvement of a veterinary ophthalmologist for case management.[5] Controversy exists about the impact of time to repositioning and patient's skull conformation on the outcome.[1,4,5] Brachycephalic animals and immediate surgical intervention have been associated with a more favorable prognosis.[1,2,4]

Further potential complications following proptosis of the globe include lateral strabismus (lateral deviation of the visual axis due to rupture of the medial extraocular muscle) (Fig. 32.5), lagophthalmos with exposure keratitis, keratoconjunctivitis sicca, neurotrophic keratitis resulting in chronic corneal ulceration, glaucoma, and phthisis bulbi.[1,3,4,6] In cases where extraocular structures are severely damaged, the globe may not survive reduction and should be enucleated (see Chapter 33).

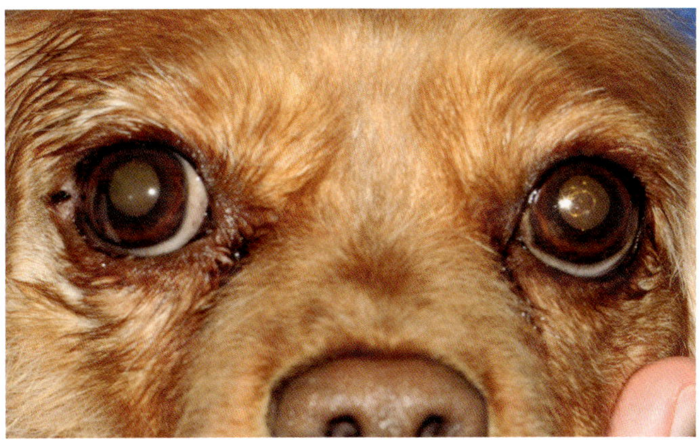

Figure 32.5 Same patient as in Figure 32.1 two weeks after repositioning of the globe and removal of the tarsorrhaphy sutures. Note the mild lateral strabismus in the right eye.

KEEP IN MIND

- Globe proptosis is an ophthalmic emergency that requires prompt surgical repositioning.
- The majority of affected animals have permanent vision loss from optic nerve damage, and lateral deviation of the eye secondary to tearing of the medial rectus muscle is common.
- Schirmer tear testing and fluorescein staining should be performed in the postoperative period to monitor for complications such as keratoconjunctivitis sicca and corneal ulceration.

References

1. Miller PE. Ocular emergencies. In: Maggs DJ, Miller PE, Ofri R (eds.). *Slatter's Fundamentals of Veterinary Ophthalmology*, 6th ed. St. Louis, MO: Elsevier Saunders; 2018. pp. 432–441.
2. Pot SA, Voelter K, Kircher PR. Diseases and surgery of the canine orbit. In: Gelatt KN (ed.). *Veterinary Ophthalmology*, vol. 2, 6th ed. Hoboken, NJ: Wiley-Blackwell; 2021. pp. 879–922.
3. Fritsche J et al. Prolapse of the eyeball in small animals: A retrospective study of 36 cases [In German]. *Tierarztl Prax.* 1996; 24(1):55–61.
4. Gilger BC et al. Traumatic ocular proptoses in dogs and cats: 84 cases (1980–1993). *J Am Vet Med Assoc.* 1995; 206(8): 1186–1190.
5. Pe'er O, Oron L, Ofri R. Prognostic indicators and outcome in dogs undergoing temporary tarsorrhaphy following traumatic proptosis. *Vet Ophthalmol.* 2020; 23(2):245–251.
6. Ali KM, Mostafa AA. Clinical findings of traumatic proptosis in small-breed dogs and complications associated with globe replacement surgery. *Open Vet J.* 2019; 9(3): 222–229.

Chapter 33
Enucleation

Maria-Christine Fischer

Enucleation is a common orbital procedure in veterinary medicine that involves the removal of the globe and surrounding tissues, including the conjunctiva, nictitating membrane, and lid margins, while preserving orbital structures like the extraocular muscles, orbital fat, and main lacrimal gland (Figs. 33.1 and 33.2a). This surgical intervention is a treatment option for advanced ocular disease processes that have resulted in a blind and painful eye or a painful eye resistant to medical management. Common indications include infected eyes, irreparable corneal or intraocular injury, severe proptosis, intractable uveitis, and intraocular neoplasia causing pain or with the potential for distant metastasis.[1–5] The decision to pursue enucleation arises from the goal of relieving suffering, eliminating the need for topical medication, and improving the overall quality of life of the patient; however all other options should be considered before enucleation, particularly for visual eyes. All enucleated globes should be submitted for histopathologic evaluation.

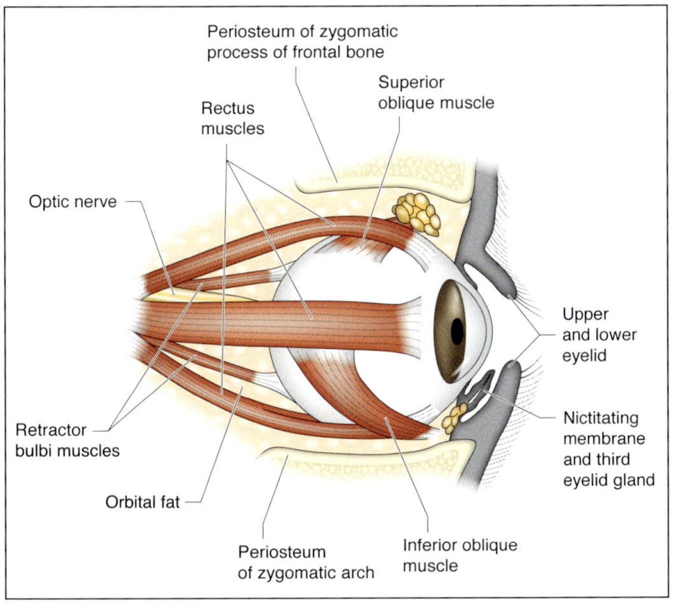

Figure 33.1 Structures of the globe.

Clinical presentation and diagnosis

The primary indications for enucleation are painful and blinding conditions, including intractable glaucoma, intraocular neoplasia, severe corneal disease (e.g., progressive corneal ulceration, keratomalacia, corneal perforation), endophthalmitis, and severe ocular trauma (including globe rupture and proptosis). Occasionally, clients opt for enucleation in cases of chronic and painful ocular surface disease that are unresponsive to treatment such as severe keratoconjunctivitis sicca.

Diagnosis of these conditions requires a complete neuro-ophthalmic and ophthalmic examination, potentially in combination with ocular ultrasound.

One of the biggest challenges in decision-making regarding enucleation is that ocular pain is easily underestimated or not perceived by owners, especially when it is chronic, as is often the case with glaucoma.[6]

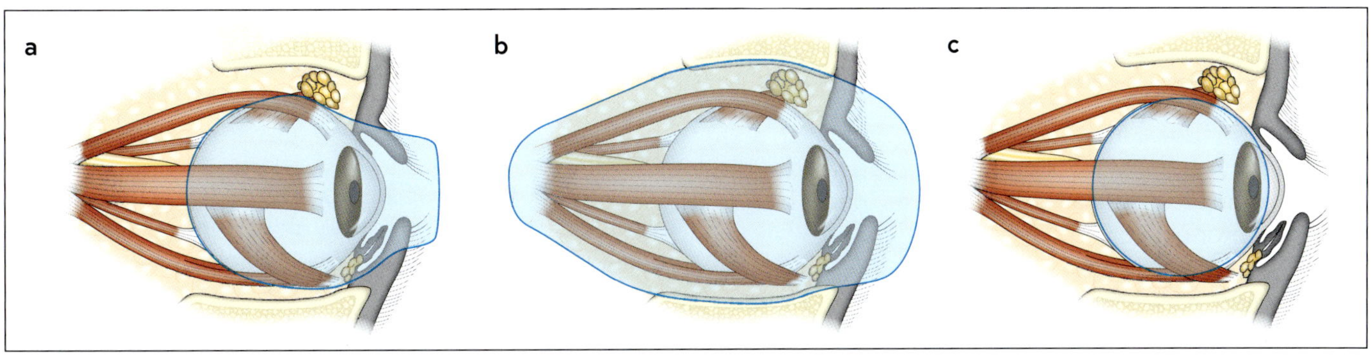

Figure 33.2 (a) Enucleation: Removal of the globe, eyelids, conjunctiva, nictitating membrane, and lacrimal gland. (b) Exenteration: Removal of the globe, eyelids, and all the orbital contents, including the periosteum. (c) Evisceration: Removal of the globe contents and placement of an intrascleral prosthesis for cosmetic reasons.

Changes in the animal's behavior are a crucial source for assessing the patient's quality of life and should be addressed when taking the clinical history.[6]

Treatment

Enucleation can be performed using two different techniques: the transpalpebral and transconjunctival approaches. The former involves accessing the eye through the eyelid skin, while the latter is performed through the conjunctiva. The transpalpebral approach is more versatile and can be used to remove glaucomatous eyes as well as globes with infection or intraocular neoplasia. The transconjunctival technique is suitable for intraocular issues like glaucoma but is unsuitable in case of neoplasia or infection not contained within the eye (e.g., melting ulcers, corneal perforations, neoplasia on the ocular surface). The transconjunctival approach has been associated with a lower relative blood loss in dogs compared to the transpalpebral approach.[7]

In addition to enucleation, two further surgical techniques for removing orbital contents can be performed, each differing in the extent of required tissue excision. These procedures are less commonly performed and therefore only briefly described.

Exenteration involves the removal of all orbital contents, including the extraocular muscles, orbital fat, lacrimal glands, and periosteum of orbital bones (Fig. 33.2b). This procedure is more invasive and is indicated when there is concern about orbital neoplasia. Skin flaps or skin grafts may be required if larger areas of periocular tissue also need to be removed.

Evisceration entails the removal of the intraocular contents only (Fig. 33.2c), leaving the fibrous tunic intact, and is typically paired with placement of an intrascleral prosthesis. Evisceration is contraindicated in cases with endophthalmitis, corneal disease, and intraocular neoplasia. It is also not recommended for cats. This procedure is primarily performed for cosmetic reasons. Long-term complications are described in almost one-third of cases.[8] Evisceration does not provide a benefit for the patient compared to enucleation.[8]

Surgical technique

Preparation of the surgical site involves clipping an area of the skin 3–5 cm wide surrounding the eyelids. The surgical site is aseptically prepared as described in Chapter 31 for eyelid lacerations.

Local anesthesia

Various regional anesthesia options, including retrobulbar, peribulbar, sub-Tenon's anesthesia, splash blocks, and the insertion of an intraorbital absorbable gelatin sponge infused with a local anesthetic, can provide comprehensive sensory blockade and pain relief during and/or after enucleation.[9] Suitable anesthetic agents include lidocaine, bupivacaine, mepivacaine, and ropivacaine, but their toxicity and doses should be taken into consideration, since systemic absorption can occur.[9]

The retrobulbar block is commonly performed; however, in the presence of orbital neoplasia or infection, it should be avoided to prevent spread of disease processes. A splash block can be applied to the orbit instead prior to wound closure.[9]

Retrobulbar block (Fig. 33.3)

The retrobulbar block provides adjunctive analgesia during enucleation by affecting the trigeminal nerve's ophthalmic branch. A ventrolateral approach is preferred for dogs,[10] using a bent 22-gauge spinal needle inserted through the lower temporal eyelid and advanced caudodorsally. Ultrasound may be used to guide the injection into the retrobulbar muscular cone (intraconally). If ultrasound is not available, a slight "popping" sensation can indicate that the orbital fascia has been pierced.[9] The needle is then advanced another 1–2 cm and 2 mL of 2% lidocaine is injected without adverse effects.[9]

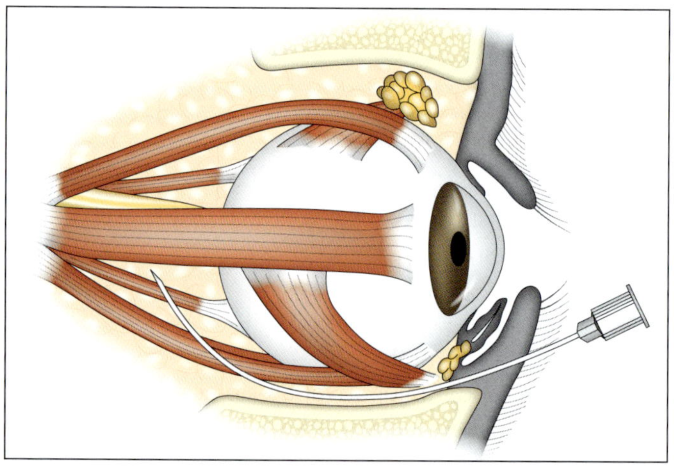

Figure 33.3 Retrobulbar nerve block. A bent 22-gauge spinal needle is inserted through the lower temporal eyelid and advanced caudodorsally. The local anesthetic is then deposited intraconally.

Splash block

For a splash block, 0.5% bupivacaine (0.1 mL/kg) is applied into the orbit following globe removal, after controlling hemorrhage and prior to placing skin sutures.[11]

Transconjunctival enucleation

1. A lateral canthotomy is performed to obtain adequate space, especially in dolichocephalic breeds. For this, a horizontal incision is made at the out-

er corner of the eye and extended laterally about 1–2 cm with Metzenbaum scissors. Some surgeons prefer to clamp that area prior to cutting, for hemostasis.

2. An eyelid speculum can be placed to improve visualization.
3. A 360-degree bulbar conjunctival peritomy is performed about 5–7 mm from the limbus with Stevens tenotomy, Metzenbaum, or Mayo scissors.
4. The sub-Tenon's plane is bluntly dissected to expose the extraocular muscles.
5. Each rectus and oblique muscle is identified and cut at the tendinous insertion to reduce hemorrhage. This can be facilitated by positioning one blade of the scissors under the muscle belly and moving the blade as anteriorly as possible to the tendinous insertion of the extraocular muscle.
6. The retractor bulbi muscle posterior to the globe is also cut.
7. Once the globe is freed from the attached tissue, the optic nerve, which is located at the posterior and ventromedial aspect of the globe, as well as the long posterior ciliary arteries and veins are cut with scissors. Care should be taken to avoid traction on the globe, as this may cause an oculocardiac reflex with reduction of the heart rate. In addition, it can lead to visual field loss and even blindness in the contralateral eye. Clamping of the optic nerve and vessels with hemostats or suture ligation is not necessary and is even contraindicated in some cases.
8. If required, hemostasis after globe removal can be achieved with direct pressure with a gauze swab for 2–5 minutes, and calcium alginate can be used in the surgical wound.[12,13]
9. The nictitating membrane and its accessory gland are excised at the base.
10. All bulbar and conjunctival tissue needs to be identified and resected completely to avoid formation of orbital cysts.
11. The eyelid margins are dissected.
12. Wound closure:
    a. The deep edges of the connective tissue are closed using 3-0 to 5-0 absorbable monofilament suture material (e.g., Monocryl) in a continuous pattern. The needle should pass through the soft tissue close to the orbital rim to reduce sinking in of the skin postoperatively. In addition, a watertight closure should be aimed for to prevent postoperative hemorrhage and swelling of the surgical site. Alternatively, techniques such as X/Y-shaped periorbital reconstruction,[14] orbital meshwork placement,[3] a Prolene or Dacron mesh,[15] or an eyelid bridge flap[16] could be considered for orbital reconstruction.
    b. The superficial layers of the subcutis are closed with 3-0 to 5-0 absorbable suture material in a simple continuous or intradermal pattern, and the knots are buried.
    c. Skin sutures are not necessary, but if required, the skin can be apposed with 3-0 to 5-0 nonabsorbable monofilament suture material on a cutting needle and in a simple interrupted pattern.
13. A pressure bandage can be placed over the surgical site for 12–24 hours to reduce postoperative swelling and bruising. For this, a gauze swab is rolled up or folded and secured in place with two or three mattress sutures, taking a skin bite above (upper eyelid region) and below (lower eyelid region).

Transpalpebral enucleation

1. The eyelids are sutured closed in a simple continuous pattern using 3-0 to 5-0 suture material of any type. Alternatively, they can be clamped with Allis tissue forceps. This step can be skipped if there is no evidence of infection.
2. An elliptical skin incision is made 3–4 mm away from the eyelid margins using a number 15 scalpel blade in two continuous movements (one for the upper eyelid and one for the lower eyelid) to achieve smooth surgical wound edges. If the eyelids are not closed, a Jaeger lid plate or the end of a scalpel handle can be inserted into the conjunctival sac to provide counterpressure and allow for an equal depth of penetration of the scalpel blade. Alternatively, the eyelid can be positioned over the orbital rim for a firmer base during the skin incision.
3. The subcutaneous tissue, orbicularis oculi muscles, and the connective tissue surrounding the eye are then sharply and bluntly dissected using Metzenbaum scissors. The dissection should be directed toward the eye approximately 8–10 mm behind the limbus. Care should be taken to ensure that the conjunctival sac stays intact to prevent infection or neoplasia from spreading. An accidental tear can be closed with a simple interrupted stitch to avoid contamination.
4. As the blunt dissection is deepened, the ligaments at the lateral and medial canthi (palpebral commissures) are identified and transected with scissors. Once they are transected, the tension on the eyelid tissue is released, and posterior dissection becomes easier.
5. Blunt and sharp dissection toward the globe is continued until no connective tissue is covering the extraocular muscles, and each rectus and oblique muscle can easily be identified.

6. The extraocular muscles are cut at the tendinous insertion to the globe to reduce hemorrhage (see step 5 of "Transconjunctival enucleation").
7. The retractor bulbi muscle posterior to the globe is also cut.
8. The optic nerve and the long posterior ciliary arteries and veins at the ventromedial aspect of the globe are sharply incised with scissors. Care should be taken to avoid traction on the globe. Clamping of the nerve and vessels with hemostats or suture ligation is not necessary and is even contraindicated in some cases.
9. The globe with the eyelids can now be removed from the orbit. It should be checked that the third eyelid and the accessory gland are contained within the conjunctival sac.
10. Hemostasis, wound closure, and optional pressure swabs are the same as for transconjunctival enucleation (see above)

Postoperative management

Postoperative care consists of systemic nonsteroidal anti-inflammatories for 5 days after surgery. Opioid drugs such as buprenorphine and methadone can be added in the immediate postoperative phase for pain relief.[1,5] Postoperative systemic antibiotics are not routinely required; there is no scientific evidence for the use of postoperative prophylactic antibiotics to prevent surgical site infections. A plastic Elizabethan collar is placed to reduce self-trauma, and the patient's activity should be restricted for 7–14 days after surgery.

Outcome

Enucleation is a routine surgery with limited intra- and postoperative complications. Intraoperatively, traction on the globe during dissection should be avoided, as this may cause an oculocardiac reflex with reduction of the heart rate.[1] In addition, it can lead to visual field loss and even blindness in the contralateral eye. The optic nerve fibers on the nasal side of each retina cross over to the opposite side of the brain via the optic nerve at the optic chiasm, and traction can damage the contralateral optic nerve fibers at the optic chiasm, especially in cats.[12]

Clamping and ligation of the optic nerve and the long posterior ciliary arteries and veins of the ophthalmic plexus prior to dissection have been described to reduce hemorrhage.[2,5,7] However, it is deemed unnecessary from a hemostatic viewpoint,[12,13] strongly recommended against by Hartley and Grundon,[4] and contraindicated in cats due to the risk of causing iatrogenic blindness.[4,12] The impact of the different techniques on blood loss has not yet been determined, but the relative blood loss has been reported to be low, with a median of 1.3% (0.1%–6.7%), in dogs, and no supportive interventions were required.[7]

The most frequent short-term complication after surgery is hemorrhage and swelling of the surgical site.[2] Mild sanguineous discharge can occur from the suture site and is typically managed using cold compresses, placing pressure bandages, applying tissue glue to seal the wound, and keeping the patient as calm as possible. Occasionally epistaxis can occur due to drainage of blood over the nasolacrimal duct.

Surgical site infection has been reported in 5% of cases after enucleation, and no specific risk factors have been identified.

Long-term complications are rare and include orbital cysts, conjunctival mucoceles, and draining fistulas, which result from inadequate removal of the caruncle at the medial canthus or from residual secretory tissues like conjunctival goblet cells and the third eyelid gland.[2,17] Brachycephalic breeds might experience orbital emphysema as a complication.[17] Additionally, an orbital sialocele was reported as a complication in enucleation surgery years after parotid duct transposition for keratoconjunctivitis sicca.[18]

Enucleation can be a daunting procedure for many owners, and some may instead elect for euthanasia of their pet. Owner education about the patient's postoperative appearance (Fig. 33.4) and quality of life helps to manage expectations. Studies have found that 90% of pet owners were satisfied after bilateral enucleation and would agree to have the procedure again, as they observed significant improvements of their dog's pain, response to facial/ocular palpation, activity levels, and overall quality of life.[6,19]

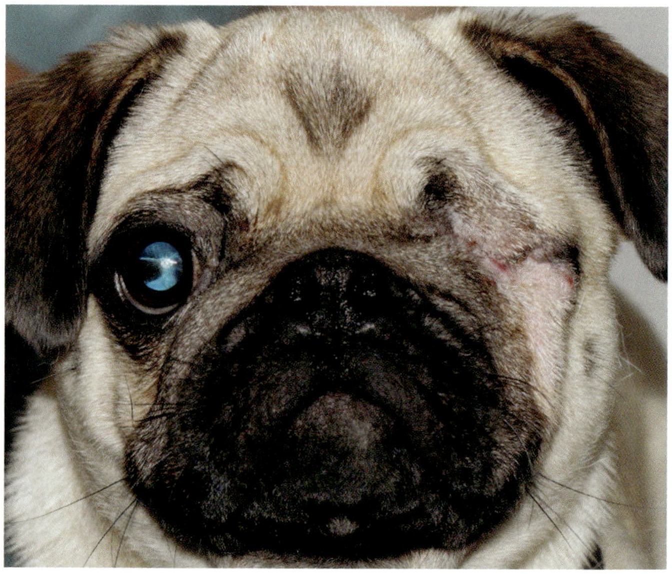

Figure 33.4 Postoperative appearance 10 days after unilateral enucleation in a Pug. Note the pigmentation of the right cornea.

KEEP IN MIND

- Two approaches for enucleation are available: transpalpebral (through the eyelid skin) and transconjunctival (through the conjunctiva).
- Traction on the globe during dissection should be avoided, as it could cause complications like oculocardiac reflex or even blindness.
- The patient's quality of life after enucleation, even bilateral, can be good.

References

1. Miller PE. Orbit. In: Maggs DJ, Miller PE, Ofri R (eds.). *Slatter's Fundamentals of Veterinary Ophthalmology*, 5th ed. St. Louis, MO: Elsevier Saunders; 2013. pp. 373–393.
2. Pot SA, Voelter K, Kircher PR. Diseases and surgery of the canine orbit. In: Gelatt KN (ed.). *Veterinary Ophthalmology*, 6th ed. Hoboken, NJ: John Wiley & Sons; 2021. pp. 907–908.
3. Cho J. Surgery of the globe and orbit. *Top Companion Anim Med.* 2008; 23(1):23–37.
4. Hartley C, Grundon RA. Diseases and surgery of the globe and orbit. In: *Equine Ophthalmology*, 3rd ed. Ames, IA: John Wiley & Sons; 2017. pp. 151–196.
5. Tobias K. *Manual of Small Animal Soft Tissue Surgery*, 2nd ed. Knoxville, TN: John Wiley & Sons; 2017. pp. 555–562.
6. Bujan JD, Boyd EJ, Pont RT. Comparing the behaviour of dogs before and after enucleation due to glaucoma. *Vet Rec.* 2021; 188(7):e53.
7. Lenihan E et al. Estimation of the intraoperative blood loss in dogs undergoing enucleation. *Vet Ophthalmol.* 2023; 26(1):19–30.
8. Barbry JB et al. Evisceration with implantation of an intrascleral silicone prosthesis in dogs: A retrospective study of 107 cases (2010–2019). *Vet Ophthalmol.* 2023. Epub ahead of print.
9. Shilo-Benjamini Y. A review of ophthalmic local and regional anesthesia in dogs and cats. *Vet Anaesth Analg.* 2019; 46(1):14–27.
10. Accola PJ et al. Development of a retrobulbar injection technique for ocular surgery and analgesia in dogs. *J Am Vet Med Assoc.* 2006; 229(2):220–225.
11. Chow DW, Wong MY, Westermeyer HD. Comparison of two bupivacaine delivery methods to control postoperative pain after enucleation in dogs. *Vet Ophthalmol.* 2015; 18(5): 422–428.
12. Donaldson D et al. Contralateral optic neuropathy and retinopathy associated with visual and afferent pupillomotor dysfunction following enucleation in six cats. *Vet Ophthalmol.* 2014; 17(5):373–384.
13. Allgoewer I, Noller CRS. Enucleation: Is ligation necessary? Proceedings of the 37th Annual Conference of the American College of Veterinary Ophthalmologists. 2006.
14. Vlachomitrou IE et al. X/Y shaped periorbital reconstructive surgery following enucleation or exenteration in dogs and cats: 24 cases (2013–2020). *J Small Anim Pract.* 2021; 62(7):580–587.
15. Spiess BM, Pot SA. Diseases and surgery of the canine orbit. In: Gelatt K, Gilger BC, Kern TJ (eds.). *Veterinary Ophthalmology*, 5th ed. Ames, IA: John Wiley & Sons; 2013. pp. 793–831.
16. Szentgali Z, Nogradi A. Improving post-operative cosmesis after enucleation in dogs and cats by using the third eyelid bridge flap technique (TEBF), May 23–26, Antwerp, Belgium, ECVO Conference. 2019; 22:1–27.
17. Ward AA, Neaderland MH. Complications from residual adnexal structures following enucleation in three dogs. *J Am Vet Med Assoc.* 2011; 239(12):1580–1583.
18. Guinan J, Willis AM, Cullen CL, Walshaw R. Postenucleation orbital sialocele in a dog associated with prior parotid duct transposition. *Vet Ophthalmol.* 2007; 10(6):386–389.
19. Hamzianpour N, Smith K, Dawson C, Rhodes M. Bilateral enucleation in dogs: A review of owner perceptions and satisfaction. *Vet Ophthalmol.* 2019; 22(5):566–576.